S0-EJQ-682

UCLA Symposia on Molecular and Cellular Biology, New Series

Series Editor, C. Fred Fox

Please contact the publisher for information about previous titles in this series.

Symposia Board

C. Fred Fox, Ph.D., Director
Professor of Microbiology, University of California, Los Angeles

Members

The members of the board advise the director in matters of policy and in identification of topics for future symposia.

Charles Arntzen, Ph.D.
Director, Plant Science and Microbiology
Dupont

Ronald Cape, Ph.D., M.B.A.
Chairman
Cetus Corporation

Ralph Christoffersen, Ph.D.
Executive Director of Biotechnology
Upjohn Company

John Cole, Ph.D.
Vice-President of Research
and Development
Triton Biosciences

Pedro Cuatrecasas, M.D.
Vice President of Research
Glaxo, Inc.

J. Eugene Fox, Ph.D.
Director
ARCO Plant Cell Research Institute

L. Patrick Gage, Ph.D.
Director of Exploratory Research
Hoffman-La Roche, Inc.

Luis Glaser, Ph.D.
Executive Vice President
University of Miami

Gideon Goldstein, M.D., Ph.D.
Vice President, Immunology
Ortho Pharmaceutical Corp.

Ernest Jaworski, Ph.D.
Director of Biological Sciences
Monsanto Corp.

Irving S. Johnson, Ph.D.
Vice President of Research
Lilly Research Laboratories

Paul Marks, M.D.
President
Sloan-Kettering Memorial Institute

David W. Martin, Jr., M.D.
Vice-President of Research
Genentech, Inc.

Hugh O. McDevitt, M.D.
Professor of Medical Microbiology
Stanford University School of Medicine

Dale L. Oxender, Ph.D.
Professor of Biological Chemistry
University of Michigan

Mark L. Pearson, Ph.D.
Director of Molecular Biology
E.I. du Pont de Nemours and Company

George Poste, Ph.D.
Vice President and Director of Research
and Development
Smith, Kline and French Laboratories

William Rutter, Ph.D.
Professor of Biochemistry
University of California, San Francisco

Donald Steiner, M.D.
Professor of Biochemistry
University of Chicago

Sidney Udenfriend, Ph.D.
Member
Roche Institute of Molecular Biology

Norman Weiner, M.D.
Vice President for Pharmaceutical
Discovery
Abbott Laboratories

Biochemical and Molecular Epidemiology of Cancer

Biochemical and Molecular Epidemiology of Cancer

Proceedings of the Abbott Laboratories-UCLA Symposium
Held in Steamboat Springs, Colorado
April 6–13, 1985

Editor

Curtis C. Harris

Laboratory of Human Carcinogenesis
National Cancer Institute
Bethesda, Maryland

Alan R. Liss, Inc. • New York

Address all Inquiries to the Publisher
Alan R. Liss, Inc., 41 East 11th Street, New York, NY 10003

Copyright © 1986 Alan R. Liss, Inc.

Printed in the United States of America

Under the conditions stated below the owner of copyright for this book hereby grants permission to users to make photocopy reproductions of any part or all of its contents for personal or internal organizational use, or for personal or internal use of specific clients. This consent is given on the condition that the copier pay the stated per-copy fee through the Copyright Clearance Center, Incorporated, 27 Congress Street, Salem, MA 01970, as listed in the most current issue of "Permissions to Photocopy" (Publisher's Fee List, distributed by CCC, Inc.), for copying beyond that permitted by sections 107 or 108 of the US Copyright Law. This consent does not extend to other kinds of copying, such as copying for general distribution, for advertising or promotional purposes, for creating new collective works, or for resale.

Library of Congress Cataloging-in-Publication Data

Abbott Laboratories-UCLA Symposium (1985 : Steamboat Springs, Colo.)

Biochemical and molecular epidemiology of cancer.

(UCLA symposia on molecular and cellular biology ; new ser., v. 40)
Some articles are reprinted from Journal of cellular biochemistry.
Includes bibliographies and index.
1. Carcinogenesis—Congresses. 2. Epidemiology—Congresses. 3. Pathology, Molecular—Congresses.
I. Harris, Curtis C., 1943–   . II. University of California, Los Angeles. III. Abbott Laboratories.
IV. Journal of cellular biochemistry. V. Title.
VI. Series. [DNLM: 1. Neoplasms—etiology—congresses. 2. Neoplasms—occurrence—congresses.
W3 U17N new ser. v. 40 / QZ 202 A132b 1985]
RC268.5.A23 1985   616.99′4071   86-2909
ISBN 0-8451-2639-3

Pages 1–110 of this volume are reprinted from the Journal of Cellular Biochemistry, Volumes 29 and 30. The Journal is the only appropriate literature citation for the articles printed on these pages. The page numbers in the table of contents, contributors list, and index of this volume correspond to the page numbers at the foot of these pages.

The table of contents does not necessarily follow the pattern of the plenary sessions. Instead, it reflects the thrust of the meeting as it evolved from the combination of plenary sessions, poster sessions, and workshops, culminating in the final collection of invited papers, submitted papers, and workshop summaries. The order in which articles appear in this volume does not follow the order of citation in the table of contents. Some of the articles in this volume were published in the Journal of Cellular Biochemistry, and they are reprinted here. These articles appear in the order in which they were accepted for publication and then published in the Journal. They are followed by papers which were submitted solely for publication in these proceedings.

Contents

Contents   xi

Contributors

Stuart A. Aaronson, Laboratory of Cellular and Molecular Biology, National Cancer Institute, Bethesda, MD 20205 [155]

John D. Adams, American Health Foundation, Valhalla, NY 10595 [191]

Peter Angel, Kernforschungszentrum Karlsruhe, Institut für Genetik und Toxikologie, D-7500 Karlsruhe 1, Federal Republic of Germany [23]

Herman Autrup, Laboratory of Environmental Carcinogenesis, The Fibiger Institute, DK-2100 Copenhagen Ø, Denmark [359]

Susan Banks-Schlegel, Laboratory of Human Carcinogenesis, Division of Cancer Etiology, National Cancer Institute, Bethesda, MD 20205 [213]

John F. Baskar, Department of Microbiology and Immunology, Lineberger Cancer Research Center, University of North Carolina at Chapel Hill, Chapel Hill, NC 27514 [323]

Frederick A. Beland, National Center for Toxicological Research, Jefferson, AR 72079, and Department of Biochemistry, University of Arkansas for Medical Sciences, Little Rock, AR 72205 [441]

Gerald Berenson, Department of Medicine, Louisiana State University, School of Medicine, New Orleans, LA 70112 [397]

Peter Biberfeld, Department of Pathology, Karolinska Institute and Hospital, Stockholm, Sweden [449]

John Bickers, Department of Medicine, Louisiana State University, School of Medicine, New Orleans, LA 70112 [397]

K. Bister, Max Planck Institut für Molekulare Genetik, Otto Warburg Labor, Berlin 33, Federal Republic of Germany [67]

Fredric Blum, Department of Environmental Medicine, New York University Medical Center, New York, NY 10016 [53]

Peter M. Blumberg, Molecular Mechanisms of Tumor Promotion Section, Laboratory of Cellular Carcinogenesis and Tumor Promotion, National Cancer Institute, Bethesda, MD 20205 [1]

Dirk Bootsma, Department of Cell Biology and Genetics, Erasmus University, 3000 DR Rotterdam, The Netherlands [387]

Dimetris C. Boumpas, Laboratory of Human Carcinogenesis, Division of Cancer Etiology, National Cancer Institute, Bethesda, MD 20892 [271]

Curtis R. Brandt, Tumor Biology Division, Fred Hutchinson Cancer Research Center, Seattle, WA 98104 [401]

Klaus D. Brunnemann, American Health Foundation, Valhalla, NY 10595 [191]

Karen Buonagura, Department of Medicine, Louisiana State University, School of Medicine, New Orleans, LA 70112 [397]

Franco M. Buonaguro, Tumor Biology Division, Fred Hutchinson Cancer Research Center, Seattle, WA 98104 [401]

William F. Busby, Jr., Massachusetts Institute of Technology, Department of Applied Biological Sciences, Cambridge, MA 02139 [233]

Peter A. Cerutti, Department of Carcinogenesis, Swiss Institute for Experimental Cancer Research, 1066 Epalinges/Lausanne, Switzerland [167]

The number in brackets is the opening page number of the contributor's article.

Lois Chandler, USC Comprehensive Cancer Center, Los Angeles, CA 90033 **[149]**

B. Chapot, Unit of Mechanisms of Carcinogenesis, International Agency for Research on Cancer, 69372 Lyon Cedex 08, France **[43]**

Karen J. Chayt, Laboratory of Tumor Cell Biology, National Cancer Institute, Bethesda, MD 20205 **[449]**

Chu Yuan-rong, Qidong Liver Cancer Institute, Jiangsu Province, China **[283]**

J.L. Cleveland, Laboratory of Viral Carcinogenesis, National Cancer Institute, NCI-Frederick Cancer Research Facility, Frederick, MD 21701 **[67]**

J. Craig Cohen, Department of Medicine, Louisiana State University, School of Medicine, New Orleans, LA 70112 **[397]**

Mark Colb, Division of Hematology/ Oncology and Cancer Research Center, Tufts-New England Medical Center, Boston, MA 02111 **[99]**

Rebecca C. Corner, Carcinogenesis Laboratory, Department of Microbiology, and Department of Biochemistry, Michigan State University, East Lansing, MI 48824-1316 **[411]**

Linda B. Couto, Laboratory of Toxicology, Department of Applied Biological Sciences, Massachusetts Institute of Technology, Cambridge, MA 02139; present address: Department of Pathology, Stanford University School of Medicine, Stanford, CA 94305 **[427]**

Michelle G. Davis, Department of Microbiology and Immunology, University of North Carolina at Chapel Hill, Chapel Hill, NC 27514 **[323]**

Richard H. Decker, Hepatitis Research, Diagnostics Division, Abbot Laboratories, North Chicago, IL 60064 **[227]**

Jan de Wit, Department of Cell Biology and Genetics, Erasmus University, 3000 DR Rotterdam, The Netherlands **[387]**

Nancy A. DiMartino, Division of Hematology/Oncology and Cancer Research Center, Tufts-New England Medical Center, Boston, MA 02111 **[99]**

Patricia A. DiNitto, Molecular Mechanisms of Tumor Promotion Section, Laboratory of Cellular Carcinogenesis and Tumor Promotion, National Cancer Institute, Bethesda, MD 20205 **[1]**

Linda M. Distlerath, Department of Biochemistry and Center in Molecular Toxicology, Vanderbilt University School of Medicine, Nashville, TN 37232 **[205]**

Zora Djurić, National Center for Toxicological Research, Jefferson, AR 72079, and Department of Biochemistry, University of Arkansas for Medical Sciences, Little Rock, AR 72205 **[441]**

Richard Doll, Imperial Cancer Research Fund, Cancer Epidemiology and Clinical Trials Unit, The Radcliffe Infirmary, Oxford OX2 6HE, United Kingdom **[111]**

Jeanne Domoradzki, Carcinogenesis Laboratory, Department of Microbiology, and Department of Biochemistry, Michigan State University, East Lansing, MI 48824-1316 **[411]**

Paul R. Donahue, Massachusetts Institute of Technology, Department of Applied Biological Sciences, Cambridge, MA 02139 **[233]**

Leon G. Epstein, Departments of Neuroscience and Pediatrics, University of Medicine and Dentistry of New Jersey, Newark, NJ 07103 **[449]**

John M. Essigmann, Laboratory of Toxicology, Department of Applied Biological Sciences, Massachusetts Institute of Technology, Cambridge, MA 02139 **[427]**

E. Kim Fifer, National Center for Toxicological Research, Jefferson, AR 72079 **[441]**

Edith Flatau, USC Comprehensive Cancer Center, Los Angeles, CA 90033; present address: Internal Medicine "B," Central Emek Hospital, Afula 18101, Israel **[149]**

T.N. Fredrickson, Laboratory of Immunopathology, National Institute of Allergy and Infectious Diseases, National Institutes of Health, Bethesda, MD 20205 **[67]**

Krystyna Frenkel, Department of Environmental Medicine, New York University Medical Center, New York, NY 10016 **[53]**

Robert C. Gallo, Laboratory of Tumor Cell Biology, National Cancer Institute, Bethesda, MD 20205 **[293,449]**

Denise A. Galloway, Tumor Biology Division, Fred Hutchinson Cancer Research Center, Seattle, WA 98104 **[401]**

Arnona Gazit, Laboratory of Cellular and Molecular Biology, National Cancer Institute, Bethesda, MD 20205 **[155]**

Brenda Gerwin, Laboratory of Human Carcinogenesis, Division of Cancer Etiology, National Cancer Institute, Bethesda, MD 20205 **[213]**

Marc T. Goodman, Cancer Research Center of Hawaii, University of Hawaii at Manoa, Honolulu, HI 96813 **[177]**

Calvert L. Green, Laboratory of Toxicology, Department of Applied Biological Sciences, Massachusetts Institute of Technology, Cambridge, MA 02139; present address: AMGen, Inc., Thousand Oaks, CA 91320-1789 **[427]**

Jerome E. Groopman, Departments of Pathology and Medicine, New England Deaconess Hospital, Boston, MA 02215 **[449]**

John D. Groopman, Boston University School of Public Health, Environmental Health Section, Boston, MA 02118 **[233]**

F. Peter Guengerich, Department of Biochemistry and Center in Molecular Toxicology, Vanderbilt University School of Medicine, Nashville, TN 37232 **[205]**

Nancy J. Haley, American Health Foundation, Valhalla, NY 10595 **[191]**

W. David Hankins, Laboratory of Experimental Carcinogenesis, National Cancer Institute, Bethesda, MD 20205 **[91]**

Mary E. Harper, Laboratory of Tumor Cell Biology, National Cancer Institute, Bethesda, MD 20205 **[449]**

Curtis C. Harris, Laboratory of Human Carcinogenesis, Division of Cancer Etiology, NCI, Bethesda, MD 20205 **[213,271]**

Stephen S. Hecht, American Health Foundation, Valhalla, NY 10595 **[191]**

Robert H. Heflich, National Center for Toxicological Research, Jefferson, AR 72079 **[441]**

Peter Herrlich, Kernforschungszentrum Karlsruhe, Institut für Genetik und Toxikologie, D-7500 Karlsruhe 1, Federal Republic of Germany **[23]**

Jan H.J. Hoeijmakers, Department of Cell Biology and Genetics, Erasmus University, 3000 DR Rotterdam, The Netherlands **[387]**

Dietrich Hoffmann, American Health Foundation, Valhalla, NY 10595 **[191]**

Robert N. Hoover, Environmental Epidemiology Branch, Division of Cancer Etiology, National Cancer Institute, Bethesda, MD 20205 **[313]**

Azhar Hossain, Laboratory of Experimental Carcinogenesis, National Cancer Institute, Bethesda, MD 20205 **[91]**

Hsia Chu-chieh, Cancer Institute, Chinese Academy of Medical Sciences, Beijing, China **[283]**

Eng-Shang Huang, Departments of Medicine, and Microbiology and Immunology, University of North Carolina at Chapel Hill, Lineberger Cancer Research Center, Chapel Hill, NC 27514 **[323]**

Mien-Chie Hung, Whitehead Institute for Biomedical Research, and Department of Biology, Massachusetts Institute of Technology, Cambridge, MA 02142 **[391]**

Shu-Mei Huong, Department of Microbiology and Immunology, University of North Carolina Chapel Hill, Chapel Hill, NC 27514 **[323]**

Hisanaga Igarashi, Laboratory of Cellular and Molecular Biology, National Cancer Institute, Bethesda, MD 20205 **[155]**

J.N. Ihle, NCI-Frederick Cancer Research Facility, LBI-Basic Research Program, Frederick, MD 21701 **[67]**

H.W. Jansen, Max Planck Institut für Molekulare Genetik, Otto Warburg Labor, Berlin 33, Federal Republic of Germany **[67]**

Peter A. Jones, USC Comprehensive Cancer Center, Los Angeles, CA 90033 **[149]**

Steven F. Josephs, Laboratory of Tumor Cell Biology, National Cancer Institute, Bethesda, MD 20205 **[449]**

Suzanne Kateley-Kohler, Carcinogenesis Laboratory, Department of Microbiology, and Department of Biochemistry, Michigan State University, East Lansing, MI 48824-1316 **[419]**

David G. Kaufman, Department of Pathology and Lineberger Cancer Research Center, University of North Carolina, Chapel Hill, NC 27514 **[33]**

William K. Kaufmann, Department of Pathology and Lineberger Cancer Research Center, University of North Carolina, Chapel Hill, NC 27514 **[33]**

Timothy Kautiainen, USC Comprehensive Cancer Center, Los Angeles, CA 90033 **[149]**

Jung-Kon Kim, Laboratory of Experimental Carcinogenesis, National Cancer Institute, Bethesda, MD 20205 **[91]**

Alfred G. Knudson, Jr., Institute for Cancer Research, Fox Chase Cancer Center, Philadelphia, PA 19111 **[127]**

Bernhard König, Molecular Mechanisms of Tumor Promotion Section, Laboratory of Cellular Carcinogenesis and Tumor Promotion, National Cancer Institute, Bethesda, MD 20205; present address: Boehringer Mannheim GmbH, Biochemica Werk Tutzing, D-8132 Tutzing, Federal Republic of Germany **[1]**

Brent E. Korba, Laboratory of Human Carcinogenesis, Division of Cancer Etiology, National Cancer Institute, Bethesda, MD 20892 **[271]**

Theodore G. Krontiris, Division of Hematology/Oncology and Cancer Research Center, Tufts-New England Medical Center, and Department of Molecular Biology and Microbiology, Tufts University School of Medicine, Boston, MA 02111 **[99]**

Mary C. Kuhns, Hepatitis Research, Diagnostics Division, Abbot Laboratories, North Chicago, IL 60064 **[227]**

Fernando Leal, Laboratory of Cellular and Molecular Biology, National Cancer Institute, Bethesda, MD 20205 **[155]**

John F. Lechner, Laboratory of Human Carcinogenesis, Division of Cancer Etiology, National Cancer Institute, Bethesda, MD 20205 **[213]**

Edward L. Loechler, Laboratory of Toxicology, Department of Applied Biological Sciences, Massachusetts Institute of Technology, Cambridge, MA 02139; present address: Department of Biology, Boston University, Boston, MA 02215 **[427]**

Christine Lücke-Huhle, Kernforschungszentrum Karlsruhe, Institut für Genetik und Toxikologie, D-7500 Karlsruhe 1, Federal Republic of Germany **[23]**

Susan A. MacKenzie, Department of Pathology and Lineberger Cancer Research Center, University of North Carolina, Chapel Hill, NC 27514 **[33]**

Veronica M. Maher, Carcinogenesis Laboratory, Department of Microbiology, and Department of Biochemistry, Michigan State University, East Lansing, MI 48824-1316 **[411,419]**

Dean L. Mann, Laboratory of Human Carcinogenesis, Division of Cancer Etiology, National Cancer Institute, Bethesda, MD 20205 **[271]**

George Mark, Laboratory of Human Carcinogenesis, Division of Cancer Etiology, National Cancer Institute, Bethesda, MD 20205 **[213]**

Lisa M. Marselle, Laboratory of Tumor Cell Biology, National Cancer Institute, Bethesda, MD 20205 **[449]**

Martha V. Martin, Department of Biochemistry and Center in Molecular Toxicology, Vanderbilt University School of Medicine, Nashville, TN 37232 **[205]**

Tohru Masui, Laboratory of Human Carcinogenesis, Division of Cancer Etiology, National Cancer Institute, Bethesda, MD 20205 **[213]**

J. Justin McCormick, Carcinogenesis Laboratory, Department of Microbiology, and Department of Biochemistry, Michigan State University, East Lansing, MI 48824-1316 **[411,419]**

James K. McDougall, Tumor Biology Division, Fred Hutchinson Cancer Research Center, Seattle, WA 98104 **[355,401]**

Assieh A. Melikian, American Health Foundation, Valhalla, NY 10595 **[191]**

H. David Mitcheson, Department of Urology, Tufts-New England Medical Center, Boston, MA 02111 **[99]**

R. Montesano, Unit of Mechanisms of Carcinogenesis, International Agency for Research on Cancer, 69372 Lyon Cedex 08, France **[43]**

H.C. Morse, III, Laboratory of Immunopathology, National Institute of Allergy and Infectious Diseases, National Institutes of Health, Bethesda, MD 20205 **[67]**

C.S. Muir, International Agency for Research on Cancer, 69372 Lyon Cedex 08, France **[135]**

Vicente Notario, Laboratory of Cellular and Molecular Biology, National Cancer Institute, Bethesda, MD 20205 **[155]**

Hannie Odijk, Department of Cell Biology and Genetics, Erasmus University, 3000 DR Rotterdam, The Netherlands **[387]**

Carl J. O'Hara, Departments of Pathology and Medicine, New England Deaconess Hospital, Boston, MA 02215 **[449]**

James M. Oleske, Departments of Neuroscience and Pediatrics, University of Medicine and Dentistry of New Jersey, Newark, NJ 07103 **[449]**

Robert F. Ozols, National Cancer Institute, National Institutes of Health, Bethesda, MD 20205 **[303]**

Joseph S. Pagano, Lineberger Cancer Research Center, School of Medicine, University of North Carolina, Chapel Hill, NC 27514 **[345]**

David R. Parkinson, Division of Hematology/Oncology and Cancer Research Center, Tufts-New England Medical Center, Boston, MA 02111 **[99]**

Malcolm C. Paterson, Health Sciences Division, Chalk River Nuclear Laboratories, Chalk River, Ontario K0J 1J0, Canada; present address: Molecular Genetics and Carcinogenesis Laboratory, Department of Medicine, Cross Cancer Institute, Edmonton, Alberta T6G 1Z2, Canada **[373]**

Miriam C. Poirier, National Cancer Institute, National Institutes of Health, Bethesda, MD 20205 **[303]**

Annette Pöting, Kernforschungszentrum Karlsruhe, Institut für Genetik und Toxikologie, D-7500 Karlsruhe 1, Federal Republic of Germany **[23]**

Richard J. Rahija, Department of Pathology and Lineberger Cancer Research Center, University of North Carolina, Chapel Hill, NC 27514 **[33]**

Hans Jobst Rahmsdorf, Kernforschungszentrum Karlsruhe, Institut für Genetik und Toxikologie, D-7500 Karlsruhe 1, Federal Republic of Germany **[23]**

U.R. Rapp, Laboratory of Viral Carcinogenesis, National Cancer Institute, Frederick, MD 21701 **[67]**

Eddie Reed, National Cancer Institute, National Institutes of Health, Bethesda, MD 20205 **[303]**

Paul E.B. Reilly, Department of Biochemistry and Center in Molecular Toxicology, Vanderbilt University School of Medicine, Nashville, TN 37232 **[205]**

Arthur D. Riggs, Department of Molecular Biology, Beckman Research Institute of the City of Hope, Duarte, CA 91010 **[9]**

Keith C. Robbins, Laboratory of Cellular and Molecular Biology, National Cancer Institute, Bethesda, MD 20205 **[155]**

Marjorie Robert-Guroff, Laboratory of Tumor Cell Biology, National Cancer Institute, Bethesda, MD 20205 **[293]**

Henry Rothschild, Department of Medicine, Louisiana State University, School of Medicine, New Orleans, LA 70112 **[397]**

Alan L. Schechter, Whitehead Institute for Biomedical Research, and Department of Biology, Massachusetts Institute of Technology, Cambridge, MA 02142 **[391]**

David A. Shafritz, Albert Einstein College of Medicine, Marion Bessin Liver Research Center, Bronx, NY 10461 **[257]**

Tsutomu Shimada, Department of Biochemistry and Center in Molecular Toxicology, Vanderbilt University School of Medicine, Nashville, TN 37232 **[205]**

Steven S. Smith, Department of Molecular Biology, Beckman Research Institute of the City of Hope, Duarte, CA 91010 **[9]**

J. Staszewski, International Agency for Research on Cancer, 69372 Lyon Cedex 08, France **[135]**

David F. Stern, Whitehead Institute for Biomedical Research, and Department of Biology, Massachusetts Institute of Technology, Cambridge, MA 02142 **[391]**

Sun Tsung-tang, Cancer Institute, Chinese Academy of Medical Sciences, Beijing, China **[283]**

Walter Troll, Department of Environmental Medicine, New York University Medical Center, New York, NY 10016 **[53]**

Steven R. Tronick, Laboratory of Cellular and Molecular Biology, National Cancer Institute, Bethesda, MD 20205 **[155]**

Diane R. Umbenhauer, Unit of Mechanisms of Carcinogenesis, International Agency for Research in Cancer, 69372 Lyon Cedex 08, France; present address: Department of Biochemistry and Center in Molecular Toxicology, Vanderbilt University School of Medicine, Nashville, TN 37232 **[43, 205]**

Lalitha Vaidyanathan, Whitehead Institute for Biomedical Research, and Department of Biology, Massachusetts Institute of Technology, Cambridge, MA 02142 **[391]**

Marcel van Duin, Department of Cell Biology and Genetics, Erasmus University, 3000 DR Rotterdam, The Netherlands **[387]**

Wim Vermeulen, Department of Cell Biology and Genetics, Erasmus University, 3000 DR Rotterdam, The Netherlands **[387]**

Masami Watanabe, Carcinogenesis Laboratory, Department of Microbiology, and Department of Biochemistry, Michigan State University, East Lansing, MI 48824-1316 **[419]**

Wei Yao-peng, Qidong Liver Cancer Institute, Jiangsu Province, China **[283]**

Robert A. Weinberg, Whitehead Institute for Biomedical Research, and Department of Biology, Massachusetts Institute of Technology, Cambridge, MA 02142 **[391]**

Andries Westerveld, Department of Cell Biology and Genetics, Erasmus University, 3000 DR Rotterdam, The Netherlands **[387]**

C.P. Wild, Unit of Mechanisms of Carcinogenesis, International Agency for Research on Cancer, 69372 Lyon Cedex 08, France **[43]**

James C. Willey, Laboratory of Human Carcinogenesis, Division of Cancer Etiology, National Cancer Institute, Bethesda, MD 20205 **[213]**

Lewis T. Williams, Howard Hughes Medical Institute, University of California, San Francisco, CA 94143 **[155]**

Vincent Wilson, USC Comprehensive Cancer Center, Los Angeles, CA 90033; present address: Laboratory of Human Carcinogenesis, National Cancer Institute, Building 37, Bethesda, MD 20205 **[149]**

Gerald N. Wogan, Massachusetts Institute of Technology, Department of Applied Biological Sciences, Cambridge, MA 02139 **[233]**

Flossie Wong-Staal, Laboratory of Tumor Cell Biology, National Cancer Institute, Bethesda, MD 20205 **[449]**

Wu Shao-ming, Cancer Institute, Chinese Academy of Medical Sciences, Beijing, China **[283]**

Ernst L. Wynder, Division of Epidemiology, Mahoney Institute for Health Maintenance, American Health Foundation, New York, NY 10017, and American Health Foundation, Valhalla, NY 10595 **[177, 191]**

George H. Yoakum, Laboratory of Human Carcinogenesis, Division of Cancer Etiology, National Cancer Institute, Bethesda, MD 20205 **[213, 271]**

Stuart H. Yuspa, National Cancer Institute, National Institutes of Health, Bethesda, MD 20205 **[303]**

Keith E. Zucker, Department of Molecular Biology, Beckman Research Institute of the City of Hope, Duarte, CA 91010 **[9]**

Preface

The primary goal of biochemical and molecular epidemiology is to identify individuals at high cancer risk by obtaining pathobiological evidence of (a) high exposure of target cells to chemical, physical, and microbial carcinogens and/or (b) increased oncogenic susceptibility due to inherited or acquired host factors.

Advances in laboratory methods have been recently developed to be used in combination with analytical epidemiology to identify individuals at high cancer risk. These methods include: (1) techniques to assess specific host susceptibility factors, (2) assays that detect carcinogens in human tissues, cells, and fluids, (3) cellular assays to measure pathobiological evidence of exposure to carcinogens, and (4) methods to measure early biochemical and molecular responses to carcinogens.

This is an important new area of emphasis consisting of multidisciplinary investigations into cancer etiology that combine epidemiological and experimental approaches. Included are efforts to incorporate already developed biochemical and molecular techniques into epidemiologic investigations and the further development and refinement of new experimental procedures into safe, accurate, reliable, and informative adjuncts to human investigations.

The potential of biochemical and molecular epidemiology to predict cancer risk on an individual basis, instead of on a population level, and prior to the onset of clinically evident cancer provides an exciting new opportunity in cancer research and prevention.

The symposium integrated plenary sessions on the fundamental aspects of carcinogenesis with lectures and workshops on the applications of both the new biotechnology and our current understanding of this multistage process to epidemiologically defined human populations. The symposium attracted an audience from diverse disciplines ranging from molecular biology to clinical medicine.

By all measures—the information presented, the intensity and vigor of discussions, and the sense of interest and excitement of participants—the symposium was successful. It is my hope that much of this has been distilled and conveyed in the series of papers and workshop summaries included in this volume.

The meeting which formed the basis for this book would not have been possible without the generous Abbott Laboratories sponsorship. Travel and subsistence expenses of speakers also were defrayed in part by Lilly Research Laboratories, Eli Lilly and Company, grant CA39223-01 from The United States Public Health Service, and an additional contribution from Abbott Laboratories. The skillful management of the symposium by Robin Yeaton, Hank Harwood, Ed Burgess and members of the symposia staff is gratefully acknowledged. In addition, I thank Chris Anderson for her efforts in the preparation of this volume. Finally, I thank the members of the advisory committee M. Bishop, P. Cerutti, C. Croce, W. Haseltine, N. Levy, J. Mulvihill, A. Skalka, and J. Tomita, who are also responsible for the success of this symposium.

Curtis C. Harris

Journal of Cellular Biochemistry 29:37–44 (1985)
Biochemical and Molecular Epidemiology of Cancer 1–8

Stoichiometric Binding of Diacylglycerol to the Phorbol Ester Receptor

Bernhard König, Patricia A. DiNitto, and Peter M. Blumberg

Molecular Mechanisms of Tumor Promotion Section, Laboratory of Cellular Carcinogenesis and Tumor Promotion, National Cancer Institute, Bethesda, Maryland 20205

The major phorbol ester receptor is the Ca^{++}-activated, phospholipid-dependent protein kinase C. Diacylglycerol stimulates protein kinase C in a fashion similar to the phorbol esters. Likewise, it inhibits phorbol ester binding competitively. Both results suggest that diacylglycerol is the/an endogenous phorbol ester analogue. Alternatively, the diacylglycerol might simply be acting to modify the phospholipid environment of the protein. If diacylglycerol were indeed functioning as an analogue, it should interact with the receptor stoichiometrically. This interaction can be quantitated by measuring the perturbation in apparent diacylglycerol binding affinity as a function of the ratio of diacylglycerol to receptor. We report here that 1,2-dioleoylglycerol interacts with the receptor with the predicted stoichiometry.

Key words: problem kinase C, diacylglycerol, competitive inhibition of phorbol ester binding, stoichiometric binding, phorbol ester receptor, [³H]phorbol 12,13-diacetate binding, tumor promotion

The biological effects of the phorbol esters appear to be mediated principally through a high-affinity receptor [1], which represents a complex between specific phospholipids, Ca^{++}, and the apoenzyme protein kinase C [2–7]. This complex is believed to play an important role in transducing the signals of extracellular messengers whose earliest effect is the enhanced breakdown of phosphatidylinositol -4,5-bisphosphate [8]. Diacylglycerol, one product of this breakdown, stimulates PKC under conditions of limiting Ca^{++} and phospholipid [9].

In analogy with the opiate receptor, the phorbol ester receptor displays high evolutionary conservation, strongly implying the existence of an endogenous analogue.

Abbreviations used: PKC, phospholipid and Ca^{++}-dependent protein kinase; [³H]PDBu, [20-³H]phorbol 12,13-dibutyrate; [³H]PDA, [20-³H]phorbol 12,13-diacetate; EGTA, ethylene glycol bis (β-aminoethyl ether)-N,N,N′,N′-tetraacetic acid.

Bernhard König's present address is Boehringer Mannheim GmbH, Biochemica Werk Tutzing, Bahnhofstrasse 9-15, D-8132 Tutzing, Federal Republic of Germany.

Received March 15, 1985; revised and accepted June 7, 1985.

© **1985 Alan R. Liss, Inc.**

Diacylglycerol is a likely candidate for such an analogue because (1) both the phorbol esters and diacylglycerols stimulate protein kinase C activity in vitro [10], and (2) both induce similar biochemical and cellular responses, including phosphorylation of a 40K protein in platelets [11,12] and a 42K protein in chicken embryo fibroblasts [13].

Kikkawa et al [14] have demonstrated that [3H]phorbol 12,13-dibutyrate binds to the complex of PKC and phosphatidylserine with a stoichiometry of approximately 1:1. Our laboratory has previously reported that 1,2-dioleoylglycerol inhibits phorbol ester binding competitively [15]; the apparent affinity was approximately 80-fold lower than that of the corresponding phorbol 12,13-dioleate [16]. As is expected for a lipophilic compound, the binding affinity of 1,2-dioleoylglycerol reflects its concentration in the lipid phase rather than its concentration averaged over the volume of the aqueous suspension. If diacylglycerol is indeed a phorbol ester analogue, it should also bind with 1:1 stoichiometry and interact at the same site on the enzyme. Neither result would be predicted if diacylglycerol simply functioned by perturbing the phospholipid bilayer. We present evidence here that diacylglycerol interacts stoichiometrically with the phorbol ester receptor/protein kinase C.

MATERIALS AND METHODS
Materials

L-α-phosphatidyl-L-serine (bovine brain), rac-1,2-dioleoylglycerol, leupeptin, phenylmethylsulfonyl fluoride, and bovine gamma globulin were from Sigma (St. Louis, MO). Diethylaminoethyl cellulose (DE-52) anion exchanger was from Whatman (Clifton, NJ). Polyethylene glycol (molecular weight—mol wt 6,000–7,500) was obtained from EM Science (Gibbstown, NJ). [3H]PDA was synthesized from 20-oxo-20-deoxy-PDA (LC Services, Waltham, MA) according to published procedures [17] and purified by high-performance liquid chromatography (HPLC) on a RP-18 column in methanol/H_2O (55:45). The specific activity of [3H]PDA was 1.49 Ci/mmol.

Purification of the Phorbol Ester Receptor

The phorbol ester aporeceptor from mouse brain cytosol was partially purified by chromatography on DE-52 as described previously [18].

[3H]PDA Binding Assay

[3H]PDA binding was assayed basically as described for [3H]PDBu [16]. The incubation mixtures contained 0.5 μg/ml of phosphatidylserine, 0.05 M Tris-Cl, pH 7.4, 100 μg/ml of DE-52 purified protein (unless indicated otherwise), 7–340 nM [3H]PDA, 3 mg/ml of bovine gamma globulin, 2 mM Ca^{++}, and 0.5 mM EGTA. (Additional chelators in the enzyme preparation [edetic acid—EDTA, EGTA] increase the total concentration of chelators to approximately 1.8 mM.) To determine the dissociation constant (K_D) for [3H]PDA, the concentration of radiolabeled phorbol ester was varied between 5 and 200 nM. To measure inhibition of phorbol ester binding, aliquots of phosphatidylserine and rac-1,2-dioleoylglycerol were mixed in chloroform, the solvent was removed under nitrogen, and the lipids were dispersed in 50 mM Tris-Cl, pH 7.4 (saturated with nitrogen) by gentle sonication. The lipids were then added to the assay mixture to give the final concentrations indicated. Nonspecific binding was measured in control samples containing at least a 150-fold molar excess of nonradioactive phorbol ester. Specific binding represents the difference between total and nonspecific binding. To determine the actual dissociation constant (K_i) for rac-1,2-dioleoylglycerol, inhibition of [^{3}H]PDA binding was measured as described above, except that the incubation mixture contained 100 μg/ml of phosphatidylserine and 0.1 mM $CaCl_2$ with a final concentration of ~1.3 mM chelators present in the enzyme preparation.

RESULTS AND DISCUSSION

Because of the insolubility of the long-chain diacylglycerols, the measurement of their direct binding to protein kinase C is difficult. Since the diacylglycerol remains in the lipid phase used to reconstitute the receptor, whether it is specifically bound or not, physical separation of the bound and free ligand is not feasible. Therefore, the approach we adopted relies on the decrease of free ligand in the lipid phase as ligand binds to the receptor. This decrease in free ligand can be detected as a shift in the apparent dissociation constant (K_{app}), expressed in terms of total ligand concentration, as a function of the ratio of ligand to receptor in the system.

The K_{app} for the diacylglycerol was determined from inhibition of radioactive phorbol ester binding according to the relationship:

$$K_{app} = \frac{I_{50}}{1 + L/K_D} \qquad (1)$$

where I_{50} = concentration of *total* diacylglycerol yielding 50% inhibition of phorbol ester binding, L = concentration of radioactive phorbol ester, and K_D = dissociation constant for phorbol ester binding. Because $I_{50} = I_{50}$(free) + I_{50}(bound) and I_{50}(bound) = n (R/2), equation 1 can be rewritten as:

$$K_{app} = K_i + \frac{n (R/2)}{1 + L/K_D} \qquad (2)$$

where K_i = actual dissociation constant for the diacylglycerol, expressed in terms of free ligand [19], R = concentration of reconstituted receptor, and n = number of diacylglycerol molecules bound per receptor molecule. The value of n can be determined by varying either R or L and measuring K_{app}.

The relatively low affinity of the diacylglycerol made it essential to optimize the assay conditions in order to get significant variation in K_{app}.

First, we maximized the concentration of receptors in the assay and minimized the concentration of phosphatidylserine. The motivation was that we had previously shown that the K_i for 1,2-dioleoylglycerol, expressed in molar concentrations, was proportional to the lipid concentration, ie, the receptor actually recognizes the concentration of diacylglycerol in the lipid phase [15]. Previous work in this laboratory had also shown that the potency of phosphatidylserine and other phospholipids to reconstitute phorbol ester binding activity was dramatically dependent on the concentration of free Ca^{++} [7]; ie, Ca^{++} reduced the requirements for phospholipids substantially. A factor limiting how much the phosphatidylserine concentration could be decreased is that 50–100 molecules of phosphatidylserine per receptor are required for reconstitution under our assay conditions.

Second, analysis was simplified provided we could restrict the increase in phorbol ester concentration (L) over the competition curve as the phorbol ester was displaced from the receptor by the diacylglycerol. This condition necessitated maintaining high concentrations of L. Because we had to measure binding activity at concentrations of L below its K_D, a phorbol ester of low binding affinity was required. We therefore synthesized and used [3H]PDA. Under our assay conditions [3H]PDA bound with a K_D of 45 ± 0.2 nM (mean ± SE, three experiments) as determined by Scatchard analysis [20] of binding data (Fig. 1). In contrast [3H]PDBu, the more usual derivative for phorbol ester binding studies, bound under similar conditions with a K_D of 0.8 ± 0.09 nM (mean ± SE, seven experiments) [7].

To determine the actual dissociation constant (K_i) for 1,2-dioleoylglycerol, inhibition of [3H]PDA binding by the diacylglycerol was measured under conditions of an excess of inhibitor over receptor. As shown in Figure 2, the measured values for inhibition of [3H]PDA binding by 1,2-dioleoylglycerol fit the theoretical curve for a competitive inhibitor. The results confirm our previously published findings

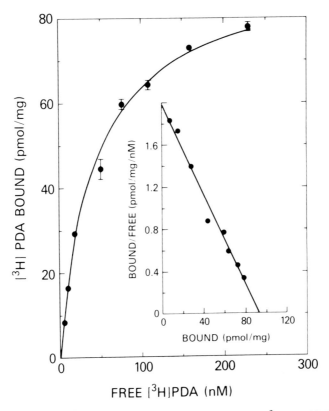

Fig. 1. Specific binding of [3H]PDA to the phorbol ester aporeceptor. [3H]PDA binding was assayed in the presence of 0.5 μg/ml of phosphatidylserine as described in Materials and Methods. Each point represents the mean value for triplicate samples. Results are representative of three independent experiments. Inset: Scatchard analysis of binding data.

using [^{3}H]PDBu and somewhat different assay conditions [15]. The measured value for the I$_{50}$ of 1,2-dioleoylglycerol was 0.75 μg/ml (see Fig. 2), and the concentration of free [^{3}H]PDA at the I$_{50}$ was 235 nM. Using these values and the K$_D$ value of 45 nM (see Fig. 1), a K$_i$ for 1,2-dioleoylglycerol of 0.12% (w/w, relative to phosphatidylserine) was determined according to equation 1.

Having determined the K$_D$ for [^{3}H]PDA binding and the K$_i$ for inhibition of phorbol ester binding by 1,2-dioleoylglycerol, we used two approaches for affecting K$_{app}$ (equation 2).

In the primary set of experiments, L was varied while R was kept constant (Fig. 3). The K$_{app}$ was shifted over a fivefold range as the [^{3}H]PDA concentration was varied from 7 nM (L/K$_D$ = 0.2) to 340 nM (L/K$_D$ = 7.6). Higher concentrations of L could not be used because of excessive nonspecific binding. The variation of K$_{app}$ with L was consistent with a direct interaction of 1,2-dioleoylglycerol with the receptor/kinase C. The data closely fit the theoretical curve calculated for a value of n = 2 and the K$_i$ of 0.12% (w/w, relative to phosphatidylserine), which was determined under conditions of a vast excess of 1,2-dioleoylglycerol over receptor. The actually determined value of n was 1.72 $\pm$ 0.11 (mean $\pm$ SE, 14 determinations). Studies on the conformation of potent and nonpotent PKC activators revealed that specific structural features are required for stimulation of the enzyme [21]. Among the diacylglycerols, 1,2-dioleoylglycerol is known to be one of the most potent PKC activators whereas the 1,3-stereoisomer is basically inactive [22]. Furthermore, Rando

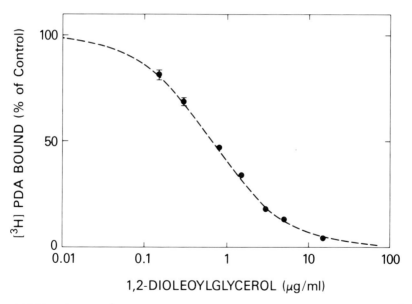

Fig. 2.   Inhibition of specific [^{3}H]PDA binding by rac-1,2-dioleoylglycerol. Specific binding of [^{3}H]PDA was measured in the presence of 100 μg/ml of phosphatidylserine and 0.1 mM Ca^{++} as described in Materials and Methods. Indicated are the mean values $\pm$ SE of triplicate determinations with duplicate determinations of nonspecific binding at each inhibitor concentration. The concentration of total [^{3}H]PDA was 255 nM; that of free [^{3}H]PDA was 235 nM at the I$_{50}$ and varied from 223–251 nM over the competition curve. The concentration of reconstituted receptor was 30.3 nM (100% = 25,000 dpm). Results are representative of three independent experiments.

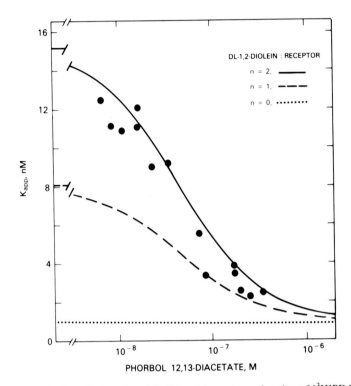

Fig. 3. Apparent binding affinity of rac-1,2-dioleoylglycerol as a function of [³H]PDA concentration. Binding of [³H]PDA to the partially purified phorbol ester aporeceptor from mouse brain was assayed as described in Materials and Methods. K_{app} values were determined at fixed concentrations of [³H]PDA (7–340 nM) by competition with varying concentrations of rac-1,2-dioleoylglycerol incorporated into phosphatidylserine (0.5 μg/ml). The concentration of reconstituted aporeceptor, determined by specific phorbol ester binding, was kept approximately constant at 13–17 nM. Each competition curve spanned at least six inhibitor concentrations, with triplicate determinations of specific [³H]PDA binding and duplicate determinations of nonspecific binding at each concentration. The K_{app} values were derived from the 50% inhibitory concentrations of rac-1,2-dioleoylglycerol in each competition curve according to equation 1 (see text). The theoretical curves for K_{app} as a function of L, indicated for n = 0 (. . . .), n = 1 (----), and n = 2 (——), were calculated according to equation 2 (see text). The R value was 14.25 ± 0.39 nM (mean ± SE, 14 experiments); the K_i value of 0.12% (w/w, relative to phosphatidylserine) measured under conditions of excess diacyglycerol over receptor (see Fig. 2) corresponds to 0.95 ± 0.04 nM (mean ± SE, three determinations) under the conditions of the present experiment.

and Young [23] reported that the stimulation of PKC by 1,2-dioleoylglycerol is stereospecific and that only the 1,2-dioleoyl-sn-glycerol is active, whereas the enantiomer, 2,3-dioleoyl-sn glycerol, is inactive. In our studies, we used the racemic mixture of 1,2-dioleoylglycerol. The active enantiomer could not be used because of considerable racemization during the sonication procedure that is required to generate uniform liposomes. Based on the concentration of the active enantiomer, the value of n is thus 0.86 ± 0.05 (mean ± SE, 14 determinations).

We were able to obtain basically the same results if the concentration of ligand (L) was kept fixed and the receptor concentration (R) was varied (Fig. 4). Increasing the receptor concentration from 2.2 to 16.4 nM led to a 3.3-fold increase in K_{app}. A plot of K_{app} versus R/2(1 + L/K_D) resulted in a linear function with a slope of

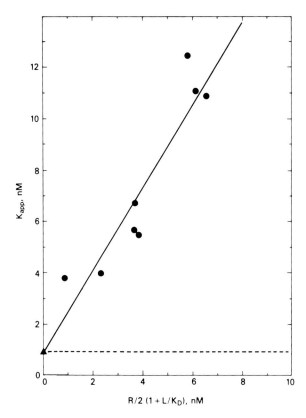

Fig. 4. Apparent binding affinity of rac-1,2-dioleoylglycerol as a function of the concentration of reconstituted receptor. The assay conditions were similar to those described in Figure 1, except that the receptor concentration was varied between 2.2 and 16.4 nM (20–100 μg/ml of DE-52 purified protein) and L was kept approximately constant between 7 and 11 nM ($1 + L/K_D = 1.15$–1.26). The Ca^{++} concentration in individual experiments was adjusted to give an approximately 0.2 mM excess over chelators (EGTA, EDTA) present in the receptor preparation. The value of n was calculated by least-squares analysis assuming the K_i value determined from Figure 2 as indicated ($\blacktriangle$). The solid line corresponds to the least squares value of n = 1.60, the dashed line corresponds to n = 0. The three data points at high receptor concentrations are derived from Figure 1.

n = 1.60 $\pm$ 0.08 (least squares $\pm$ SE, eight determinations). Once again, based on the concentration of the active enantiomer of 1,2-dioleoylglycerol, a value of n close to one was obtained (n = 0.8).

The stoichiometric interaction of 1,2-dioleoylglycerol with the phorbol ester receptor corroborates the indirect evidence that diacylglycerols are endogenous phorbol ester analogues. The experiments obviously cannot address the issue of whether other classes of endogenous analogues of phorbol esters exist. Other classes of structurally dissimilar exogenous analogs of phorbol esters are known, including the indole alkaloids dihydroteleocidin B and lyngbyatoxin, and the polyacetate aplysiatoxin [24]. As we have discussed elsewhere, competitive binding activity does not mean that compounds will function identically [15]. Marked differences in the pharmacokinetic behavior of phorbol esters and diacylglycerols would be predicted.

The stoichiometric binding of diacylglycerol to the phorbol ester receptor/ protein kinase C enhances the likelihood that pharmacological antagonists can be designed. Given the important role postulated for protein kinase C in signal transduction, such compounds could be of considerable interest.

ACKNOWLEDGMENTS

We thank Dr. S.H. Yuspa for careful reading of the manuscript.

REFERENCES

1. Blumberg PM, Dunn JA, Jaken S, Jeng AY, Leach KL, Sharkey NA, Yeh, E: In Slaga TJ (ed): "Mechanisms of Tumor Promotion," Vol 3. Boca Raton, Florida: CRC press, 1984, pp 143–184.
2. Ashendel CL, Staller JM, Boutwell RK: Biochem Biophys Res Commun 111:340, 1983.
3. Sando JJ, Young MC: Proc Natl Acad Sci USA 80:2642, 1983.
4. Niedel JE, Kuhn LJ, Vandenbark GR: Proc Natl Acad Sci USA 80:36, 1983.
5. Leach KL, James ML, Blumberg PM: Proc Natl Acad Sci USA 80:4208, 1983.
6. Parker PD, Stabel S, Waterfield MD: EMBO J 5:953, 1984.
7. König B, DiNitto PA, Blumberg PM: J Cell Biochem 27:255, 1985.
8. Berridge MJ: Biochem J 220:345, 1984.
9. Nishizuka Y: Nature 308:693, 1984.
10. Castagna M, Takai Y, Kaibuchi K, Sano K, Kikkawa U, Nishizuka Y: J Biol Chem 257:7847, 1982.
11. Sano K, Takai Y, Yamanishi J, Nishizuka Y: J Biol Chem 258:2010, 1983.
12. Kaibuchi K, Takai Y, Sawamura M, Hoshijima M, Fujikura T, Nishizuka Y: J Biol Chem 258:6701, 1983.
13. Gilmore T, Martin GS: Nature 306:487, 1983.
14. Kikkawa U, Takai Y, Tanaka Y, Miyake R, Nishizuka Y: J Biol Chem 258:11442, 1983.
15. Sharkey NA, Leach KL, Blumberg PM: Proc Natl Acad Sci USA 81:607, 1984.
16. Sharkey NA, Blumberg PM: Cancer Res 45:19, 1985.
17. Kreibich G, Hecker E: Z Krebsforsch 74:448, 1970.
18. Kikkawa U, Takai Y, Minakuchi R, Inohara S, Nishizuka Y: J Biol Chem 257:13341, 1982.
19. Cheng YC, Prusoff WH: Biochem Pharmacol 22:3099, 1973.
20. Scatchard G: Ann NY Acad Sci 51:660, 1949.
21. Brasseur R, Cabiaux V, Huart P, Castagna M, Baztar S, Ruysschaert JM: Biochem Biophys Res Commun 127:969, 1985.
22. Couturier A, Bazgar S, Castagna M: Biochem Biophys Res Commun 121:448, 1984.
23. Rando RR, Young N: Biochem Biophys Res Commun 122:818, 1984.
24. Sugimura T: Gann 73:499, 1982.

Journal of Cellular Biochemistry 29:337–349 (1985)
Biochemical and Molecular Epidemiology of Cancer 9–21

Purification of Human DNA (Cytosine-5-)-Methyltransferase

Keith E. Zucker, Arthur D. Riggs, and Steven S. Smith

Department of Molecular Biology, Beckman Research Institute of the City of Hope, Duarte, California 91010

We have developed a facile procedure for the purification of DNA methyltransferase activity from human placenta. The procedure avoids the isolation of nuclei and the dialysis and chromatography of large volumes. A purification of 38,000-fold from the whole cell extract has been achieved. The procedure employs ion exchange, affinity, and hydrophobic interaction chromatography coupled with preparative glycerol gradient centrifugation. A protein of 126,000 daltons was found to copurify with the activity and was the major band seen in the most highly purified material after SDS gel electrophoresis. This observation, coupled with an observed sedimentation coefficient of 6.3S, suggests that the enzyme is composed of a single polypeptide chain of this molecular weight. Hemimethylated DNA was found to be the preferred substrate for the enzyme at each stage in the purification. The ratio of the activity of the purified product on hemimethylated to that on unmethylated M13 duplex DNA was about 12 to 1. Thus, the purified activity has the properties postulated for a maintenance methyltransferase. The availability of highly purified human DNA methyltransferase should facilitate many studies on the structure, function, and expression of these activities in both normal and transformed cells.

Key words: DNA methyltransferase, 5-methylcytosine, hydrophobic interaction chromatography, maintenance methylase

DNA (cytosine-5-)-methyltransferase (E.C.2.1.1.37) has been partially purified from several mammalian sources [1–6]; however, in no case has the enzyme been purified to homogeneity. The low yields of even the partially purified enzyme limit most *in vitro* studies. As a result, very few of the properties of this important mammalian enzyme have been unambiguously determined. In most studies, the rate of transfer of methyl groups from S-adenosyl-L-methionine (SAM) to hemimethylated native DNA was found to be considerably higher than that to unmethylated native DNA [3,7–10]. Thus, the enzymes possess the properties of the "maintenance methy-

Abbreviations used: Tris, tris(hydroxymethyl) aminomethane; EDTA, ethylenediamine tetraacetic acid; TCA, trichloroacetic acid; PEI, poly(ethylene-imine); SDS, sodium dodecyl sulfate.

Received April 17, 1985; revised and accepted August 2, 1985.

© **1985 Alan R. Liss, Inc.**

lases" whose existence was originally suggested by Holliday and Pugh [11] and by Riggs [12] as part of a proposal for the somatic inheritance of patterns of DNA methylation at d[CG] doublets. According to these hypotheses fully methylated d[CG] doublets in duplex DNA would give rise to two hemimethylated daughter strands in nascent DNA and the maintenance methylase(s) would rapidly replace the missing methyl groups, thereby regenerating the parental pattern in both daughter cells. Since the time of these proposals it has been convincingly demonstrated that hemimethylated DNA, constructed *in vitro*, is converted to fully methylated DNA *in vivo* following transfection into mammalian cells [13]. Moreover, methylation patterns applied *in vitro* are somatically inherited following transfection [14,15].

Available evidence indicates that methylation patterns can set limits on the transcriptional potential of both normal and transformed cells. A strong negative correlation exists between DNA methylation at critical sites within or near a gene and the potential for the expression of that gene. This has lead to the suggestion that loss of DNA methylation is a necessary but not a sufficient condition for gene expression [16,17]. For recent reviews on these topics see Doerfler [18], Riggs and Jones [19], Nyce et al [20], and Cooper [21].

Abnormal methylation patterns associated with transformed cells have been reported [22–26]. In general, DNA from these cells has been found to be hypomethylated compared to normal tissue, suggesting that at least a transient interruption in normal maintenance methylation often occurs during the generation of transformed cells. Clearly, a key control point in processes associated with oncogenic transformation and normal development might be the DNA methyltransferase(s) that appear(s) to be responsible for somatic inheritance of methylation patterns in DNA. Other cell lineage-specific alterations in methylation pattern [27,28] appear to involve *de novo* methylation and thus might originate with modulation of the activity or specificity of the DNA methyltransferases. To begin to understand the processes that control and modulate DNA methylation patterns, detailed studies of the biochemistry and molecular biology of the enzymes must be performed. However, none of the currently available isolation schemes provide a convenient method for the preparation of amounts of highly purified material. In this report we describe a procedure for the large-scale purification of the enzyme from human placenta.

MATERIALS AND METHODS
DNA Methyltransferase Assay

The standard DNA methyltransferase assay was carried out in polypropylene microcentrifuge tubes in a final volume of 0.10 ml containing 50 mM Tris-acetate, pH 7.8; 10 mM Na_2EDTA; 1.0 mM dithiothreitol; 0.01 mg/ml RNase A; 2.0 μM S-adenosyl-L-[^{3}H]methionine (5–15 Ci/mmol, Amersham Corp. Arlington Heights, IL); 10% (v/v) glycerol; and 0.167 mg/ml heat-denatured *Micrococcus lysodeikticus* DNA (Sigma Chemical Co., St. Louis, MO). After preincubating the mixture for 15 min at 37°C, the reaction was initiated with less than 3 μl of the enzyme preparation. Incubation was continued at 37°C for 1 hr, and the reaction was stopped by placing the tube on ice after an equal volume of 100 mM Tris-acetate, pH 8.0, was added. The resulting mixture was extracted with an equal volume of phenol/chloroform/isoamyl alcohol (25:24:1). One hundred forty microliters of the aqueous phase was removed and immediately precipitated with 5.0 ml of 5% (w/v) TCA containing 5.0

mM sodium pyrophosphate in a 5.0-ml polypropylene tube. Precipitates were collected on GF/C filters (Whatman Inc., Clifton, NJ) and washed three times with 5.0 ml of 2% TCA containing 5.0 mM sodium pyrophosphate. Filters were soaked for 20 min in a tray containing 5% TCA, 5 mM sodium pyrophosphate (about 10 ml per filter) at room temperature, and then rewashed twice as described above. A final wash with 5.0 ml of 100% ethanol dehydrated the filters, which were then dried in an oven at 160°C for 5 min and counted in 10 ml of a tolulene-based scintillation fluid. All sets of assays in which differences in salt concentration were introduced by the enzyme preparation were adjusted with NaCl to the highest salt concentration in the series [29]. After the phosphocellulose-batch step, phenol extration was omitted. A unit of activity is that amount of enzyme that will incorporate-1 pmole of [^{3}H]methyl groups into TCA-insoluable material in 1 hr under the above conditions in a reaction mixture containing 30 mM NaCl. To make direct comparisons of the data with those previously reported by other investigators, we also assayed the enzyme from fractions I through VII under the reaction conditions and with the substrates reported by Pfeifer et al [3] and Wang et al [8].

Enzyme Solubilization

All purification steps were carried out at 4°C unless otherwise indicated. Four full-term placentas were collected shortly after delivery. After removal of the cord and outer membrane, the remaining material was minced with scissors and added to an equal volume of a twofold concentrated solution of buffer A (50 mM Tris-acetate, pH 7.8; 0.1 mM Na$_2$EDTA; 10 mM 2-mercaptoethanol; 25% glycerol). This crude cell suspension was homogenized in a Waring CB-6 Commercial Blender for 10 min. Cell debris was removed by centrifugation at 8,700g for 10 min. PEI (Polymin P, BASF, Ludwigshafen, Federal Republic of Germany) was added to the supernatant (fraction I) to a final concentration of 0.015% using a 10% solution neutralized with HCl as previously described [29]. After 10 min on ice, a precipitate formed. The supernatant fluid (fraction II) was collected by centrifugation at 18,000g for 30 min.

Phosphocellulose Adsorption and Elution

Phosphocellulose (Whatman, P11) was precycled as described by the manufacturer and equilibrated with 0.10 M NaCl in buffer A. Fraction II was mixed with 0.20 volumes of packed phosphocellulose. The mixture was stirred for 30 min, filtered through a sintered glass funnel under vacuum, and washed with at least five column-volumes of equilibration buffer. The methyltransferase was eluted by adding 100 ml of 0.40 M NaCl in buffer A per placenta and the eluate was collected by filtration. This step was repeated once more and the eluates pooled to give fraction III.

Hydroxylapatite Chromatography

Fraction III was mixed with 0.12 volume of packed hydroxylapatite (Bio-gel HTP, Bio Rad Laboratories) that had been equilibrated with 10 mM potassium phosphate in buffer A. The suspension was stirred for 30 min and then loaded into a column. The column was washed with five column-volumes of equilibration buffer and then a six column-volume linear gradient from 10 mM to 500 mM potassium phosphate in buffer A was used to elute the enzyme. Fractions having significant methyltransferase activity were pooled and dialyzed for 12 hr against 25 volumes of

50 mM NaCl in buffer A to give fraction IV. This material could be stored at $-20°C$ for up to 1 week without significant loss of activity. We found it convenient to store material at this stage and have successfully carried out the purification steps described below using the pooled material from two to ten placentas. When the scale of the procedure was changed, column and gradient sizes were proportionally altered.

Cibacron Blue Agarose Chromatography

Fraction IV from four placentas was applied to a 40-ml (2.5 cm $\times$ 8 cm) column of Cibacron blue agarose (Bethesda Research Laboratories) equilibrated with 50 mM NaCl in buffer A. After washing with five column-volumes of equilibration buffer, a ten column-volume linear gradient from 50 mM to 2.0 M NaCl in buffer A was applied. Fractions having methyltransferase activity were pooled to give fraction V.

Hydrophobic Interaction Chromatography

Fraction V was adjusted with 5.0 M NaCl to 1.50 M NaCl in buffer A and applied to a 40-ml (1.4 cm $\times$ 27 cm) column of dodecyl agarose (Sigma Chemical Co.) equilibrated with the same buffer. The enzyme was eluted with three column-volumes of buffer A containing 1.5 M NaCl. Fractions with significant activity were pooled and immediately applied to a 2.0-ml hydroxylapatite column equilibrated with 10 mM potassium phosphate in buffer B (50 mM Tris-acetate, pH 7.8; 0.10 mM Na_2EDTA; 10 mM 2-mercaptoethanol; 2.0% glycerol). The column was washed with five column-volumes of equilibration buffer and then the methyltransferase was eluted with 0.50 M potassium phosphate in buffer B to yield fraction VI.

Glycerol Gradient Centrifugation

Fraction VI was applied to two linear glycerol gradients (5 to 25% glycerol) in 50 mM Tris-acetate, pH 7.8; 0.10 mM Na_2EDTA; 10 mM 2-mercaptoethanol; and 0.50 M potassium phosphate (12 ml each). Centrifugation was carried out in a Beckman SW 40Ti rotor for 40 hr at 40,000 rpm. Equal-sized fractions (about 0.5 ml each) were collected from the gradients by puncturing the bottom of the tube. Fractions containing significant enzyme activity were pooled from all gradients to give fraction VII.

Analytical Heparin Sephrose Chromatography

Fraction VII was dialyzed for 12 hr against 50 mM NaCl in buffer A and then applied to a 0.50-ml column of heparin sephrose prepared by the method of Iverius [30] and equilibrated with the dialysis buffer. After washing with five column-volumes of the equilibration buffer, the enzyme was eluted with a 5-ml linear gradient from 0.05 M to 2.0 M NaCl in buffer A.

Protein Assays

Protein concentrations were determined by the method of Bradford [31] using bovine serum albumin as standard. PEI does not interfere with this method of protein determination [unpublished observations].

Hemimethylated DNA Synthesis

Hemimethylated DNA was synthesized *in vitro* by the method of Gruenbaum et al [32] using single-stranded M13 phage DNA. Double-stranded unmethylated DNA was synthesized by the same procedure except that dCTP was used instead of 5-methyl dCTP.

Protein Gel Electrophoresis

The procedures used for sodium dodecyl sulfate slab gel electrophoresis were those of Laemmli [33], with modifications described by Smith and Braun [29]. Dilute protein samples were concentrated by TCA precipitation [29] prior to gel electrophoresis.

RESULTS AND DISCUSSION
Enzyme Solubilization and Poly(ethylene-imine) Treatment

Existing methods for the purification of the methyltransferases from eukaryotic sources have been useful in the characterization of the activity. However, many studies on the structure and function of the enzyme require large amounts of highly purified material. Nuclear isolation and extraction procedures employing high speed centrifugation and dialysis steps prior to column chromatography are part of most published purification procedures [2,3,34]. This sets practical limits on the scale of the purification. The solubilization procedure described here removes these constraints.

Homogenization of placental tissue in buffer A followed by low speed centrifugation to remove cell debris yielded a slightly turbid crude extract. Considerable nucleic acid was solubilized by this procedure. Agarose gel electrophoresis showed that both RNA and DNA were present. Salt extracted from the placental tissue raised the conductivity of fraction I to that of 0.1 M NaCl in buffer A. We compared the enzyme prepared by the method described above with that prepared from nuclei isolated by the method of Wang et al [8]. Detectable activity was considerably higher in these crude extracts than it was in those prepared from isolated nuclei (see Table I). Although the crude extract prepared from isolated nuclei was more highly enriched in methyltransferase than the crude extract prepared by the present procedure, the isolation of nuclei was very time consuming and did not lend itself to larger scale work.

Since it is possible to solubilize substantially more enzyme without the use of nuclear isolation or high salt, the bulk of the enzyme may be loosely associated with the nucleus. This is consistent with the results of Sano et al [4], who reported localizing most of the activity in the cytoplasmic fraction from bovine thymus.

TABLE I. Preparation of Crude Extracts*

Method	Volume (ml)	Activity (U)	Specific activity (units/mg protein)
Low salt whole cell homogenization	621	46,700	1.25
High salt extraction of nuclei	119	29,322	159

*Whole human placentas were dissected and divided into equal portions. One portion was used for the preparation of a crude extract by high salt extraction from isolated nuclei using the method of Wang et al [8]; the other portion was used to prepare a crude extract by the homogenization of whole cells as described in this report. Total enzyme activity and total protein concentration were determined on the crude extracts. The values presented represent the values obtained from a single placenta and are average values obtained for three independent experiments.

PEI treatment efficiently removed nucleic acid from the low salt crude extracts as judged by agarose gel electrophoresis on samples of fraction II (data not shown). However, it also irreversibly inactivated the enzyme at higher concentrations. The optimal amount for removal of nucleic acid was determined by adding increasing amounts of 10% solution of PEI to 1.0-ml aliquots of a representative crude extract [35]. Since the addition of excess PEI resulted in loss of enzyme activity, we found it advisable to determine the optimal PEI concentration required when new lots were prepared. Calibration for each placental preparation has not been necessary.

Phosphocellulose Batch Adsorption and Elution

Because of the large volumes involved at this stage in the purification, batch adsorption and elution is advantageous. Analytical column chromatography of fraction II on phosphocellulose showed that the DNA methyltransferase eluted as a single wide peak at approximately 0.24 M NaCl in buffer A (data not shown). Thus, the enzyme could be adsorbed directly from fraction II to phosphocellulose equilibrated with buffer A containing 0.10 M NaCl. The minimum amount required to adsorb the maximum amount of enzyme was estimated experimentally. Only two thirds of the activity could be removed from the supernatant with excess phosphocellulose. The minimum amount required to adsorb this amount of activity was 0.20 ml packed column material per milliliter of fraction II.

Batch elution with 0.40 M NaCl in buffer A was necessary to recover the bound enzyme. Additional enzyme could not be removed with higher salt washes. This purification step removed more than 99% of the total protein while activating the enzyme to yield over 100% of the total activity found in fraction II, making it a valuable initial step.

Hydroxylapatite Batch Adsorption and Chromatography

Adsorption of fraction III onto hydroxylapatite was also done in batch to facilitate rapid manipulation of large volumes. As much as 1.50 M NaCl in buffer A does not prevent the binding of the DNA methyltransferase to this matrix. Fraction III contained only 0.40 M NaCl and could be bound to hydroxylapatite without dilution or dialysis to lower the salt, making it a convenient purification step. The enzyme from 1.0 ml of fraction III was bound quantitatively by 0.12 ml packed hydroxylapitite.

Analytical column chromatography showed that the DNA methyltransferase could be eluted as a single peak of activity ranging from 0.15 to 0.25 M potassium phosphate in buffer A (data not shown). Extensive washing followed by gradient elution were necessary to obtain maximal purification with hydroxylapatite. The resulting eluate (fraction IV) was purified approximately threefold over that of fraction III, with quantitative recovery of the enzyme activity. The large concentration of enzyme activity that resulted at this step facilitated manipulations at subsequent stages in the purification.

Dye-Ligand Chromatography

The results of chromatography on Cibacron blue agarose have not been previously reported for the human enzyme. Gradient elution resulted in a single symmetrical peak at about 1.10 M NaCl in buffer A. The enzyme was enriched about fivefold by this chromatographic step with a yield of slightly over 100%. Fraction V consists of at least 100 different polypeptide chains (as shown in Fig. 4), suggesting that considerable further purification is required at this point. When we tested column matrices that had been successfully used to purify the enzyme in other published procedures, no more than a threefold purification beyond fraction V was obtained. Affinity steps like DNA cellulose and S-adenosyl-L-homocysteine agarose also gave little purification at this stage.

Hydrophobic Interaction Chromatography

Chromatography of fraction V on hydrophobic interaction columns of increasing carbon chain lengths revealed that a chain length of 12 carbons was useful for DNA methyltransferase purification. In experiments like that shown in Figure 1, the enzyme was applied to the column at 1.5 M NaCl. Under these conditions, the material that did not bind tightly to the column contained more than 80% of the input activity and was highly purified. Two major peaks of protein are seen in the weakly bound material. One class of protein, including DNA methyltransferase, eluted after about 3.5 column-volumes, whereas a second class of protein eluted after about seven column-volumes. However, more than 90% of the input protein was retained by the

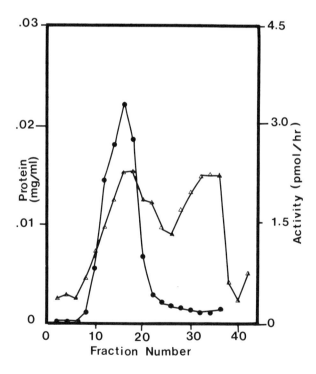

Fig. 1.   Dodecyl agarose chromatography. The pooled active fractions from the Cibacron blue agarose column (fraction V) were adjusted to 1.5 M NaCl in buffer A and applied to a 1.4 cm × 27 cm column of dodecyl agarose equilibrated with the same buffer. After the sample was applied, the column was washed with three column-volumes of the same buffer. Fractions (8 ml) were collected at a flow rate of 40 ml/hr. (△), Protein concentration; (●), methyltransferase activity.

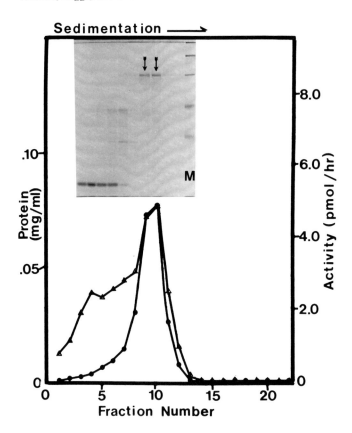

Fig. 2. Preparative glycerol gradient sedimentation. DNA methyltransferase (0.9 ml of fraction VI) was layered onto a 5 to 25% glycerol gradient (12 ml) in 50 mM Tris-acetate, pH 7.8; 0.10 mM Na$_2$EDTA; 10 mM 2-mercaptoethanol; and 0.5 M potassium phosphate and sedimented as described in Materials and Methods. The gradients were fractionated into about 23 equal 0.5-ml fractions. Total activity and protein were determined for each of the fractions in the gradient. ($\triangle$), Protein concentration; ($\bullet$), methyltransferase activity. Inset: SDS gel electrophoretic profile for fractions 3 through 12 from the gradient. The last lane on the right of the photograph (M) contained molecular weight markers as follows: myosin, 205,000; β-galactosidase, 116,000; bovine serum albumin, 66,000; and ovalbumin, 45,000. The two peak fractions are marked with vertical arrows.

column. These columns were not reused. Alternatively, the enzyme could be bound at salt concentrations just above 1.5 M and eluted with a gradient to lower salt.

When the chromatography is carried out at high salt, as shown in Figure 1, dialysis of fraction V can be avoided. Further, because the enzyme does not bind to the column, it is possible to perform this step very rapidly. Since more than 90% of the protein is removed and the volume increases slightly, the methyltransferase emerges from the column at very low protein concentration. It does not store well at this stage and should be concentrated immediately. Hydroxylapatite provides a rapid concentration method. The specific activity of the enzyme actually decreases about 40% after this concentration step. The overall purification obtained over the Cibacron blue pool is still tenfold. It is possible to elute the enzyme from hydroxylapatite in a buffer containing only 2% glycerol, permitting direct loading of fraction VI onto the glycerol gradients.

TABLE II. Large-Scale Purification of DNA Methyltransferase From Human Placenta*

Fraction	Volume (ml)	Total units (U)	Total protein (mg)	Specific activity (U/mg)	Yield purification %	Fold	Activity ratio
Fraction I, crude extract	2,640	206,400	137,000	1.50	100	1.0	—
Fraction II, PEI	2,452	141,200	122,400	1.20	68	0.77	—
Fraction III, phosphocellulose	1,372	168,000	932	180	81	120	10.4
Fraction IV, hydroxylapatite	170	168,400	343	490	82	328	8.9
Fraction V, Cibacron blue	87	173,600	68	2,600	84	1,690	5.2
Fraction VI, dodecyl-HAP[a]	2.0	34,360	1.5	24,000	17	15,200	10.0
Fraction VII, glycerol gradient	2.9	15,680	0.27	58,000	7.6	38,300	12.3

*All data are averages for three independent preparations. The activity ratio is defined as the enzyme activity on hemimethylated duplex M13 RF DNA divided by the enzyme activity on unmethylated duplex M13 RF DNA under the conditions described in Materials and Methods.

[a]Dodecyl-HAP, pooled material after dodecyl agarose chromatography and hydroxylapatite concentration.

Size Fractionation Using Glycerol Gradient Centrifugation

The last step in the purification procedure involved size fractionation of fraction VI. A typical glycerol gradient profile is shown in Figure 2. The DNA methyltransferase activity sedimented at a rate faster than any other protein in the mixture. Fraction VII showed a purification of about 2.5-fold with slightly less than 50% of the total activity retained, on average. Analytical glycerol gradients using internal marker enzymes confirmed the results of Pfeifer et al [3] by showing that the DNA methyltransferase had a sedimentation coefficient of approximately 6.3S (data not shown). The specific activity of the peak fractions in glycerol gradients from independent preparations was constant. Moreover, this peak was resolved from other protein in the profile and appears to be composed largely of active enzyme.

Evidence for Enzyme Purity

The specific activity of the most highly purified enzyme was 58,000 units mg of protein under the standard assay conditions. The specific activity of fraction VII was also determined using the reaction conditions described by Wang et al [8] or by Pfeifer et al [3] in one experiment. The resulting values were 123,000 units mg of protein using the *de novo* substrate and reaction conditions employed by Wang et al [8] and 60,800 units/mg under the conditions employed by Pfeifer et al [3]. Thus, the enzyme described here is more than 28-fold higher in specific activity than that obtained with these two alternative preparation methods. Storage of fraction VII at −20°C resulted in the loss of 50% of the activity in 8 weeks. The purification is summarized in Table II. The final product (fraction VII) was purified 38,000-fold over crude extracts, with an apparent 8% recovery of the total enzyme activity.

An SDS polyacrylamide gel analysis of the steps in the purification is shown in Figure 3. Increasing purification is seen with each step in the procedure. Fraction VII

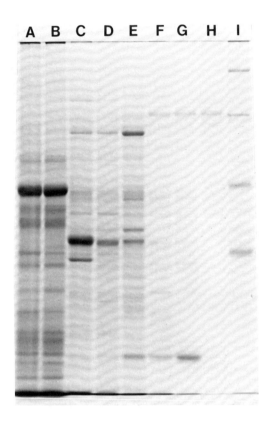

Fig. 3. Polyacrylamide sodium dodecyl sulfate slab gel electrophoresis of the fractions obtained in the purification of DNA methyltransferase. Sodium dodecyl sulfate slab gel electrophoresis and staining conditions were as described in Materials and Methods. The gel shown contains 10% polyacrylamide. Lane A) 250 μg fraction I; lane B) 250 μg fraction II; lane C) 50 μg fraction III; lane D) 50 μg fraction IV; lane E) 50 μg fraction V, lane F) 20 μg pooled dodecyl agarose peak; lane G) 20 μg fraction VI; lane H; 8.0 μg fraction VII. Lane I molecular weight markers: myosin, 205,000; β-galactosidase, 116,000; bovine serum albumin, 66,000; and ovalbumin, 45,000.

shows one major band of protein at about 126,000 daltons, suggesting it is a major component of the enzyme.

Additional evidence for purity is seen from the elution profile for fraction VII on heparin sepharose (Fig. 4). This matrix gives a fivefold purification of enzyme from fraction IV. Total protein and enzyme activity from fraction VII chromatographed on heparin sepharose. Neither protein nor activity were detected in the flowthrough or wash fractions. Moreover, the SDS polyacrylamide gel profile of the pooled peak fractions from this profile show no detectable difference between this material and that of fraction VII (data not shown), suggesting that the enzyme was very highly purified before chromatography on heparin sepharose.

Maintenance and *De Novo* Enzyme Activity

The ratio of enzyme activity on DNA that contains hemimethylated sites to that on double-stranded unmethylated DNA was determined for each stage in the purification. The results (Table II) show that the DNA methyltransferase has a clear

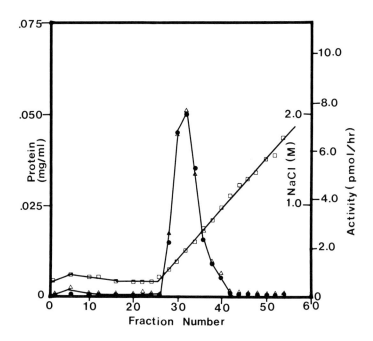

Fig. 4. Cochromatography of total protein and enzyme activity. Peak fractions from the glycerol gradient were pooled (fraction VII), dialyzed against buffer A containing 50 mM NaCl, and applied to a 0.50-ml column of heparin sepharose. After washing the column with five column-volumes of equilibration buffer, it was eluted with a linear gradient from 50 mM to 2.0 M NaCl in buffer A (5.0 ml total). Fractions (0.20 ml) were collected at a flow rate of 1.0 ml/hr. (□), NaCl concentration; (△), protein concentration; (●), methyltransferase activity.

preference for hemimethylated DNA. Activity ratios for fractions I and II could not be determined accurately. The observation of the relatively low activity ratio for fraction V was reproducible.

The results of analytical chromatography and sodium dodecyl sulfate gel electrophoresis on fraction VII also suggest that the enzyme is nearly homogeneous. The SDS gel profile of fraction VII shows that it is composed primarily of a single polypeptide chain of 126,000 daltons. If the enzyme is a typical globular protein, then the observed sedimentation coefficient of 6.3S suggests that it is composed of a single polypeptide chain. However, two additional minor bands of 57,000 and 66,000 account for about 5% of the total protein based on the results of densitometric scanning of Coomassie-stained gels. These two bands were also seen in gels after analytical heparin sepharose column chromatography. Gels stained with silver by the method of Merril et al [35] showed no additional bands.

The DNA methyltransferase purified by this procedure was able to catalyze both the *de novo* and maintenance methylation reactions. Both catalytic activities copurify with the 126,000-dalton polypeptide, and both are demonstrable at each stage in the purification. This result strengthens suggestions [3,8,34,36] that these activities reside on the same enzyme molecule. The maintenance activity of the most highly purified material, as measured by the rate of transfer of methyl groups to hemimethylated M13 duplex DNA, is about 12-fold higher than the *de novo* activity on unmethylated M13 duplex DNA. At each stage in the purification, the rate of maintenance methylation was higher than the *de novo* rate by an average factor of 9.4.

Since this enzyme may carry out *de novo* methylation *in vivo* and since it seems likely that the selectivity of this process must be highly regulated, it is possible that the reaction conditions could be optimized *in vitro* to permit higher rates of activity on double-stranded duplex DNA. The availability of the enzyme in pure form and in relatively large amounts should permit studies of this type on both the maintenance and *de novo* activities. Moreover, studies of the structure, function, regulation, and expression of DNA methyltransferase activities can now be performed.

ACKNOWLEDGMENTS

This work was supported by the following grants from the N.I.H.: S07RR05841 (S.S.S.), GM32863 (S.S.S.), GM312163 (A.D.R.), and CA2652905 (J.R. Benfield). We also acknowledge support from the Council for Tobacco Research U.S.A., Inc. (grant 1571 to S.S.S.). In addition, we thank Sally Wilkins for technical assistance.

REFERENCES

1. Kalousek F, Morris NR: J Biol Chem 244:1157, 1969.
2. Roy PH, Weissbach A: Nucleic Acids Res 2:1669, 1975.
3. Pfeifer GP, Grunwald S, Boehm TLM, Drahovsky D: Biochim Biophys Acta 740:323, 1983.
4. Sano H, Noguchi H, Sager R: Eur J Biochem 135:181, 1983.
5. Adams RLP, Davis T, Fulton J, Kirk D, Qureshi M, Burdon RH: Curr Top Microbiol Immunol 108:143, 1984.
6. Ruchirawat M, Becker FF, Lapeyre J: Biochemistry 23: 5426, 1984.
7. Adams RLP, McKay EL, Craig LM, Burdon RH: Biochim Biophys Acta 561:345, 1979.
8. Wang RYH, Huang L, Ehrlich M: Nucleic Acids Res 12:3473, 1984.
9. Gruenbaum Y, Cedar H, Razin A: Nature 295:620, 1982.
10. Jones PA, Taylor SM: Nucleic Acids Res 9:2933, 1981.
11. Holliday R, Pugh JE: Science 187:226, 1975.
12. Riggs AD: Cytogenet Cell Genet 14:9, 1975.
13. Stein R, Gruenbaum Y, Pollack Y, Razin A, Cedar H: Proc Natl Acad Sci USA 79:61, 1982.
14. Wigler M, Levy D, Perucho M: Cell 24:33, 1981.
15. Pollack Y, Stein R, Razin A, Cedar H: Proc Natl Acad Sci USA 77:6463, 1980.
16. Van der Ploeg, LTH, Flavell RA: Cell 19:947, 1980.
17. Busslinger M, Hurst J, Flavell RA: Cell 34:197, 1983.
18. Doerfler W: Annu Rev Biochem 52:93, 1983.
19. Riggs AD, Jones PA: Adv Cancer Res 40:1, 1983.
20. Nyce J, Weinhouse S, Magee PN: Br J Cancer 48:463, 1983.
21. Cooper DN: Hum Genet 64:315, 1983.
22. Lapeyre J, Becker FF: Biochem Biophys Res Commun 87:698, 1979.
23. Smith SS, Yu JC, Chen CW: Nucleic Acids Res 10:4305, 1982.
24. Feinberg AP, Vogelstein B: Biochem Biophys Res Commun 111:47, 1983.
25. Tolberg ME, Smith SS: FEBS Lett 176:250, 1984.
26. Cheah MS, Wallace CD, Hoffman RM: J Natl Canc Inst 73:1057, 1984.
27. Chapman V, Forrester L, Sanford J, Hastie N, Rossant J: Nature 307:284, 1984.
28. Jahner D, Stuhlmann H, Stewart CL, Harbers K, Lohler J, Simon I, Jaenisch R: Nature 298:623, 1982.
29. Smith SS, Braun R: Eur J Biochem 82:309, 1978.

30. Iverius PH: Biochem J 124:677, 1971.
31. Bradford, MM: Anal Biochem 72:248, 1976.
32. Gruenbaum Y, Cedar H, Razin A: Nucleic Acids Res 9:2509, 1981.
33. Laemmli UK: Nature 227:680, 1970.
34. Bolden A, Ward C, Siedlecki JA, Weissbach A: J Biol Chem 259:12437, 1984.
35. Merril CR, Switzer RC, Van Keuren ML: Proc Natl Acad Sci USA 76:4335, 1979.
36. Grunwald S, Drahovsky D: Int J Biochem 16:883, 1984.

Journal of Cellular Biochemistry 29:351–360 (1985)
Biochemical and Molecular Epidemiology of Cancer 23–32

12-O-Tetradecanoylphorbol-13-Acetate (TPA)-Induced Gene Sequences in Human Primary Diploid Fibroblasts and Their Expression in SV40-Transformed Fibroblasts

Peter Angel, Hans Jobst Rahmsdorf, Annette Pöting, Christine Lücke-Huhle, and Peter Herrlich

Kernforschungszentrum Karlsruhe, Institut für Genetik und Toxikologie, Postfach 3640, D-7500 Karlsruhe 1, Federal Republic of Germany

We have isolated cDNA sequences from TPA-treated primary human fibroblasts, which indicate RNA species that are coordinately regulated after treatment of these cells with either ultraviolet light, mitomycin C, the UV-induced factor EPIF, or TPA. The levels of RNA are elevated in Bloom syndrome (cells of two out of three patients). After transformation with SV40 one of the sequences is overexpressed while another one is reduced. Both genes maintain their inducibility by the agents mentioned.

Key words: human genetic stress response, Bloom syndrome, metallothionein IIa, UV-induced extracellular protein-inducing factor, cDNA cloning

The complete transformation of primary fibroblasts into tumor cells has been dissected into several genetic steps. The first step—immortalization—can be imitated by the experimentally induced expression of any one of a number of genes [1–5] and can be induced by treatment with carcinogens [7]. Immortalized cells become tumorigenic if transfected by one member of a second group of genes [1–7] or if treated with a tumor promoter [8]. These observations suggest that the process of complete transformation requires at least two steps. The involvement of additional steps is likely, eg, the complete transformation of immortalized cells by carcinogens seems to require two events, a frequent and a rare one [9].

Although current views implicate constitutive expression of a number of genes in the transformed cell [10–14], it is conceivable that carcinogens and tumor pro-

Received April 30, 1985, revised and accepted July 24, 1985.

© **1985 Alan R. Liss, Inc.**

moters act by inducing transient functions, eg, a mutator function. This possibility may be supported by the spontaneously elevated mutation rate in the human cancer risk disease Bloom syndrome [15,16].

We have observed earlier that skin fibroblasts from patients with Bloom syndrome express a number of proteins at an elevated rate which normal cells express only when treated with a tumor promoter or with a carcinogen [17,18]. We have used molecular hybridization and cDNA cloning techniques to define RNA sequences that change in abundance after TPA (12-O-tetradecanoylphorbol-13-acetate) treatment. We show that these RNAs are coordinately induced by either carcinogen or TPA treatment and that their expression is elevated spontaneously in cells from two of three patients with Bloom syndrome. Upon transformation of human skin fibroblasts with SV40, the expression of one of the sequences remains elevated. This RNA codes for metallothionein and its elevated expression appears to confer better surviving ability after gamma-ray, X-ray or α-ray treatment. Another RNA species coding for a secreted protein is reduced in the transformed cell. Inducibility by TPA or by the UV-induced factor EPIF [18] is maintained.

MATERIALS AND METHODS
Cells and Culture Conditions

Most cells and their origin have been described [17,18]. SV40-transformed normal human fibroblasts (GM 637) and Xeroderma pigmentosum group A fibroblasts (XP12 Ro) were obtained from JE Cleaver (San Francisco, CA); XPGM 2994 were from the Human Genetic Mutant Cell Repository (Camden, NJ). The cells were grown in monolayers using Dulbecco's minimal essential medium supplemented with 15% fetal calf serum and antibiotics. The pH was maintained at 7.2 and the temperature at 37°C. To ensure optimal growth conditions, cells were seeded at $5 \times 10^5/10$-cm petri dish and the experiments performed 72 hr later.

RNA Purification

Cells were lysed in 7 M urea, 2% SDS, 0.35 M NaCl, 1 mM EDTA, 10 mM Tris HCl, pH 8.0, and the nucleic acids were extracted several times with phenol-chloroform. The RNA was obtained as pellet by centrifugation through CsCl [19]. The RNA pellet was taken up in 10 mM Tris HCl, pH 7.5, and precipitated by ethanol. Poly A$^+$ RNA was purified on oligo-dT-celulose [20].

cDNA Library and Screening

Double-stranded cDNA [21] was synthesized from 10 μg of poly A$^+$ RNA isolated from normal human fibroblasts (Berlin-2) which had been treated with 20 ng/ml TPA for 8 hr. The presence of induced RNAs was tested by in vitro translation in a reticulocyte system. The double-stranded cDNAs were tailed with oligo-dC and inserted into the dG-tailed Pst I site of pBR 322. After annealing, the constructs were transformed into competent Escherichia coli C 600. About 1,200 tetracycline-resistant, ampicillin-sensitive colonies were obtained from 30 ng recombinant plasmid. Individual colonies were grown on L-broth agar plates containing tetracycline at 15 μg/ml and transferred to nitrocellulose by toothpicks. Triplicate filters were prepared. The transferred bacterial clones were permitted to grow to colonies of 2 mm diameter. One filter was stored at 4°C in a sealed bag. The cells on the other two filters were lysed with 10% SDS and the DNA denatured and adsorbed to the filters using 0.5 M NaOH, 1.5M NaCl [21]. The filters were transferred consecutively to 1.5M NaCl, 0.5 M Tris, pH 8.0, and to 0.18 M NaCl, 10 mM NaH_2PO_4, pH 7.4, 1 mM EDTA. The filters were then dried, baked at 80°C for 2 hr, and washed at 65°C in 50 mM Tris HCl, pH 8.0, 1 M NaCl, 1 mM EDTA, 0.1% SDS for 2 hr to remove cell debris. Prehybridization was carried out at 42°C for 6 hr. The mixture contained 50% formamide, 0.9 M NaCl, 50 mM NaH_2PO_4, pH 7.4, 5 mM EDTA, 0.1% SDS, bovine serum albumin, ficoll, and polyvinyl pyrrolidone each, 100 μg/ml small, denatured salmon sperm DNA, 1 μg/ml poly A. One filter was hybridized with radioactive, single-stranded cDNA prepared from poly A^+ RNA of nontreated growing cells, the other with cDNA to RNA from TPA-treated cells. The hybridization mixture contained 2×10^6 cpm ^{32}P-cDNA in 1.5 ml of prehybridization buffer. Incubation was at 42°C for 14 hr. The filters were washed three times at room temperature with $2 \times$ SSC, 0.1% SDS and two times at 68°C with $1 \times$ SSC, 0.1% SDS, dried, and put on film (Kodak X-Omat AR) using an intensifier screen. For the screening see Results and Figure 1.

Dot Blot RNA Hybridizations

Dot blot hybridizations were performed essentially according to Kafatos et al [22]. The required amount of total or poly A^+ RNA was dried in a vacuum centrifuge, taken up in 20 μl 50% formamide, 6% formaldehyde, $1 \times$ TBE (90 mM Tris, 90 mM boric acid, 2.5 mM EDTA pH 8.0), heated at 37°C for 15 min and then at 65°C for 3 min, diluted with 180 μl $10 \times$ SSC, and spotted onto nitrocellulose filters. After baking at 80°C, the filters were prewashed twice at 65°C in $4 \times$ SSC, 0.02% each of bovine serum albumin, ficoll, and polyvinyl pyrrolidone, 0.1% SDS, and 3.3% PiPPi (100% PiPPi is 200 ml 1 M NaH_2PO_4 + 300 ml 1 M Na_2HPO_4 + 200 ml 7.5% $Na_4P_2O_7$ + 300 ml H_2O). To the second wash 20 μg/ml salmon sperm DNA were added. Hybridization was performed at 65°C in $4 \times$ SSC, 10 mM EDTA, 0.1% SDS, 20 μg/ml salmon sperm DNA, and 50 ng/ml nick-translated probe DNA (specific activity 3×10^7–10^8 cpm/μg DNA) for 18 hr. The filters were washed at 65°C consecutively in $2 \times$ SSC, $1 \times$ SSC, and $0.5 \times$ SSC containing 0.1% SDS, 3.3% PiPPi, and were dried and put on film using an intensifier screen.

UV and TPA treatment, in vitro translation, two-dimensional (2D) gel electrophoresis, the preparation of EPIF, and the technique of surviving colony count have been described elsewhere [17,18,23].

RESULTS

The Isolation of cDNA Clones Complementary to TPA-Induced mRNA Species

The TPA-induced mRNAs were quite abundant and could be detected by in vitro translation without difficulty. The translation products have been resolved by two-dimensional gel electrophoresis (Fig 3. in Schorpp et al [18]. An example of the actual RNA preparation used for cloning is shown in Figure 1. We prepared cDNA clones starting from poly A^+ RNA of TPA-treated human fibroblasts and isolated those that hybridized to RNA species that showed an altered abundance after TPA treatment. This was achieved by differentially hybridizing to radioactive total cDNA that had been prepared using either poly A^+ RNA from TPA-treated or from control

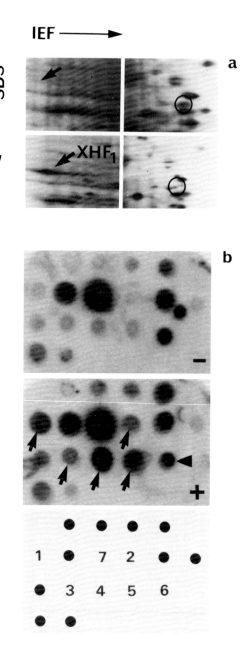

Fig. 1. Screening of the cDNA library. Poly A$^+$ RNA was prepared from logarithmically growing human skin fibroblasts (Berlin-2) and from a parallel culture that had been treated with 20 ng/ml TPA for 8 hr. a) Poly A$^+$ RNA (0.2 μg) was added to 10 μl of a reticulocyte lysate and incubated in the presence of ^{35} S-methionine (4 mCi/ml final conc.) at 30°C for 1 hr. Total protein was resolved by 2-D PAGE [17]. Two regions from the autoradiograms were selected: the area resolving protein XHF1 and an area from the acidic region showing a spot that is reduced. The upper panels were from control cells, the lower panels from TPA-treated cells. The RNA coded also for the other inducible proteins (not

cells. The abundant sequences that have been investigated further have been numbered 1 to 6 (Fig. 1). Clone 7 hybridized equally well to both probes and has been used as a standard clone. Clones 1, 2, 4, and 5 hybridized strongly to cDNA prepared from TPA-treated cells, while clone 3 was labeled only slightly more intensively than to control cDNA. Clone 6 showed a reduced hybridization signal with cDNA made from TPA-treated cells.

The cDNA clones were characterized by hybrid-promoted translation and sequencing experiments to be described elsewhere [24]. Clones 1, 4, and 5 select RNA that codes for the secreted protein XHF 1 [17,18] (Fig. 1). Clone 3 represents part of the metallothionein IIa gene sequence [25].

Coordinate Regulation by TPA, UV, MMC, and EPIF

The cDNA clones indicate RNA species that are rapidly induced by TPA in primary fibroblasts except for clone 6 RNA, which is reduced. The increased levels of RNA at 8 hr after TPA were determined by dot blot hybridizations (Fig. 2). The increases were already detectable at 2 hr after TPA (not shown). As anticipated by the data on the protein level [18], ultraviolet light (UV), mitomycin C (MMC), or the induced extracellular protein-inducing factor EPIF induced similar changes in RNA abundance as did TPA. Examples are shown in Figures 2 and 4. The RNA complementary to cDNA clone 7 did not respond to any of the agents, nor did actin mRNA. The coordinate regulation by carcinogenic and cocarcinogenic agents is an astonishing observation because it suggests that both groups of agents share a mechanism of action although it does not imply that this action is related to the assumed roles in carcinogenesis.

Elevated RNA Levels in Cells From Patients With Bloom Syndrome

Cells from patients with the autosomal recessive genetic disease Bloom syndrome are characterized by chromosomal instability. The instability is detected as a high spontaneous rate of sister chromatid exchanges [26] or mutations [15,16]. Presumably as a consequence of chromosomal instability the patients run an increased risk of developing cancer [26]. Skin fibroblasts from Bloom patients were examined for their content in RNA sequences complimentary to the cDNA clones isolated. Cells from two of three patients had extraordinarily high levels of the RNA species without any treatment (Fig. 3). The fact that one Bloom patient differed in this respect suggests that the phenotypic entity may fall into different complementation groups. The obvious speculation that the spontaneous chromosome instability and the elevated expression of TPA-inducible RNAs are part of an endogenous state of "tumor promotion" cannot be further substantiated at this time, and we realize that alternative interpretations are possible (see notes of caution in Mallick et al [17]). Since all

---

shown) [17,18]. b) Double-stranded cDNA was synthesized from 10 μg of poly A$^+$ RNA from TPA-treated cells. The cDNAs were tailed with oligo-dC and inserted into the dG-tailed Pst I-site of pBR 322. Examples are shown of the 1,200 tetracycline-resistant, ampicilline-sensitive E coli C 600 colonies that had been obtained by transformation with cDNA plasmids. After lysis of the cells and binding of the DNA, the nitrocellulose filters were hybridized to ^{32}P-cDNA synthesized from the cytoplasmic poly A$^+$ RNA present in either nontreated cells (−) or TPA-treated cells (+; 20 ng/ml for 8 hr). Clones 1, 4, and 5 were more abundant in the TPA-cDNA probe, clones 2 and 3 were slightly more abundant, while clone 6 was reduced in the TPA probe. Clone 7 mRNA was present in equal amounts in both probes. Dots mark other colonies that have not been examined further.

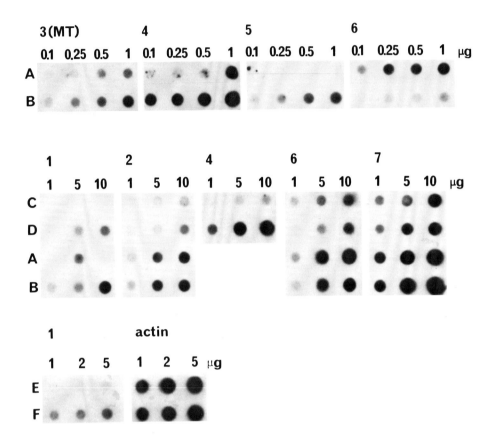

Fig. 2.   TPA, UV, and MMC regulate mRNA abundance. Normal human fibroblasts (Berlin-2) were treated with 20 ng TPA/ml for 8 hr (B) or harvested in the logarithmic growth phase (A). Fibroblasts from a patient with Cockayne's syndrome (GM 1856) were UV-irradiated (9 J/m^2) (D) or nonirradiated (C) and harvested 48 hr later. SV40-transformed normal human fibroblasts (GM 637) were treated with 1 μg/ml mitomycin C (F) for 8 hr or nontreated (E). The amounts of total RNA indicated (second and third rows) or poly A$^+$ RNA (first row) were dotted onto nitrocellulose and probed with nick-translated gene probes. The cDNA clones appear as numbers above each set. A pipetting error occurred at the "5 μg spot" of 1A. This signal should be added to the 5 μg spot of 1B. For all experiments, clone 7 and actin served as control hybridizations. Examples are shown: clone 7 in row 2 and actin in row 3. Responses following MMC treatment were also observed for the cDNA clones not shown here. UV inductions done with normal human fibroblasts required larger dose but resulted in similar increases of RNA.

biopsy specimens were, to our knowledge, from peripheral skin, differences owing to site of biopsy are not likely [27]. We hope of course that the cloned sequences may help to clarify these points.

Expression of TPA-Inducible Sequences in Transformed Cells

Although the gene products mediating the cancerogenesis-promoting effect of TPA may not be among the cloned sequences, we were interested to investigate whether transformation influenced the expression of these genes. We chose SV40

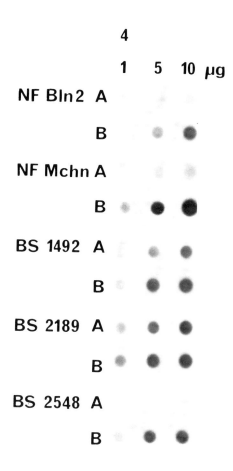

Fig. 3.   Elevated expression of clone 4 (XHF1)-mRNA in two out of three Bloom cells. Cell lines of normal human fibroblasts and of Bloom syndrom fibroblasts were either untreated (A) or treated with 20 ng TPA/ml for 8 hr (B). The indicated amounts of total RNA were dotted onto nitrocellulose filters and probed with [32] P-labeled clone 4 cDNA. Normalization of the dots were as in Figure 2.

transformation of skin fibroblasts because we had obtained the aforementioned data using the normal counterpart of these cells. Both SV40-transformed normal fibroblasts and SV40-transformed fibroblasts from a patient with Xeroderma pigmentosum (group A) had threefold higher metallothionein RNA levels than the corresponding nontransformed primary fibroblasts. The noninduced abundance of XHF1-RNA, however, was fivefold lower in both transformed cells than in the primary fibroblasts (Fig. 4). Both transformed and nontransformed cells respond to TPA (not shown) or EPIF (Fig. 4) to the same degree. Thus, in these two pairs of cells transformation had a differential effect on the genes examined. We do not know whether the cells were isogenic, since they were not from the same individual. It cannot be determined at this point whether the sequences described are involved in transformation since normal and transformed cells differ in many respects. Our working hypothesis is that XHF1 represents an extracellular differentiation function that is lost by transformation and that increased metallothionein RNA levels cause growth advantage. Suggestive

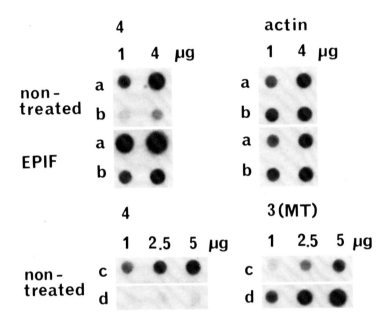

Fig. 4. Expression and inducibility of XHF 1 and metallothionein mRNA in primary and SV40-transformed human fibroblasts. Upper panel: Primary Xeroderma pigmentosum cells (group A, XPGM 2994, a) or SV40-transformed XP cells (XP12 Ro, b) were either untreated or treated with EPIF (from UV-irradiated XPGM 2994 cells 48 hr after irradiation) for 8 hr. The indicated amounts of RNA were dotted on nitrocellulose and probed with [32] P-labelled clone 4 cDNA or mouse α-actin cDNA, respectively. Lower panel: RNA was prepared from both normal human fibroblasts (NF Mchn, c) and SV40-transformed normal human fibroblasts (GM 637, d). The indicated amounts of RNA were probed with [32] P-labeled clone 4 cDNA and clone 3 cDNA (metallothionein cDNA). Note that exposure periods were tenfold longer than in Figure 3 to visualize expression of clone 4 mRNA in transformed cells.

support for this hypothesis comes from survival curves: Transformation of normal and Xeroderma fibroblasts led to increased resistance toward ionizing or α-radiation (Fig. 5).

DISCUSSION

It would not be surprising if transformed cells expressed other genes than normal cells. The transforming factor acts in a pleiotropic manner. This is reflected on the transcript level and has been used to characterize transformation-specific sequences [28–31]. One set of such transcripts is activated by transformation with SV40 [30] as is metallothionein RNA described in this paper. It thus appears that SV40 transformation and a tumor promoter regulate the same gene. Similarly, the protein MEP is elevated by either transformation or TPA [31]. Coordinate regulation by carcinogenic and cocarcinogenic agents does not, however, necessarily extend to SV40 transformation since the TPA-inducible gene for XHF1 responded in an opposite direction.

The TPA-inducible genetic program resembles vaguely the SOS response in E coli. We have called the program a stress response. The SOS response is essentially

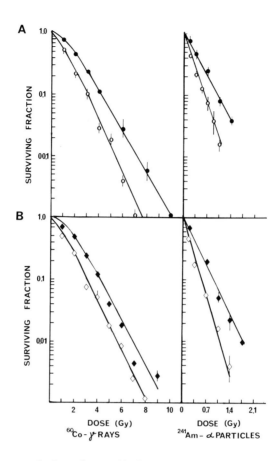

Fig. 5. Survival curves of primary human skin fibroblasts (open symbols) or SV40-transformed human fibroblasts (closed symbols) after exposure to either ^{60} Cobalt-gamma rays or ^{241} Americium-alpha particles. A) Cells derived from a healthy individual. B) Cells derived from a patient suffering from Xeroderma pigmentosum (group A). The data represent mean values of two to three independent experiments each ± standard error. A third pair of nontransformed and transformed skin fibroblasts gave similar results (not shown).

transient in nature but may lead to permanent genetic changes, eg, mutations [32]. The same dichotomy must be envisaged for the action of TPA. We have given evidence elsewhere that the stress response includes a gene amplifying function [33]. This exemplifies the transient nature of the stress response. Maintained expression of a carcinogen or tumor promoter-induced gene in transformed cells is a new facet of the response.

REFERENCES

1. Rassoulzadegan M, Naghashfar Z, Cowie A, Carr A, Grisoni M, Kamen R, Cuzin F: Proc Natl Acad Sci USA 80:4354, 1983.
2. Land H, Parada LF, Weinberg RA: Nature 304:596, 1983.
3. Jenkins JR, Rudge K, Currie GA: Nature 312:651, 1984.
4. Eliyahn D, Raz A, Gruss P, Givol D, Oven M: Nature 312:646, 1984.

5. Parada LF, Land H, Weinberg RA, Wolf D, Rotter V: Nature 312:649, 1984.
6. Van den Elsen P, de Pater S, Houweling A, Van der Veer J, Van der Eb A: Gene 18:175, 1982.
7. Newbold RF, Overell RW: Nature 304:648, 1983.
8. Connan G, Rassoulzadegan M, Cuzin F: Nature 314:277, 1985.
9. Kennedy AR, Cairns J, Little JB: Nature 307:85, 1984.
10. Slamon DJ, de Kernion JB, Verma IM, Cline MJ: Science 224:256, 1984.
11. Campisi J, Gray HE, Pardee AB, Dean M, Sonenshein GE: Cell 36:241, 1984.
12. Hayward WS, Neel BG, Astrin SM: Nature 290:475, 1981.
13. Nusse R, van Ooyen A, Cox D, Fung YKT, Varmus H: Nature 307:131, 1984.
14. Rothberg PG, Erisman MD, Diehl RE, Rovigatti UG, Astrin SM: Mol Cell Biol 4:1096, 1984.
15. Warren ST, Schultz RA, Chang CC, Wade MH, Trosko JE: Proc Natl Acad Sci USA 78:3133, 1981.
16. Vijayalaxmi, Evans HJ, Ray JH, German J: Science 221:851, 1983.
17. Mallick U, Rahmsdorf HJ, Yamamoto N, Ponta H, Wegner R-D, Herrlich P: Proc Natl Acad Sci USA 79:7886, 1982.
18. Schorpp M, Mallick U, Rahmsdorf HJ, Herrlich P: Cell 37:861, 1984.
19. Ullrich A, Shine J, Chirgwin J, Pictet R, Tischer E, Rutter WJ, Goodman HM: Science 196:1313, 1977.
20. Aviv H, Leder P: Proc Natl Acad Sci USA 69:1408, 1972.
21. Maniatis T, Fritsch EF, Sambrook J: "Molecular Cloning. A Laboratory Manual." Cold Spring Harbor, NY: Cold Spring Harbor Laboratory, 1982.
22. Kafatos FC, Jones CW, Efstratiadis A: NAR 7:1541, 1979.
23. Lücke-Huhle Comper W, Hieber L, Pech M: Radiat Environ Biophys 20:171, 1982.
24. Angel P, Pöting A, Mallick U, Rahmsdorf HJ, Schorpp M, Herrlich P: Mol Cell Biol (submitted).
25. Karin M, Richards RI: Nature 299:797, 1982.
26. German J: In German J (ed): "Chromosome Mutation and Neoplasia." New York: Alan R. Liss, Inc., 1983, p 347.
27. Thompson RG, Nickel B, Finlayson S, Meuser R, Hamerton JL, Wrogemann K: Nature 304:740, 1983.
28. Groudine M, Weintraub H: Proc Natl Acad Sci USA 77:5351, 1980.
29. Yamamoto M, Maehara Y, Takahashi K, Endo H: Proc Natl Acad Sci USA 80:7524, 1983.
30. Scott MRD, Westphal K-H, Rigby PWJ: Cell 34:557, 1983.
31. Donerty PJ, Hua L, Liau G, Gal S, Graham DE, Sobel M, Gottesman MM: Mol Cell Biol 5:466, 1985.
32. Herrlich P, Mallick U, Ponta H, Rahmsdorf HJ: Hum Genet 67:360, 1984.
33. Lücke-Huhle C, Herrlich P: "Proceedings of the ASJ-Meeting on Radiation Carcinogenesis." Corfu (in press), 1985.

Journal of Cellular Biochemistry 30:1–9 (1986)
Biochemical and Molecular Epidemiology of Cancer 33–41

Quantitative Relationship Between Initiation of Hepatocarcinogenesis and Induction of Altered Cell Islands

William K. Kaufmann, Susan A. MacKenzie, Richard J. Rahija, and David G. Kaufman

Department of Pathology and Lineberger Cancer Research Center, University of North Carolina, Chapel Hill, North Carolina 27514

We have quantified the initiation of hepatocytic neoplasms and the induction of altered cell islands in regenerating livers of rats given a single treatment with one of three carcinogens before or during the peak of DNA synthesis after partial hepatectomy. For up to 20 wk after treating livers during the peak of DNA synthesis with methyl(acetoxymethyl)nitrosamine (DMN-Ac), hepatocytic neoplasms were not seen. Thereafter, in rats fed the liver tumor promoter, phenobarbital, neoplasms emerged continuously so that by 60 wk after initiation, livers held an average of 5.5 neoplasms. Islands of cellular alteration, identified by their abnormal retention of glycogen on fasting, also appeared to emerge continuously between 20 and 60 wk after initiation. By 60 wk, promoted livers contained about 10,000 islands. In DMN-Ac-initiated, phenobarbital-promoted livers, neoplasms and islands maintained a constant numerical relationship over time with about 1,450 islands emerging for every neoplasm that emerged. This ratio of islands to neoplasms differed according to the type of carcinogen used to initiate hepatocarcinogenesis and depending on whether promotion with phenobarbital was included. In livers initiated with DMN-Ac but not promoted with phenobarbital, the ratio of islands to neoplasms was about 7,750:1. In livers initiated by treatment with $(\pm)$-$7\alpha,8\beta$-dihydroxy-$9\beta,10\beta$-epoxy-7,8,9,10-tetrahydrobenzo[a]pyrene at the peak of DNA synthesis and then promoted with phenobarbital, the ratio of islands to neoplasms was 7,200:1. In livers exposed to gamma rays at the peak of DNA synthesis in regenerating livers and promoted, no neoplasms were seen in our sample although islands could be enumerated. Evaluation of another group of rats irradiated during the prereplicative phase of regeneration revealed two neoplasms in nine treated livers and a ratio of islands to neoplasms of greater than 12,000:1. Thus, when comparing livers treated once with carcinogen and then promoted, this ratio of islands to neoplasms differed considerably according to the carcinogen being tested. These results suggest that the induction of glycogen-retaining hepatocyte islands may not be a quantitative measure of the initiation of hepatocarcinogenesis.

Received April 17, 1985; revised and accepted September 5, 1985.

© **1986 Alan R. Liss, Inc.**

Key words: hepatocarcinogenesis, initiation, promotion, neoplasm, altered-cell island

The initiation phase of carcinogenesis is phenomenologically defined as that process whereby susceptible target cells are irreversibly altered by a subthreshold dose of carcinogen so that upon subsequent application of a noncarcinogenic stimulus (ie, promotion) neoplasms are produced [1,2]. However, suprathreshold doses of carcinogen or repetitive low doses typically induce benign and malignant neoplasms without the need for the promoting stimulus. Both the initiation of hepatocarcinogenesis by a subthreshold dose of carcinogen [3] and the induction of neoplasms directly by a suprathreshold dose of carcinogen [4,5] appear to require two elements [6]; (1) damage to DNA, and (2) proliferation of damaged cells. Seemingly, during the replication and division of hepatocytes with damaged DNA, irreversible alterations are produced that dispose these cells to neoplasia.

We are interested in identifying the factors that may influence the initiation of hepatocarcinogenesis. In a study of the relationship of the cell division cycle to the susceptibility of proliferating hepatocytes to initiation by the chemical carcinogen, DMN-Ac, we found the S phase to be a period of maximal sensitivity [3]. Hepatocytes in G_1 appeared to be significantly less sensitive, suggesting that prereplicative DNA repair reduces cellular risk of initiation by this chemical.

Recent studies suggest that initiation of hepatocarcinogenesis might be monitored in short-term assays that quantify hepatocytic islands of cellular alteration [7]. These islands are induced by hepatocarcinogens and display a variety of morphological, biological, and biochemical abnormalities (see [8,9] for reviews). To date, there have been few studies in which the yields of islands estimated by morphometric techniques are compared with the yields of hepatocytic neoplasms induced under the same conditions in the same livers. Here we describe the results of our preliminary efforts to quantify hepatocytic neoplasms and islands of cellular alteration in livers that were treated once with a hepatocarcinogen given before or during the peak of hepatocyte DNA synthesis after partial hepatectomy. We reasoned that if altered cell islands represent the clonal progeny of initiated hepatocytes, as some have suggested [8], then treatments with carcinogens that induce equivalent numbers of islands also should produce equivalent yields of neoplasms after promotion.

METHODS

Male F344 rats were obtained from Charles River Breeding Laboratories (Kingston, MA) at about 6 wk of age. They were acclimated for 1 wk and weighed 100 g at the time of treatment. Rats were treated with the chemical carcinogens during the peak of DNA synthesis 18–20 hr after a two-thirds partial hepatectomy [4]. DMN-Ac of greater than 98% purity was synthesized by Dr. G. Muschik, Program Resources, Inc., NCI-FCRF (Frederick, MD) by the method of Roller et al [10]. DMN-Ac was dissolved in phosphate-buffered saline, pH 5.5, immediately before use. $(\pm)$-7α,8β-dihydroxy-9β,10β-epoxy-7,8,9,10-tetrahydrobenzo[a]pyrene (BPDE) synthesized at Midwest Research Institute (Kansas City, MO) and of greater than 99% purity, was dissolved in anhydrous dimethylsulfoxide (silylation grade from Pierce Chemical Co., Rockford, IL). Immediately before administration, 25 μl of this solution was mixed with 0.5 ml of Steroid Suspending Vehicle (Armour Pharmaceutical Co., Kankakee, IL), and the mixture was then drawn into a syringe. Aqueous solutions of carcinogen were administered directly into the hepatic portal vein (at 5 ml per kg body weight) as previously described [4]. For treatment with gamma radiation, rats were anesthetized with brevital and placed in a restraining apparatus with 3/8 inch of lead shielding the upper and lower thirds of the body. The middle third of the rat containing the regenerating liver remnant was not shielded. Irradiation from above and below was performed with a Gammacell 40 Cesium 137 source at a dose rate of 1.4 GY per min. For the dose-response study, irradiation was performed at 18 hr after partial hepatectomy. Another group of rats was irradiated at 4 hr after partial hepatectomy during the prereplicative phase of liver regeneration [4]. Three wk after treatment with carcinogen, rats were fed a Purina chow diet containing 0.05% phenobarbital. Some DMN-Ac-treated rats were fed the Purina chow diet alone.

At intervals after treatment, groups of rats were sacrificed for analysis of hepatocytic neoplasms and altered cell islands. One week before sacrifice, phenobarbital was removed from the diet. Rats were fasted for 24 hr before sacrifice to deplete livers of glycogen. After removal of the liver, a 1-cm^2 slice (2-mm thick) of the right lateral lobe was frozen on solid CO_2, and 8-μm-thick sections were cut on a cryostat. Sections were stained with periodic acid and the Schiff reagent (PAS) and counterstained with hematoxylin. The diameters of glycogen-storage islands seen in transections were measured with an eyepiece micrometer. The numbers of islands per liver were estimated according to the stereologic method of Pugh et al [11] as described in [12]. The remaining liver was fixed in formalin, then cut at 1–2 mm intervals to identify neoplasms. All gross identifications were confirmed by subsequent histologic analysis as previously described in detail [4].

RESULTS
Time-Course of Hepatocarcinogenesis in DMN-Ac-Treated Rats

In DMN-Ac-treated rats fed a diet containing 0.05% phenobarbital, yields of hepatocytic neoplasms increased continuously after a latency of 20 weeks (Fig. 1). By 60 wk after treatment, livers contained an average of 5.5 neoplasms, both nodules and carcinomas. In these animals, the numbers of glycogen-storage islands also appeared to increase continuously between 20 and 60 wk after treatment (Fig. 2). By 60 wk, livers were estimated to contain about 10,000 of these islands. For this 60-wk group, the diameters of liver neoplasms identified in histologic sections were measured (n = 33). The volumes of these neoplasms were estimated assuming that the neoplasms were spheroids. Within individual livers neoplasms were estimated to occupy from 1–20% of the liver volume with an average of 5% of the liver occupied by neoplasm. Consequently, for the estimation of island numbers in nonneoplastic tissue, the use of the total liver volume [12] did not significantly alter the results. In the rats fed the diet containing phenobarbital as promoter, neoplasms and islands appeared to maintain a constant numerical relationship over time, with one neoplasm emerging for every 1,450 islands (Fig. 1, insert). In treated rats not fed the promoter the islands emerged later, but by 45 and 60 wk their numbers approximated those seen in promoted rats (Fig. 2). However, the yields of hepatocytic neoplasms were significantly less in rats fed control diet than in rats fed phenobarbital-containing diet (Fig. 1). At 45 and 60 wk after treatment with DMN-Ac, the ratios of yields of neoplasms for promoted versus nonpromoted rats were 6.1 and 8.3, respectively. The ratio of islands to neoplasms in nonpromoted livers (7,750:1, Table I) was somewhat

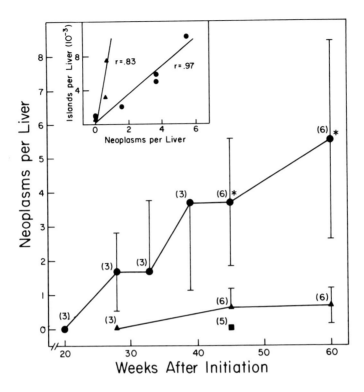

Fig. 1. Kinetics of emergence of hepatocytic neoplasms following initiation with DMN-Ac. The mean yields of hepatocytic neoplasms ($\pm$SD) were enumerated in groups of rats (numbers in parentheses) at various times after treatment with 0.1 mmole/kg DMN-Ac. (●), DMN-Ac-treated rats fed diet containing 0.05% phenobarbital; (▲), DMN-Ac-treated rats fed control diet; (■), hepatectomized rats fed diet containing 0.05% phenobarbital.(*), $P < .025$ for carcinogen-treated rats fed phenobarbital diet vs carcinogen-treated rats fed control diet (Student's t test). Insert: For each experimental time-point, the average yields of neoplasms were plotted against the estimated yields of glycogen-storage islands as illustrated in Figure 2. (Reprinted from [12] with permission.)

less than the 11,000:1 value that was calculated previously by linear regression [12]. No hepatocytic neoplasms and few glycogen-storage islands were seen in solvent-treated control rats fed the phenobarbital-containing diet for 42 wk.

Dose-Responses for Initiation of Hepatocarcinogenesis by DMN-Ac, BPDE, and Gamma Radiation

Rats were treated once with DMN-Ac, BPDE, or gamma radiation at the peak of DNA synthesis after partial hepatectomy, then 3 wk after treatment, phenobarbital was added to their diet at 0.05%. Based on the results of the time-course study described above, animals were held for 39–45 wk after treatment with carcinogen to allow sufficient time for expression and growth of islands and neoplasms. Dose-response curves for induction of glycogen-storage islands and for initiation of neoplasms are shown in Figure 3. Whereas a single dose of all three carcinogens appeared to be able to induce islands of cellular alteration, the carcinogens varied in their abilities to induce neoplasms. At doses of carcinogen that induced approximately

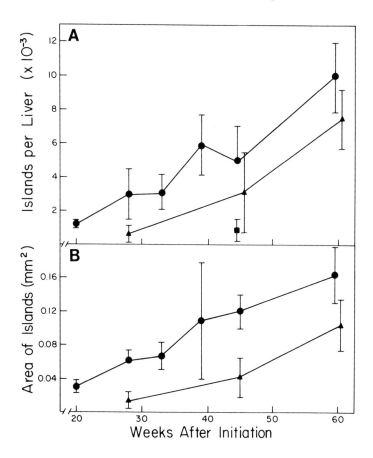

Fig. 2.   Kinetics of emergence of glycogen-storage islands following initiation with DMN-Ac. A) The mean yields of islands displaying abnormal retention of glycogen upon fasting (±SD) were estimated from transections by quantitative stereology. Symbols are as in Figure 1. B) The mean areas of islands (±SD) at various times after initiation. Symbols are as in Figure 1. (Reprinted from [12] with permission.)

TABLE I. Island to Neoplasm Ratio

Carcinogen	Protocol	Dietary phenobarbital	Rats	No. per liver[a] Islands	Neoplasms	Ratio[b]
DMN-Ac	Time-course	+	37	2,986	2.05	1,456
		−	15	3,430	0.47	7,751
DMN-Ac	Dose-response	+	15	3,827	2.67	1,433
BPDE	Dose-response	+	9	4,828	0.67	7,206
Gamma rays	Dose-response	+	6	2,650	0	(>15,900)
Gamma rays	6 Gy at 4 hr after partial hepatectomy	+	9[c]	2,694	0.22	12,245

[a]The average Nos. of induced islands and neoplasms were determined for the data presented in Figures 1–3.
[b]Ratio = the average No. of islands per liver divided by the average No. of neoplasms.
[c]Six livers in this group were evaluated to determine the average Nos. of glycogen-storage islands.

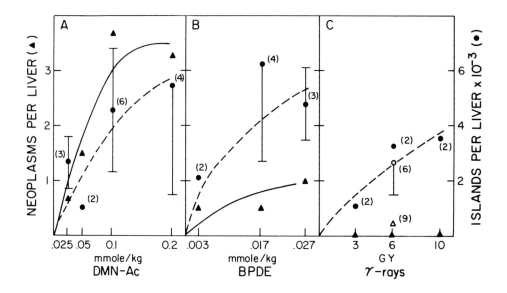

Fig. 3.   Dose-responses for initiation of hepatocytic neoplasms and for induction of glycogen-storage islands following a single treatment with carcinogen. The yields of neoplasms (triangles) and islands (circles) were enumerated in livers of rats fed 0.05% phenobarbital for 36–42 wk after a single initiating treatment with various doses of (A) DMN-Ac, (B) BPDE, or (C) gamma radiation. In parentheses are the numbers of livers analyzed at each experimental point. In C, the open symbols depict yields of islands and neoplasms in a group of rats irradiated at 4 hr after partial hepatectomy. Error bars enclose one standard deviation about the mean.

equal numbers of islands, DMN-Ac produced several neoplasms per liver, BPDE produced 0.5–1 neoplasm per liver, and for the sample of livers treated at the peak of DNA synthesis in regenerating livers, gamma rays failed to induce any neoplasms. This result is summarized in Table I in which the total number of induced islands in our sample was compared with the total number of induced neoplasms. As noted above, the ratio of islands to neoplasms was about 1,450:1 for DMN-Ac-treated livers. For BPDE-treated livers, this ratio was about 7,200:1. The ratio could not be computed for the gamma-irradiated livers owing to the lack of induced neoplasms. These results suggested a lower limit of about 16,000:1 for this ratio in livers irradiated at the peak of DNA synthesis after partial hepatectomy. In another experiment, the timing of irradiation after partial hepatectomy was varied. In a group of nine rats irradiated with 6 Gy at 4 hr after partial hepatectomy and then promoted with phenobarbital, two hepatocytic neoplasms were observed 45 wk after irradiation. The average number of glycogen-storage islands estimated for livers in this group was 2,694 (n = 6, SD 1,186). Consequently, the computed ratio of islands to neoplasms was 2694/0.22 or 12,245 in this group of irradiated livers (Table I).

DISCUSSION

Islands of histochemically altered hepatocytes are generally seen in livers soon after an exposure to a carcinogen that produces hepatocytic neoplasms after a longer observation period [12,13]. Consequently, it appears that the observation of such islands long after a test compound had decayed gives at least qualitative evidence of initiating activity [7,8]. Our current results confirm observations that islands appear in far greater numbers that neoplasms [12–15] and demonstrate that for livers treated with DMN-Ac, islands are produced in a constant ratio to initiated hepatocytes of about 1,450:1. However, in livers treated with BPDE or gamma rays and then promoted with phenobarbital, the observed ratios of the yields of induced islands of glycogen retention to hepatocytic neoplasms were 7,200:1 and 12,200:1, respectively. These results suggest that the population of glycogen storage islands may not be the progeny of initiated hepatocytes.

Previous studies have shown that phenobarbital may increase the frequency of observation of islands of cellular alteration following a single initiating treatment with chemical carcinogens [14]. Our results discussed in more detail in [12] suggested that at 28 wk after treatment with DMN-Ac, promoted livers contained about five times as many islands as nonpromoted livers. However, at 45 and 60 wk after treatment, the numbers of islands in promoted and nonpromoted livers were nearly equivalent. Others have reported results similar to these [15,16] or results indicating that island frequencies were not appreciably affected by the promoter [17]. It has recently been reported that in some islands of cellular alteration, expression of gamma glutamyl-transpeptidase may be reversibly induced by phenobarbital [18]. In the absence of the promoter, these islands, although present, would not be scored owing to the lack of marker enzyme activity. Altered cell islands that display abnormal retention of glycogen on fasting presumably have a defect in the complex pathways of carbohydrate metabolism, such as a deficiency in glucose-6-phosphatase. Expression of this deficiency may not be affected by the inductive effects of phenobarbital. Our studies suggest that phenobarbital may speed the initial emergence and growth of altered cell islands expressing the glycogen-storage phenotype, but it does not affect the numbers of these islands that ultimately appear in damaged livers. In contrast, the promoter does not appear to speed the emergence or growth of neoplasms [19], but rather it enhances the expression of the neoplastic phenotype by initiated cells that would otherwise remain latent.

Ionizing radiation has been reported to increase the incidence of hepatic neoplasia when administered to mice with regenerating livers [20,21]. We also are aware of a preliminary report of the induction of altered cell islands in regenerating livers of rats exposed to ionizing radiation and 3-aminobenzamide [22]. To our knowledge, there have been no previous reports of radiation-induced hepatic neoplasia in the rat. The results of an extensive analysis of hepatocarcinogenesis in gamma-irradiated livers are currently being quantified and will be presented elsewhere. Our preliminary results suggest that gamma radiation is indeed capable of inducing altered cell islands and initiating hepatocytic neoplasia. However, in comparison to BPDE and DMN-Ac, this radiation appears to be less efficient in producing initiated hepatocytes that can be promoted to form neoplasms. Neoplasms initiated by gamma rays may have an unusually long latency so that they might not be readily detected as a result of our study design. This possibility would require that in the initiated cell populations that are produced by different carcinogens there are differences that affect the speed with which initiated cells can be promoted to form neoplasms. Alternatively, gamma rays may be able to induce efficiently only a subset of the genetic alterations that initiate hepatocarcinogenesis in the rat. Support for this concept may be found in the recent observation that, in combination with the treatment of neonatal rats with diethylnitrosamine, gamma radiation produced a synergistic increase in the frequency of altered cell islands [23].

DMN-Ac and BPDE both appeared to be effective initiators of hepatocarcinogenesis when given as a single dose after partial hepatectomy. When viewed on a molar basis, BPDE appeared to be a more efficient inducer of islands of cellular alteration than DMN-Ac. However, in the absence of information on the levels of specific DNA adducts produced in damaged livers and of the effects of these adducts on oncogenetic alterations, comparisons of relative efficiencies of induction of islands or initiation of neoplasms must be viewed with caution. A more thorough analysis of the effects of dose of carcinogen and of the time after treatment on the yields of induced islands and neoplasms also is required before comparisons of carcinogenic effectiveness can be attempted.

In summary, we found that in livers given a single treatment with one of three known carcinogens followed by promotion with phenobarbital there were carcinogen-dependent differences in the ratios of yields of islands of cellular alteration to yields of neoplasms. Comparison of the hepatocellular alterations induced by the three carcinogens evaluated here may reveal a specific subset of alterations associated with elevated risk of developing cancer in the liver. The present results suggest that the cellular alteration(s) associated with retention of glycogen on fasting may not be directly associated with the formation of initiated cells that can be promoted to form neoplasms.

ACKNOWLEDGMENTS

We are grateful to Michael Judge and Scott Stroup for their excellent technical assistance in these studies. This work was supported by PHS grant △CA32238 awarded by the National Cancer Institute, DHHS. D.G.K. was the recipient of a Research Career Development Award (△CA00431) from the NCI. R.J.R. was supported by an Environmental Pathology training grant (△ES07017) from the NIEHS.

REFERENCES

1. Berenblum I, Shubik PA: Br J Cancer 3:384, 1949.
2. Boutwell RK: Prog Exp Tumor Res 4:207, 1964.
3. Kaufmann WK, Kaufman DG, Rice JM, Wenk ML: J Cell Biochem 8A:137, 1983.
4. Kaufmann WK, Kaufman DG, Rice JM, Wenk ML: Cancer Res 41:4653, 1981.
5. Craddock VM, Frei JV: Br J Cancer 30:503, 1974.
6. Grisham JW, Kaufman DG, Kaufmann WK: Syn Survey Path Res 1:49, 1983.
7. Tatematsu M, Hasegawa R, Iwaida K, Tsuda H, Ito N: Carcinogenesis 4:381, 1983.
8. Pitot HC, Sirica AE: Biochim Biophys Acta 605:191, 1980.
9. Bannasch P, Mayer D, Hacker HJ: Biochim Biophys Acta 605:217, 1980.
10. Roller PP, Shimp DR, Keefer LK: Tetrahedron Let 25:2065, 1975.
11. Pugh TD, King JH, Koen H, Nychka D, Chover J, Wahba G, He Y, Goldfarb S: Cancer Res 43:1261, 1983.
12. Kaufmann WK, MacKenzie SA, Kaufman DG: Am J Pathol 119:171, 1985.
13. Peraino C, Staffeldt EF, Carnes BA, Ludeman VA, Blomquist JA, Vesselinovitch SD: Cancer Res 44:3340, 1984.
14. Pitot HC, Barsness L, Goldsworthy T, Kitagawa T: Nature 271:456, 1978.
15. Kitagawa T, Sugano H: Gann 69:679, 1978.
16. Herren SL, Pereira MA: Envir Health Perspect 50:123, 1983.

17. Moore MA, Hacker HJ, Kunz HW, Bannasch P: Carcinogenesis 4:473, 1983.
18. Sirica AE, Jicinsky JK, Heyer EK: Carcinogenesis 5:1737, 1984.
19. Peraino C. Staffeldt EF, Haugen DA, Lombard LS, Stevens FJ, Fry RJM: Cancer Res 40:3268, 1980.
20. Cole LJ, Nowell PC: Science 150:1782, 1965.
21. Wiley AL, Vogel HH, Clifton KH: Radiat Res 54:284, 1973.
22. Enomoto K, Dempo K, Oyamada M, Suzuki J, Sakurai T, Mori M: Proc Am Assoc Cancer Res 25:125, 1984.
23. Peraino C, Grdina D, Carnes B: Proc AACR 26:74, 1985.

Journal of Cellular Biochemistry 30:171–179 (1986)
Biochemical and Molecular Epidemiology of Cancer 43–51

Monitoring of Individual Human Exposure to Aflatoxins (AF) and N-Nitrosamines (NNO) by Immunoassays

C.P. Wild, D. Umbenhauer, B. Chapot, and R. Montesano

Unit of Mechanisms of Carcinogenesis, International Agency for Research on Cancer, 69372 Lyon Cedex 08, France

Highly sensitive immunoassays have been used to quantitate aflatoxins (AF) and N-nitrosamines (NNO) in human body fluids and tissues, respectively. This approach was taken in order to quantitate environmental exposure to these agents at an individual level to facilitate the investigation of their role in the etiology of human cancer. In order to analyse AF in human urine, an immunopurification step has been developed by using AF-specific antibody bound to AH-Sepharose 4B gel in a small (4-ml gel volume) affinity column prior to enzyme-linked immunosorbent assay (ELISA). The ELISA can be used to quantitate aflatoxin B_1 (AFB$_1$) over the range 0.01 ng/ml to 10 ng/ml and the assay system has been validated by using human urine samples spiked with AFB$_1$ over this concentration range. In addition, 29 urine samples from the Philippines have been analysed and found to contain a range of levels from zero to 4.25 ng/ml AFB$_1$ equivalent with a mean of 0.875 ng/ml. This compared with a mean of 0.066 ng/ml AFB$_1$ equivalent in samples from France.

Radioimmunoassay of O^6-methyldeoxyguanosine (O^6-medG) has been performed on human oesophageal and cardiac stomach mucosal DNA from tissue samples obtained during surgery in Linxian County, People's Republic of China, an area of high risk for both oesophageal and stomach cancer. Using the methodology described and having 1 mg of hydrolyzed DNA allows the detection of approximately 25 fmol O^6medG per mg DNA. Of the 37 tissue samples analyzed from Linxian County, 17 samples had levels of O^6-medG ranging from 15 to 50 fmol/mg DNA, ten showed higher levels up to 160 fmol/mg DNA, and the

Abbreviations used: AF, aflatoxins; NNO N-Nitrosamines; ELISA, enzyme-linked immunosorbent assay; RIA, radioimmunoassay; O^6-medG, O^6-methyldeoxyguanosine; O^6-AT, O^6-alkylguanine DNA alkyltransferase; PHC, primary hepatocellular carcinoma; HBV, hepatitis B virus; AFB$_1$-N7-G, 8,9-dihydro-8(N^7-guanyl)-9-hydroxy aflatoxin B$_1$; AFB$_1$-FAPY, 8,9-dihydro-8-(N^7-formyl-2′,5′,6′,-triamino-4′-oxo-N^5-pyrimidyl)-9-hydroxy aflatoxin B$_1$.

D. Umbenhauer's present address is Department of Biochemistry, Vanderbilt University School of Medicine, Nashville, TN 37232.

Received July 24, 1985; revised and accepted September 26, 1985.

© **1986 Alan R. Liss, Inc.**

remaining ten samples were below the limit of detection. For comparison, 12 tissue samples were obtained from hospitals in Europe and all showed levels below 45 fmol O^6-medG/mg DNA with seven below the limit of detection. All tissue samples from Linxian County showed normal levels of O^6-alkylguanine DNA alkyltransferase when compared to levels in other parts of the world.

The approaches described appear promising for assessing the role of AFB_1 in the etiology of human liver cancer and of nitrosamines as possible causative agents in oesophageal or stomach cancer.

Key words: N-nitrosamines, aflatoxins, ELISA, RIA, human environmental exposure monitoring

Epidemiology has been successful in identifying various agents or types of exposures as responsible for the induction of some human cancers. However, this has occurred mainly in situations where the exposure was very high or the type of cancer detected was of unusual occurrence in the general population. The low sensitivity of epidemiological studies is such that is is difficult to ascertain the etiology of human cancer when this is of multifactorial origin or the result of exposure to relatively low levels of carcinogens. In these situations, the determination of an association between the environmental occurrence of certain carcinogens and a given tumour in man appears more and more problematic. The possibility of quantitating a low-level environmental exposure to a particular carcinogen at an individual level appears to be a promising approach for establishing such an association. The considerations outlined above apply particularly to the role of aflatoxin B_1 in the etiology of liver cancer and of N-Nitrosamines (NNO) as causative agents of some human cancers.

With these two groups of carcinogens an increased understanding of their intracellular fate has helped to determine which are the most desirable end-points for measurement of individual human exposure. These may be measurement of the carcinogen itself, or a degradation product or measurement of a specific reaction product in either body fluids or tissues. The development of antibodies highly specific for carcinogens or carcinogen reaction products [1–5] and their application in extremely sensitive immunoassays have provided the necessary methodology for such measurements. In our laboratory, we have been concentrating on the application of immunoassays to quantitate at an individual level (1) aflatoxins (AF) in human body fluids and (2) the presence in human tissues of DNA adducts derived from exposure to NNO. We briefly report here the development of such methodologies and their application.

Aflatoxin, a potent hepatocarcinogen in several animal species [6], has been implicated epidemiologically along with hepatitis B viral (HBV) infection, as having a causal role in human primary hepatocellular carcinoma (PHC) [7–9]. In this paper we report data which established a method for measuring the presence of AF in human urine samples and include data from samples obtained from the Philippines, a country with a known presence of AF and associated high incidence of PHC [10]. In addition, we present results showing the detection of O^6-methyldeoxyguanosine (O^6-medG), a promutagenic alkylation adduct from NNO [11], in oesophageal and cardiac stomach DNA from individuals from Linxian County, People's Republic of China. This population has a high incidence of oesophageal and gastric cancer [12] and there is evidence of environmental exposure to NNO [13]. These two studies illustrate the adequate sensitivity and practical feasibility of such an approach for monitoring human environmental exposure.

DETERMINATION OF AFLATOXINS IN HUMAN URINE BY ELISA

The production and characterization of the the the rabbit polyclonal antibody used in the immunoassay for AF have been previously reported in detail [14] and the ELISA method used is a modification of that described by Martin et al [15]. The standard inhibition curve for AFB$_1$ shown in Figure 1 is linear over the range 1.6–1,600 fmol (0.01–10 ng/ml) AFB$_1$ with a 50% inhibition value of 115 fmol (0.7 ng/ml). For comparison, the sensitivity of the ELISA for the human urinary metabolites AFM$_1$ [16], AFP$_1$ [J.D. Groopman personal communication], and the AF-DNA adducts also found in human urine [17] are shown. Although the assay requires 9-, 390-, 43-, and 23-fold more AFM$_1$, AFP$_1$, AFB$_1$-N7-G, and AFB$_1$-FAPY, respectively than AFB$_1$ to give 50% inhibition, the assay sensitivity for these compunds is among the highest available [5]. These data illustrate the broad specificity of this antibody, which also included recognition of AFB$_1$-conjugated compounds [14].

An affinity column was produced by binding the antibody to AH-Sepharose 4B gel (Pharmacia), thus allowing the extraction of AF from urine samples as a method of purification prior to ELISA. The ability of the affinity column to bind AFB$_1$ was measured by two methods by using [^{3}H]AFB$_1$ and unlabelled AFB$_1$. Initially 2 pmol [^{3}H]AFB$_1$ in 5 ml PBS was loaded onto the mini-column and bound AF eluted with 1 M acetic acid, pH 2.5. The radioactivity in fractions from the column was determined and analysis showed that 89% of radioactivity was bound prior to acid elution. HPLC analysis showed that unbound radioactivity in a breakthrough peak was due to presence of tritiated water. Similar levels of retention were obtained by using

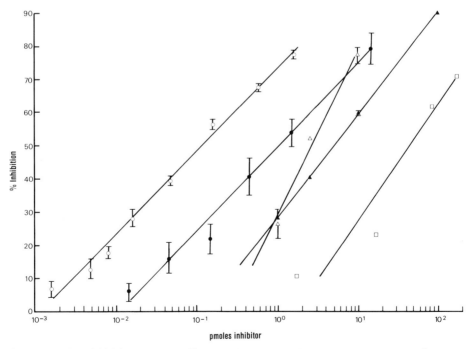

Fig. 1.   Standard inhibition curve for (○) AFB$_1$ in ELISA including cross-reactivity of (●)AFM$_1$; (□)AFP$_1$; (△)AFB$_1$-FAPY; and (▲)AFB$_1$-N7-G in the assay.

[^{3}H]AFB$_1$ in human urine samples which were precipitated with ethanol prior to immunopurification.

In order to examine the reproducibility and validity of the assay system, a human urine sample was split into 5-ml aliquots and spiked with AFB$_1$ or AFM$_1$ (0.01–10 ng/ml). A good correlation (Fig. 2) was seen between the ELISA determination, following immunopurification on the affinity column, and the quantity of AFB$_1$ in the spiked sample. In contrast, preliminary data show that recovery of AFM$_1$ was 6% at 10 ng/ml and 29% at 1 ng/ml AFM$_1$.

In order to further determine the reproducibility of the assay system, a urine sample obtained from the Philippines, identified as positive for AF contamination, was split into nine fractions of 5 ml which were then processed and assayed individually. The mean value determined was 1.48 ± 0.27 ng/ml AFB$_1$ equivalent with a % inhibition range in the ELISA of 48–55.1% (samples diluted 2/5 in PBS for assay).

A preliminary study of 29 urine samples for the Philippines was performed to test the sensitivity of the assay in terms of AF levels present environmentally. Of the 29 samples analysed seven showed inhibition values <30% in the ELISA with an overall range from zero to 4.25 ng/ml AFB$_1$ equivalent (see Discussion) and a mean of 0.875 ng/ml. This compared with a mean of 0.066 ng/ml in nine urine samples collected in Lyon, France, with six of those nine giving inhibitions <30%.

PRESENCE OF O^6-METHYLDEOXYGUANOSINE IN HUMAN TISSUE DNA

DNA (2–12 mg) was extracted from tissues obtained from Linxian County, People's Republic of China, and from European areas of low oesophageal cancer and the presence of O^6-medG determined by RIA [18]. The results [19] presented as fmol O^6-medG/mg DNA show (Fig. 3) the presence of the promutagenic lesion O^6-medG in DNA of oesophageal mucosa, cardiac stomach mucosa, and oesophageal tumour tissue from Linxian County. The majority of samples had O^6-medG levels lower than 50 fmol/mg but in ten samples (eight non-tumour oesophagus; two cardiac stomach) levels of 60–160 fmol of O^6-medG/mg DNA were quantitated. In comparison, tissues from Europe showed levels always less than 45 fmol/mg DNA with seven out of 13 below the limit of detection (< 20% inhibition in RIA).

The relatively high levels of O^6-medG detected in the tissues from Linxian County were compared with the levels of O^6-alkylguanine DNA alkyltransferase (O^{6}AT) present in those tissues (Table I) determined in an in vitro repair assay [20]. The data show that there is no evidence of any deficiency in the population for O^6-AT activity when compared with oesophagus from other parts of the world, nor is there evidence that the repair activity in the oesophagus is lower than other tissues of the gastrointestinal tract.

DISCUSSION

As previously shown in preliminary work by other investigators [21,5], the two studies presented here show that the antibodies available to carcinogens and carcinogen adducts can be used in assays which attain sufficient sensitivity to quantitate environmental levels of target antigens in human tissues and body fluids. Several points, however, in relation to methodology and the choice of end-point to be measured arise from the data we have presented and warrant discussion.

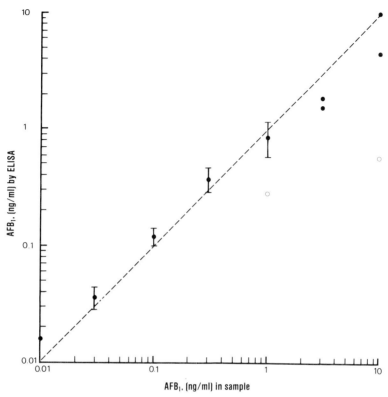

Fig. 2. Correlation study of known quantities of (●)AFB$_1$ or (○)AFM$_1$ spiked into human urine samples and measured by ELISA following immunopurification. Each point represents the mean ±SE of three or four individually processed samples except where data points are given as single points, in which case each point represents one determination.

Clearly for routine screening of exposure (eg, field studies) it is necessary to assay in a non-invasive way and to this end urine samples, and blood, are prime candidates. The initial problem we encountered in the AF study however is a common one, ie, nonspecific interference in the ELISA by urinary constituents. This has been overcome as described here, and similarly by Groopman et al [22], by the use of an immunopurification step with an antibody affinity column which specifically extracts AF-related components. Having thus removed nonspecific factors, however, one is still likely to be faced with a number of different AF products in the assay sample due to the complex metabolism and excretion of the carcinogen. For example AFB$_1$ [23], AFM$_1$ [16], AF-DNA adducts [17], and AFP$_1$ [J.D. Groopman, personal communication] have been identified in human urine whilst some AF water-soluble conjugates have been identified in primate [24] and may be present in man. Examination of the antibodies available to AF [5] shows that the production of an antibody with the extreme specificity obtained for O^6-alkylguanine adducts [18,25,26] has not been achieved. In addition, these antibodies have not been fully characterized in terms of their cross-reactivity with water-soluble AF conjugates which (1) may be present in urine samples and (2) may be recognized by many of the antibodies which are

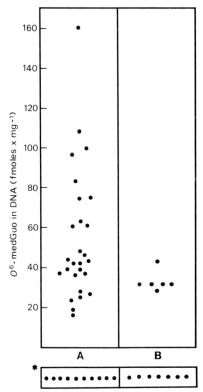

Fig. 3. O[6]-methyldeoxyguanosine content of DNA in human oesophageal and cardiac stomach tissue samples, and in samples of oesophageal tumour tissue fron Linxian County, People's Republic of China (A), and Europe (B) measured by competitive radioimmunoassay. Inhibition values of less than 20% were considered negative and are listed in the boxes marked with an asterisk [from 19].

raised to AF conjugates. It follows therefore that the measurement made by immunoassay with the methods described above will be an integration of the absolute quantity of, and the antibody affinity for, each of the AF components present.

At the present time this screening approach permits the assessment of a population for a positive AF exposure, and presumably increases the sensitivity of analysis by measuring a number of AF components together, but care is needed in making population comparisons unless it can be demonstrated that the relative quantities of the various human urinary AF metabolites are constant. This becomes even more important when inter-study comparisons are made where different antibodies have been used and this may explain the large reported differences in AF levels in, for example, Gambia and the People's Republic of China [see 5].

We present the data on the Philippines urine samples as ng/ml AFB_1 equivalent due to the fact that the antibody recognises at least AFM_1 and AFB_1 (Fig. 2) and indeed initial HPLC fractionation of some of the Philippines urine samples, after the immunopurification step, suggests that a major proportion of the ELISA inhibition we measured was by unidentified water-soluble AF conjugates [Wild, unpublished data]. However, because of the lack of characterization of these products we are as

TABLE I. O^6-Methylguanine DNA Alkyltransferase Activity in Human Tissues

| Tissue | No. of samples | fmol O^6-meG removed/mg protein | | |
		Mean	Range	Reference
Linxian County, PRC[b]				
Oesophagus-normal	8	190	87–246	
Oesophagus-tumour	5	326	122–447	[19]
Stomach	15	199	81–257	
Other studies				
Oesophagus	3	217	184–283	[34]
Stomach	5	200	145–250[a]	[35]
	14	730	360–1000	[36]
	7	460	180–1190	[37]
Small intestine	12	210	18–740[a]	[35]
Colon	10	261	135–413	[36]
	10	140	29–280[a]	[35]
	4	350	60–550	[37]
Rectum	3	360	220–470	[37]

[a]Data derived from Figure 2, reference 35.
[b]People's Republic of China.

yet unable to say if they are a major urinary AF component in absolute quantities. The identification of such products and detailed analysis of their cross-reactivity with our antibodies should allow the optimisation of an ELISA for their measurement and a concomitant increase in sensitivity.

In contrast to the somewhat incomplete picture of AF metabolism in vivo, the characterization of the metabolism and reactivity of NNO is much better understood [27]. We have detected the presence of O^6-medG in DNA from oesophageal tissue obtained through surgery from a population in Linxian County at high risk of oesophageal cancer. This observation is particularly significant in view of the pro-mutagenic nature of this lesion, which is considered as having an important role in the multistage process of carcinogenesis [11]. Because of this point, the approach described here represents a valuable integration of laboratory and epidemiological studies for the identification of causes of human cancer. The immunovisualisation of such adducts described recently [28] could eventually permit their determination at a cellular and macromolecular level.

In view of the efficient O^6-AT repair process for O^6-medG [29], which is present in normal quantities in these tissue samples (Table I), our measurement reflects an integrated response of reaction and repair of this lesion in the DNA at the target site. The O^6-medG lesion is present in the DNA despite a large excess of repair protein and it is important to emphasize that our data will be an underestimation of total exposure. The levels determined therefore probably reflect either a persistent fraction of a fairly recent exposure or the accumulation of adducts in regions of DNA which are repaired less efficiently. The latter may include DNA which is in a conformation resistant to repair [30] or DNA in a subpopulation of cells with an O^6-AT repair deficiency such as that seen in some human tumour cell lines in culture [31]. The latter deficiency would be masked by our examination of activity of total tissue protein extracts for O^6-AT activity.

In parallel to these studies, it may be desirable to quantitate a more stable alkylation adduct, where the dose-response relationship would not be complicated by efficient adduct repair. Experimental studies in rats have shown [32] that another promutagenic lesion, O^4-ethylthymidine, although formed initially in quantities three-to fourfold less that O^6-ethyldeoxyguanosine, accumulates to levels 50-fold higher after 11-wk chronic administration of diethylnitrosamine. This lesion may therefore also be an appropriate end-point for exposure monitoring being both relatively persistent and implicated in tumorigenesis [33].

In conclusion, the methodologies described to assess human exposure to AF or NNO appear a very promising tool to be used in epidemiological studies aiming at the determination of the role of these carcinogens in the etiology of human cancer.

ACKNOWLEDGMENTS

The authors would like to acknowledge Dr. N. Munoz for supplying the urine samples from the Philippines. We also thank P. Collard-Bianchi and K. Zouhair for the preparation of the manuscript. The work reported in this paper was undertaken during the tenure of research training fellowships awarded by the International Agency for Research on Cancer to C.P. Wild and D. Umbenhauer.

REFERENCES

1. Muller R, Rajewsky MF: J Cancer Res Clin Oncol 102:99, 1981.
2. Strickland PT, Boyle JM: Prog Nucleic Acid Res Mol Biol 31:1, 1984.
3. Poirier M: J Natl Cancer Inst: 67:515, 1981.
4. Kriek E, Den Engelese L, Scherer E, Westra JG: Biochim Biophys Acta 738:181, 1984.
5. Garner RC, Ryder R, Montesano R: Cancer Res 45:922, 1985.
6. Wogan GN: In Okuda K, Peters RL (eds): "Hepatocellular Carcinoma." New York: John Wiley and Sons, Inc., 1976, pp 25–42.
7. Peers FG, Linsell CA: Br J Cancer 27:473, 1973.
8. Van Rensburg SJ, Cook-Mozaffari P, Van Schalkwijk DJ, Van der Watt JJ, Vincent TJ, Purchase IF: Br J Cancer 51:713, 1985.
9. "IARC Monographs on the Evaluation of the Carcinogenic Role of Chemicals to Humans, Vol 10." Lyon: International Agency for Research on Cancer, 1976.
10. Bulatao-Jayme J, Almero EM, Castro CA, Jardeleza TH, Salamat LA: Int J Epidemiol 11:112, 1982.
11. Pegg A: Cancer Invest 2:223, 1984.
12. Yang CS: Cancer Res 40:2633, 1980.
13. Lu SH, Ohshima H, Bartsch H: In O'Neill IK, Von Borstel RC, Miller CT, Long J, Bartsch H (eds): "N-Nitroso-Compounds: Occurrence, Biological Effects and Relevance to Human Cancer." IARC Scientific Publ No 57. Lyon: International Agency for Research on Cancer, 1985, pp 947–953.
14. Sizaret P, Malaveille C, Montesano R, Frayssinet C: J Natl Cancer Inst 69:1375, 1982.
15. Martin CN, Garner RC, Tursi F, Garner JV, Whittle HC, Ryder RN, Sizaret P, Montesano R: In Berlin A, Draper M, Hemminki K, Vainio H (eds): "Monitoring Human Exposure to Carcinogenic and Mutagenic Agents." IARC Scientific Publ No 59. Lyon: International Agency for Research on Cancer, 1984, pp 313–321.
16. Campbell TC, Caedo JP, Bulatao-Jayme J, Salamat L, Engel RW: Nature 227:403, 1970.
17. Autrup H, Bradley KA, Shamsuddin AKM, Wakhisi J, Wasunna A: Carcinogenesis 4:1193, 1983.
18. Wild CP, Smart G, Saffhill R, Boyle JM: Carcinogenesis 4:1605, 1983.
19. Umbenhauer D, Wild CP, Montesano R, Saffhill R, Boyle JM, Huh N, Kirstein U, Thomale J, Rajewsky MF: Int J Cancer 36:661, 1985.
20. Hall J, Bresil H, Montesano R: Carcinogenesis 6:209, 1985.
21. Perera F., Poirier MC, Yuspa SH, Nakayama J, Jaretzki A, Curnen MM, Knowles DM, Weinstein IB: Carcinogenesis 3:1405, 1982.
22. Groopman JD, Trudel LJ, Donahue PR, Marshak-Rothstein A, Wogan GN: Proc Natl Acad Sci USA 81:7728, 1984.

23. Yang G, Nesheim S, Benavides J, Veno I, Campbell AD, Pohland A: In Preusser R (ed) : "Medical Mycology." Zentralblatt Bukt Suppl 8. Stuttgart: Gustat Fischer Verlag, 1980.
24. Dalezios J, Wogan GN, Weinreb SM: Science 171:584, 1971.
25. Muller R, Rajewsky MF: Cancer Res 40:887, 1980.
26. Saffhill R, Stickland PT, Boyle JM: Carcinogenesis 3:547, 1982.
27. Lawley, PD: In Searle CD (ed): "Chemical Carcinogens." ACS Monograph 182. Washington DC: 1984, pp 325–484.
28. Nehls P, Rajewsky MF, Spiess E, Werner D: Embo J 3:327, 1984.
29. Yarosh D: Mutat Res 145:1, 1985.
30. Boiteux S, Laval F: Carcinogenesis 6:805, 1985.
31. Day RS III, Ziolkowski CHJ, Scudiero DA, Meyer SA, Mattern MR: Carcinogenesis 1:21, 1980.
32. Swenberg JA, Dryoff MC, Bedell MA, Popp JA, Huh N, Kirstein U, Rajewsky MF: Proc Natl Acad Sci USA 81:1692, 1984.
33. Singer B: Cancer Invest 2:233, 1984.
34. Grafstrom RC, Pegg AE, Trump BF, Harris CC: Cancer Res 44:2855, 1984.
35. Myrnes B, Giercksky KE, Krokan H: Carcinogenesis 4:1565, 1983.
36. Kyrtopoulos SA, Vrotsou B, Golematis, B, Bonatsos M, Lakiotis G: Carcinogenesis 5:943, 1984.
37. Myrnes B, Norstrank K, Giercksky KE, Sunneskog C, Krokan H: Carcinogenesis 5:1061, 1984.

Journal of Cellular Biochemistry 30:181–193 (1986)
Biochemical and Molecular Epidemiology of Cancer 53–65

Copper Ions and Hydrogen Peroxide Form Hypochlorite From NaCl Thereby Mimicking Myeloperoxidase

Krystyna Frenkel, Fredric Blum, and Walter Troll

Department of Environmental Medicine, New York University Medical Center, New York, New York 10016

Sea urchins have elaborated multiple defenses to assure monospermic fertilization. In this work, we have concentrated on a study of the mechanism(s) by which hydrogen peroxide (H_2O_2) prevents polyspermy in *Arbacia punctulata*. We found that it is not H_2O_2 but probably hypochlorous acid/hypochlorite ($HOCl/OCl^-$) derived from H_2O_2 that is toxic to the supernumerary sperm. The spermicidal activity of H_2O_2 is potentiated by at least one order of magnitude by cupric ions (Cu^{2+}). This increased toxicity is not due to the formation of hydroxyl radicals ($\cdot OH$) because $\cdot OH$ scavengers did not counteract the activity of Cu^{2+}. Moreover, substitution of Cu^{2+} by ferrous ions (Fe^{2+}), which are known to cause formation of $\cdot OH$ from H_2O_2, had no effect on fertilization even at 10^2–10^3 times higher concentrations. In contrast, 3-amino-1,2,4-triazole (AT), an $HOCl/OCl^-$ scavenger, totally reversed the toxic effects of Cu^{2+}. Furthermore, we found that $HOCl/OCl^-$ is generated in solutions of H_2O_2 and Cu^{2+} in the presence of 0.5 M NaCl and that its accumulation is abolished by AT. Thus it is possible that the antifertility properties of copper are due to its ability to mediate formation of $HOCl/OCl^-$. $HOCl/OCl^-$ generated by Cu^{2+} from H_2O_2 and Cl^-, a low concentration of exogenously added $HOCl/OCl^-$, or increased concentrations of H_2O_2 has similar inhibitory effects on the fertilization process in sea urchins. Therefore, we suggest that polyspermy is prevented by the action of a myeloperoxidase that affects the formation of $HOCl/OCl^-$ from the Cl^- present in sea water through reaction with H_2O_2 generated by the newly fertilized egg.

Key words: sea urchins, copper ions, hydrogen peroxide, hypochlorous acid/hypochlorite, myeloperoxidase, spermicidal activity

The prevention of polyspermy is a complicated process [1]. Multiple defenses are necessary because fertilization by more than one sperm leads to an asymmetrical cleavage, which inevitably ends in the death of the embryo. In sea urchins, different mechanisms have developed to prevent polyspermic fertilization. The permanent block consists of raising a fertilization envelope (FE) that is totally impenetrable to

Received April 17, 1985; revised and accepted October 22, 1985.

© **1986 Alan R. Liss, Inc.**

the sperm. However, it takes up to 1 min to complete its formation. To protect eggs from supernumerary sperm during the time needed for completion of FEs, other, faster responses exist. These include a rapid, sodium-dependent electrical depolarization of the egg plasma membrane [2,3], various secretory products released by the egg's cortical granules [1,4], production of arachidonic acid oxidation products [5], and release of H_2O_2 [6–8].

In this work, we have concentrated on a study of the mechanism(s) by which H_2O_2 prevents polyspermy. It already has been shown that removal of H_2O_2 by incubation with catalase causes 100% polyspermy in *Arbacia punctulata* [6]. Similarly, soybean trypsin inhibitor, which prevents the release of H_2O_2 from eggs [6,9], also causes polyspermy [10]. These findings confirm the importance of H_2O_2 release to assure a monospermic fertilization. We have recently observed that Cu^{2+} interfered with the fertilization process by potentiating the effects of H_2O_2 [11]. H_2O_2 is generated by sea urchin eggs in response to a successful entry of the first sperm through the egg's membrane [6,7]. Transition metal ions are known to interact with H_2O_2. These interactions often lead to formation of more reactive activated oxygen species, such as $\cdot OH$ [12–16]. We thought it would be important to determine which (if any) active oxygen species is formed during the interaction of Cu^{2+} with H_2O_2 and, if possible, to determine its effect on fertilization.

The first hypothesis was that Cu^{2+} generates spermicidal $\cdot OH$ from H_2O_2. However, $\cdot OH$ scavengers did not counteract the activity of Cu^{2+}. Moreover, when Cu^{2+} was substituted by Fe^{2+}, which is known to cause formation of $\cdot OH$ from H_2O_2, Fe^{2+} had no effect on fertilization even at concentrations 10^2–10^3 times higher than that of Cu^{2+}. We then postulated that $HOCl/OCl^-$ was generated from H_2O_2 by Cu^{2+}. Exogenously added buffered $HOCl/OCl^-$ inhibited fertilization, whereas both the scavengers of $HOCl/OCl^-$ and catalase counteracted the activity of Cu^{2+} by increasing fertilization and polyspermy. We also found that $HOCl/OCl^-$ is indeed produced by the interaction of Cu^{2+} with H_2O_2 and Cl^- by using the formation of taurine chloramine as a measure of generated $HOCl/OCl^-$.

Based on these results, we concluded that the toxicity of Cu^{2+} ions to the fertilization process is due to the formation of $HOCl/OCl^-$ from Cl^- ions, which are present in high concentration in sea water and can be oxidized by H_2O_2 produced by the fertilized egg. Myeloperoxidase (MPO), an enzyme known to generate $HOCl/OCl^-$ from Cl^- and H_2O_2 by activated neutrophils [17–20], may be among the peroxidases present in gametes. Therefore, we suggest that $HOCl/OCl^-$ is generated by gametes through an MPO-mediated process as one of several mechanisms developed by sea urchins to prevent polyspermy.

MATERIALS AND METHODS
Materials

Arbacia punctulata sea urchins were supplied by the Marine Biological Laboratory (MBL) and kept in large glass tanks with flowing fresh sea water. Sea water was centrally distributed into MBL laboratories and filtered through Whatman No. 1 paper prior to use. Catalase, taurine, 3-amino-1,2,4-triazole, hydrogen peroxide, and mannitol were obtained from Sigma (St. Louis, MO), sodium hypochlorite from Aldrich (Milwaukee, WI) and Chelex 100 from Bio-Rad Laboratories (Rockville Centre, NY).

Methods

Fertilization experiments. Eggs and sperm were obtained by injection of 0.5 M KCl into the coelomic cavity of *A punctulata* as described by Coburn et al [6]. Fertilization was monitored microscopically and assessed by timing, morphology, and symmetry of cleavage. Standard experiments consisted of approximately 1×10^5 eggs fertilized with 1×10^7 sperm in 2 ml of filtered sea water. This ratio of eggs to sperm usually resulted in $\geq 90\%$ fertilization. Gametes were treated with different reagents for 30 sec just prior to fertilization.

Determination of HOCl/OCl$^-$ formation. Although HOCl/OCl$^-$ has a characteristic absorption at 292 nm, and therefore can be directly measured spectrophotometrically, its molar extinction coefficient of 3.5×10^2 is too low to be of use when only small amounts are present. Moreover, since H_2O_2 is produced during fertilization of sea urchins, the small amounts of HOCl/OCl$^-$ (if formed) would be readily reduced by H_2O_2 back to Cl$^-$ and thus would go undetected. To circumvent these potential shortcomings, the method used by Weiss et al [18] for determination of HOCl/OCl$^-$ generated by another complex cellular system, human neutrophils, was adopted for this work. In this method, taurine is present in the reaction mixture and efficiently reacts with HOCl/OCl$^-$ as soon as it is formed. The resultant taurine chloramine is neither reduced nor oxidized by H_2O_2. However, its extinction coefficient of 3.98×10^2 is also too low and would not afford the required sensitivity. Since 1 mol of chloramine retains 2 mol oxidizing equivalents, its concentration can be sensitively determined by its ability to oxidize 2 mol of either 5-thio-2-nitrobenzoic acid to 1 mol of the disulfide or 2 mol of I$^-$ to I$_3^-$ [17,18]. Both methods show increased extinction coefficients of the products with $\epsilon = 1.36 \times 10^4$ for the former and $\epsilon = 2.29 \times 10^4$ for the latter. The oxidation of I$^-$ was chosen because it has an ϵ almost twice as high as the other method. Overall, by using formation of taurine chloramine (from taurine and HOCl/OCl$^-$), and by coupling it with the oxidation of I$^-$ to I$_3^-$, the sensitivity of the spectrophotometric method is increased by almost two orders of magnitude.

All assays were carried out in polypropylene tubes at $4°C$. Glass distilled water and buffers were passed through Chelex 100 to remove adventitious transition metal ions. A standard reaction mixture of 1 ml consisted of 0.01 M taurine dissolved in 0.01 M potassium phosphate and 0.5 M NaCl buffer, pH 7.4, and was incubated with various concentrations of H_2O_2 and $CuCl_2$ for 10 min, after which time the reaction was stopped by the addition of 50 μg catalase. Catalase was included to prevent reduction of HOCl/OCl$^-$ by excess H_2O_2 [17–19]. After 5 min, KI was added to the final concentration of 20 mM, and, after an additional 5 min, absorbance at 350 nm, or spectra of liberated I_2 were recorded (Beckman, Model DU7). In other experiments, AT was incubated together with H_2O_2 and $CuCl_2$, or varying concentrations of NaOCl were used instead of H_2O_2 and $CuCl_2$. Appropriate blanks were prepared that contained all components except the one whose concentration was varied.

Two molecules of taurine chloramine are needed to liberate one I_2. Therefore, the measured amount of I_2 was multiplied by two to give an estimate of taurine chloramine formation. The standard curve of taurine chloramine formation by the exogenously added HOCl/OCl$^-$ was constructed. The efficiency of this reaction at different concentrations was used to calculate the total amount of HOCl/OCl$^-$ formed by $Cu^{2+}/Cl^-/H_2O_2$ mixtures and the percent of Cu^{2+} or H_2O_2 conversion to taurine chloramine.

RESULTS

The effects of Cu^{2+} ions on fertilization of *A punctulata* sea urchins are shown in Figure 1. The most pronounced inhibition of fertilization occurred between 1 and 5×10^{-7} M Cu^{2+}. In different experiments, values for inhibition by 6×10^{-7} through 1×10^{-6} M Cu^{2+} varied between 70% and 100%. As can be seen in Figure 1, addition of catalase restored fertilization even when the concentration of Cu^{2+} ions was as high as 10^{-4} M. These results show that in order to exert its activity Cu^{2+} must interact with H_2O_2.

Table I shows the effects on fertilization of Cu^{2+} alone, H_2O_2 alone, and their combination as measured by percent initial cleavage (at 45 min) and percent FEs. During the normal fertilization process, these two measures have the same values. However, with exposure to toxic agents, either cleavage or both cleavage and formation of FEs can be inhibited. For this reason, the occurrence of both was evaluated. Cu^{2+} alone had the strongest effect on eggs. Both cleavage and FEs were virtually abolished. Pretreatment of eggs with H_2O_2 inhibited cleavage at a higher concentration (5×10^{-4} M) but did not interfere with the formation of FEs. Pretreatment of eggs with a mixture of Cu^{2+} and H_2O_2 abolished both cleavage and the formation of FEs. When sperm were incubated with either Cu^{2+} or H_2O_2 prior to mixing with eggs, there was practically no effect on fertilization except at higher H_2O_2 concentrations (5×10^{-4} M) when some inhibition of cleavage occurred. However, mixtures of Cu^{2+} and H_2O_2 at all H_2O_2 concentrations tested, greatly reduced cleavage and abolished formation of FEs. These results indicate that another damaging agent might be formed from H_2O_2 by the action of Cu^{2+}. Since sperm do not produce H_2O_2, Cu^{2+} alone does not impair their ability to fertilize eggs. However, eggs are known to generate H_2O_2 [6,7]; therefore, Cu^{2+}-induced toxicity to eggs is probably caused by interaction with the endogenously formed H_2O_2. This is corroborated by the finding that incubation with catalase counteracted the effects of Cu^{2+} (Fig. 1).

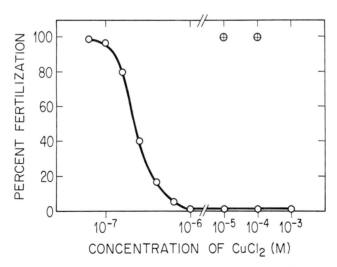

Fig. 1.   Effect of Cu^{2+} on fertilization of *Arbacia punctulata* (○) and of Cu^{2+} in the presence of 1 mg catalase/ml (⊕).

TABLE I. Effects of Cu^{2+} Alone, H_2O_2 Alone, and Cu^{2+} in the Presence of H_2O_2 When Either Eggs (E) or Sperm (S) Were Pretreated Prior to Fertilization

Treatment	Pretreated gametes	Fertilization envelope (%)	Cleavage (%)
Control	—	100	100
Cu^{2+}	E	1–2	1–2
H_2O_2 (M)	S	>95	>95
5×10^{-5}	S	100	100
1×10^{-4}	E	100	>95
	S	100	100
5×10^{-4}	E	100	60
	S	100	40–80
1×10^{-3}	S	>95	0
H_2O_2/Cu^{2+a}(M)			
5×10^{-5}	S	0	30
1×10^{-4}	S	0	6
5×10^{-4}	E	0	0
	S	0	0

[a]$Cu^{2+} = 1 \times 10^{-6}$ M.

TABLE II. Determination of Whether Spermicidal Activity of H_2O_2 Is Mediated by $\cdot OH$ Radicals: Effects of Cu^{2+}, Fe^{2+}, and Cu^{2+} in the Presence of Mannitol, an $\cdot OH$ Scavenger, on Fertilization

Treatment	Percent cleavage	
	−mannitol	+ 0.1 M mannitol
Control	96	87
Cu^{2+}(M)		
1×10^{-7}	95	88
2×10^{-7}	95	87
4×10^{-7}	85	20
8×10^{-7}	35	0
Control	80	
Fe^{2+}(M)		
1×10^{-7}	90	
1×10^{-6}	83	
1×10^{-5}	92	
1×10^{-4}	92	

Transition metal ions such as Fe^{2+} are known to produce $\cdot OH$ from H_2O_2 in a Haber-Weiss reaction [12–14]. It has been assumed that Cu^{2+} also interacts with H_2O_2 in a similar manner. To test whether $\cdot OH$ radicals were generated, eggs were fertilized in the presence of Cu^{2+} and mannitol, an $\cdot OH$ scavenger [19,21]. Even at 0.1 M, mannitol did not reverse Cu^{2+}-induced inhibition of fertilization. On the contrary, it actually potentiated the toxic effects of Cu^{2+}, as can be seen in Table II. These results indicate that $\cdot OH$ radicals are not formed by the action of Cu^{2+} and therefore could not be responsible for its toxic effects. To prove definitively whether $\cdot OH$ are or are not involved in H_2O_2-induced effects on fertilization, eggs were fertilized in the presence of Fe^{2+} ions. As can be seen in Table II, Fe^{2+} ions did not inhibit cleavage even at concentrations 10^2–10^3 times higher than that of Cu^{2+} ions, thus eliminating $\cdot OH$ as a possible damaging agent.

It has been found that, like neutrophils, sea urchin eggs release arachidonic acid, oxidize it, and form prostaglandins and other cyclooxygenase-derived metabolites [5]. The inactivation of excess sperm by H_2O_2 released by a fertilized egg has been likened to the peroxidatic killing of bacteria by neutrophils [22,23]. It is known that neutrophils have several pathways that utilize H_2O_2 generated during the respiratory (oxidative) burst [20]. Among them, the MPO-halide-H_2O_2 system is prominent in inactivation of bacteria [20,23]. MPO catalyzes the oxidation of halide ions (mostly chloride since they are the most abundant) by H_2O_2 with the formation of the very powerful oxidant $HOCl/OCl^-$ [17,18,20,24]. Fertilization of sea urchin eggs occurs in sea water, which has a very high concentration of Cl^- ions (0.5–0.6 M). Therefore, we investigated the possibility that the MPO-halide-H_2O_2 system is responsible for the inactivation of the supernumerary sperm and that the interaction of Cu^{2+} with H_2O_2 in the presence of Cl^- mimics the MPO system. It is already known that the inactivation of a sperm by H_2O_2 is catalyzed by a peroxidase [6,7]. However, it is not certain whether this particular peroxidase is located in the egg or in the sperm, although the most recent evidence points to the latter [23,25].

To determine whether $HOCl/OCl^-$ could be formed by the interaction of Cu^{2+} with H_2O_2 released by the fertilized egg, fertilization was carried out in the presence of Cu^{2+} and AT, which is known to scavenge $HOCl/OCl^-$ [18]. Although AT also inhibits ovoperoxidase, this enzyme is thought not to participate in sperm inactivation [25]. As Table III shows, there is a dramatic reversal of Cu^{2+}-induced inhibition of fertilization as measured by both cleavage and FE formation. Furthermore, eggs fertilized in the presence of 10^{-5} or 10^{-6} M Cu^{2+} and 10 mM AT and left over night showed no apparent toxic effects.

To determine whether AT acted on the Cu^{2+}-induced intermediate or mediated H_2O_2-induced inhibition of fertilization, either eggs or sperm were preincubated with H_2O_2 in the presence or absence of 10 mM AT. In both cases, there were no significant

TABLE III. Effect of 3-amino,1,2,4-triazole on Cu^{2+}-Mediated Inhibition of Fertilization

Treatment	Fertilization envelope (at 5 min postfertilization, %)	Cleavage (at 45 min post-fertilization, %)
Control	99	99
AT (mM)		
10	100	96
100	99	92
Cu^{2+} (M)		
1×10^{-6}	0	0
5×10^{-6}	0	0
1×10^{-5}	0	0
Cu^{2+} (M) + AT (mM)		
$1 \times 10^{-6} + 1$	—	94
$1 \times 10^{-6} + 10$	99	99
$5 \times 10^{-6} + 10$	99	99
$1 \times 10^{-5} + 1$	—	94
$1 \times 10^{-5} + 10$	>95	99
$1 \times 10^{-6} + 100$	99	99

changes in H_2O_2 effects on fertilization, as measured by initial cleavage and FEs, proving that AT interacted with the Cu^{2+}-induced intermediate and scavenged it in situ before it could inactivate the sperm. These findings indicate that $HOCl/OCl^-$ might indeed have been formed through $Cu^{2+}/Cl^-/H_2O_2$ interaction. Next, we tested the influence of exogenously added $HOCl/OCl^-$ on fertilization. When sperm were pretreated with 7×10^{-4} M $HOCl/OCl^-$ buffered with sea water and then diluted to 1.7×10^{-5} M upon addition to the eggs there was no fertilization. When $HOCl/OCl^-$ was diluted to 7×10^{-6} M, fertilization, as measured by the formation of FEs, occurred at the level of 97% showing that there was no permanent effect on the sperm's ability to penetrate the egg's plasma membrane. However, there was no cleavage. Preexposure of eggs to $HOCl/OCl^-$ led to 60% fertilization, again with no apparent cleavage. The effects of the sea water-buffered $HOCl/OCl^-$ on cleavage were similar to those of Cu^{2+} and H_2O_2, thus strengthening the hypothesis that $HOCl/OCl^-$ is the active intermediate.

Hypochlorous acid/hypochlorite produced by the $MPO/Cl^-/H_2O_2$ system in stimulated neutrophils is known to interact with taurine, which is present in the cells, forming taurine chloramine [17,18]. If $HOCl/OCl^-$ is generated by $Cu^{2+}/Cl^-/H_2O_2$, then it also should interact with taurine. Taurine (1 and 10 mM), which by itself is relatively nontoxic, potentiated the toxic effects of Cu^{2+} and further inhibited fertilization from 66% (Cu^{2+} alone) to 28% and 3%, respectively. If taurine chloramine was formed, it would act as another powerful oxidizing agent. It has been shown that chloramines and chloramides are actually formed by the $MPO/Cl^-/H_2O_2$ system through $HOCl/OCl^-$ as an intermediate [17,18,26] and that they cause fragmentation of peptides and oxidation of bacterial components [17]. These destructive changes can be prevented by washing bacteria, which removes the chloramine derivatives [17]. Therefore, the results showing the potentiation of Cu^{2+} toxicity by taurine and the return of a capability to fertilize (as measured by FE formation) by diluting out $HOCl/OCl^-$ from pretreated sperm again point to the possibility that $HOCl/OCl^-$ is formed by the interaction of Cu^{2+} with H_2O_2.

To show unambiguously that $HOCl/OCl^-$ can be generated, H_2O_2 was incubated with Cu^{2+} and Cl^- ions in the presence of taurine. As soon as it is formed, $HOCl/OCl^-$ interacts with taurine producing taurine chloramine [17,18]. Chloramine has a characteristic absorption maximum at 250 nm; however, its molar extinction coefficient of about 400 is too low for quantitative analysis. Since it is a powerful oxidizing agent, it was allowed to oxidize KI to I_3^-, whose maximum is at 350 nm with a molar extinction coefficient of 2.29×10^4 [17,18]. Figure 2 shows that incubation of H_2O_2 with Cu^{2+} and Cl^- ions (——) generated the same product as commercially available $HOCl/OCl^-$ (- - - -). The formation of this product was abolished when any of the three substrates was omitted from the reaction mixture. When incubation was carried out in the presence of 10 mM AT, an $HOCl/OCl^-$ scavenger [18], there was no absorption at 350 nm either. To determine whether $\cdot OH$, a strong oxidizing agent, would also cause production of I_3^-, Cu^{2+} was substituted by Fe^{2+}, which is known to generate $\cdot OH$ from H_2O_2. Since there was no absorption maximum at 350 nm, it is concluded that in this system, $\cdot OH$ is not capable of generating I_3^-. All these results paralleled the findings obtained during fertilization of sea urchins. Therefore, it is concluded that Cu^{2+} indeed generated $HOCl/OCl^-$ from H_2O_2 in the presence of Cl^- ions and thereby mimics the action of myeloperoxidase.

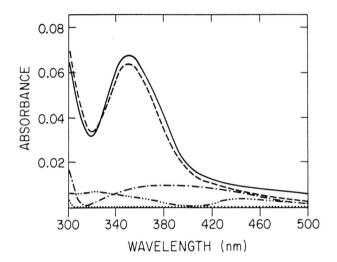

Fig. 2.   Generation of I_3^- by taurine chloramine obtained by incubation of taurine dissolved in 0.01 M phosphate, 0.5 M NaCl buffer, pH 7.4, with: 1) synthetic 15 nmole $HOCl/OCl^-$/ml (- - - -), 2) 100 nmole Cu^{2+}/ml and 100 nmole H_2O_2/ml (——), 3) 100 nmole Cu^{2+}/ml in the absence of H_2O_2 ($\cdots$), 4) 100 nmole H_2O_2/ml in the absence of Cu^{2+} (-··-), 5) 100 nmole Cu^{2+} and 100 nmole H_2O_2 in the absence of Cl^- (-····-).

Figure 3 shows that formation of $HOCl/OCl^-$ is linear between 10 and 100 nmole H_2O_2/ml reaction mixture when 100 nmole of Cu^{2+} is used and that it can be extrapolated to 0. Similarly, it is linear between 10 and 100 nmole Cu^{2+}/ml when 100 nmole H_2O_2 is used, but its slope is different. The lowering of Cu^{2+} concentration below 10 nmole/ml still results in measurable formation of $HOCl/OCl^-$. However, these values are located on a line with a different slope, which can be linearly extended to 0. These results suggest that there is no threshold for $HOCl/OCl^-$ formation even when minute amounts of H_2O_2 and Cu^{2+} are present. Figure 3 also shows that, when the synthetic $HOCl/OCl^-$ is used, formation of taurine chloramine coupled with oxidation of KI is also linear. However, under the conditions of this assay, the reaction did not go to completion. The yield of this reaction varied from 50% when 5 nmole $HOCl/OCl^-$/ml was used to 30% at higher concentrations (Table IV). The same reaction yields were assumed for $HOCl/OCl^-$ generated by a Cu^{2+}/ Cl^-/H_2O_2 system. As Figure 4 shows, approximately 20% of H_2O_2 is converted into $HOCl/OCl^-$ by 100 nmole Cu^{2+}/ml regardless of H_2O_2 concentration. In contrast, when the concentration of H_2O_2 used for the reaction was held constant at 100 nmole/ ml and that of Cu^{2+} was varied, the percent of H_2O_2 converted into $HOCl/OCl^-$ also varied from >50% for low concentrations of Cu^{2+} (2.5–10 nmole) down to 20% for 100 nmole Cu^{2+}. The comparison of the percent conversion into $HOCl/OCl^-$ by varying concentrations of H_2O_2 and Cu^{2+} shows that low concentrations of Cu^{2+} generate $HOCl/OCl^-$ more efficiently than low concentrations of H_2O_2. Further-more, it seems that concentrations of Cu^{2+} higher than equimolar concentrations of H_2O_2 would suppress production of $HOCl/OCl^-$.

It is possible that the generation of $HOCl/OCl^-$ during interaction of Cu^{2+} with H_2O_2 and Cl^- involves reduction of Cu^{2+} to Cu^+. In such cases, $HOCl/OCl^-$, which is a strong oxidizing agent, might reoxidize some of the Cu^+ back to Cu^{2+}.

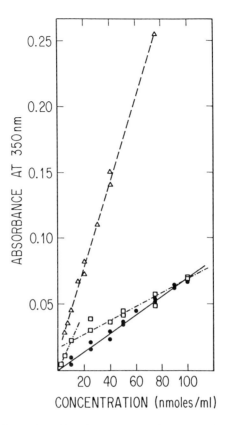

Fig. 3.   Generation of I_3^- by taurine chloramine obtained by incubation of taurine dissolved in 0.01 M phosphate, 0.5 M NaCl buffer, pH 7.4, with varying concentrations of: 1) synthetic HOCl/OCl$^-$ ($\triangle$), 2) H_2O_2 in the presence of 100 nmole Cu^{2+}/ml ($\bullet$), and 3) Cu^{2+} in the presence of 100 nmole H_2O_2/ml ($\square$).

Thus, in the presence of taurine, both production of taurine chloramine and reoxidation of Cu^+ may compete for HOCl/OCl$^-$. Therefore, the measured value would represent a net formation of HOCl/OCl$^-$. To determine the feasibility of this hypothesis, we had to prove that HOCl/OCl$^-$ is capable of oxidizing Cu^+ in the presence of taurine. Incubation of buffered HOCl/OCl$^-$ (15, 30, or 60 nmole/ml) with Cu^+ (100 nmole/ml) and taurine (10 μmole/ml) in 0.01 M phosphate, 0.5 M NaCl, pH 7.4 buffer resulted in about 20% inhibition of taurine chloramine formation, whereas the same amount of Cu^{2+} was without effect. Preincubation of the same concentrations of HOCl/OCl$^-$ and Cu^+ at 4°C for 10 min prior to addition of taurine resulted in 85%, 59%, and 53% reduction of taurine chloramine formation, respectively. These results show that HOCl/OCl$^-$ has a potential to oxidize Cu^+ in a dose-dependent manner. The amount of Cu^+ oxidized apparently depends on the ratio of HOCl/OCl$^-$ to Cu^+ in the absence of taurine. When taurine is present in the incubation mixture from the beginning of the incubation, the percent of Cu^+ that can be oxidized remains constant. When H_2O_2 (100 nmole/ml) was incubated with Cu^+, Fe^{2+}, or Fe^{3+} (100 nmole/ml) and taurine (10 μmole/ml) in the same buffer, there was no generation of taurine chloramine. All these results prove that it is Cu^{2+} that is needed to generate

TABLE IV. Efficiency of Taurine Chloramine Formation From Synthetic HOCl/OCl⁻ and Taurine

Amount of HOCl/OCl⁻ used (nmole)	$A_{350} \times 10^{-3a}$	HOCl/OCl⁻ equivalents measured (nmole)[b]	Reaction efficiency[c]
5	29.0	2.53	0.51
7.5	37.5	3.28	0.44
10	47.0	4.10	0.41
15	62.5	5.46	0.36
20	78.5	6.86	0.34
25	95.0	8.30	0.33
30	111.0	9.70	0.32
40	145.0	12.66	0.31
50	176.0	15.37	0.31
75	257.0	22.45	0.30

[a]A_{350} values were obtained from Figure 3 ($\triangle$).
[b]Iodine formation was calculated from molar extinction coefficient $\epsilon = 2.29 \times 10^4$ at 350 nm. To obtain HOCl/OCl⁻ equivalents, that value was multiplied by 2 because two molecules of taurine chloramine derived from two molecules of HOCl/OCl⁻ are needed to produce one molecule of iodine.
[c]Reaction efficiency was obtained by dividing HOCl/OCl⁻ equivalents by the amount of HOCl/OCl⁻ actually used.

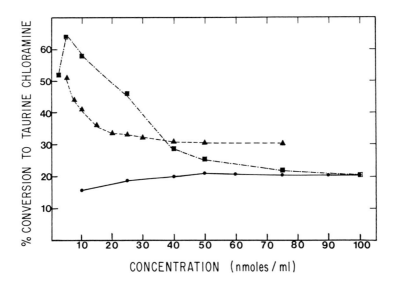

Fig. 4.   Efficiency of conversion of taurine to taurine chloramine by HOCl/OCl⁻. Reactions were carried out in 0.01 M phosphate, 0.5 M NaCl buffer, pH 7.4, with varying concentrations of: 1) synthetic HOCl/OCl⁻ ($\blacktriangle$), 2) H_2O_2 in the presence of 100 nmole Cu^{2+}/ml ($\bullet$), and 3) Cu^{2+} in the presence of 100 nmole H_2O_2/ml ($\blacksquare$).

HOCl/OCl⁻ from H_2O_2 and Cl⁻ and that during such a process Cu^{2+} is reduced to Cu^+. In turn, some of this Cu^+ is reoxidized to Cu^{2+} by HOCl/OCl⁻, thus lowering the final yield of HOCl/OCl⁻.

DISCUSSION

It has been known for a long time that copper is an essential element for normal metabolism [27] and that it also plays a role in inflammation [28,29]. It is thought that some of its effects are due to interference with the biosynthesis of prostaglandins [30] and also with the ability to form complexes with a variety of ligands [28,29]. There are a number of postulated mechanisms that attempt to explain the various activities of copper. Among others, it is suggested that copper effectively scavenges the superoxide anion radical [31–33], which is associated with inflammation [34,35]. Depending on the valence, it is supposed to convert superoxide to either molecular oxygen (Cu^{2+}) or to H_2O_2 (Cu^+ and Cu^{2+}) [36,37]. Therefore, we originally anticipated that the effect of Cu^{2+} on the fertilization of sea urchins was also due to its superoxide dismutase-mimetic capability. To our surprise, instead of generating H_2O_2, Cu^{2+} caused its disappearance. In this work, we proved that Cu^{2+} interacts with H_2O_2 in the presence of Cl^- and forms $HOCl/OCl^-$, a product known to be formed by MPO from H_2O_2 and Cl^-. Thus, we show that, in addition to mimicking superoxide dismutase, it also is capable of mimicking myeloperoxidase.

Sea urchins have developed multiple defenses to prevent polyspermic fertilization [1]. We and others have previously shown that rapid generation of H_2O_2 by the newly fertilized egg is a very effective defense mechanism [6,7]. The unresolved question left was how this H_2O_2 interferes with the ability of supernumerary sperm to refertilize the egg. It appears that the amount of H_2O_2 formed is very high—10 pmole H_2O_2 per egg [7]. Since 0.1 ml of packed eggs ($\sim 1 \times 10^5$) produces 1 μmole H_2O_2, then 10^{-5} μmole would be generated by one egg in a volume of 1×10^{-6} ml. This means that the initial concentration of H_2O_2 at the egg's membrane is as high as 10 mM. In our experiments, we have used an average of 1×10^5 eggs in 2 ml of sea water. Upon fertilization, these eggs would generate 1 μmole H_2O_2, a 5×10^{-4} M final concentration. When eggs were pretreated with H_2O_2 for 30 sec prior to addition of sperm, the inhibition of fertilization was observed starting with 5×10^{-4} M H_2O_2 (Table I), the same concentration as is generated by the eggs to prevent polyspermy [7]. Similar results were obtained upon preincubation of sperm. When gametes were treated with H_2O_2 in the presence of 1×10^{-6} M Cu^{2+}, the effects of H_2O_2 were potentiated and manifested one order of magnitude sooner.

In all experiments, we have found that Cu^{2+}/H_2O_2-induced effects on fertilization seemed to be qualitatively the same as those of H_2O_2 alone but occurred at lower concentrations of H_2O_2. These findings indicate that the actual mechanism of H_2O_2-mediated prevention of polyspermy is the same as that artificially created by the Cu^{2+}/H_2O_2 system.

Since the fertilization process occurs outside sea urchins in sea water [1], we propose that the Cl^- ions present in high concentrations (0.5–0.6 M) participate in a formation of the active intermediate, $HOCl/OCl^-$, upon reaction with H_2O_2. However, the formation of $HOCl/OCl^-$ from H_2O_2 and Cl^- requires a mediation by myeloperoxidase [17,18,20,26]. This enzyme has not been identified in sea urchins as yet, although there is evidence that the antipolyspermic activity of H_2O_2 is mediated by peroxidase [23,25]. Spermicidal activity present in mammalian systems has been shown to be mediated by peroxidase as well [38].

In our in vitro assays, we used concentrations of Cu^{2+}, H_2O_2, and Cl^- similar to those in the fertilization experiments. In the presence of an excess H_2O_2, 2.5×10^{-6} M Cu^{2+} caused formation of 1.3×10^{-6} M $HOCl/OCl^-$ from 1×10^{-4} M H_2O_2 (Table V). Assuming linearity at low concentrations, 1×10^{-6} M Cu^{2+} used in fertilization experiments might have caused formation of 0.5×10^{-6} M $HOCl/OCl^-$ from 5×10^{-4} M H_2O_2. Preincubation of sperm with exogenous $HOCl/OCl^-$

TABLE V. Rates of Conversion of Cu^{2+}/Cl^-/H_2O_2 Into HOCl/OCl^- When Either H_2O_2 or Cu^{2+} Is In Limiting Amounts

Amount of H_2O_2 or Cu^{2+} used (nmole)	A_{350} $\times 10^{-3a}$	HOCl/OCl^- equivalent measured (nmole)[b]	Reaction efficiency[c]	Total HOCl/OCl^- formed (nmole)[d]	Percent conversion to HOCl/OCl^{-e}
H_2O_2/100 nmole Cu^{2+}					
10	7.5	0.66	0.41	1.6	16.0
25	18.0	1.57	0.33	4.8	19.2
40	28.5	2.49	0.31	8.0	20.0
50	36.0	3.14	0.30	10.5	21.0
60	42.5	3.71	0.30	12.4	20.7
75	53.0	4.63	0.30	15.4	20.5
90	63.5	5.55	0.30	18.5	20.6
100	70.0	6.11	0.30	20.4	20.4
Cu^{2+}/100 nmole H_2O_2					
2.5	4.5	0.39	0.3	1.3	52.0
5	11.0	0.96	0.3	3.2	64.0
10	20.0	1.75	0.3	5.8	58.0
25	31.0	2.71	0.3	9.0	36.0
40	39.0	3.41	0.3	11.4	28.5
50	44.0	3.84	0.3	12.8	25.6
75	57.0	4.98	0.3	16.6	22.0
100	69.5	6.07	0.3	20.2	20.2

[a]A_{350} values were obtained from Figure 3 for H_2O_2 (●) and for Cu^{2+} (□).
[b]The same as footnote b in Table IV.
[c]Values taken from the appropriate positions in Table IV.
[d]Values of "total HOCl/OCl^- formed" were obtained by dividing "HOCl/OCl^- equivalents measured" by the appropriate reaction efficiency.
[e]Percent conversion to HOCl/OCl^- was calculated by dividing "total HOCl/OCl^- formed" by the amount of the reagent (H_2O_2 or Cu^{2+}) used and multiplying by 100.

did not inhibit its ability to penetrate the egg's membrane as assessed by the presence of FEs when the concentration of HOCl/OCl^- was 7×10^{-6} M. However, at that concentration, there was still no cleavage. It therefore appears that the exogenous HOCl/OCl^- is as effective as inhibitory concentrations of H_2O_2 but at concentrations 10^2–10^3-fold lower than that of H_2O_2.

We have shown that Cu^{2+} mimics myeloperoxidase because it forms HOCl/OCl^- from H_2O_2 and Cl^-. It is possible that this process is among those responsible for the known antifertility properties of copper [39,40]. Furthermore, HOCl/OCl^- reoxidizes Cu^+, again similarly to MPO, which is oxidized by the same product. In the absence of scavenging agents, HOCl/OCl^- is reduced by Cu^+. However, in the presence of scavengers such as primary amines and even NH_4^+ ions, it preferentially forms chloramines, which are also powerful oxidizing agents [17,18,24]. Since HOCl/OCl^- generated by Cu^{2+} from H_2O_2 and Cl^-, exogenous HOCl/OCl^-, and higher concentrations of H_2O_2 all have similar inhibitory effects on the fertilization process in sea urchins, we suggest that it is myeloperoxidase that mediates formation of HOCl/OCl^- from endogenous H_2O_2 to prevent polyspermy.

ACKNOWLEDGMENTS

These studies were supported by NIH grants CA-16060 (W.T.) and BRSG SO7 RR05399-23 (K.F.) and the New York University School of Medicine Honors Program (F.B.). The authors wish to thank Catherine Bearce and Kazimierz Chrzan for excellent technical assistance. Part of this work was performed in the Marine Biological Laboratory, Woods Hole, MA, and was published as an abstract in Biol Bull 167:517, 1984.

REFERENCES

1. Schuel H: Biol Bull 167:271, 1984.
2. Jaffe LA: Nature 261:68, 1976.
3. Schuel H, Schuel R: Dev Biol 87:249, 1981.
4. Epel D: Curr Topics Dev Biol 12:186, 1978.
5. Schuel H, Traeger E, Schuel R, Boldt J: Gamete Res 10:9, 1984.
6. Coburn M, Schuel H, Troll W: Dev Biol 84:235, 1981.
7. Boldt J, Schuel H, Schuel R, Dandekar PV, Troll W: Gamete Res 4:365, 1981.
8. Aranov C, Eisen M, Zimmerman M, Troll W: Biol Bull 161:333, 1981.
9. Sinsheimer P, Coburn M, Troll W: Biol Bull 159:469, 1980.
10. Longo FJ, Schuel H: Dev Biol 34:187, 1973.
11. Blum F, Bearce C, Frenkel K, Troll W: Biol Bull 167:517, 1984.
12. Fridovich I: Annu Rev Pharmacol Toxicol 23:239, 1983.
13. Youngman RJ: TIBS 9:280, 1984.
14. Green MJ, Hill HAO: In Packer L (ed): "Methods in Enzymology, Vol 105." New York: Academic Press, 1984, pp 3–22.
15. Troll W, Frenkel K, Wiesner R: JNCI 73:1245, 1984.
16. Troll W, Frenkel K, Teebor G: In Fujiki H, et al (eds): "Cellular Interactions by Environmental Tumor Promoters." Tokyo: Japan Sci Press, Utrecht: VNU Sci Press, 1984, pp 207–218.
17. Thomas EL: Infect Immun 23:522, 1979.
18. Weiss SJ, Klein R, Slivka A, Wei M: J Clin Invest 70:598, 1982.
19. Rosen H, Klebanoff SJ: J Clin Invest 58:50, 1976.
20. Babior BM: N Engl J Med 298:659, 1978.
21. Levitz SM, Diamond RD: Infect Immun 43:1100, 1984.
22. Foerder CA, Klebanoff SJ, Shapiro BM: Proc Natl Acad Sci USA 75:3183, 1978.
23. Klebanoff SJ, Foerder CA, Eddy EM, Shapiro BM: J Exp Med 149:938, 1979.
24. Weiss SJ, Lampert MB, Test ST: Science 222:625, 1983.
25. Boldt J, Alliegro C, Schuel H: Gamete Res 10:267, 1984.
26. Harrison JE, Schultz J: J Biol Chem 251:1371, 1976.
27. Evans GW, Johnson WT: In Sorenson JRJ (ed): "Inflammatory Diseases and Copper." Clifton, New Jersey: Humana Press, 1982, pp 3–15.
28. Sorenson JRJ: In Sorenson JRJ (ed): "Inflammatory Diseases and Copper." Clifton, New Jersey: Humana Press, 1982, pp 289–301.
29. Lewis AJ, Smith WE, Brown DH: In Sorenson JRJ (ed): "Inflammatory Diseases and Copper." Clifton, New Jersey: Humana Press, 1982, pp 303–318.
30. Boyle E, Freeman PC, Goudie AC, Mangan FR, Thompson M: J Pharm Pharmacol 28:865, 1976.
31. Halliwell B: FEBS Lett 56:34, 1975.
32. Milanino R, Passarella E, Velo GP: Adv Inflam Res 1:281, 1979.
33. Kensler TW, Trush MA: Environ Mutagen 6:593, 1984.
34. Goldstein BD, Witz G, Amoruso M, Troll W: Biochem Biophys Res Commun 88:854, 1979.
35. Salin ML, McCord JM: J Clin Invest 56:1319, 1975.
36. Brigelius R, Spötl R, Bors W, Lengfelder E, Saran M, Weser U: FEBS Lett 47:72, 1974.
37. deAlvare LR, Goda K, Kimura T: Biochem Biophys Res Commun 69:687, 1976.
38. Smith DC, Klebanoff SJ: Biol Reprod 3:229, 1970.
39. Zipper J, Medel M, Prager R: Am J Obstet Gynecol 105:529, 1969.
40. Tatum HJ: Am J Obstet Gynecol 112:1000, 1972.

Journal of Cellular Biochemistry 30:195–218 (1986)
Biochemical and Molecular Epidemiology of Cancer 67–90

Interaction Between *Raf* and *Myc* Oncogenes in Transformation In Vivo and In Vitro

J.L. Cleveland, H.W. Jansen, K. Bister, T.N. Fredrickson, H.C. Morse, III, J.N. Ihle, and U.R. Rapp

Laboratory of Viral Carcinogenesis, National Cancer Institute (J.L.C., U.R.R.), NCI-Frederick Cancer Research Facility, LBI-Basic Research Program (J.N.I.), Frederick, Maryland 21701, Max Planck Institut fur Molekulare Genetik, Otto Warburg Labor, Berlin 33, Federal Republic of Germany (H.W.J., K.B.), and Laboratory of Immunopathology, National Institute of Allergy and Infectious Diseases, National Institutes of Health, Bethesda, Maryland 20205 (T.N.F., H.C.M.)

3611 MSV, a *raf*-oncogene-transducing murine retrovirus, induces fibrosarcomas and erythroid hyperplasia in newborn mice after a latency of 4–8 wk. In contrast, new recombinant murine retroviruses carrying the *myc* oncogene (J-3, J-5 construct viruses) do not induce tumors before > 9 wk. A combination of both oncogenes in an infectious murine retrovirus (J-2) induces hematopoietic neoplasms in addition to less prominent fibrosarcomas and pancreatic adenocarcinoma 1–3 wk after inoculation. The hematologic neoplasms consist of immunoblastic lymphomas of T and B cell lineage and erythroblastosis. If animals were inoculated with a variant of the J-3 virus, which induces altered foci in cultures of NIH 3T3 cells, carcinoma developed in the pancreas with a 2–6 mo latency. In parallel to the synergistic action of both oncogenes on hematopoietic cells in vivo, we find that *raf*-oncogene-induced transformation of bone marrow cells in culture is enhanced by the addition of *myc*, which by itself does not transform these cells when grown in standard media. We conclude that concomitant expression of *raf* and *myc* oncogenes in hematopoietic and epithelial cells alters their respective transforming activities. The contribution of v-*myc* in this synergism was examined by use of a series of recombinant murine retroviruses capable of expressing the avian v-*myc* to study the effect of altered *myc* expression on hematopoietic/lymphoid cells. With either interleukin 3- or interleukin 2-dependent cell lines, introduction of the recombinant viruses abrogated the requirement for IL 3 or IL 2 for growth, and associated with this was the suppression of c-*myc* expression. The findings suggest that *myc* is a component in the signal transduction pathway for IL 3 and IL 2 and support an autoregulatory mechanism of c-*myc* expression. In contrast to v-*myc*, expression of v-*raf* in primary lymphoid/hematopoietic cells has an immortilizing function without abrogating the requirement for IL 3 for growth. This suggests that v-*raf* and v-*myc* affect different components of growth regulation, as, for example, commitment (v-*myc*) and cell cycle progression (v-*raf*).

Key words: *raf, myc*, oncogene, synergism

Received May 29, 1985; revised and accepted October 7, 1985.

Published by Alan R. Liss, Inc., 1986

During the past several years, evidence has been accumulating which suggests that activation of cellular protooncogenes is the common denominator for tumor induction by chemical and biological carcinogens. Protooncogenes are a subset (~0.1%) of cellular genes which, after incorporation into retroviruses, or upon specific alteration within the cell in structure [1–4] or regulation [3,5], are capable of inducing tumorous growth.

Protooncogenes control the growth and affect the differentiation of eukaryotic cells. Long before the discovery of viral oncogenes and their cellular homologs [6], it was clear that malignantly transformed cells were genetically altered in regard to their growth factor requirements for propagation in culture [7,8]. Moreover, the fact that cells transformed by oncogene-transducing mammalian retroviruses were blocked for the binding of epidermal growth factor [9], and released transforming growth factors into the culture medium [10,11], suggested early on that several oncogenes might cause transformation by affecting the signal transmission pathway of growth factors. At least four of the approximately 25 known oncogenes derive from components of the growth factor signal transduction pathway: *erb*B, which derives from a portion of the receptor gene for epidermal growth factor (EGF) [12]; *sis*, which is homologous to part of the gene for platelet-derived growth factor (PDGF) [13–15]; *fms*, which is related to the receptor for colony-stimulating factor, CSF-1 [16]; and *myc*, which can relieve the requirement of fibroblasts for PDGF [17] and myeloid and lymphoid cells for IL-3 and IL-2, respectively [41,85]. Moreover, *myc* is induced [5] along with c-*fos* [18–20] and r-*fos* [21] by PDGF.

Recent findings have demonstrated that oncogenes may act synergistically in specific combinations when assayed with primary fibroblast cells in culture [22,23]. To examine the possible interaction of the *raf* and *myc* oncogenes in vivo in the development of tumors, we have used naturally occurring and recombinant murine retroviruses carrying *raf* and *myc* or only *myc* oncogenes. Several types of data suggest possible interaction of the *raf* and *myc* oncogenes in some tumors. A subclass of the small cell lung carcinomas, the small cell/large cell (SC/LC) carcinomas which have a particularly poor prognosis, have amplified *myc* gene DNA [24] and also express the c-*raf*-1 gene [25]. In addition, both familial renal carcinoma [26] and transfected DNA from primary stomach cancer [27] show translocations or rearrangements of the c-*raf*-1 locus, respectively, and presumably express c-*myc*. Moreover, the avian homolog of v-*raf*, v-*mil*, is naturally linked to v-*myc* in the carcinoma virus MH2 [28–32] where it presumably contributes to carcinoma induction since avian acute leukemia viruses which only contain v-*myc* have a much lower incidence of this tumor type [33,34]. It therefore became important to test the effect of v-*myc* on the oncogenicity of 3611 MSV. Our findings provide the first evidence for a synergistic action between the *raf* and *myc* oncogenes during lymphoma induction in vivo and suggest a mechanism that may underlie this phenomenon. The synergistic action of these two oncogenes has also been demonstrated in vitro where immortalization of primary murine bone marrow [84] or fetal liver cultures [Y. Weinstein, J. Cleveland, U. Rapp, J.N. Ihle, in preparation] requires expression of both *onc* genes.

The contributions of *raf* and *myc* to this synergism have been studied in vitro by examining their effects on hematopoietic/lymphoid cell differentiation, immortalization, and factor dependence for growth. With either interleukin 3 (IL 3)- or interleukin 2 (IL 2)-dependent cell lines, the viruses expressing v-*myc* alone were capable of abrogating the requirement of IL 3 or IL 2 for growth. Associated with this abrogation was the suppression of c-*myc* expression.

EFFECT OF *RAF/MIL*- AND *MYC*-TRANSDUCING VIRUSES ON NIH 3T3 CELLS

In order to investigate potential interactions between the v-*raf* and v-*myc* onco-genes, we have made constructs [40,41] between DNA from p3611 MSV, pMH2, and pMC29 such that either or both genes were part of a transmissible viral genome (Fig. 1). To determine the biological activity of the various viruses, cloned DNAs were cotransfected with helper virus DNA (leuk strain of M-MuLV) onto NIH 3T3 fibroblast cells. Transfected cells were observed for the development of transformed foci and production of virus particles by assay for reverse transcriptase in the culture medium. Since neither of the two *myc* recombinants pHWJ-3 and pHWJ-5 induce foci of morphologically transformed cells, DNA from these constructs was cotrans-fected with a neomycin resistance marker (pSV2neo). Clones of antibiotic-resistant cells were examined for v-*myc* expression by immunoprecipitation with *myc*- and p30-specific antibodies and virus stocks were prepared from positive cells by rescue

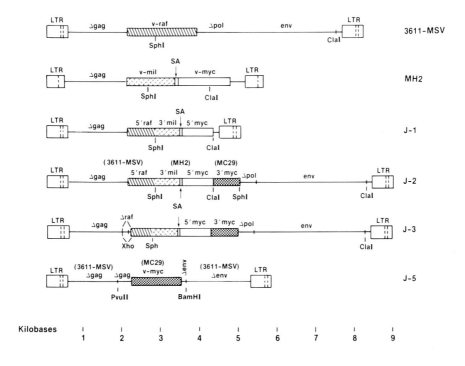

Fig. 1. Genomic organization of the defective viruses 3611-MSV and MH2 and of the construct viruses J-1 through J-5. Important restriction enzyme sites are indicated and the sizes of the various viruses are shown in kilobases. The origin of specific v-*onc* sequences in the constructs is indicated by specific shadings: ▨,3611-MSV v-*raf*; ▩, MH2 v-*mil*; ▢, MH2 v-*myc*; ▥, MC29 v-*myc*. SA indicates presence of splice acceptor sequences present in MH2 v-*myc*.

with ecotropic and amphotropic helper viruses (M-MuLV and 4070 A MuLV). All three v-*myc* recombinant viruses, J-2, J-3, and J-5, were produced at similar levels by helper-virus-infected cultures as determined by dot blot hybridization of viral RNA with a v-*myc*-specific DNA probe. In agreement with the hybridization data, indirect immunofluorescence assays for v-*myc* protein in acutely infected NIH 3T3 cells showed that all three viruses were produced at comparable titers of infectious virus.

In contrast to pHWJ-3 and pHWJ-5, constructs pHWJ-1 and pHWJ-2 do induce foci on NIH 3T3 cells. The fact that pHWJ-1 was transforming provided the first evidence for biological activity of the v-*mil* gene in MH2. Sequence comparisons between v-*mil* and v-*raf* have shown previously [32] that v-*mil* differs in 19 positions in its amino acid sequence from v-*raf*. Our transfection data show that 17 of these changes are compatible with transformation since they are located 3' of the Sph I site at which the v-*mil* fragment was joined with v-*raf* in pHWJ-1 (Fig. 1). The morphology of transformed foci induced by J-1 virus differs, however, from those induced by 3611 MSV in that the foci are more flat and transformed cells are more commonly interspersed with nontransformed cells (Fig. 2). Addition of the hybrid MH2-MC29 v-*myc* gene to the hybrid v-*raf/mil* gene in pHWJ-2 has a dramatic effect on the fibroblast-transforming activity of the virus (Fig. 2). Foci of morphologically transformed cells are very dense, homogeneous, and consist of less elongated cells. We conclude that the 5' half of MH$_2$ v-*myc* is biologically active and that concomitant expression of v-*raf/mil* and v-*myc* in NIH 3T3 fibroblast cells alters their transformed phenotype.

PATHOGENICITY IN NEWBORN NFS/N MICE

High-titer virus stocks of J-1 and -2 were prepared by cloning cells from individual foci and stocks of J-3 and -5 by rescue of transfected, neomycin-resistant cells with ecotropic and amphotropic helper MuLV as described above [40]. The tumor-inducing potential of construct viruses J-1 to J-5, as well as that of 3611 MSV and helper virus controls, was determined by intraperitoneal inoculation of newborn NFS/N mice. Consistent with the differential ability of these viruses to transform

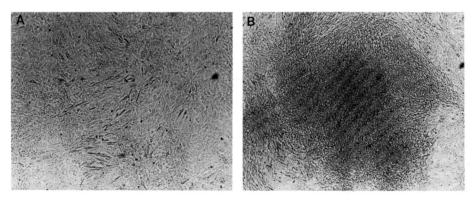

Fig. 2. Morphology of representative NIH/3T3 cell foci induced by J-1 (panel A) and J-2 (panel B). Conditions for infection were as previously described [38]. Comparison was between foci from dishes containing a comparable number of foci. Reproduced from previously published figure [40].

fibroblasts in culture, we observed a striking difference in their ability to induce tumors in newborn mice (Table I); 3611 MSV induced sarcomas and less frequent erythroid hyperplasia with a latency of 4–8 wk. Viruses derived from pHWJ-3 and -5 did not produce tumors with a latency < 9 wk, at which time the M-MuLV helper-virus-produced disease began. V-*myc* recombinant virus-specific RNA was present in such tumor cells (data not shown). Recently, using Cas-Br-M-MuLV as helper virus for infections with J-3 or J-5 we have again observed T cell lymphomas with a latency of 1½–4 mo, a disease which is not characteristic of Cas-Br-M-MuLV-infected animals [54]; therefore, the v-*myc*-transducing retroviruses do indeed appear to cause T cell lymphomas [Morse, Hartley, Yetter, Frederickson, Majumdar, Cleveland, and Rapp, submitted]. In contrast, the dual-oncogene-transducing virus J-2 induced lymphomas and erythroblastosis which killed the mice after an average latency of 2–3 wk, depending on the helper virus used (leuk M-MuLV or 4070 A, respectively). Viruses with the same in vitro and in vivo transforming properties as the input viruses were recovered from tumors induced by 3611 MSV, J-1, and J-2. We conclude from the pathogenicity pattern that concomitant expression of v-*raf* and v-*myc* in hemato-poietic cells has a synergistic effect on the transformation of these cells in vivo.

Recently we have isolated a variant virus from the spleens of mice which were originally inoculated with J-3 virus. This virus induces altered foci (less transformed than J-2) on NIH 3T3 cells and upon injection into newborn mice causes immuno-blastic lymphomas and adenocarcinoma of the pancreas with a latency of 2–6 mo [unpublished results]. Analysis of this variant virus indicates that this virus likely arose by recombination of the J-3 virus with the c-*raf*-1 locus; protein analysis

TABLE I. Tumor Development in Newborn NSF Mice*

Virus	Incidence	Latency (wk)	Pathology
3611			
M-MuLV	30/30	4–8	Fibrosarcoma, erythroid hyperplasia
4070	22/22	4–10	
J-1			
MuLV	20/20	7–10	Fibrosarcoma, erythroid hyperplasia
J-2			
M-MuLV	18/18	1–3	Lymphoma (T+B), erythroblastosis,
4070	12/12	2–4	fibrosarcoma,
			adenocarcinoma of pancreas,
			liver, and lung
J-3			
M-MuLV	12/12	9–16	Lymphoma (T)
4070	5/5	16	Lymphoma (T)
J-5			
M-MuLV	11/11	9–16	Lymphoma (T)
4070	8/8	16	Lymphoma (T)
Helper			
M-MuLV	20/20	9–16	Lymphoma (T)
4070	0/20	>52	N/A

*Newborn NFS/N mice were inoculated intraperitoneally with $2–5 \times 10^4$ focus-forming units (FFU) of 3611, J-1, or J-2 virus, and $1–2 \times 10^3$ v-*myc* fluorescence-inducing units (FIU) of J-3 or J-5 virus. Inoculated mice were observed for tumor growth and autopsied at late stages of disease. Tumors were evaluated by light microscopic examination of hematoxylin-eosin-stained tissue sections. NA = nonapplicable. Modified from previously published data [40].

indicates this recombination event allows the variant to make a gag-*raf* fusion protein unlike J-3, which makes no detectable *raf* products (data not shown).

HISTOPATHOLOGY AND FMF ANALYSIS OF TUMORS INDUCED BY J-2 AND CONTROL VIRUSES

Lesions induced in mice inoculated with J-2 virus consist of lymphoma, erythroblastosis, sarcoma, and dysplasia progressing to frank carcinoma, of pancreatic acinar cells [40]. Usually, neonatally inoculated mice have advanced lymphomas and erythroblastosis at 1–3 wk of age. By this time, sarcomatous growths are also seen in some animals. Pancreatic lesions appear sporadic, but since they are only discernable by histologic examination, the incidence may be higher than currently appreciated. Representative examples for the various histological lesions are shown in Figure 3.

Neoplasms appearing in mice inoculated with the 3611 virus are restricted to sarcoma, which may be very large, occurring in muscles and spleen (Fig. 3A). Erythroid hyperplasia is observed in the early stages after inoculation, but rarely progresses, being restricted to the splenic red pulp spared by sarcomatous growth and small foci within the hepatic periportal areas where they also occur in J-2 virus-infected mice (Fig. 3C).

Sarcomas induced by either J-1 or J-2 (Fig. 3B) are similar to 3611 MSV-induced sarcomas but are characteristically smaller and spread diffusely through both the red and white pulp. The sarcomas of J-2 virus-inoculated mice which develop sarcomas are comparable in tumor size to age-matched J-1 virus-inoculated mice. These findings suggest that the development of sarcomas induced by v-*raf* in 3611 MSV is not accelerated by the combination with v-*myc* in J-2 virus.

Erythroblastosis is evidenced in J-2-inoculated mice by the uniform population of basophilic erythroblasts and, to a minor extent, more mature erythroid precursors in spleen. Extensive stasis of erythroblasts is observed in the hepatic sinusoids (Fig. 3D), a characteristic of erythroleukemia induced by other MuLV [55]. Usually, the hematocrit is only moderately reduced by the time this lesion has become prominent, indicating a differentiative capacity for these erythroblasts.

Lymphomas occur as uniform enlargements of all lymph nodes and of the splenic periarteriolar sheaths. In nodes, there are fairly uniform sheets of large lymphoid cells characterized by a prominent central nucleus and a thick nuclear membrane (Fig. 3E). These morphological features identify the neoplastic cells as immunoblasts. Within the hepatic parenchyma, foci of immunoblasts are seen (Fig. 3D) and diffuse stasis of these cells is also observed within the alveolar walls of the lung. In advanced cases, immunoblasts are present in peripheral blood in large numbers.

Pancreatic dysplasia is observed as isolated groups of distorted acini formed by very large, palely staining cells containing large vesicular nuclei. Acini surrounding these dysplastic foci are usually unaffected (Fig. 3F). Pancreatic carcinoma caused by the variant J-3 virus is illustrated in Figure 3G and shows extensive dysplasia of the pancreas.

To type the cells that make up the lymphomas, we analyzed J-2 virus-induced tumors by cell sorting and fluorescence assays [42,43] for lineage-specific cell surface markers [40]. Spleens and lymph nodes from neonatally J-2-infected NFS/N mice characteristically contain large populations of blast cells. In spleens, two populations

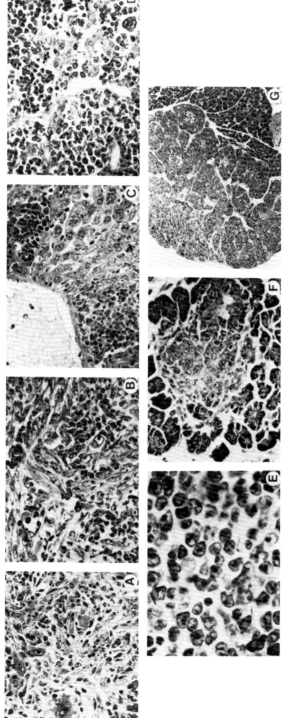

Fig. 3. Lesions of mice inoculated neonatally with J-2, 3611 MSV, or the J-3 variant viruses. Panel A) Sarcomatous lesions in the spleen of a 3611-infected mouse were composed of fusiform cells and irregularly shaped giant cells. These splenic growths were very well vascularized and affected mice sometimes died from hemorrhages due to splenic rupture. Panel B) Sarcomatous lesion in the spleen of a J-2-infected mouse showed a more diffuse type of growth pattern, possibly representative of early stages in the development of this lesion. Erythroblasts, the most prominent feature in spleens of J-2-infected mice, can be seen intermixed with the sarcoma cells. Panel C) A section for the liver of a J-2-infected mouse with a focus of erythroid precursors at the upper right and one of myeloid precursors at the lower left. Panel D) A section from the liver of a J-2-infected mouse showing extensive stasis of erythroblasts within the sinusoids at the upper left and one of immunoblasts at the lower left. Panel E) Immunoblastic lymphoma in the lymph node of a J-2-infected mouse. Panel F) A focus of dysplastic acinar cells in the pancreas of a J-2-infected mouse. Note the presence of mitotic figures and the large vesicular nuclei of the dysplastic cells. Panel G) Adenocarcinoma of the pancreas caused by the J-3 variant showing extensive dysplasia of the pancreas. Modified from previously published figure [40].

of blast cells can be distinguished by their reactivity with antibody to the panlympho-cyte antigen, Ly 5. Ly 5^+ blasts comprise 8–56% of spleen cells whereas the remaining blast cells are Ly 5^-, in contrast to a normal NFS spleen with 95% Ly 5^+ cells. As spleen cells from mice with erythroleukemias induced by other MuLV can be either Ly-5$^-$ or Ly-5$^+$ whereas all lymphomas are Ly-5$^+$ [55,56], the results of these analyses are consistent with the histologic studies which showed a predominance of erythroblasts over immunoblasts in spleens of mice infected with J-2.

Lymph node cells from J-2-infected mice were always > 95% Ly-5$^+$ and contained varying proportions of blast cells (40–95%) and residual normal Ly-5$^+$ lymphocytes; Ly-5$^-$ blasts were never observed. These results support the histologic findings that nodes from mice infected with J-2 contain varying proportions of immunoblasts and normal cells but contain no erythroblasts.

To determine the cellular origins of the Ly 5$^+$ immunoblasts detected in lymphoid tissues of infected mice, the cells were reacted with antibodies to the T-cell antigen Thy-1 and the B-cell lineage antigens sIg and Ly-5(B220). FMF analysis of these populations demonstrated that they are variably composed of T- and B-lineage immunoblasts. Spleen cells from J-2-infected mice also contain mixtures of Thy-1$^+$ and Ly-5(B220)$^+$, sIg$^-$ blast cells. We conclude that J-2 virus induces blast cells in several hematopoietic lineages including Ly-5$^-$ erythroblasts and Ly-5$^+$ immuno-blasts of both T- and B-cell origin.

The combined results of histological and FMF studies of mice infected with J-2 at birth show that they die of immunoblastic lymphomas and fulminating erythroblas-tosis after an average latency of 2 wk. In addition to these advanced neoplasms, all mice had early sarcomas of the spleen (Fig. 3B) and some developed pancreatic acinar dysplasia (Fig. 3F) and frank carcinoma. The rapidity with which the erythro-blastosis and lymphomas develop is unparalleled in studies of other rapidly transform-ing viruses including all of the mammalian single oncogene transducing viruses.

These findings contrast strikingly with the relatively prolonged courses of disease in mice infected with 3611 MSV (6-wk average latency), J-1, J-3, or J-5 virus (> 9 wk latency). Mice inoculated with the first two viruses often died from splenic rupture due to the extensive growth of splenic sarcomas and exhibited numerous sarcomas. The latter animals had no evidence of sarcomas of skeletal and visceral muscles. Mice infected with the J-3 and J-5 constructs rescued with M-MuLV died with T-lineage lymphomas with latency similar to that of the helper virus [40]. However, using several different helper viruses we have recently demonstrated a role for v-*myc* in the development of these lymphomas [Morse et al, submitted].

GROWTH PROPERTIES OF TUMOR-DERIVED CELLS IN CULTURE

Earlier studies have demonstrated that hematopoietic cells from tumors of mice infected as newborns with 3611 MSV and expressing *gag-raf* fusion proteins require interleukin 3 (IL 3) for maintenance of growth in culture (Table II) [Rapp and Ihle, unpublished data, 37,40]. Similarly, infection of fetal liver and bone marrow cells with 3611 MSV in vitro yields permanently growing cultures which retain their dependence on IL 3 [37,40,41]. In contrast to growth requirements of hematopoietic cells from tumors induced by v-*raf*-transducing virus (and v-H-*ras*-transducing virus), cells transformed in vivo by virus carrying both v-*raf* and v-*myc* oncogenes grow independent of IL 3 or any other lymphokine supplement (Table II). In parallel to the

TABLE II. Frequency of Establishing Long-Term Lines[*]

Virus	Oncogene	In vivo primary tumors		In vitro HPT cultures	
		+IL 3	−IL 3	+IL 3	−IL 3
None	—	0/10	0/10	0/3	0/3
3611	*raf*	10/10	0/10	3/3	0/3
HaSV	*ras*	3/3	0/3	10/10	0/10
J-2	*raf/mil* + *myc*	10/10	10/10	2/2	2/2

[*]For tumor induction, newborn NSF/N mice were inoculated with 3611 MSV, Harvey SV, and J-2 virus as described previously [37]. Infection of hematopoietic tissue cells (HPT) in culture included fetal liver (3611 MSV, Harvey SV, and J-2) and bone marrow (3611 MSV, J-2). Culture medium was supplemented with IL 3 at 20 μm/ml. IL, interleukin.

synergistic action of *raf* and *myc* in vivo, we have recently demonstrated that co-expression of these two oncogenes induces the selective proliferation of murine bone marrow cells [84] and fetal liver cells [Cleveland, Rapp, Ihle, and Weinstein, in preparation] in the absence of specific growth factor (GF) supplements. Interestingly, in parallel to our results in vivo, in vitro infections of fetal liver cultures with J-2 have given rise to several different lineages of GF-independent, immortalized cells including pre-B cells, mast cells, and myeloid stem cells. In contrast, cells infected with *raf*- or *myc*-only virus did not transform hematopoietic cells in the absence of GF. The high plating efficiency of J-2 tumor-derived hematopoietic cells in regular medium in culture made it possible to use standard radiolabeling techniques for detection of v-*raf*- and v-*myc*-specific protein (see below).

EXPRESSION OF V-*RAF*- AND V-*MYC*-SPECIFIC PRODUCTS IN CELLS TRANSFORMED IN VIVO AND IN VITRO

Expression of the v-*raf* or v-*raf/mil* hybrid oncogene could readily be distinguished from expression of its cellular counterpart because of its linkage to viral *gag* protein. In the case of v-*myc*, expression of the viral oncogene protein was more difficult to establish in tumor cells because of the similarity in size and antigenicity of viral and cellular *myc* protein. We therefore determined the presence of virus-specific RNA as well as the expression of viral oncogene proteins in infected cells.

RNAs from infected fibroblasts and from cell cultures of J-2 virus-induced mouse tumors were analyzed by Northern blot hybridization [40]. RNAs from J-2 virus-transformed fibroblasts and cell cultures derived from J-2 virus-induced tumors hybridized with U3-LTR and *env* probes revealed a genomic species of 7.6 kb and a subgenomic RNA of 5.6 kb. No 3.0-kb *env* subgenomic RNA was detectable. Presumably insertion of additional v-*myc* sequences into this construct abrogates normal splicing of this RNA. These RNAs also hybridized with the v-*myc* and *raf* cDNA probes [40]. Interestingly, hybridization of Northern blots of J-2 virus-infected fibroblast or tumor cells with a c-*myc* probe does not show detectable levels of c-*myc* RNA. In contrast, blots from control fibroblast and 3611 MSV-infected fibroblast cells show readily detectable levels of c-*myc* transcripts [unpublished data].

The translation of v-*raf*- and v-*myc*-specific RNA into v-*raf*- and v-*myc*-specific proteins in infected fibroblast cell lines was established by immunoprecipitations of labeled cell lysates with antibodies directed against MuLV p30, v-*raf*, and v-*myc* (Fig. 4). The first three lanes of Figure 4, panel A, show the *gag-raf* fusion proteins

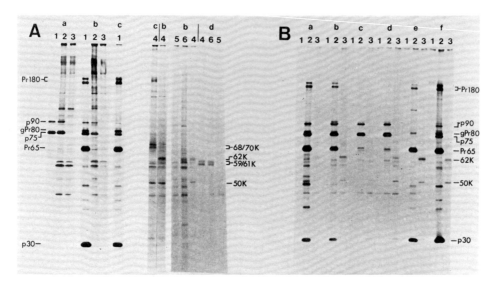

Fig. 4. SDS-PAGE analysis of *gag*-, *raf/mil*-, and *myc*-related proteins in cells transformed in vitro and in vivo by J-2 construct virus. Boiled SDS lysates of cells labeled with ^{35}S-methionine were prepared [51,52] and immunoprecipitation was performed by using aliquots of lysates containing identical amounts of radioactivity [30]. A) Comparison of proteins precipitated from the following cell lines: (a) 3611B3, (b) NIH/J-2 (M-MuLV), (c) NIH/J-1 (M-MuLV), (d) MH2-A103NP. Precipitation was done with the following antisera: lanes 1) anti-p30*gag*, lanes 2) anti-*raf*(SP63), lanes 3) anti-*raf*(SP63) preadsorbed to SP63 peptide, lanes 4) anti-*myc* [53], lanes 5) anti-*myc*C (IgG) preadsorbed to *myc*C peptide, lanes 6) anti-*myc*C (IgG) without peptide block. Fluorographs were exposed for 3–10 days. The positions of the *gag-raf/mil* products p75 and p90, and those of the helper-virus-encoded proteins Pr180 *gag-pol*, gPr80*gag*, and Pr65*gag* are indicated to the left. Proteins precipitated by anti-*myc* sera are indicated in kilodaltons to the right. B) Analysis of proteins from cells derived from mouse tumors induced by J-2. Precipitation was performed with normal goat serum (lanes 1), goat-anti-p30*gag* (lanes 2), and anti-*myc* (lanes 3) from the following tumor cell lines: (a) spleen A, (b) spleen C, (c) spleen D, (d) thymus C, (e) submaxillary lymph node A, (f) NIH/J-2 (M-MuLV). The exposure time of the fluorograph was 5 days. Reproduced from previously published figure [40].

p75 and p90 in fibroblasts transformed by 3611 MSV. These proteins are also expressed in fibroblasts transformed with J-2 and J-1 viruses carrying the *raf/mil* hybrid gene (panel A, lanes b 1–3 and lane c 1, respectively). These lanes also show additional virus structural proteins precipitated by anti-p30 as expected for helper-virus-producing cells. Expression of v-*myc* was determined by immunoprecipitation with two different anti-*myc* sera, a synthetic peptide serum [51] and a serum raised against *myc* protein produced in *Escherichia coli* [53]. v-*myc*-specific bands corresponding to a 62K protein were detected only in J-2 virus-transformed cells (panel A, lanes b 4–6). The 62-kD protein is considered to be the product of v-*myc* since (1) it is detected by both sera, (2) precipitation with v-*myc* peptide serum was competed by synthetic peptide, and (3) its presence was restricted to J-2 virus-infected cells. The v-*myc*-specific proteins in MH2-transformed chicken cells are slightly smaller at 59/61K (panel A, d 4–6).

Cells from tumors induced by J-2 virus all express p75/90 v-*raf/mil*-specific proteins [38,39] with the exception of cells from submaxillary lymph node (panel B, lane e 2). In agreement with this observation, we found by infectious center assays that only 0.04% of these cells released focus-forming virus, as compared to 60% for spleen A (lane a), 20% for spleen C (lane b), 100% for thymus C (lane d), and 100% for spleen D (lane C). Spleen D and thymus C show the lowest levels of helper-virus-specific proteins. Variable levels of a 62K *myc* protein band were detected in all the tumors presented in Figure 4B. We conclude that v-*raf* and v-*myc* are expressed in J-2 virus-infected fibroblast lines and the majority of J-2-induced tumors.

MECHANISMS OF *RAF* AND *MYC* SYNERGISM: ROLE OF *MYC* IN ABROGATING SPECIFIC GROWTH FACTOR REQUIREMENTS

The majority of neoplasms caused by the dual oncogene virus J-2 were of hematopoietic/lymphoid lineage. To assess the contribution of *raf* and *myc* in these neoplasms, we examined the effects of these recombinant retroviruses on two growth-factor-dependent lymphoid and hematopoietic cell lines requiring either interleukin 2 (IL 2) or interleukin 3 (IL 3) for viability.

IL 2 is required for the proliferation of antigen-activated mature T cells [reviewed in 58] while IL 3 induces the proliferation and differentiation of early hematopoietic/lymphoid stem cells [reviewed in 59,60]. A number of IL 2-dependent cytotoxic T cell lines have been established. Although the frequency of establishing lines suggests that an immortalizing event is required [61], once established, the cell lines continue to depend on IL 2 for growth. For our experiments we used an SV 40-specific, H-2Kb-restricted, cytotoxic T cell line (CTB6) from C57BL/6J mice [36] (provided by Dr. Barbara Knowles, Wistar Institute, Philadelphia, Pennsylvania).

IL 3-dependent cell lines have been isolated from primary retrovirus-induced lymphomas [54,62] and from long-term bone marrow cultures [63,64]. As above, the frequencies for establishing lines suggest that an immortalizing event may be required. For our studies we used the FDC-P1 cell line, which has properties of early myeloid lineage cells [63,65]. These cells differ from normal IL 3-responsive cells in their limited capacity to differentiate, but have a normal diploid karyotype.

To evaluate the effects of v-*myc* expression, we used the constructs shown in Figure 1 and, in addition, another recombinant (HF) containing the complete MC29 v-*myc* cloned into the *gag* gene of Moloney leukemia virus [85]. In the absence of IL 3, FDC-P1 cells rapidly lose viability and factor-independent variants have not been obtained [63,65,66]. However, when the cells which had been exposed to the J-2 virus were cultured in the absence of IL 3, factor-independent cells were obtained. Factor-independent cell lines were not obtained with FDC-P1 cells alone, with cells exposed to 3611 MSV [*raf*, 37,41], HaSV [H-*ras*, 37], FBR [*fos*, unpublished data] (see Table III), or to helper virus (data not shown). When the factor-independent cells were assayed, transforming virus was detectable. Similarly when CTB6 cells were exposed to the J-2 or HF viruses and cultured in the absence of IL 2, factor-independent cell lines were obtained which replicated transforming virus. To evaluate the contribution of the v-*raf*/v-*mil* oncogene, FDC-P1 cells were exposed to the J-3 virus or the HF virus. In both cases, factor-independent FDC-P1 cell lines were obtained when cells were cultured in the absence of IL 3.

To characterize the cells, we examined representative lines for the expression of the v-*raf*/*mil* and/or v-*myc* oncogenes by Northern blot analysis (Fig. 8). In uninfected NIH 3T3, FDC-P1, or CTB6 cells there are no detectable v-*myc* hybridizing RNAs (Fig. 5A), whereas there was a 3.1-kb RNA detected with the *raf* probe

TABLE III. Isolation of Factor Independent Lines*

Virus	Oncogene	CTB6 (T)		FDPC-1 (myeloid)	
		+IL 2	−IL 2	+IL 3	−IL 3
None	−	+	−	+	−
3611	raf	+	−	+	−
HaSV	ras	NT	NT	+	−
J-2	raf + myc	+	+	+	+
J-3	myc	+	+	+	+
HF(J-5)	myc	+	+	+	+
FBR	fos	+	−	+	−

*The indicated cell lines were infected with the various viruses in the presence of polybrene (25 μM) in IL 3 (FDC-Pl cells [35]) or IL 2 (CTB6 cells [36]). Following infection, the FDC-Pl or CTB6 cells were maintained in media supplemented with IL 3 or IL 2 [37] for 4 days and cultured in media with or without factors for 4 wk. During this period the majority of the cells died out and factor-independent cells emerged. NT, not tested.

(Fig. 5B). This RNA has the expected size of the endogenous c-raf-1 gene mRNA and was observed at comparable levels in all infected cell lines. The 7.6- and 7.4-kb genomic RNAs of the J-2 and J-3 viruses, respectively, were readily detectable using v-myc and raf probes in infected NIH 3T3 cells, in FDC-P1 cells infected with the J-2 or J-3 viruses, or CTB6 cells infected with the J-2 virus. With the v-myc probe, major subgenomic RNAs of 6.3 and 6.1 kb for the J-2 and J-3 viruses, respectively, were also observed. In FDC-P1 cells infected with the HF virus there was a major 6.4-kb RNA which hybridized with the v-myc probe but not with the raf probe, consistent with the structure of the viral genome. In addition, there was a major subgenomic RNA of 5.1 kb whose origin is not known. Similar anomalous transcripts have been observed with other recombinant retroviruses [67].

The Northern blot data suggested differences in the levels of viral RNA. To quantitatively evaluate differences, dot blot analysis was done. As shown in Figure 5C, FDC-P1 cells infected with either the J-2 or J-3 virus had approximately a ten-fold higher level of v-myc hybridizing RNA than that observed with fibroblasts. In CTB6 cells infected with the J-2 virus, there was approximately a 100-fold higher level of RNA. The basis for these differences is not known although Southern blot analysis suggests that it is not due to multiple integrated proviruses (data not shown) and therefore may be due to lineage-specific effects on the enhancer sequences of the virus [68].

We also examined the cell lines for expression of the v-myc and v-raf/mil proteins. By immunoprecipitation all the lines examined expressed the v-myc protein of 62 kD comparable to that seen in infected fibroblasts and at levels similar to that of c-myc in FDC-P1 cells grown in the presence of IL 3 (data not shown). Because of the cross reactivity of the anti-myc sera with mouse c-myc protein and the similarity in the sizes in c-myc and v-myc proteins [69,70], the identification of myc protein as viral relies on the observation that none of the infected lines contains c-myc RNA (see below). With either FDC-P1 or CTB6 cells infected with the J-2 virus the expected gag-(v-raf/mil) fusion protein of 75 kD [38] was detectable by immunoprecipitation (data not shown).

To evaluate the factor dependence, ^{3}H-thymidine incorporation assays were used. As shown in Figure 6A, parental FDC-P1 cells required approximately 0.2 ng/ml of IL 3 for half-maximal activity. In contrast, J-2, J-3, or the HF virus-infected

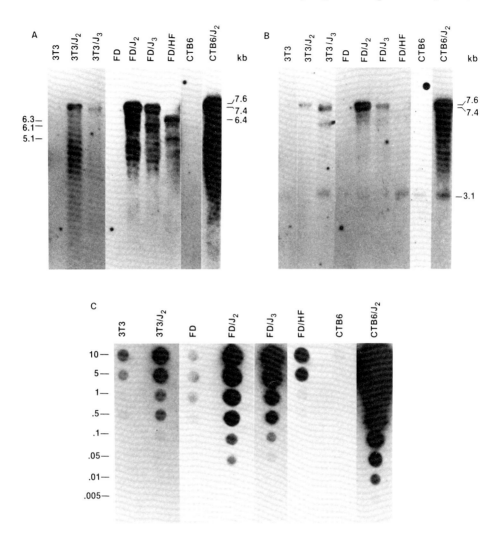

Fig. 5. Northern analysis of recombinant retroviruses in factor-independent cell lines. Polysome-associated RNA was prepared as described [45] and poly A RNA was selected by two cycles of oligodeoxythymidilic cellulose chromatography. The RNA (10 μg) was denatured by glyoxalation [46], separated electrophoretically in 1.2% agarose, blotted onto nitrocellulose (Schleicher & Schuell), and hybridized under stringent conditions [44] with ^{32}P-labeled nick-translated [47] DNA probes. A) V-*myc* hybridizations. For a v-*myc* probe, the 1.4-kbp PstI/AhaIII fragment (Oncor, Incorporated, Gaithersburg, MD) of the MC29 provirus was used [48,49]. The intensity of hybridization between the various samples varies considerably; lanes 1–3 and 8 were exposed for 3 days whereas lanes 4–7 and lane 9 were exposed for 20 hr. Recombinant retroviral genome-sized RNAs are indicated at the right; subgenomic RNAs are indicated in the left margin. Sizes are given in kilobases and were determined from ^{32}P-labeled, denatured Hind III fragments of bacteriophage lambda DNA. B) *Raf* hybridizations. The blot shown in (A) was stripped [44] and hybridized as above with 2.9-kbp human *raf* cDNA probe [Bonner et al, in press]. The exposure of all the samples was 3 days. The 3.1-kb transcript is the endogenous *raf* mRNA. C) Quantitative analysis of v-*myc* RNA levels in factor-independent cell lines. Poly A RNA, isolated from the indicated cell lines, was denatured by treatment with formamide/formaldehyde [44] and loaded onto wells of a dot blot apparatus (Schleicher & Schuell). The amount of poly A RNA (μg) in each well is indicated at the left margin. Hybridizations were done with the v-*myc* probe as in (A) and blots were exposed for 20 hr.

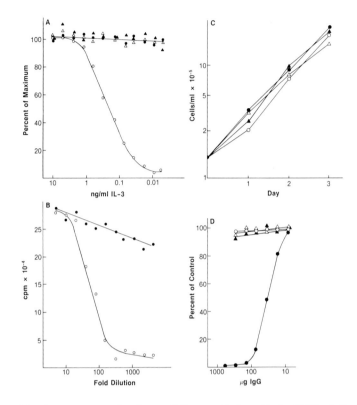

Fig. 6. Proliferative responses of various cell lines to IL 3 or IL 2. A) The indicated cells were obtained from exponentially growing cultures and were pelleted and resuspended twice in RPMI-1640 containing 10% FCS. In 96-well microtiter plates appropriate dilutions of purified IL 3 were made in wells containing 0.05 ml of RPMI-1640 with 10% FCS to which 0.05 cells (10^5) were added. The cells were incubated for 24 hr at 37°C after which 1 μCi of ^{3}H-thymidine was added per well and the cells were incubated for an additional 6 hr at 37°C. The cells were harvested with an automated cell harvester. IL 3 was purified to apparent biochemical homogeneity as previously described [82]. The results are plotted as the percentage of maximal ^{3}H-thymidine incorporation seen in the presence of excess IL 3. The cell lines examined included the parental FDC-P1 cells (○—○) and FDC-P1 cells infected with the J-2 (●—●), J-3 (△—△), or HF (▲—▲) viruses. B) The experiments were as in (A) except that the cells were incubated for 48 hr prior to pulsing with ^{3}H-thymidine. The IL 2 was partially purified from conditioned media from PMA-induced EL-4 cells as previously described [83]. The cells examined included the parental CTB6 cells (○—○) and CTB6 cells infected with the J-2 virus (●—●). C) Growth curves for control and infected FDC-P1 cells. The growth curves were obtained by seeding the cells at 5×10^5 cells/ml in RPMI-1640 containing 10% FCS in the presence or absence of IL 3. Viable cell numbers were determined at the indicated times. The cells examined included the parental FDC-P1 cells (○—○) which were grown in the presence of IL 3 (20 units/ml) or J-2 (●—●), J-3 (△—△) or HF (▲—▲) infected FDC-P1 cells which were grown in the absence of IL 3. D) Lack of inhibition of growth by antisera against IL 3. The indicated cells were obtained from exponentially growing cultures and were pelleted and resuspended twice in RPMI-1640 containing 10% FCS. In 96-well microtiter plates, twofold dilutions of immune or control protein A Sepharose-purified IgG were made in 0.05 ml of RPMI-1640 containing 10% FCS. For the parental FDC-P1 cells 0.01 ml of IL 3 (2 units) was added to each well. The samples were incubated for 2 hr at 37°C and the cells (10^5) in 0.05 ml were added. The cells were incubated for 24 hr at 37°C and pulsed with ^{3}H-thymidine as in Figure 4. The cell line examined included the parental FDC-P1 cells (○—○) and J-2 (●—●), J-3 (△—△) and HF (▲—▲) infected FDC-P1 cells. The preparation and characteristics of the immune IgG have been previously described [71].

cells showed no dependency on IL 3. Similarly the J-2-infected CTB6 cells showed a vastly decreased requirement for IL 2 (Fig. 6B). As shown in Figure 6C, the growth curves and the doubling times were comparable for each of the virus-infected FDC-P1 cell lines in the absence of IL 3 and for the parental cell line grown in the presence of IL 3.

One mechanism for the abrogation of factor dependence is the production of a requisite growth factor. However, with none of the infected cell lines did we detect mitogenic activity for the parental cell lines in conditioned media (data not shown). In the assay for IL 3, the lack of detectable activity indicates concentrations of less than approximately 0.02 ng/ml. Another approach was to examine the effect of an antiserum [71] against IL 3. As shown in Figure 6D, the immune IgG inhibited the IL 3-dependent proliferation of the parental FDC-P1 cells but had no effect on J-2, J-3, or HF virus-infected cells. In agreement with these results, Northern hybridization with IL 3 cDNA as probe demonstrated that none of the FDC-P1 factor-independent cell lines produced IL 3 mRNA (data not shown).

The absence of a requirement for IL 3 suggests that the expression of IL 3 receptors might be altered. To evaluate this, the ability to bind ^{125}I-labeled IL 3 was determined. The FDC-P1 cells infected with the J-2, J-3, or the HF virus bound iodinated IL 3 at levels comparable to the uninfected parental cells (data not shown).

The retention of receptors for IL 3 raised the question of whether IL 3 could alter the expression of c-*myc*. This was of interest since the rapid loss of viability in the absence of IL 3 has not allowed a direct analysis of IL 3-induced expression of c-*myc*. As shown in Figure 7A, c-*myc* RNA was detectable in the parental FDC-P1 cells grown in IL 3. However, no c-*myc* was detectable in the virus-infected cell lines grown in the presence or absence of IL 3. To determine whether the absence of c-*myc* RNA was due to low levels under steady-state conditions, cells were examined at various times after exposure to IL 3. As shown in Figure 7B, no c-*myc* RNA was detected at 30 min, 2 hr, or 72 hr in culture. To determine whether the absence of c-*myc* RNA was a general property of cells infected with the recombinant viruses, we examined the cloned, producer-fibroblast cell lines. As shown in Figure 7C, c-*myc* RNA was readily detectable in the control fibroblasts but was not detected in the infected cells.

To determine whether the abrogation of a requirement for IL 3 affected tumorigenicity, the J-3- and HF-infected cells were tested for tumor formation in *nu/nu* mice, since neither of these viruses induces tumors over the time period examined [40]. As shown in Table IV, the parental FDC-P1 cells were not tumorigenic as previously described [35]. In contrast, FDC-P1 cells infected with the J-3 or the HF virus did induce tumors.

The ability of v-*myc* expression to abrogate the requirements for IL 3 or IL 2 supports the hypothesis that these growth factors regulate *myc* expression. This is consistent with the observation that IL 2 can be shown to increase c-*myc* transcription in normal, lymphoid cells [K. Kelly, personal communication]. Thus it appears that c-*myc* acts as a central relay for the transmission of signals from several distinct (competence-inducing) growth factors including PDGF, IL 3, and IL 2. Consistent with our speculation on the induction of autonomous growth by a combination of progression (v-*raf*)- and competence (v-*myc*)-inducing factors is our finding that lymphoid cells from J-2 virus-induced tumors could be readily grown in culture without addition of specific lymphokines.

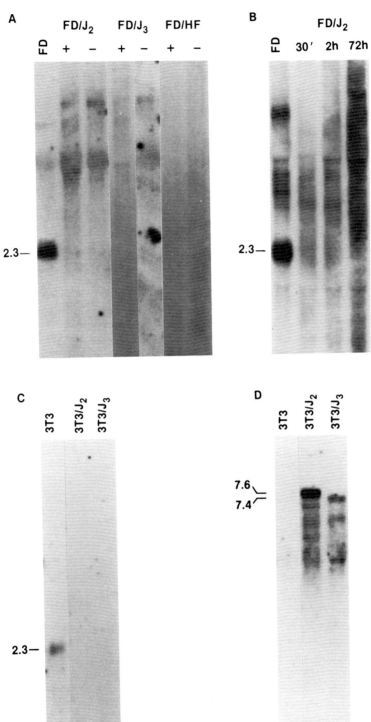

Fig. 7

It was surprising that we were unable to induce c-*myc* expression in the infected FDC-P1 cells with IL 3 even though these cells retained receptors for this ligand. The absence of c-*myc* in these cells seems likely due to a regulatory effect of v-*myc* on c-*myc* expression as suggested by the observation that infected fibroblasts, J-2-transformed pre-B cells, and myeloid cells from fetal liver (data not shown) also have no detectable c-*myc* RNA. The specific suppression of c-*myc* expression is suggested by the lack of comparable effect on c-*raf* (and c-*abl* and c-*myb*, not shown) expression. The inability to induce c-*myc* expression is not due to alteration of the endogenous loci as determined by Southern blot analysis of EcoRI-restricted DNAs (data not shown). The ability of an activated c-*myc* locus to negatively regulate the normal allele has been suggested by other studies [75–77]. The mechanisms for this effect are not known but may involve the interaction of the *myc* protein or a *myc*-induced protein with potential regulatory sequences defined by sensitivity to DNAase I [77]. Experiments are currently in progress to assess the DNAase I sensitivity of these sites in the c-*myc* loci of infected FDC-P1, CTB6, and NIH 3T3 cells.

Recent studies have demonstrated that tumorigenesis requires multiple events. In hematopoietic tumors such as myeloid tumors, stages of tumor progression have been described [78,79]. For example, murine myelogenous leukemias appear blocked in differentiation but often require IL 3 for growth in vitro [54,62] and some HTLV-1-induced cutaneous T cell lymphomas require IL 2 for growth [80,81]. In these cases, the activation of c-*myc* can be envisioned as one potential mechanism for the progression to a factor-independent phenotype. This type of role for c-*myc* activation may also occur in other lineages including B-cells in which there is a high incidence of altered c-*myc* expression associated with transformation.

TABLE IV. Tumorigenicity of Recombinant Retrovirus Infected FDC-Pl Cells in NU/NU Mice*

Cell line	Tumors/total	Average latency (days)
FDC-Pl	0/5	>60
FDC-Pl (J-3)	5/5	28
FDC-Pl (HF)	5/5	30

*Nu/nu BALB/c mice of 4–6 wk of age were inoculated intraperitonealy with 2×10^6 cells. Morbid mice were killed and examined microscopically for evidence of tumors.

Fig. 7. A) C-*myc* expression in FDC-P1 lines in the presence (+) and absence (−) of IL 3. Total RNA was prepared and polyA-containing RNA was selected by oligo d[T] cellulose chromatography. The RNA (15 μg) was denatured, electrophoresed, blotted, and hybridized as in Figure 2. The c-*myc* probe was the 5.6-kbp BamHI fragment of the mouse genomic c-*myc* [75]. B) Time course examining c-*myc* expression. Total RNA was prepared from FDC-Pl (J-2) cells at the indicated times after the addition of IL 3 and polyA RNA was analyzed as above. The autoradiographs were overexposed to detect c-*myc* transcripts. C,D) *Myc* expression in NIH/3T3 lines. PolyA RNA (15 μg) was prepared from the indicated cell lines and analyzed by Northern blot hybridization. C-*myc* hybridization is shown in C in which exposure of the autoradiographs was for 1 wk. V-*myc* hybridization is shown in D and the exposure of the autoradiograph was for 3 days.

CONTRIBUTIONS OF *RAF* TO SYNERGISM

The role of *raf* in the synergy between *myc* and *raf* has been more difficult to define. The properties of the *raf* oncogene group, a multigene family, are summarized in Table V. The viral oncogene v-*raf* was originally isolated by our group from mouse cells by retrovirus transduction [38,39] into the defective virus 3611 MSV. Subsequently, we have identified the putative oncogene v-*mil*, of the avian carcinoma virus MH$_2$, as being homologous to v-*raf* [32]. The normal c-*raf*-1 polypeptide has a MW of 74 kD (Fig. 8E,F) and is a phosphoprotein (Fig. 8C,D) with associated in vitro autophophorylating protein kinase activity (Fig. 8A,B).

The function of the cellular homolog of v-*raf*, c-*raf*-1, in this synergism is unknown although we do know c-*raf*-1 is a cytosolic protein and we have detected Ser/Thr-specific protein kinase activity for the transforming versions of c-*raf*-1 [72]. All of the transforming forms of c-*raf*-1, ie, v-*raf* containing 37 kD of *raf*, v-*mil* containing 40 kD of *raf*, and an LTR-activated version of c-*raf*-1 containing 50 kD of

TABLE V. The *Raf* Oncogene Family

A: Genes homologous to v-*raf*	
Transduced as the transforming gene, v-*raf*, of 3611 MSV	Isolated from a mouse with lung and peritoneal tumors induces fibrosarcoma/histiocy toma in newborn mice
Avian homolog of v-*raf* (v-*mil*) is part of MH2	An avian carcinoma virus which also contains v-*myc*
Member of the *src* family	Has associated *ser/thr* specific protein kinase activity
Two genes in man, an active gene c-*raf*-1 and a pseudogene c-*raf*-2	The active gene maps on chromosome 3 at p25; site is specifically altered in small cell lung carcinoma, ovarian carcinoma, familial renal carcinoma, and mixed salivary gland tumors
Active gene has 17 exons	11 exons homologous to v-*mil* and 9 exons to v-*raf*; 5 additional coding exons at 5' end spread over another 15 kb
	A 3.4-kb mRNA in human lymphocytes, fetal liver, and placenta is colinear with v-*raf*
One of the gene products is 74 kD	Liver and placental mRNAs code for a 648AA protein which contains no transmembrane region
The 74 kD c-*raf*-1 protein from NIH 3T3 is phosphorylated in *ser/thr*	

B: Genes related to v-*raf*	
There are at least two different active *raf*-related genes which are closely related to each other	These are designated δ-*raf*-1 and δ-*raf*-2 and are distinguishable by in situ hybridization to human metaphase chromosomes
δ-*raf*-1	δ-*raf* is located on mouse and human chromosome X, in man at Xp12
Isolated from spleen cDNA library using v-*raf*	
Expression is tissue specific	Is transcribed as a 2.4 kb mRNA
Homology between δ-*raf* and c-*raf*-1 is 69% for DNA and 74% for amino acid sequences	Homology is highest in the kinase domain
δ-*raf* recombinant retrovirus transforms NIH 3T3 cells	Induces sarcomas in newborn NFS/N mice
δ-*raf*-2	Located on human chromosome 7 near the centromere

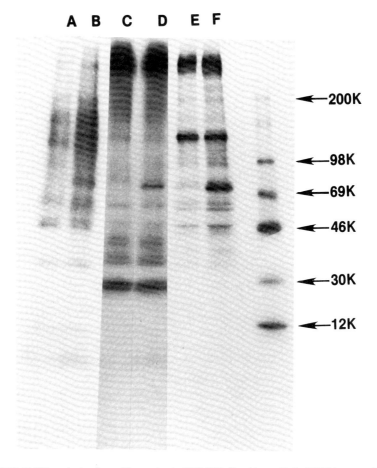

Fig. 8.   SDS-PAGE analysis of c-*raf*-1 proteins in NIH/3T3 fibroblasts. Boiled SDS lysates of unlabeled cells (A,B) and of cells labeled with ^{35}S-orthophosphate (C,D) or with ^{35}S-methionine (E,F) were prepared and immunoprecipitation carried out as previously described [38]. In vitro kinase assay of immunoprecipitated c-*raf*-1 (A,B) was performed as published [38]. Precipitation was done with anti-c-*raf*-1 (SP63) antisera with (A,C,E) or without (B,D,F) peptide block. The exposure time of the fluorograph was 2 days.

raf, are truncated at their amino terminus. Therefore, the truncated portion of the c-*raf* protein may correspond to a binding site for a regulatory ligand which may normally activate the protein.

Whatever its exact function in the cell it is clear that transforming versions of c-*raf*-1 can immortalize hematopoietic cells without affecting specific growth factor requirements (see Table II) and that, in addition to transforming NIH/3T3 fibroblasts, v-*raf* is capable of morphologically transforming primary rat and human embryo fibroblasts [25]. Furthermore, v-*raf*-transformed fibroblasts share with cells transformed by other acute transforming retroviruses the loss of EGF binding activity and the release of transforming growth factor (TGF) α and TGFβ into the culture medium [unpublished data]. Moreover, secretion of TGFs can be demonstrated without concentration of culture fluid by seeding a single transformed nonproducer cell together with 10^5 untransformed FRE rat fibroblasts cells into soft agar where recruitment of soft agar growth can be observed in the vicinity of the large colony of virus-transformed cells (Fig. 9). These data suggest that *raf* affects different components of growth regulation than those affected by *myc*.

CONCLUSIONS

We have shown here that combination of the oncogenes v-*raf* and v-*myc* in a murine retrovirus accelerates tumor induction relative to v-*raf*- or v-*myc*-transducing viruses by a factor greater than three. The spectrum of cell types that make up the tumor mass is shifted from the predominantly fibroblastic and erythroid populations observed in v-*raf*-induced tumors to erythroblasts and lymphoid cells of T and B lineages. In addition to the lymphomas and erythroblastosis which generally are the cause of deaths of inoculated mice, fibrosarcomas and pancreatic dysplasia also develop. However, carcinoma of the ovary, which appears to be typical of the avian retrovirus MH2 [33,34] containing the avian homolog of v-*raf* in addition to v-*myc*, have not been observed. Using a J-3 variant, however, we have observed carcinomas of the liver, lung, and pancreas [unpublished results]. This is the first molecular analysis of a mammalian carcinoma virus. Lymphoid/hematopoietic cells from tumors produced by the dual-oncogene-containing virus J-2 grow in regular culture medium whereas cells from tumors induced by v-*raf* alone require IL 3 for growth. In contrast to the complementation observed between oncogenes for transformation of primary fibroblasts in vitro [24,25], synergism between v-*raf* and v-*myc* in vivo appears to exclude fibroblasts and be restricted to cells of the hematopoietic system and endodermal epithelium. This synergy in hematopoietic cells was also evident in vitro where immortalization of GF-independent lines derived from fetal liver or bone marrow required expression of both oncogenes.

What may be the basis for the synergism between *raf* and *myc*? A dissection of factors involved in the growth regulation of BALB/3T3 fibroblast cells [78,79] has led to the identification of two categories of signals, competence signals (acting early in G1 phase) and progression signals (which act later on G1 phase of the cell cycle), both of which are required for cell population to proceed. Analogous combinations of factors may be required for growth regulation of hematopoietic cells as well. In the fibroblast system, progression factors include epidermal growth factor (EGF) and presumably also transforming growth factor α (TGFα), which acts through the same receptor [11]. Fibroblast cells transformed by v-*raf* share with cells transformed by v-*mos*, v-*fes*, v-*abl*, and v-*ras* the loss of EGF binding activity and the induction of growth factor secretion including TGF α [9,10]. We therefore suggest that v-*raf*, directly or indirectly, provides progression signals to these cells. Interestingly, constitutive expression of the EGF-specific progression signal is associated with development of erythroleukemia in birds infected with the v-*erb*B-transducing virus AEV [6] and may therefore be the basis for the erythroid hyperplasia induced by 3611 MSV. Does v-*raf* also provide competence signals? A hallmark of the competence-inducing factor PDGF is its ability to induce transient transcription of the cellular protooncogenes *myc* [5] and *fos* [20] but not *raf* or *ras*. Moreover, *myc* can partially substitute for PDGF [16] and thus may act as a central transmitter of its competence signal. Transformation of fibroblast cells with v-*raf* is not generally associated with increased expression of *myc* [Rapp, unpublished]. It is therefore tempting to speculate that the

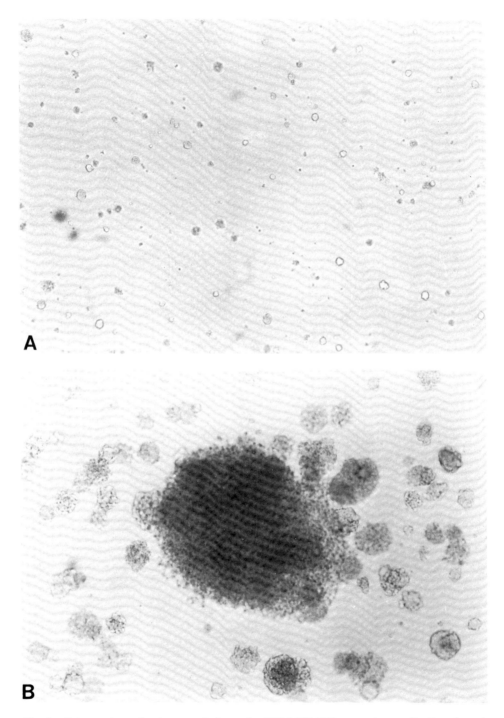

Fig. 9. Release of transforming growth factors by 3611 MSV FRE nonproducer cells. Transformed nonproducer cells were mixed (panel B) with untransformed FRE cells at a ratio of $1/10^5$. Cells were suspended in 0.3% noble agar in DMEM substituted with 10% FCS and seeded on top of 5 ml 0.5% agar base in 60-mm petri dishes. Colonies were scored after 10 days. Growth of untransformed FRE cells is shown in panel A.

basis for the observed synergism between v-*raf* and v-*myc* is the combination of signals for progression and competence. However, the competence factor PDGF is presumably not important for growth regulation of lymphoid cells. Since we have demonstrated that infection of interleukin 3- or interleukin 2-dependent lymphoid cells [85] with v-*myc* recombinant retroviruses abrogates both growth factor requirements, these factors may be the functional equivalent of PDGF in hematopoietic and lymphoid cell lineages.

ACKNOWLEDGMENTS

This research was sponsored by the National Cancer Institute, DHHS, under contract No. NO1-CO-23909 with Litton Bionetics, Inc. The contents of this publication do not necessarily reflect the views or policies of the Department of Health and Human Services, nor does mention of trade names, commercial products, or organizations imply endorsement by the U.S. Government.

REFERENCES

1. Der CJ, Krontins TG, Cooper GM: Proc Natl Acad Sci USA 79:3637, 1979.
2. Reddy EP, Reynolds RK, Santos E, Barbacid M: Nature 300:149, 1982.
3. Taub R, Kirsch I, Morton C, Wendir G, Swan D, Tronick S, Aaronson S, Leder P: Proc Natl Acad Sci USA 79:7837, 1982.
4. Taparowsky E, Suarad Y, Fasano O, Shimizu K, Goldfarb M, Wigler M: Nature 300:762, 1982.
5. Kelly K, Cochran BH, Stiles CD, Leder P: Cell 35:603, 1983.
6. Bishop JM: Ann Rev Biochem 52:301, 1983.
7. Temin HM: In "Growth Regulating Substances for Animal Cells in Culture," The Wistar Symposium Monograph No. 7:103, 1967.
8. Temin HM: J Cell Physiol 75:107, 1970.
9. De Larco JE, Todaro GJ: Proc Natl Acad Sci USA 75:4001, 1978.
10. Todaro GJ, De Larco JE, Marquardt H, Bryant ML, Sherwin SA, Sliski AH: In Sato GH, Ross R (eds): "Hormones and Cell Culture, Book A, Cold Spring Harbor Conferences on Cell Proliferation, 6, New York: Cold Spring Harbor, 1979, pp 113–127.
11. Marquardt H, Hunkapiller MW, Hood LE, Twardzik DR, De Larco JE, Stephenson JR, Todaro GJ: Proc Natl Acad Sci USA 80:4684, 1983.
12. Downward J, Yarden Y, Mayes E, Scrace G, Totty N, Stockwell P, Ullrich A, Schlessinger J, Waterfield MD: Nature 207:521, 1984.
13. Waterfield MD, Scrace T, Whittle N, Stroobant P, Johnsson A, Wasteson A, Westermark B, Heldin C-H, Huang JS, Deuel TF: Nature 304:35, 1983.
14. Doolittle RF, Hunkapiller MW, Good LE, Devare SG, Robbins KC, Aaronson SA, Antoniades HN: Science 221:275, 1983.
15. Johnsson A, Heldin CH, Wasteson A, Westermark B, Deuel TF, Huang JS, Seeburg DH, Gray E, Ullrich A, Scrace G, Stroobant P, Waterfield MD: Embo J 3:921, 1984.
16. Sherr CJ, Rettenmier CW, Sacca R, Roussel MF, Look AT, Stanley ER: Cell 41:665, 1985.
17. Armelin HA, Armelin CS, Kelly K, Stewart T, Leder P, Cochran BH, Stiles CD: Nature 310:655, 1984.
18. Muller R, Bravo R, Burckhardt J: Nature 312:20, 1984.
19. Greenberg ME, Ziff EB: Nature 311:433, 1984.
20. Kruijer W, Cooper J, Hunter T, Verma IM: Nature 312:711, 1984.
21. Cochran BH, Zullo J, Verma I, Stiles CD: Science 226:1080, 1984.
22. Land H, Parada LF, Weinberg RA: Nature 304:596, 1983a.
23. Land H, Parada LF, Weinberg RA: Science 222:771, 1983b.
24. Little CD, Nau MM, Carny DN, Gazdan AF, Minna JD: Nature 306:194, 1984.
25. Rapp UR, Bonner TI, Cleveland JL: In: Gallo RC, Stehelin D, Varnier OE (eds): "Retrovirus in Human Pathology." In press.

26. Patterson et al: Proc Natl Acad Sci USA (in press).
27. Shimuzu K, Nakatsu Y, Sekiguchi M, Hokamura K, Tamaka K, Terada M, Sugimara T: Proc Natl Acad Sci USA 82:5641, 1985.
28. Coll J, Righi M, de Taisne C, Gegonne A, Stehelin D: Embo J: 2:2189, 1983.
29. Jansen H, Lurz R, Bister K, Bonner TI, Mark GE, Rapp UR: Nature 307:281, 1984.
30. Jansen HW, Patschinsky T, Bister K: J Virol 48:61, 1983.
31. Jansen HW, Ruckert B, Lurz R, Bister K: Embo J 2:1969, 1983.
32. Sutrave P, Bonner TI, Rapp UR, Jansen HW, Patschinsky T, Bister K: Nature 309:85, 1984.
33. Alexander RW, Moscovici C, Vogt PK: J Natl Cancer Inst 62:359, 1979.
34. Carr JG: Br J Cancer 14:77, 1960.
35. Dexter TM, Garland J, Scott D, Scolnick E, Metcalf D: J Exp Med 152:1036, 1980.
36. Pan S, Knowles BB: Virol 125:1, 1983.
37. Ihle JN, Keller J, Rein A, Cleveland J, Rapp U: In: "Cold Spring Harbor Symposium Papers." Cancer Cells 3:211, 1984.
38. Rapp UR, Reynolds FH Jr, Stephenson JR: J Virol 45:914, 1983a.
39. Rapp UR, Goldsborough MD, Mark GE, Bonner TI, Groffen J, Reynolds FH Jr, Stephenson JR: Proc Natl Acad Sci USA 80:4218, 1983b.
40. Rapp UR, Cleveland JL, Fredrickson TN, Holmes KL, Morse HC III, Patschinsky T, Jansen HW, Bister K: J Virol 55:23, 1985.
41. Rapp UR, Bonner TI, Moelling K, Jansen HW, Bister K, Ihle J: In: "Recent Results in Cancer Research." In press.
42. Davidson WF, Fredrickson TN, Rudikoff EK, Coffman RL, Hartley JW, Morse HC III: J Immunol 133:744, 1984.
43. Morse HC III, Chused TM, Boehm-Truitt M, Mathieson BJ, Sharrow SO, Hartley JW: J Immunol 122:443, 1979.
44. Thomas PS: Proc Natl Acad Sci USA 77:5201, 1980.
45. Stringer JR, Holland LE, Swanstrom RI, Rivo K, Wagner EK: J Virol 21:889, 1977.
46. McMaster CK, Carmichael GG: Proc Natl Acad Sci 74:4835, 1977.
47. Rigby PWJ, Drachmann M, Rhodes C, Berg P: J Mol Biol 133:237, 1979.
48. Lautenberger JA, Schultz RA, Garon CF, Tsichlis PN, Papas TS: Proc Natl Acad Sci 78:1518, 1981.
49. Vennstrom B, Mascovici C, Goodman HM, Bishop JM: J Virol 39:625, 1981.
50. Leder P, Battey J, Lenoir G, Moulding C, Murphy W, Potter H, Stewert T, Taub R: Science 222:765, 1983.
51. Patschinsky T, Walter G, Bister K: Virology 136:348, 1984.
52. Cooper JA, Hunter T: J Biol Chem 258:1108, 1983.
53. Bunte T, Donner P, Pfaff E, Reis B, Greiser-Wilke I, Schaller H, Moelling K: Embo J 3:1919, 1984.
54. Holmes KL, Palaszynski E, Fredrickson TN, Morse HC III, Ihle JN: Proc Natl Acad Sci USA (in press).
55. Silver JE, Fredrickson TN: J Exp Med 158:493, 1983.
56. Fredrickson TN, Langdon WY, Hoffman PM, Hartley JW, Morse HC III: J Natl Cancer Inst 72:447, 1984.
57. Hwang L-HS, Park J, Gilboa E: Mol Cell Biol 4:2289, 1984.
58. Smith KA: Immunol Rev 51:337, 1980.
59. Ihle JN: In: "Contemporary Topics in Molecular Immunology." 1985, Vol. 10, p 93.
60. Ihle JN, Weinstein Y: In: "Recognition and Regulation in Cell-Mediated Immunity." In press.
61. Nabholz M, Conselmann A, Acuto O, Norhm M, Haas W, Phlif H, VonBoehmer H, Hengartner H, Mach JP, Engers H, Johnson JP: Immunol Rev 51:125, 1980.
62. Ihle JN, Rein A, Mural R: In: "Advances in Viral Oncology." 1984, Vol. 4, p 95.
63. Dexter TM, Garland J, Scott D, Scolnick E, Metcalf D: J Exp Med 152:1036, 1980.
64. Greenberger JS, Gans P, Davisson P, Moloney W: Blood 53:987, 1979.
65. Ihle JN, Keller J, Greenberger S, Henderson L, Yetter RA, Morse HC III: J Immunol 129:1377, 1982.
66. Ihle JN, Rebar L, Keller J, Lee JC, Hapel A: Immunol Rev 63:101, 1981.
67. Vennstrom B, Kahn P, Adkins B, Enrietto P, Hayman MJ, Graf T, Luciw P: Embo J 3:3223, 1984.
68. Celander D, Haseltine WA: Nature 312:159, 1984.

69. Hann SR, Eisenman RN: Mol Cell Biol 4:2486, 1984.
70. Patschinsky T, Walter G, Bister K: Virol 136:348, 1984.
71. Bowlin TL, Scott AN, Ihle JN: J Immunol 133:2001, 1984.
72. Moelling K, Heimann B, Beimling P, Rapp UR, Sander T: Nature 312:558, 1984.
73. Cochran BH, Reffel AC, Stiles CD: Cell 33:939, 1983.
74. Stiles CD, Capone GT, Scherr CD, Antoniades HN, Van Wyk JJ, Pledge WJ: Proc Natl Acad Sci USA 76:1279, 1979.
75. Taub R, Moulding C, Battey J, Murphy W, Vasicek T, Lenoir GM, Leder P: Cell 36:339, 1984.
76. Rabbitts TH, Forster P, Hamlyn P, Baer R: Nature 309:592, 1984.
77. Siebenlist U, Henninghausen L, Battey J, Leder P: Cell 37:381, 1984.
78. Graf T, Ade N, Beug H: Nature 275:496, 1978.
79. Heard JM, Fichelson S, Sola B, Martial MA, Varet B, Levy JP: Mol Cell Biol 4:216, 1984.
80. Poiesz BJ, Ruscetti FW, Mier JW, Woods AM, Gallo RC: Proc Natl Acad Sci USA 77:6815, 1980.
81. Hoshino H, Esumi H, Miwa M, Shimoyama M, Minato K, Tobinai K, Hirose M, Watanabe S, Inada N, Kinoshita K, Ichimaru M, Sugimura T: Proc Natl Acad Sci USA 80:6061, 1983.
82. Farrar JJ, Fuller-Farrar J, Simon PL, Hilfiker ML, Stadler BM, Farrar WL: J Immunol 125:2555, 1980.
83. Ihle JN, Keller J, Henderson L, Klein F, Palaszynski EW: J Immunol 129:2431, 1982.
84. Blasi E, Mathieson BJ, Varesio H, Cleveland JL, Borchert P, Rapp UR: Nature 318: 667, 1985.
85. Rapp UR, Cleveland JL, Brightman K, Scott A, Ihle JN: Nature 317: 434, 1985.

Journal of Cellular Biochemistry 30:311–318 (1986)
Biochemical and Molecular Epidemiology of Cancer 91–98

Treatment of a Fatal Transplantable Erythroleukemia by Procedures That Lower Endogenous Erythropoietin

Azhar Hossain, Jung-Kon Kim, and W. David Hankins

Laboratory of Experimental Carcinogenesis, National Cancer Institute, Bethesda, Maryland 20205

The in vitro growth of primary erythroleukemia cells has been examined in the presence and absence of the hormone erythropoietin (EPO). Although these leukemic cells had previously been considered to be hormone-independent, addition of EPO was found to be essential for maximum growth in culture. Erythroid colonies that grew in the presence of EPO were leukemogenic when returned to mice. Influence of EPO on the in vivo growth of leukemic cells was indicated by our findings that (1) administration of the hormone caused a more severe leukemia and rapid death, and (2) transfusion of red blood cells, which lowers endogenous EPO, led to decreased spleen size and increased survival of leukemic mice. We suggest from our results that hormone-associated therapy might be efficacious in the treatment of this and, perhaps, other leukemias.

Key words: leukemia, antihormone therapy, hormone-associated therapy, erythropoietin

More than eight decades ago, Beatson noted that oophorectomy had beneficial effects for some women with breast cancer [1]. This was one of the first suggestions that some tumors are dependent on hormones for their growth. Subsequent studies demonstrated that approximately one-third of breast cancer patients showed a marked improvement upon administration of compounds that were antagonistic to or reduced the effectiveness of estrogen. In addition, the development of animal models for the induction, analysis, and treatment of mammary and prostatic cancers [2] led to successful antisteroid treatment of prostatic cancers. Yet, despite the initial excitement generated by these discoveries, hormone-associated therapy is today rarely considered as a primary treatment of other solid tumors or leukemias. Factors that may have contributed to the lack of widespread application of antihormone therapy include 1) the unequivocal success of chemotherapy, radiotherapy, and surgery in a few specific cancers, 2) lack of demonstration of efficacy of antihormone therapy in other animal cancers, and 3) a general opinion in the medical community that most tumors are autonomous and hormone-independent.

Received May 31, 1985; revised and accepted October 22, 1985.

© **1986 Alan R. Liss, Inc.**

Our laboratory has studied growth, differentiation, and hormone sensitivity of virus-transformed hemopoietic cells over the past several years. Unexpected observations, made during these studies, led us to propose a model of carcinogenesis that, if accurate, has conceptual and practical implications for the diagnosis and therapy of human cancer. Briefly, this model [3,4] holds that transforming events leading to cancer can provide a heritable growth/survival advantage to tumor cells without blocking their ability to differentiate or altering other fundamental cellular properties. The model also suggests that, excepting a growth advantage, the properties of tumors are just reflections of normal cell properties at or subsequent to the developmental stage at which the oncogenic transformation occurred. One prediction of this model is that most, if not all, tumor populations retain sensitivity to, and a requirement for, natural, physiologic growth factors for their survival and/or proliferation.

As one test of this prediction, we have assessed the erythropoietin (EPO) sensitivity of highly tumorigenic erythroleukemia cells. This report presents our preliminary results, which indicate that the leukemic erythroid progenitors do require EPO for growth in vitro and that survival of leukemic mice can be markedly extended by hormone-associated therapy in vivo.

MATERIALS AND METHODS

Derivation of Transplantable Erythroleukemia Cell Lines

Erythroleukemia cell lines were derived by the procedure of Oliff et al [5]. A total of eight transplantable lines were derived from eight individual leukemic mice. These lines have been passaged, approximately once each month, for the past 2 yr. At each passage, a single cell suspension was prepared from one leukemic spleen. Of this suspension, 1 million cells were inoculated intravenously into ten adult (6–8 wk old) mice. Within 2–4 wk, a fatal leukemia developed in the recipients. Chromosomal marker studies of Oliff et al [5] have indicated that transplantable erythroleukemia lines, derived by similar methodology, were clearly of donor origin.

In Vitro Culture of Erythroleukemia Cells

At random passages in vivo, the enlarged spleens containing leukemic cells were removed and single cell suspensions prepared. The cells were incubated in Iscove's modified Dulbecco's MEM containing 2% methylcellulose and 30% fetal calf serum and 0.021 mM β-mercaptoethanol, as described by Mager et al [6]. EPO, where indicated, was added to give a final concentration of 0.3 U/ml. Three different preparations of EPO were used in this study: sheep plasma EPO from Connaught Laboratories (Toronto, Ontario, Canada); human urinary EPO from the National Heart, Blood, and Lung Institute (Bethesda, MD); and murine EPO produced by murine erythroleukemia cells as previously described [7]. Methylcellulose cultures were incubated at 37°C in an atmosphere of 5% CO_2 and 95% air. Cultures were monitored on an inverted scope at a magnification of ×40.

Immunofluorescence

Spectrin immunofluorescence assays were performed as previously described [8]. Colonies picked from culture dishes were suspended in phosphate-buffered saline containing 20% fetal calf serum and spun onto glass slides using a Shandon cytocentrifuge. The antisera against spectrin was a generous gift from Dr. John Portis (Rocky

Mountain Laboratories, Hamilton, MT). The ability of this antiserum to recognize spectrin was confirmed by immunoprecipitation and PAGE, as described by Koury et al [9].

Hypertransfusion

Transfusion of mice was as described by Oliff et al [5]. Briefly, each transfused mouse received weekly intraperitoneal injections (1 ml) of a suspension prepared to contain 80% packed red blood cells from syngeneic exbreeder mice.

RESULTS

Stimulation of Erythroleukemia Cell Growth In Vitro by EPO

To test whether erythroleukemia cells retained erythropoietin sensitivity, we cultured primary spleen cells from leukemic mice with and without the hormone. It should be noted that, under the culture conditions employed herein, virtually no erythroid cell growth is observed in cultures of normal spleen cells even in the presence of EPO. As for the leukemic spleen, very few cells were observed without EPO, whereas in the presence of EPO numerous large, tightly packed colonies appeared. Although some small colonies were occasionally present in cultures without added EPO, Figure 1 is representative of the hormone's effects on leukemia cell proliferation in vitro. Since the EPO preparation employed for Figure 1 was quite impure (specific activity 15 U/mg), we cannot be sure that the stimulatory agent is authentic EPO. However, similar results were obtained when we used 0.3 U/ml of partially purified human urinary EPO or partially purified murine EPO produced by erythroleukemia cells [7]. Nonetheless, it is still possible that the stimulatory effects are due to a contaminant in the EPO preparation.

To optimize the conditions for culture of these cells, a dose-response experiment was performed; the results are shown in Figure 2. Spleen cells were cultured in the methylcellulose colony assay as described for Figure 1. Although the number of colonies definitely increased with increasing EPO, precise quantitation was difficult owing to the fact that the colonies were suspended at different viewing levels throughout the methylcellulose. Therefore, total nucleated cell counts were determined following recovery of the cells from methylcellulose by centrifugation. A plateau was observed at ~ 0.1–0.3 U/ml. Consequently, an EPO concentration of 0.3 U/ml was chosen for subsequent experiments.

Characterization of Leukemic Cells That Grew in the Presence of EPO in Culture

The colonies that developed in the EPO-treated cultures were removed with a micropipette, pooled, and centrifuged onto glass slides using a cytocentrifuge. Slides were stained with Wright stain or benzidine stain or were assayed for the presence of spectrin by indirect immunofluorescence (Table I). The vast majority of the cultured cells exhibited blastic morphology resembling proerythroblasts and were positive for spectrin. Nevertheless, very little evidence of terminal differentiation was observed; virtually all cells grown in the presence of EPO were benzidine-negative.

Next, EPO-induced colonies were pooled and inoculated into adult syngeneic mice, and the recipients were monitored for 3 mo. Adults were chosen because newborn mice are sensitive to induction of erythroleukemia by virus that may be

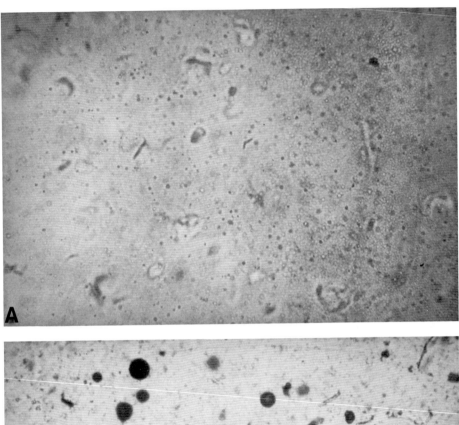

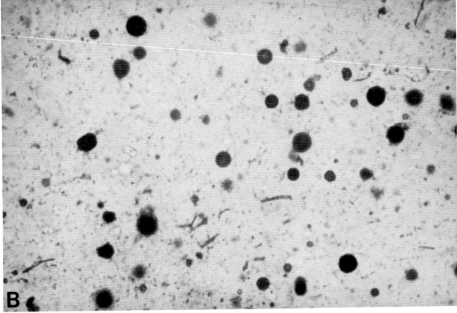

Fig. 1.   Effect of EPO on leukemia cell growth in vitro. Spleen cells from passage 5 of transplantable erythroleukemia line 19 were seeded at a concentration of 1 million cells/ml in methylcellulose as described in Materials and Methods. Connaught step III erythropoietin was added to half the cultures (B) and the remainder (A) received an equivalent amount of Hanks' balanced salt solution. Photographs were made in situ using a Leitz inverted microscope at a magnification of ×25.

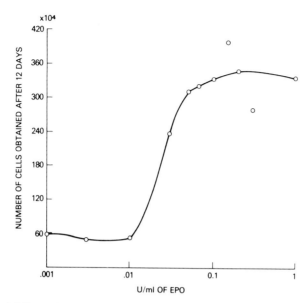

Fig. 2.   Effect of different doses of EPO on leukemia cell growth in culture. Cultures were prepared as in Figure 1 except that the final concentration of EPO was varied as indicated. On day 12, cells were collected by centrifugation, and the number of nucleated cells per plate was determined.

TABLE I. Characteristics of Cells That Grew in Culture in the Presence of Erythropoietin

Line	Morphology	Hemoglobin-positive	Spectrin-positive	Tumorigenic deaths/recipients
EL-16	Erythroid	No	Yes	10/10
EL-17	Erythroid	No	Yes	10/10
EL-18	Erythroid	No	Yes	8/8
EL-19	Erythroid	No	Yes	8/8
EL-20	Erythroid	No	Yes	10/10

produced by the leukemic cells. In control experiments, 15 daily injections of conditioned medium from erythroleukemia cultures did not induce erythroleukemia in adult mice within 3 mo. In contrast, inoculation of pooled colonies from the EPO-treated cultures produced a fatal leukemia within 3 months after inoculation. This tumorigenicity was a characteristic of all the colonies tested (Table I). These results indicate that the cells stimulated to proliferate and form colonies were erythroid and demonstrate that the EPO-stimulated erythroblasts were malignant in that they induced a fatal leukemia.

In Vivo Influence of EPO on Erythroleukemia Development

The apparent requirement for EPO for in vitro growth of the erythroleukemia cells led us to test the possibility that tumor growth in vivo is also modulated by EPO (Fig. 3). Tumor cells were inoculated and recipient mice were hypertransfused at weekly intervals throughout the course of the leukemia development. As can be seen from a comparison of groups A and B, the hypertransfusion led to a significant extension ($P = 0.001$) in the survival times of the leukemic mice. Thus mice that

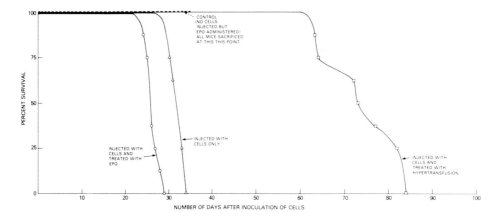

Fig. 3. Effect of hypertransfusion or EPO administration on the survival of mice with erythroleukemia. One million cells from transplantable erythroleukemia line EL-19 were injected intravenously into each 50 adult mice. The mice were divided into four groups. Group A (△) received no further treatment. Group B (□) received weekly transfusions of 1 ml per mouse of reconstituted blood containing 80% red blood cells. Group C (○) was transfused as B, but each mouse also received daily intraperitoneal injections of 0.2 unit of Connaught step III erythropoietin. All mice were monitored and the spleens palpated each day. Group D (---) was a control for group C. These mice received daily injections of EPO but had not been inoculated with leukemic cells. None of the mice in group D died during the monitoring period.

were hypertransfused lived two to three times longer than those that did not receive red blood cell transfusions.

The increased survival times were most likely mediated through a reduction of endogenous EPO as a result of the transfusion. However, since leukemic mice were severely anemic, we considered the possibility that hypertransfusion had simply corrected the anemia and thereby increased survival. Two experimental findings argue against this contention. First, palpation of recipient mice 25 days after inoculation revealed that spleens from transfused mice were considerably smaller than those of untreated mice. This provides circumstantial evidence that the leukemic cells grow more slowly in the transfused mice. An illustration of this difference in spleen is shown in Figure 4. Second, simultaneous administration of EPO plus hypertransfusion led to more rapid leukemia and survival times similar to those of untreated recipients (groups B and C were significantly different at P = 0.001). That is, the transfusions were of little survival value when mice were simultaneously administered exogenous EPO.

DISCUSSION

In the present study, we investigated the effects of a hormone, erythropoietin, on transformed erythroid cells that produce a rapid and fatal leukemia when inoculated into syngeneic mice. We found that addition of EPO to cultures of the leukemic cells produced dramatic effects on their proliferation. In fact, little if any growth occurred in the absence of added hormone. This observation of EPO sensitivity in vitro led us to examine the influence of EPO on leukemia cell growth in vivo. Considerable

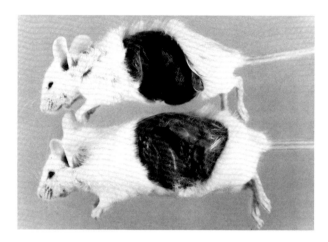

Fig. 4.   Effect of transfusion of spleen size in erythroleukemic mice. On day 25 of the experiment described in the legend to Figure 3, one mouse from group A (top, untreated) and one from group B (bottom, hypertransfused) were sacrificed, and the spleens and livers were exposed and photographed.

evidence was obtained that EPO dramatically stimulated the proliferation or viability of erythroleukemia cells in the animal as well as in culture.

Such growth-promoting effects of EPO on leukemic cells are interesting for three reasons. First, EPO is a hormone usually associated with an induction of terminal erythroid differentiation. Although EPO in this study caused extensive proliferation, the stimulated erythroid cells did not exhibit hemoglobin synthesis or nuclear condensation, which are characteristic of terminal red blood cell development. Although these results do not argue against a differentiative role for EPO, they do emphasize a possible role for the hormone in stimulating proliferation, and perhaps ensuring viability, of erythroid progenitors.

Second, these results provide an example of erythroleukemia cells that have become tumorigenic without losing their sensitivity to a growth factor that presumably regulates the growth of the antecedent normal erythroid progenitors. Several investigators have suggested that tumor cells lose their requirement for natural growth factors. Shrader and Crapper [10], for example, recently associated the abrogation of requirement for exogenous lymphoid growth factors with a truly malignant phenotype. In earlier reports [3,4], we proposed a model of carcinogenesis that suggests that normal cells can become transformed by acquisition of a heritable growth advantage without an arrest in differentiation or abrogation of growth factor requirements. Most of the evidence cited in support of the model was derived from observations that hemopoietic cells, transformed in vitro or in vivo by any of a number of retroviruses, were able to continue terminal maturation and retained sensitivity to physiologic hormones [11,12]. However, in that these primary transformants did not induce tumors upon inoculation into mice, it could be argued that they were not truly malignant cells but had only received a growth stimulation. In the present study, however, the erythroleukemia cells stimulated to proliferate in vitro induced a fatal leukemia in 100% of the mice receiving these cells. Therefore, the present experiments provide additional support for the notion that truly malignant cells retain sensitivity to physiologic growth factors.

Third, the present experiments suggest that at least one type of murine leukemia is treatable by procedures that lower an endogenous hormone. It should be noted that our encouraging results were obtained under experimental conditions (eg, number of cells inoculated, transfusion schedule, etc) that were arbitrarily chosen. It can be anticipated that even longer survival times could be achieved by optimization of the treatment regimen. Our current extension of these studies includes preparation of hormone-related therapeutic reagents such as 1) neutralizing monoclonal antibodies against EPO and 2) competitive analogs of EPO.

The experiments in this study were designed to test the hypothesis [3,4] that apparently autonomous leukemic cells retain hormone sensitivity and therefore respond to antihormone therapy. As an extension of this hypothesis, it is possible that other mouse and human leukemias also retain sensitivity to physiologic growth factors and are treatable on that basis. Furthermore, in addition to breast and prostatic cancers, solid tumors of the lung, colon, liver, brain, and other tissues may retain sensitivity to external growth factors. Accordingly, experiments are in progress in our laboratory to assess the hormone sensitivities of such tumors in primary cultures. In this regard, it is noteworthy that bombesin, a newly identified growth factor, not only stimulated normal human epithelial cells [3] but also increased the colony-forming efficiency of cells derived from small cell carcinomas of the lung [4].

ACKNOWLEDGMENTS

We thank Kyung Chin for laboratory assistance and Ellen Hankins for help in manuscript preparation. The authors also wish to thank Dr. Charles B. Huggins at the University of Chicago for stimulating discussions relating to hormone-associated therapy of cancer.

REFERENCES

1. Beatson GT: Lancet 2:104, 162, 1909.
2. Huggins CB: "Experimental Leukemia and Mammary Cancer." Chicago: University of Chicago Press, 1979.
3. Hankins WD, Kaminchik J, Luna J: In Stamatoyannopoulos G, Nienhuis AW (eds): "Globin Gene Expression and Hematopoietic Differentiation." New York: Alan R. Liss, Inc., 1983 pp 245–261.
4. Hankins WD: JNCI 70:725, 1983.
5. Oliff A, Ruscetti S, Douglas EC, Scolnick EM: Blood 58:244, 1981.
6. Mager DL, Mak TW, Bernstein A: Proc Natl Acad Sci USA 78:1703, 1981.
7. Tambourin P, Casadevall M, Choppin J, Heard JM, Fichelson S, Wending F, Hankins WD, Varet B: Proc Natl Acad Sci USA 80:7678, 1983.
8. Furth ME, Scolnick EM: J Virol 48:125, 1983.
9. Koury MJ, Bondurant MC, Duncan DT, Krantz SB, Hankins WD: Proc Natl Acad Sci USA 79:635, 1982.
10. Schrader JW, Crapper RM: Proc Natl Acad Sci USA 80:6892, 1983.
11. Hankins WD, Kost TA, Koury MJ, Krantz SB: Nature 276:506, 1978.
12. Hankins WD, Scolnick EM: Cell 26:91, 1981.
13. Willey JC, Lechner JF, Harris CC: Exp Cell Res 153:245, 1984.
14. Carney D, Oie H, Moody T, Gazdar AF, Minna JD: Science 214:1246, 1985.

Journal of Cellular Biochemistry 30:319–329 (1986)
Biochemical and Molecular Epidemiology of Cancer 99–109

Human Restriction Fragment Length Polymorphisms and Cancer Risk Assessment

Theodore G. Krontiris, Nancy A. DiMartino, Mark Colb, H. David Mitcheson, and David R. Parkinson

Division of Hematology/Oncology and Cancer Research Center (T.G.K., N.A.D., M.C., D.R.P.) and Department of Urology (H.D.M.), Tufts-New England Medical Center, and Department of Molecular Biology and Microbiology, Tufts University School of Medicine, (T.G.K.), Boston, Massachusetts 02111

The polymorphic restriction fragments of the human Ha-*ras* locus, produced by the variable tandem repetition (VTR) of a short consensus sequence, fall into three classes based on allelic frequencies. Alleles of the "rare" class (individual frequencies <0.5%) have been detected only in white blood cell and tumor DNA of cancer patients. This phenomenon is independent of ethnic origin. No significant association of rare alleles with cancer patients has been demonstrated at an independent tandem repeat locus, VTR4.1. The results suggest that the Ha-*ras* restriction fragment length polymorphism is useful in cancer risk assessment.

Key words: oncogenes, Ha-*ras*, restriction fragment length polymorphism, human genetics, cancer risk assessment

The recent advances in molecular biology have had a major impact on our understanding of the pathogenesis of cancer. At the same time, concepts that have been applied to the diagnosis of genetic diseases hold promise for the analysis of inherited susceptibility to cancer. One of the most important of these concepts is the restriction fragment length polymorphism (RFLP). When restriction endonucleases were employed in the structural analysis of DNA, it was shown that hereditary variations such as deletions, insertions, and even point mutations could be reproducibly demonstrated by this approach [reviewed in 1]. Thus polymorphic changes in DNA sequence could result in altered restriction fragment length as detected by digesting DNA with the appropriate enzyme and then subjecting the products to agarose gel electrophoresis. These migration differences were first detected in cloned

Abbreviations used: RFLP, restriction fragment length polymorphism; WBC, white blood cell; VTR, variable tandem repeat; GU, genito-urinary.

Received September 3, 1985; revised and accepted November 11, 1985.

© 1986 Alan R. Liss, Inc.

DNA; but, with the advent of Southern blotting, polymorphisms in genomic DNA also became accessible. The key maneuver in this type of analysis is choosing the proper restriction endonuclease. This is largely a matter of trial and error, although certain enzymes with CpG in the recognition sequence (MspI and TaqI, for example) more frequently reveal RFLPs [2].

DNA polymorphisms detected by restriction endonucleases fall into one of two categories. In the first, called *site polymorphism,* the recognition site for a given enzyme in a particular region of DNA either appears or disappears as the result of point mutation. Two phenotypes are therefore possible: the two different fragment sizes generated by the site-present and site-absent alleles. Such a polymorphism, based on the specific sequence of one restriction endonuclease, will be revealed only by that enzyme. In the second category, called *insertion/deletion polymorphisms,* variation in fragment length is the result of insertion or deletion of DNA sequences. This polymorphism will be detected by any restriction endonuclease that possesses recognition sites tightly spanning the region of sequence alteration. Since the insertions or deletions can assume a continuum of lengths, more than two alleles are possible.

RFLPs in human DNA were first described in the β-globin gene cluster [3,4]. These were site polymorphisms identified within the δ-globin gene [3] and near the β-globin gene [4]. The clinical significance of these results was immediately appreciated; the β-globin RFLP was associated with the sickle trait. Insertion/deletion polymorphism in human DNA was first demonstrated in a region with unknown function [5]. Since that time, insulin [6], ζ-globin [7], and Ha-*ras* [8–11] have all been linked to polymorphisms of the insertion/deletion type.

The list of DNA polymorphisms associated with disease loci continues to expand. These data currently provide the basis for many active investigations on the utility of RFLPs in both prenatal diagnosis and risk assessment. In addition to the diagnostic applications, RFLPs promise to revolutionize human genetic mapping. Botstein et al [12] have pointed out that the systematic collection of 150–400 independent probes for polymorphic regions of human DNA should provide a definite set of genetic markers with which to map the entire genome. A cooperative effort on the international level is now being organized [13].

Because of the highly polymorphic nature of the human Ha-*ras* gene, we analyzed the distribution of allelic restriction fragments in cancer patients and cancer-free controls. Our results suggest the Ha-*ras* RFLP may prove useful in determining cancer risk. Here we report updated results from a continuing study [first described in 11].

MATERIALS AND METHODS
Study Population and Sample Collection

Unrelated whites, without a personal or first-degree family history of cancer, comprised the control or normal population referred to below. Cancer patients, again unrelated whites, were enlisted from the New England Medical Center Hospitals. These patients demonstrated a variety of tumors, including carcinomas of the head and neck, breast, lung, and lower gastrointestinal tract, sarcomas, melanomas, acute and chronic lymphocytic and nonlymphocytic leukemias, and Hodgkin's and non-Hodgkin's lymphomas.

WBC were separated from peripheral blood by dextran sedimentation and frozen at $-20°C$ until further use. Discarded tumor tissue from surgical resection or biopsy was frozen in liquid nitrogen or dry ice-ethanol and stored at $-70°C$.

Southern Blotting

DNA was extracted from WBC or tumor tissue, digested with restriction endonuclease, fractionated on agarose gels, and transferred to nitrocellulose as previously described [11]. Radiolabeled probe, utilizing the human Ha-*ras* plasmid pEC [14], was prepared by nick-translation [15] and employed in filter hybridization [18] as described by Der et al [19].

Isolation of VTR4.1

The 990 bp MspI fragment of pEC, which contains the Ha-*ras* variable tandem repeat (VTR), was nick-translated, and the resulting probe was used to screen a human phage library [3] by standard methods of in situ hybridization [17]. Filters were hybridized at $50°C$ in $5×$ SET ($1×$ SET = 0.15 M NaCl, 1 mM EDTA, 20 mM Tris pH 8) and washed several times at room temperature and $37°C$ in $2×$ SET. One phage of approximately 200,000 screened demonstrated a strong signal. The phage was isolated, after which the region of homology to the Ha-*ras* VTR was identified and subcloned. DNA sequencing of the subclone revealed the tandem repetition of a 35 bp consensus sequence. [M. Colb, B. Mermer, and T.G. Krontiris, in preparation]. The region, designated VTR4.1, has been used as probe in the survey of human DNAs as described in Results.

RESULTS

Approximately 1,000 bp downstream from the polyadenylation signal of the human Ha-*ras* gene is a region of tandemly repeated nucleotides [9]. A 28 bp consensus sequence is aligned head-to-tail from 30 to 100 times. This VTR is the basis for the Ha-*ras* polymorphism [8–11].

The enzyme combination MspI/HpaII has sites closely flanking the Ha-*ras* VTR; digestion occurs about 115 bp upstream and 50 bp downstream. The remainder of the Ha-*ras* sequences recognized by the probe are digested so extensively that they are not seen under the gel conditions we use. (The isoschizomers are employed together to reduce the effect of DNA methylation on digestion.) Southern blots of over 350 WBC and tumor DNA preparations have revealed at least 24 fragments with distinct gel migration patterns (Table I, Fig. 1).

Four of the fragments revealed by MspI/HpaII (MH) digestion were quite common, accounting for $\sim93\%$ of the total number analyzed (Table I). The individual frequencies in this group ranged from 7% to 65%. Another five alleles occurred at intermediate frequencies, from 0.5% to 1.5% for each allele. Finally, we detected

TABLE I. Distribution of Ha-*ras* Alleles

Class	Members	Frequency
Common	a1, a2, a3, a4	0.07–0.65
Intermediate	a1.1, a1.2, a1.3, a4.1, a5	0.005–0.015
Rare	Total of 15	<0.005

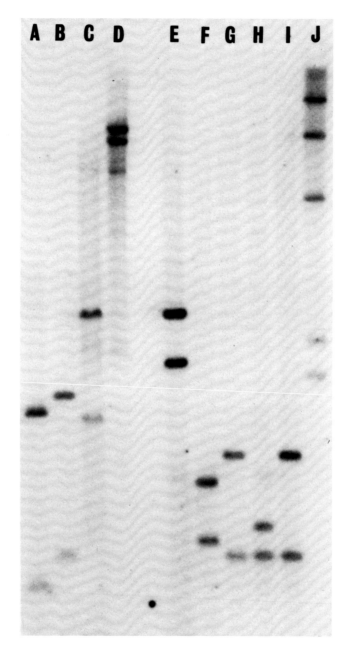

Fig. 1.   Polymorphic fragments of the Ha-*ras* gene. WBC DNA was digested and blotted as described in Materials and Methods. Probe was the nick-translated 6.6 kb BamHI fragment of pEC. Lanes A–D represent the MspI/HpaII/PstI (A), MspI/HpaII (B), PstI (C), and BamHI (D) digests of a WBC DNA with a1 and a2.2 allelic fragments. Lanes E–I are the MspI/HpaII digests of a marker DNA with a3 and a4 fragments (E), a leukemia DNA with a1.1 and a1.4 fragments (F), a marker DNA with a1 and a2 fragments (G and I), and a leukemia DNA with a1 and a1.2 fragments (H). J is HindIII-digested and end-labeled λDNA; the 23 kb band is poorly visualized here.

a large class with at least 15 different members. Each of these fragments represented < 0.5% of the total.

Figure 1 shows examples of several alleles in the intermediate and rare categories. Lane E contains the MH digest of a DNA with the common a3 and a4 alleles. Lanes G and I have the MH digest of one with the common a1 and a2 alleles. The MH digest of DNA in lane B demonstrates the rare allele a2.2 as the upper band and common allele a1 as the lower band. Lanes F and H, also MH digests, demonstrate unusual alleles present in two acute myelogenous leukemia DNAs. Two unusual fragments in these lanes are in the intermediate class: a1.1 the lower band in F and a1.2 the upper band in H. The upper band in F is the rare allele a1.4.

When the MH digest reveals an unusual fragment, we repeat the digest with several enzymes to rule out partial digestion and MH site polymorphism. For example, lanes B–D in Figure 1 are the MH, PstI, and BamHI digests of the DNA with the a2.2 allele. Note that two prominent bands representing the Ha-*ras* gene are present in each digest.

Figure 1 also demonstrates the resolution of our gels. From Ha-*ras* sequence data [9], we have determined that the MspI/HpaII site 5′ to the tandem repeat is 113 bp from the PstI site also on that side (itself 3 bp from the start of the tandem repeat). Lane A is an MspI/HpaII/PstI triple digest adjacent to the MH digest in lane B. This shows the migration difference produced by 115 bp in the region of a1 (lower pair of fragments in A and B) as well as in the region of a3 (upper pair of fragments). Since the Ha-*ras* tandem repeat monomer is 28 bp long, we are capable of discerning differences of two repeat units (lane F, lower fragment) and, occasionally, even of one repeat unit. Such resolution is diminished, of course, in higher-molecular-weight regions near a3 and a4.

When we analyzed the distribution of common, intermediate, and rare alleles in cancer patients and cancer-free controls, we found that rare alleles appeared only in cancer patients (Tables II and V). Intermediate alleles also occurred more frequently in cancer patients, although this association was not as strong as that observed for rare alleles.

We have observed rare restriction fragments in first-degree relatives of cancer patients. This indicates that unusual Ha-*ras* alleles are transmitted in a mendelian fashion and, at least for the cases we have observed, do not arise de novo in cancer patients. As an example, Figure 2 shows a pedigree from a large kindred with the Von Hippel Lindau syndrome. We have studied nearly 100 members of the family; the pedigree in Figure 2 is being presented because it illustrates the pattern of transmission of one rare allele, a2.2, and one intermediate allele, a1.2. Cross-hatched symbols indicate affected individuals. The index case, indicated by the arrow, was

TABLE II. Comparison of Rare Alleles in Control and Cancer DNAs*

DNA source	Common alleles	Intermediate alleles	Rare alleles	Probability
Control WBC	311	11	0	—
Tumors + pt. WBC	394	27	31	<0.001
Pt. WBC	241	19	24	<0.001
Tumors	153	8	7	<0.01

*Probability by χ^2 (2 df). Comparisons are control WBC vs Tumor + pt. (patient) WBC; control WBC vs pt. WBC; and control WBC vs tumor.

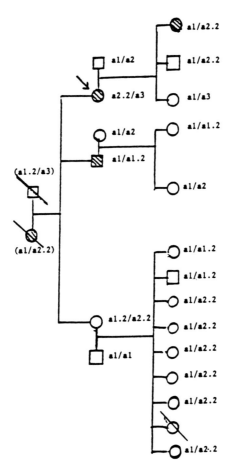

Fig. 2.   Pedigree from a kindred with the Von Hippel Lindau syndrome. See text for details.

noted to have the rare allele a2.2. The genotypes in generation I were deduced both from sibs in the VHL kindred and from the progeny shown here. Although the number of genotypes is small, we can certainly conclude that both rare and intermediate alleles do not necessarily arise de novo in cancer patients. Both the a2.2 and a1.2 alleles are present in multiple sibs of generation II and were transmitted to progeny of generation III.

   The ethnic composition of control and cancer populations could obviously be an important source of bias in our study. Data on the ethnic group/national origin of study entrants were collected and monitored to determine if ethnic imbalance materially influenced our results (Table III). The four grandparents of each entrant were classified by ethnic group/nationality. The number of grandparents in each ethnic category was determined and this figure expressed as a percentage of the total number of grandparents. Four additions were made to the "unknown" category when no ethnic data were available for a given individual. The distribution of rare alleles among these groups is given in Table III. In seven instances, an allele appeared in an individual with grandparents in two ethnic groups; in these cases, the alleles were

TABLE III. Distribution of Rare Alleles by Ethnic Group/Nationality

Group	Percent of grandparents		Rare alleles	
	Cancer	Control	Cancer	Control
Unknown	35.8	27.4	11	0
Irish	14.0	27.3	3	0
Italian	14.3	7.7	4	0
English	5.7	7.6	3	0
Jewish	7.6	9.2	5	0
German	3.7	3.9	2	0
Scottish	3.6	2.0	2	0
French	3.0	2.2	0	0
Polish	1.9	4.0	1	0
Portuguese	2.4	0.9	1	0
Russian	0.2	1.2	0	0
Estonian	0.0	0.5	0	0
Ukranian	0.4	0.0	1	0
Lithuanian	0.9	0.9	0	0
Swedish	1.0	0.5	1	0
Norwegian	0.0	0.2	0	0
Danish	0.2	0.5	1	0
Finnish	0.2	0.5	0	0
Austrian	0.0	0.5	0	0
Swiss	0.0	0.2	0	0
Greek	1.3	0.5	0	0
Albanian	0.2	0.0	0	0
Lebanese	0.4	0.0	0	0
Armenian	0.4	0.0	1	0
Syrian	0.4	0.0	1	0
AmIndian	0.0	0.7	0	0
Canadian	1.1	0.9	0	0
Spanish	0.0	0.1	0	0
Hungarian	0.0	0.5	0	0
Dutch	0.4	0.1	1	0

listed under both ethnic groups. Several considerations support the conclusion that allele distribution is unaffected by ethnic composition.

First, the number of rare alleles in each ethnic group, including "unknown" is proportional to the representation of that ethnic group in the "cancer" sample. No single ethnic group, including "unknown," is contributing a disproportionate number of rare alleles. Therefore, even a great disparity in the ethnic composition of "cancer" and "control" would not be expected to bias the results. Corroborating evidence for this conclusion is found in the "Irish" category. There, an excess of Irish entries has recently accumulated in the "control" group. Despite this difference, rare alleles still predominate in the "cancer" group. So, when the sample is skewed in the "Irish" category by 1:2, "cancer" to "control," the alleles are still 3:0 in the opposite direction. Similarly, there is a slight excess of Italian patients in the "cancer" group, but, once again, the number of unusual alleles is proportional to the number of Italian grandparents. Second, when rare alleles appear more than once, they appear in more than one ethnic group. The allele a2.2, for example, has appeared in a patient with four Irish grandparents and a patient with four Armenian grandparents.

Bladder carcinoma is potentially a useful tumor model for the interaction of environmental and host susceptibility factors. Ha-*ras* gene activation by mutation is prominent in this tumor type. Also, environmental carcinogens play a prominent etiologic role. The mutation of Ha-*ras* by ultimate carcinogens has been observed [20]. Finally, bladder cancer patients are at greater risk for developing a second primary tumor in a different tissue. We have been blotting WBC DNA from patients with bladder cancer, nonbladder GU malignancies (mostly prostate and renal), and nonmalignant GU disease (mostly infertility and benign prostatic hypertrophy). As is shown in Table IV, there is a much greater prevalence of unusual Ha-*ras* alleles in patients with bladder malignancy.

These results are particularly interesting because of the nature of the alleles detected. Eight of 13 are within one to three tandem repeat monomers of the a1 allele (monomer length 28 bp). The others migrate very near a2 (one), and a3 (two), or a4 (two). Thus, in contrast to most rare alleles, which are quite distinct from the common alleles (see again lane B in Fig. 1), the unusual alleles associated with bladder carcinoma are grouped around specific deviations from the common alleles. Most of them appear identical to the intermediate alleles a1.1 and a1.2. Because of this clustering, we have considered the possibility that "bladder" alleles did not arise from changes in tandem repeat length but rather from clustered point mutations resulting in MH site polymorphisms. Such an outcome would, of course, imply hypermutability of the Ha-*ras* gene near its VTR. We are now conducting detailed restriction mapping of the WBC DNAs displaying these alleles to distinguish MH site polymorphism from minor VTR changes.

Approximately 40% of patients from families with prominent histories of cancer demonstrate rare alleles. However, our preliminary linkage data indicate that Ha-*ras* is not identical to, nor closely linked to, the disease locus in several cancer syndromes. Although we must be careful about generalizing from the cancer family results, the emerging picture is that Ha-*ras* is not the primary determinant of disease in patients with rare alleles. Therefore, the two broadest alternatives for the association phenomenon are 1) that the Ha-*ras* gene, its VTR, or a closely linked gene tangentially participates in the pathogenesis of a given tumor in a patient with a rare fragment—say, through the intervention of a germline mutant Ha-*ras* gene during tumor progression, or 2) the that Ha-*ras* locus is irrelevant to pathogenesis, the VTR being merely a marker for genomic instability—say, increased sister chromatid exchange—in those people destined to get cancer. The investigation of the former possibility requires cloning and characterizing rare allelic fragments. To pursue the latter possibility, we have begun to isolate clones representing other tandem repeat loci and to perform population studies with them. In this way, we can compare the population genetics of VTRs to determine if the Ha-*ras* phenomenon is unique or global. If the phenomenon is global, we would systematically collect and characterize VTRs for their use as a battery of predictive markers.

TABLE IV. Unusual Ha-*ras* Alleles in Bladder Carcinoma

	Unusual alleles/total patients
Bladder cancer	13/31
Nonbladder GU cancer	2/20
Benign GU disease	1/25

We have cloned another tandem repeat using the Ha-*ras* VTR as probe. The clone, designated VTR4.1, recognizes a locus independent from Ha-*ras*. The enzyme HaeIII just spans the repeat region, which consists of head-to-tail arrays of a 35 bp consensus sequence. Therefore, we have used this enzyme to digest and Southern blot nearly all of the DNAs screened in the Ha-*ras* population study. (The VTR4.1 survey employed about 20 DNA samples not screened in the Ha-*ras* survey, and vice versa.) Six of the seven fragments detected with this probe are shown in Figure 3. The seventh (a7) is an apparent deletion of a large segment of the VTR in a cancer-free individual. The fragment counts and frequencies (we have not yet formally demonstrated allelism with all fragments of VTR4.1) are listed in Table V; fragments with an asterisk (*) have been detected only in cancer patients. Unlike that of the Ha-*ras* gene, polymorphic variation of VTR4.1 is relatively restricted. There is no significant accumulation of rare fragments in cancer patients. Therefore, this locus does not demonstrate the same population behavior.

DISCUSSION

Our survey of Ha-*ras* restriction fragments in cancer patients and cancer-free controls has revealed a marked inequality in the distribution of fragments with allelic

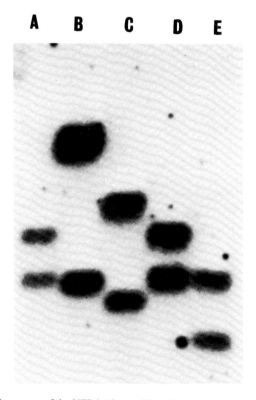

Fig. 3.   Polymorphic fragments of the VTR4.1 locus. Five WBC DNAs were digested with HaeIII and blotted. Probe was the nick-translated VTR4.1 tandem repeat. DNAs possessing fragments corresponding to alleles a1 and a4 (lanes A and D), a1 and a5 (B), a2 and a3 (C), and a1 and a6 (E) are shown. a3 is the upper band of lane C.

TABLE V. Comparison of Allele Distribution at Two Distinct
VTR Loci*

| Ha-*ras* | | 4.1 | |
Allele	No.	Allele	No.
a1	493	a1	651
a2	86	a2	89
a3	70	a3	26
a4	56	a4	2
a1.2	15	a5*	2
a1.1	8	a6*	1
a4.1	7	a7	1
a5	4		
a1.3	4		
a2.2*	3		
a3.2*	3		
a0.1*	2		
a2.01*	2		
a1.4*	2		
a3.1*	2		
a2.02*	1		
a2.1*	1		
a2.11*	1		
a2.12*	1		
a4.2*	1		
a3.3*	1		
a3.4*	1		
a2.015*	1		
a2.025*	1		
a>1*	2		
a>2*	1		
a>3*	4		
a>4*	1		
Total	774		772

*The asterisk (*) indicates alleles detected only in DNAs from tumors
or patient WBC. a > 1 designates unusual fragments migrating
between a1 and a2; a > 2, between a2 and a3; a > 3, between a3
and a4; and a > 4, above a4. These fragments do not appear to
comigrate with intermediate alleles but have not yet been further
characterized.

frequencies below 0.5%. These rare alleles have thus far been observed only in
cancer patients. From studies with first-degree relatives and kindreds, as summarized
above, it is likely that the mode of transmission for rare alleles is truly mendelian. It
is quite possible that these alleles arise over much shorter time periods than one would
ordinarily expect genetic variation to occur. Jeffreys et al [17] reported the de novo
appearance of a new allele at another tandem repeat locus. Perhaps such repeats are
more unstable in high-risk groups. In any event, once a new *ras* fragment appears,
its mode of inheritance is apparently uncomplicated.

We have also shown that the ethnic distribution in our study populations is
unlikely to affect our conclusions. First, no ethnic group with a demonstrably low
frequency of rare alleles is overrepresented in the "control" group. Second, no ethnic
group with a demonstrably high frequency of rare alleles is overrepresented in the
"cancer" group.

The high degree of polymorphism and the association of many rare alleles with cancer patients was not observed with another tandem repeat locus, VTR4.1. At the present time, we cannot ascribe this difference to some intrinsic feature of Ha-*ras* (thereby favoring a direct role of this region in pathogenesis) or to the unsuitability of VTR4.1. We will continue to search for an independent VTR locus as polymorphic as Ha-*ras* to repeat this type of comparison. A population analysis with insulin, which does have as many allelic fragments as *ras,* is being contemplated. We would prefer, however, to conduct the initial studies with unlinked markers (Insulin, like Ha-*ras*, is on 11p).

We have recently obtained molecular clones of the common (a1) and unique (a2.1) allelic fragments from the WBC DNA of a patient with familial melanoma. Studies are now in progress to determine if phenotypic differences between the clones can be detected. This approach, together with continuing population studies, may lead to an understanding of the molecular genetic basis of cancer risk.

ACKNOWLEDGMENTS

This work was supported by the American Institute for Cancer Research and by NIH grant CA37866 as well as by the Laub Memorial Fund of the New England Medical Center Hospitals. N.A.D. and M.C. were supported by postdoctoral training grants HL07437 and CA09429, respectively. T.G.K. is a fellow of the John A. and George L. Hartford Foundation.

REFERENCES

1. Nathans D, Smith H: Annu Rev Biochem 44:273, 1975.
2. Barker D, et al: Cell 36:131, 1984.
3. Lawn RM, et al: Cell 15:1157, 1978.
4. Kan YW, Dozy AM: Proc Natl Acad Sci USA 75:5631, 1978
5. Wyman AR, White R: Proc Natl Acad Sci USA 77:6754, 1980.
6. Bell GI, et al: Nature 295:31, 1982.
7. Goodbourn SEY, et al: Proc Natl Acad Sci USA 80:5022, 1983.
8. Goldfarb M, et al: Nature 296:404, 1982.
9. Capon DJ, et al: Nature 302:33, 1983.
10. White R, et al: Nature 313:101, 1985.
11. Krontiris TG, et al: Nature 313:369, 1985.
12. Botstein D, et al: Am J Hum Genet 32:314, 1980.
13. Marx JL: Science 229:150, 1985.
14. Chang EH, et al: Nature 297:479, 1982.
15. Maniatis T, et al: Proc Natl Acad Sci USA 72:1184, 1975.
16. Maniatis T, et al: "Molecular Cloning". Cold Spring Harbor, NY: Cold Spring Harbor Laboratory, 1982.
17. Jeffreys AJ, et al: Nature 314, 67, 1985.
18. Southern EM: J Mol Biol 98:503, 1975.
19. Der CJ, et al: Proc Natl Acad Sci USA 79:3637, 1982.
20. Marshall C, et al: Nature 310:586, 1984.

Biochemical and Molecular Epidemiology of Cancer 111–125 (1986)

Cancer: A World-Wide Perspective

Richard Doll

Imperial Cancer Research Fund, Cancer Epidemiology and Clinical Trials Unit, The Radcliffe Infirmary, Oxford OX2 6HE, United Kingdom

I have long believed that the practical prevention of cancer would be advanced more quickly were there closer collaboration between those who study the conditions under which the disease occurs in man and those who seek to understand the mechanism by which the progeny of a cell escape from control, multiply uselessly, and distribute themselves about the body. The time when laboratory research workers seemed to think that leukemia was the most common form of cancer is long past, and the main facts about the incidence of the different types, and the ways in which it varies throughout the world, are now well known. Even newspapers and television like to describe the hot spots of esophageal cancer in China and are quick to announce that cancer of the lung has overtaken cancer of the breast as the leading cause of fatal cancer in women in yet another American state, and there can be few who are interested in cancer who do not have a fairly clear idea of the qualitative importance of the established causes of the principal types. I thought, therefore, that I would review only briefly the problems that cancer presents in different parts of the world and expand on three fields in which epidemiology and laboratory science overlap: namely, the role of genetic susceptibility in determining the risk of disease, the practical measures for prevention, and the use of biological markers in identifying human hazards.

WORLD-WIDE FREQUENCY

Any quantitative estimate of the total burden of different types of cancer on a world scale is, of necessity, only very approximate; there are no reliable figures for the incidence of the disease in many large populations. Parkin, Stjernswärd, and Muir [1], have, however, provided an intelligent guess at what the burden is likely to be using the best available data for each of the 24 geographical areas for which population estimates and projection are regularly produced by the United Nations. These varied, of course, in quality from the precise figures for incidence with a high proportion of cases histologically confirmed that have been collected by long estab-

Received May 8, 1985.

© **1986 Alan R. Liss, Inc.**

lished registries to hospital series for the proportions of cancers of different types that had to be converted to national rates from general knowledge of the relationship between cancer mortality and total mortality in different populations at various stages of development. On this basis, Parkin and colleagues were able to suggest figures for 12 of the most common types and for cancers of all sites combined excluding cancer of the skin.

These 12 types are listed in Table I. Three it will be noted (oral-pharyngeal tumors, lymphatic tumors, and leukemia) are not specific types of cancer but groups that include cancers with different causes varying in incidence in different places. Other cancers that are common in some areas had to be omitted. Skin cancer was omitted entirely because it is so rarely fatal that its incidence is seldom accurately recorded, and cancers of pancreas, larynx, ovary, corpus uteri, and penis were omitted as individual types (though included in the total) because of diagnostic difficulties or because the data were too few to allow estimates to be made.

Most data were available for a period in the mid-1970s, and the results shown in Table II are those estimated for 1975. The figures must, however, be appreciably greater by now; not only is the world population growing (from a little over 4 billion in 1975 to a projected figure of 5.2 billion in 1990), but the demographic changes that have followed the reduction of infant and childhood mortality are producing progressively greater proportions of persons in the middle and older age groups among whom cancer is more likely to occur. Age-specific incidence rates of some of the cancers

TABLE I. Types of Cancer for Which Incidence Is Estimated [1]

Mouth and pharynx	Prostate
(lip, tongue, buccal cavity, salivary gland,	Bladder
nasopharynx, pharynx)	Lymphatic tissue
Esophagus	(Hodgkin's, non-Hodgkin's, myeloma)
Stomach	Leukemia
Colon and rectum	(chronic myeloid, chronic lymphatic, acute
Liver	myeloid, adult T-cell, other acute lymphatic)
Lung	
Breast	
Cervix uteri	

TABLE II. Estimated Numbers of Cancers Occurring Worldwide in 1975 [1]

Type of cancer	No. in thousands
Stomach	682
Lung	591
Breast	541
Colon/rectum	507
Cervix	459
Mouth/pharynx	340
Esophagus	296
Liver	259
Lymphatic	221
Prostate	198
Bladder	176
Leukemia	170

Other sites (by subtraction) = 1,430; all sites other than skin = 5,870.

are changing too, the most notable being those for gastric and lung cancer, which are, respectively, decreasing and increasing nearly everywhere. According to the International Agency for Research on Cancer [2], the number of new cases of lung cancer will have been more than 1 million in 1984 and the lung already will have displaced the stomach as the leading site for the development of the disease.

The importance of the individual types varies, of course, from one population to another because of differences in the age distribution of the population, differences in exposure to carcinogenic agents, and differences in susceptibility that might be either genetic or acquired. If allowance is made for demographic factors, which are of interest, in relation to cancer, only insofar as they affect the need for clinical care, the other factors cause a range of age-specific risks that is less than fivefold only when the cancer is uncommon everywhere, and they often cause a range of 100-fold or more as in the case of cancers of the esophagus, liver, and penis, nonmelanomatous cancers of the skin, Burkitt's lymphoma, and Kaposi's sarcoma.

The 19 types listed in Table III are so common in some populations that, in the absence of other causes of death, 1% or more of men or women would develop the disease by 75 yrs of age, and five are sometimes so common that under the same conditions they would affect 10% of men or women by the same age. All vary at least sixfold when comparisons are made at the ages for which even the data from cancer registries in poor countries are likely to be reasonably reliable. These types, it will be noted, include ten of the 12 types studied by Parkin et al [1]. The two remaining types (lymphatic tumors and leukemia) are, however, omitted; they are groups of several etiologically distinct diseases, none of which is individually common enough anywhere to meet the criteria for inclusion. Of these 19 types that are common some-

TABLE III. Range of Incidence Rates for Common Cancers

Type of cancer	Sex	High incidence population	Highest cumulative incidence	Ratio of highest and lowest rates[a]
Skin (chiefly nonmelanoma)	M	Australia, Queensland	>20	>200
Esophagus	M	Iran, northeast	20	300
Lung	M	England	11	35
Stomach	M	Japan	11	25
Cervix uteri	F	Columbia, Coli	10	15
Prostate	M	US black	9	40
Liver	M	Maputo (part)	8	100
Breast	F	Canada, British Columbia	7	7
Colon	M	US, Connecticut	3	10
Corpus uteri	F	US, Los Angeles	3	30
Buccal cavity	M	India, Bombay	2	25
Rectum	M	Denmark	2	20
Bladder	M	US, Connecticut	2	6
Ovary	F	Denmark	2	6
Nasopharynx	M	Singapore, Chinese	2	40
Pancreas	M	New Zealand, Maori	2	8
Larynx	M	Brazil, Sao Paulo	2	10
Pharynx	M	India, Bombay	2	20
Penis	M	Uganda (part)	1	300

[a]At 35–64 years of age, standardized for age.

where, only one is so evenly distributed that 1% of one sex would always be affected: that is, cancer of the breast.

The cumulative incidence of all types of cancer varies, in contrast, somewhat less, the range recorded by the IARC [3] for 70 populations being less than fivefold, whereas the ratio of the incidence recorded for the two sexes varied only betweeen 0.7 and 1.8 to 1 and was mostly between 1.0 and 1.3 to 1 despite the existence of several prevalent cancers limited to one sex. This degree of variation in the incidence of all types of cancer combined is, as Julian Peto (personal communication) pointed out, slightly more than would be obtained if hypothetical registries were created by allocating one of the observed incidence rates, or one of the observed sex ratios, for each type of cancer to each registry at random. Some of the variation, however, must be due to a failure to pick up all cases in some of the less developed populations, particularly those occurring in old age, and the simplest interpretation of this degree of variation is that the incidence of each type is determined independently of the others.

GENETIC SUSCEPTIBILITY

There are, therefore, no grounds for the hypothesis that Cramer [4] put forward 50 years ago: namely, that the proportion of the population susceptible to cancer is relatively small, that practically all who are susceptible develop it, and that the effect of exposure to different agents is to determine only the site and the age at which the cancer appears. I mention the hypothesis, however, because it seems to have an extraordinary vitality and keeps being resurrected. In fact, it is not needed to explain the observations that gave rise to it and, for at least two reasons, is patently untrue.

First, family studies have never shown any evidence of familial excess of cancers of all types, not even among the families of patients with *xeroderma pigmentosum*. Familial clustering of cases is usually limited to particular types of cancer or, in a few exceptional cases, to a few types specifically associated with each other. Second, industrial hazards that have caused a particular type of cancer in 30–50% of exposed men have never been accompanied by any reduction in the age-specific incidence of other types, which has continued to be the same as in the nonexposed population.

Genetic susceptibility to a particular type of cancer, however, is another matter. Differences in this type of susceptibility account for some of the differences in incidence between population groups—certainly for some of the differences in skin cancer and (to a small extent) for gastric cancer through differences in blood group distribution and possibly for some of the differences in chronic lymphatic leukemia, which is so rare in Chinese, Japanese and Indians irrespective of the conditions under which they live. However, the evidence of changing incidence rates with time and on migration and the close correlation between the incidence of individual types of cancer with aspects of lifestyle, both across national boundaries and between social groups within them, make it difficult to believe that hereditary determinants of susceptibility are responsible for most of the recorded differences in incidence.

Two sets of observations seem at first sight to rule out any major differences in susceptibility to the development of the common cancers, but more detailed analyses suggest that this deduction is unjustified.

First, it has long been known that most of the common cancers show some degree of familial clustering but that the risk among sibs of probands is seldom more than twice that in the general population, and we cannot exclude the possibility that an excess of this degree is due to a common environment. This was certainly not excluded in the one large study that reported familial clustering of lung cancer in that the allowance for smoking habits was incomplete [5]. Even childhood cancers, which might be expected to have a large genetic component, show only a weak tendency for familial clustering, as is illustrated by the experience of some 15,000 families in Britain among whom one or more children developed cancer earlier than 15 yrs of age, ie, the majority of affected families in the country over a 20-yr period [6]. If we exclude data for twins and for children with cancers with a simple genetic basis, such as retinoblastoma and *xeroderma pigmentosum* the total cancer risk among sibs of affected children was about 2/1,000, ie, about twice normal, and the relative risk for the same type of cancer as the probands varied beween 1 and 7 (Table IV).

Such small relative differences are, however, consistent with large differences in susceptibility [7,8]. Consider for example a recessive gene that increases the risk of a particular cancer 50-fold in homozygotes. The relative risk in the sibs of probands would be just over fourfold if the population frequency of the gene was approximately 10% and less (and possibly much less) if the gene frequency was either higher or lower. Even in identical twins the relative risk could be small (as it is for most common cancers), as is shown in Table V, depending again on the population frequency of the gene. Also, similar analyses show that the observed relative risk

TABLE IV. Pairs of Siblings Developing Cancer in Childhood [6]

Type of cancer	Ratio of numbers observed and expected with these types of cancer						
	Leukemia	Lymphoma	Central nervous system	Neuro-blastoma	Wilm's	Bone	Other
Leukemia	2.3	2.9			1.2		
Lymphoma		5.4			0.6		
Central nervous system			2.9	2.5	1.2	5.0	3.1
Neuroblastoma				7.5	—	—	5.4
Wilm's					—	—	—
Bone						—	—
Other							3.6

TABLE V. Risk of Cancer in Relatives of Probands Relative to Unit Risk in General Population: Susceptibility Determined by Recessive Gene [8]

Incidence in homozygotes relative to unit incidence in others	Gene frequency					
	0.01		0.10		0.50	
	Identical twin	Sibling	Identical twin	Sibling	Identical twin	Sibling
2	1.00	1.00	1.01	1.00	1.12	1.05
10	1.01	1.00	1.67	1.20	2.44	1.60
50	1.24	1.06	11.7	4.16	3.56	2.07
100	1.96	1.24	25.5	8.24	3.77	2.15
∞	10^4	2,550	100	30.3	4.00	2.25

would be compatible with a mixture of susceptibilities ranging up to 100-fold. It follows therefore that, whereas some of the observed examples of familial clustering could be due to a common environment, other examples could well reflect major variations in the genetic susceptibility of different individuals, particularly, perhaps, the excess of breast cancer in the families of women who develop bilateral disease earlier than 50 yrs of age [8].

The other set of observations that might be regarded as militating against the possibility of such variation is the steady increase in the incidence of cancer with a power of age that is observed in most populations for most of the common cancers other than those of the organs of reproduction. This rules out the possibility that cancer occurs only in a small proportion of highly susceptible people, the rest being not susceptible at all. If it did, the age-specific incidence rate would have to cease increasing with age once a substantial proportion of the population had already developed the disease, and this does not generally happen until after 80 yrs of age, when the diagnosis of cancer is too incomplete to justify use of the data, provided, that is, that circumstances have been stable for long enough for both the young and the old to have been regularly exposed to the same carcinogenic agents to the same extent from the same initial age.

Only one set of data that I am aware of shows a flattening of the curve relating incidence to age in a high-risk population under these conditions: namely, that showing the incidence of hepatocellular carcinoma in parts of Mozambique, where the population is exposed to extremely large amounts of aflatoxin. According to Van Rensburg et al [9], the incidence in these groups ceases to rise after 40 yrs of age and eventually decreases, whereas in lower-risk populations the incidence continues to rise into old age. Cancer incidence data for old age groups in developing countries is, of course, liable to be deficient, but this has been allowed for by Van Rensburg and colleagues, and the shapes of the curves are notably different for high- and low-risk populations in the same country. In this case, however, the factor determining susceptibility is presumably not genetic but is acquired as a result of childhood infection with the hepatitis B virus.

Many sets of national data for other types of nonreproductive cancer have at some time shown a reduction in the rate of increase in mortality in old age, but this has nearly always ceased to occur, at least in those under 80 yrs of age, as diagnostic standards have improved. Sometimes too a peak incidence has been observed between 60 and 65 yrs of age, as happened with lung cancer following the introduction of cigarette smoking, but this is a cohort effect that has disappeared progressively with time and there is no suggestion that the pool of susceptibles is nearing exhaustion up to 80 yrs of age, even in men who smoke 25 cigarettes or more per day, despite the fact that more than 30% of them would develop the disease by this age in the absence of other causes of death.

These observations, however, do not rule out the possibility that susceptibility varies as much as 50-fold. This, as Julian Peto [8] has shown, is consistent with a progressive increase in incidence with age, at least until a cumulative incidence has been produced as great as that currently observed for cancer of the lung. With a cumulative incidence of this order and 1% of the population 50 times as susceptible to the disease as the rest, the susceptible group would be virtually extinct by 50 yrs of age, but the inflection in the curve relating incidence to age would be extremely small. If 10% were susceptible, the inflection would be large, but it would occur at the end of the human life span, when recorded rates for many cancers show a comparable decline that could well be due to underdiagnosis. If 50% were susceptible, the falling in incidence would be gross, but it would not occur until the cohort had reached the age of 100 yrs. With the cumulative incidence rates that are actually observed, a high-risk subgroup would have to suffer a 100-fold greater risk for its elimination to produce an incidence pattern that was detectably different from that in a homogeneous population.

The small effect of even gross heterogeneity has been demonstrated particularly neatly in an animal experiment in which benzo(a)pyrene was applied regularly to the skin of outbred Swiss mice [10]. A crude analysis showed that the incidence of tumors varies as a power of the duration of regular treatment in the same way as the incidence of lung cancer in humans varies with the duration of cigarette smoking and the incidence of skin cancer varies with the duration of exposure to ultraviolet light. However, when Parish [11] reanalyzed the data to assess separately the incidence of first, second, third, and fourth tumors among animals that had previously shown, respectively, zero, one, two, or three tumors, she found that there was substantial heterogeneity among the animals in their susceptibility to tumor induction. After each period of exposure, the incidence of second tumors in mice that had already developed one tumor was substantially higher than that of first tumors in mice that had developed no tumors previously, and the incidence of third and fourth tumors in mice that had developed two or three tumors was higher still. Moreover, once exposure had been long enough for a high incidence rate to be achieved (ca 5% per wk) the increase in rate with further exposure fell off below the rate to be expected with the normal power law. When, however, the constant in the normal relationship:

$$\text{weekly incidence} = \text{constant} \times \text{some power of duration of exposure} \quad (1)$$

was replaced by a random term for each mouse representing susceptibility, a good fit to a typical fifth power relationship was obtained not only for first tumors but also for all subsequent ones. Precise description of the distribution of susceptibility is not possible with these data, but the fit obtained is compatible with a log normal variation spanning a range of more than 100-fold.

We see from this experiment that gross differences in susceptibility to tumor induction are compatible with an apparent power law relationship for the rate of induction of first tumors until the incidence rate approaches 5% per week in mice, corresponding to approximately 5% per year in humans, and even cigarette smokers regularly smoking 25–40 cigarettes per day fail to achieve a lung tumor incidence rate of quite 2% per year by 80 years of age.

Genetic differences in physiological function could be responsible for differences in susceptibility, for example, the differences that have been observed in the efficiency of ciliary action in clearing atmospheric pollutants from the bronchi [13], but the most promising results have come from the study of variations in human capacity to metabolize exogenous chemicals. In vitro studies have shown interindividual variations in microsomal monooxygenase (MMO) levels and DNA binding for the liver, lung, colon, esophagus, and placenta, and for several types of cell, and twin and family studies have shown that genetic factors are primarily responsible for maintaining at least some of the variation. It still has to be shown, however, that any of these are closely related to the risk of developing cancer in humans.

One observation that is not in doubt is that induced levels of aryl hydrocarbon hydroxylase (AHH) are frequently high in cigarette smokers with lung cancer but not in patients with solid tumors or childhood leukemia. This association between lung cancer and high AHH levels is reminiscent of the finding that in mice genetically regulated variations in MMO inducibility largely determined susceptibility to the induction of cancer by many chemicals [14]. In humans, however, several physiological and environmental factors have been found to influence the level of such enzymes in mitogen-activated human lymphocytes, including age, season, and smoking habits [15,16], and it remains uncertain whether the high AHH levels in lung cancer patients are the cause of the disease or are confounded with it.

Another, and perhaps more promising, observation is the association between lung cancer and the ability to metabolize debrisoquine. A study of 245 lung cancer patients and 232 sex- and age-matched smoking controls found that extensive metabolizers were proportionally more frequent in the cancer patients (78.8% vs 27.8%) whereas poor metabolizers were very much less frequent (1.6% vs 9.0%) [17]. Similar excesses were not found in bladder cancer patients who were occupationally exposed in the dye-manufacturing industry [18] nor in patients with tumors of the large bowel [17].

A third association has been reported between bladder cancer and N-acetyl transferase activity. Animal studies suggest that hepatic N-acetyl transferase activity can be a rate-limiting step in the detoxification of the arylamines that cause bladder cancer [19], and this could be of importance in human cancer if the carcinogenic metabolites of arylamines to which workers in the dye industry and cigarette smokers are exposed are nonacetylated. However, the human data are conflicting. Small, statistically nonsignificant excesses of slow acetylators have been found in two series of bladder cancer patients [20,21], and a subset of one series showed a highly significant excess of slow acetylators in patients with occupational exposure to benzidene ($P < 0.001$) but no excess in cigarette smokers [21].

Such observations encourage the belief that knowledge of differences in susceptibility might help to unravel the mechanism of carcinogenesis, and it is probably for this reason that such knowledge is most worth pursuing. However, this might also enable high-risk groups to be identified among whom disease is liable to occur at particularly young ages and on whom prophylactic advice could be most usefully focused. It is unlikely, however, ever to lay to rest the concern expressed by Rauscher [22] and so frequently repeated that "Scientists are still unable to explain . . . why some heavy smokers apparently are resistant to the development of lung cancer . . . or why some vinyl chloride workers develop angiosarcoma of the liver" any more than advances in physics will explain why a particular uranium atom failed to decay.

CAUSES OF CANCER
Measures for Prevention

The most immediate need, therefore, is still to discover carcinogenic agents that can be avoided, and we still have very little idea of any such agents for half of the 12 types of cancer, each of which, according to Parkin et al [1], affects between 150,000 and 700,000 people every yr. For the other half, however, we can already visualize major reductions in risk, amounting in some cases almost to total elimination (Table VI).

TABLE VI. Measures for the Prevention of Leading Cancers on a National Scale

Measures for prevention	Type of cancer
Reduction of smoking and limitation of tar yield	Lung
	Mouth, pharynx, larynx, and esophagus
	Bladder, possibly kidney
	Pancreas
Reduction of chewing mixtures of betel, tobacco, and lime	Mouth and pharynx
Reduction of alcohol consumption	Mouth, pharynx, larynx, and esophagus
Elimination of bilharziasis (schistosoma haematobium)	Bladder
Immunization against hepatitis B virus	Liver
Reduction of aflatoxin in food	Liver
?Immunization against EB virus	Nasopharynx (in S. Chinese)
?Immunization against human papilloma virus	Cervix

TABLE VII. Incidence of Lung Cancer in Female Nonsmokers: Chinese and Other Women [23]

Area	Annual rate per 100,000			
	Chinese	Japanese	White	Hawaiian
Shanghai	18.4	—	—	—
Hong Kong	15.2	—	—	—
Hawaii	20.5	7.4	—	7.3
Japan, Miyagi	—	7.5	—	—
Los Angeles	—	—	7.5	—

The practical benefit to be expected from reducing the consumption of alcohol and tobacco and of the types of quid that are commonly chewed in much of Asia and the East Indies is too well known to need elaboration. Two points, however, are worth noting.

First, the total elimination of smoking would reduce the incidence of lung cancer to very low levels almost everywhere. Some few occupational hazards have caused substantial increases in nonsmokers (including exposure to asbestos and bischloromethyl ether), but the only large group among whom the rates in nonsmokers are known to be raised is that of Chinese women, for whom it is more than doubled irrespective of where they live [23] (Table VII). This presumably is due to some cultural characteristic, such as the use of the wok for cooking, rather than to genetic susceptibility, as the rates in Chinese men are similar to those in other ethnic groups.

Second, it is unrealistic to believe that whole populations will abandon smoking altogether within a few yrs. It is therefore important to discover whether it is possible to obtain substantial benefit by other means. That it is possible is shown most clearly by the reduction in mortality from lung cancer in Britain, where the death rate has fallen by two-thirds in men aged 30–39 yrs and is declining in men at all ages up to 75 yrs. This substantial fall began well before there was any material reduction in the amount of tobacco smoked in the corresponding sex and age groups and seems most likely to have been due largely to the reduction in the tar yield of the cigarettes smoked. That the effect should have been so much more marked in Britain and Finland (where the trends have been similar) than in many other countries can be explained by the fact that smoking habits had stabilized in these countries earlier than elsewhere, so that the mortality rate in men up to 50 yrs of age had already reached a plateau before tar yields began to be reduced, whereas in many other countries, including the US, the effects of tar reduction have been largely cancelled by the delayed effect of the increase in consumption that continued throughout the 1950s. Progressive restriction of the maximum yield of tar per cigarette might, therefore, be a valuable ancillary measure, particularly in China, Denmark, and the USSR., where the mean tar deliveries per cigarette are still 25–30 mg: that is, similar to those that were common in Britain and the US before 1960.

The other measures for the prevention of cancer listed in Table VI include two for the prevention of cancer of the liver. Either can be expected to reduce the high incidence of the disease in many parts of Africa and Asia to little more than that observed in North America and Europe, as it seems likely that two agents act synergistically. The evidence to inculpate the hepatitis B virus is, perhaps, stronger than that to inculpate aflatoxin, but neither alone can account for the geographical distribution of the disease. Immunization is likely to be the most reliable method in the long run, but it will take decades to show an effect, and the reduction of aflatoxin in the diet might conceivably be quicker acting.

The two other types of immunization that are listed in Table VI are more speculative. A vaccine against the EB virus has been developed using viral surface antigen (gp 340) incorporated into artifical liposomes, that induces virus-neutralizing antibodies in the cottontop tamarin monkey, one of the only two animals known to be fully susceptible to experimenal infection with the virus [24]. If it proves to be protective against infectious mononucleosis in humans (as the hepatitis B vaccine has been against hepatitis) it will certainly be worth trying in South China, Singapore, and Hong Kong, where nasopharyngeal cancer is always associated with infection with the virus and is one of the most common types. Whether a vaccine can be developed against the human papilloma virus remains to be seen, but the evidence that two or more types of the virus (certainly types 16, 18, and possibly some others) are involved in the production of cervical cancer, which will be reviewed elsewhere in this volume, is now very strong indeed.

If these various viruses (the hepatitis B virus, the EB virus, and some types of the papilloma virus) are, as I believe, causal factors in the production of human cancer, it is important to note that they all share a feature in common with the virus that causes adult T-cell leukemia/lymphoma: namely, that the cancers produced—with one exception discussed below—seldom appear until many years after infection has occurred. This suggests that other factors are also required before the clinical disease is indicated. In the case of the hepatitis virus, this appears to be exposure to aflatoxin, which is a powerful liver carcinogen in its own right in laboraory experiments. In the case of the EB virus, it might well be some chemical in the rotted, salted fish that is a favorite food of the Southern Chinese and is given to babies on weaning that helps to produce nasopharyngeal cancer [25], and occasionally it is intensive suppression, given, for example, to facilitate organ transplantation, that leads to the appearance of non-Hodgkin's lymphoma. However, there are as yet no clues to the other factors that contribute to the appearance of cervical cancer and adult T-cell leukemia/lymphoma. The one exceptional situation, when a long latent period does not seem to be required, follows infection with the EB virus in childhood in some tropical areas where Burkitt's lymphoma appears in a very small proportion of cases within 2–10 yrs.

These measures to which I have briefly referred, plus the elimination of bilharziasis in Egypt, Tanzania, and Malawi, might perhaps reduce the global risk of all cancers, other than cancer of the skin, by some 20%, but they would still leave very high risks of esophageal cancer in parts of central Asia, China, and perhaps also East and South Africa, as well as high and widspread risks of cancers of the stomach, large bowel, and breast.

Many clues to the causes of these cancers exist, some of which are summarized in Table VIII, but in no case is the evidence, in my opinion, sufficient to justify a national program for prevention. The evidence relating a low-fiber diet to the risk of cancer of the large bowel is, perhaps, the strongest, but a definite conclusion is unlikely to be reached until methods for the estimation of the many different types of dietary fibers have been agreed upon internationally and the physiological effects of each type established. Figures obtained by precise methods that exclude all starch reduce the negative correlation that has been reported between colon cancer and the pentose fraction, predominant in cereals, and it now seems that the closest negative correlation is with total nonstarch polysaccharides, to which vegetables make a major contribution [26,27].

The relation betwen the fat content of the diet and the risk of breast cancer, which is so clear between countries and is an attractive explanation of the trend in breast (and large bowel) cancer in Japan, remains uncertain when comparisons are made between individuals with and without the disease. Unlike myocardial infarction, the incidence of the disease is not correlated with such markers of fat intake as blood cholesterol [28] and obesity. The latter was thought to be correlated, but the association with obesity was with increased mortality, and this, it now seems, is due to a higher fatality rate in obese people once the disease has occurred rather than to an increased incidence [29]. The most promising clue to the cause of the disease is the relation that has been observed between incidence and the 17 β-estradiol (E_2) available in the blood (that is, free estradiol and estradiol bond to albumin). This is reduced after the first pregnancy, which has long been known to reduce the risk when pregnancy occurs early in life, and it is lower in Japanese women with a low risk of developing the disease than in the high-risk British. The difference between the national groups has been missed until recently, because it is not due to a difference in the concentration of sex hormone binding globulin (SHBG), which is almost identical in the two groups, but to a difference in the proportion of estradiol that is actually

TABLE VIII. Measures Possibly of Value for Prevention of Leading Cancers

Measure	Type of cancer
Dietary	
Increased fiber	Colon, rectum
Reduced fat	Breast, colon, rectum
Increased fruit	Stomach
Reduced nitrates	Stomach
	Esophagus (China)
Improved preservation of food	
Refrigeration	Stomach
Medication	
Vitamin A, β-carotene	Multiple sites
Vitamin C, E	
Vitamin B_2, B_6, B_{12}, folic	
acid	
Selenium	

bound to the globulin, a much lower proportion being bound in the British women (ca 30%) than in the Japanese (ca 50%) [30]. It is difficult, however, to see how this is going to lead to any practicable means of prevention, unless the proportions bound to the two types of protein are determined by, say, some dietary factor.

For the rest, I have listed a variety of vitamins and trace elements, deficiencies of which have been related to one or another type of cancer or, in the case of vitamin A complex, to epithelial cancers as a class. All are currently being investigated either in cohort studies in which serum banks are being utilized to provide information about the physiological state of people who subsequently develop cancer or remain cancer-free or in controlled trials to find out if prescription of the anticancer agent will reduce the risk of cancer in healthy people or will cause regression of premalignant changes.

A remarkable example of the latter is provide by the study that Hennekens et al [31] are carrying out in Boston, in which 22,000 US doctors are collaborating by taking tablets that contain either β-carotene or a placebo (and, as it happens, also aspirin and a placebo in attempt to see whether a small dose of aspirin will reduce the risk of vascular disease). The evidence on which the trial was based has been strengthened by the Stich et al [32] report of the effect of dietary additives on the proportion of cells showing micronuclei in buccal smears taken from betel and tobacco chewers in the Philippines. The proportion showing micronuclei reflects the frequency of chromatid breaks and translocations and can be taken as an index of the prevalence of the carcinogen to which the subjects are exposed. In men who chew the local mixtures of betel and tobacco, the proportion is about eight times higher than in men who neither chew nor smoke. After 9 weeks of administration of vitamin A or β-carotene, the percentage of micronucleated cells fell substantially (from 4.0% to 1.7% and from 3.4% to 1.2% respectively), whereas no reduction as observed with a placebo (3.4% to 3.3%) or with canthaxanthin, which resembles β-carotene in being an excellent quencher of singlet oxygen but is not converted to retinol. It cannot, of course, be assumed that a reduction in the micronuclei count necessarily implies a reduced risk of cancer, which can be determined only by longer-term studies on a larger scale, nor does it follow that similar results would be obtained in Western populations on a fuller diet. Indeed, the further evidence that has been obtained in the last few years in Norway [33], Britain (Wald, personal communication), and the US [34] has tended to weaken rather than to strengthen the negative correlations that had been reported between the vitamin A/β-carotene index of foods and the risk of lung cancer and between blood retinol levels and cancer incidence in general.

Use of Biological Markers

If epidemiologists are to contribute further to the discovery of the causes of cancer, they are, I think, most likely to do so if biochemists, pathologists, and molecular biologists are able to define biological markers that reflect the extent to which individuals have been exposed to suspect agents, thus enabling incidence to be related to objective measures instead of to descriptions that are seldom quantitative, often incomplete, and sometimes biased. One splendid example of such a marker is the evidence of viral infection, which has provided a clear picture of the importance of the hepatitis B carrier state in the etiology of cancer of the liver. Using such data, Beasley [35] was able to show that the risk of developing the disease is several hundred times greater in carriers of the virus than in noncarriers, and this is impossible to explain on any grounds other than that the virus is a cause of the disease. Now we can look forward to similar data to test the relationship between infection with specific types of the human papilloma virus and cervical cancer.

Another potentially useful marker is the frequency of stable abnormalities in the chromosomes of lymphocytes, which provides a measure of the extent of past exposure to ionizing radiations and possibly also to some mutagenic chemicals. Large numbers of cells need to be examined if exposure to small doses is to be detected, but counting such abnormalities could provide a useful technique to test, for example, the hypothesis that the excess of childhood leukemia observed around the British nuclear processing plant in Windscale is due not to chance but to a gross underestimate of the dose that local children have, in one way or another, received.

These are, however, special cases, and we shall have to learn much more about the mechanisms of carcinogenesis before it becomes practicable to measure changes in DNA that have been caused by specific chemical carcinogens in the sufficiently distant past to allow for an induction period that is commonly measured in decades. For the time being, we have to be content with markers of recent exposure that can be used to characterize high-risk groups or to pick out individuals at high risk, that is, if repetition shows that the results for a given individual are sufficiently constant for him or her to be allocated consistently to the same group. To be useful epidemiologically, such tests should not cause discomfort (except perhaps in very high-risk areas such as in Linxian, where people may even tolerate the taking of esophageal smears). In practice, this means that the tests are limited to the examination of serum, urine, feces, and saliva, hair and nail clippings, and cells from blood or smears from accessible organs. All these materials can be preserved in biological banks, which can be used in the future to test new hypotheses; the few that already exist are being used to test the predictive value of blood levels of trace elements, vitamins, and hormones. Among these banks, the most notable is the extraordinary collection of serum samples that has been obtained from randomly selected populations in the many counties of China that experience gross differences in the incidence of cancers of the esophagus, stomach, liver, nasopharynx, lung, and cervix (R. Peto, personal communication). Valuable though such banks already are, they will become progressively more valuable as new tests are developed to measure exposure, like the measurement of O^6-methyl-2^1-deoxyguanosine in DNA [36] and of metabolites of aflatoxin B_1 in urine [37].

One simple test that has been developed in Oxford [38] provides the means for measuring nitrates and nitrites in tissue fluids on a large scale, and this is enabling us to investigate the relationship between exposure to nitrates with a consequent risk of in vivo nitrosation and the risk of developing gastric cancer. So far, our studies have been limited to the comparison of people living in high- and low-risk areas in Britain and to men employed in the manufacture of nitrate fertilizers. The results, in brief, show either no relationship at all or an inverse relationship, due presumably to the fact that the main source of nitrates in the British diet is vegetables, which might contain some protective factors [39,40].

EPILOGUE

It seems, then, from this review, that the immediate outlook is for an increase in the incidence of cancer in the world as a whole, resulting primarily from the increasing proportion of old people in the populations of the developing countries and secondily to the spread of the high risk of cancers of the lung, breast, and large bowel that are currently associated with a high standard of living. Soon, however, we can expect to see a reduction in age-specific risks by the application of measures that are already clear. If it is possible to develop effective vaccines against the viruses that have been found to play a crucial part in the development of some of the common cancers, the total reduction worldwide might be as much as 20% and more, of course, in countries where tobacco-related cancers already cause a high proportion of all cancer deaths.

To those who are devoting their energy to the discovery of the causes of cancer, this rate of progress must seem disappointingly slow. From a historical perspective, however, the rate is seen to have accelerated so rapidly in the last 40 yrs that it is difficult to believe that avoidable causes of all the principal cancers will not soon be discovered and that it will be long before we can reduce the risk of developing cancer by 75 yrs of age, in the absence of other causes of death, from one in three or four, as it is now, to less than one in ten.

REFERENCES

1. Parkin DM, Stjernswärd J, Muir CS: Bull WHO 62:163, 1984.
2. International Agency for Research on Cancer: "Tobacco Smoking. IARC Monographs on the Evaluation of the Carcinogenic Risk of Chemicals to Humans." Lyon: IARC, Vol 38, 1985.
3. Waterhouse J, Muir C, Correa P, Powell J (eds): "Cancer Incidence in Five Continents." Lyon: IARC, Vol 3, 1976.
4. Cramer W: Lancet 1:1, 1934.
5. Tokuhata GK, Lilienfeld AM: J Natl Cancer Inst 30:289, 1963.
6. Draper GJ, Heaf MM, Wilson, LMK: J Med Genet 14:81, 1977.
7. Lilienfeld AM: Cancer Res 25:1330, 1965.
8. Peto J: In: "Banbury Report 4. Cancer Incidence in Defined Populations." Cold Spring Harbor, NY: Cold Spring Harbor Laboratory, 1980, pp 203–213.
9. Van Rensburg SJ, Cook-Mozaffari P, Van Schalkwyk DJ, Van der Watt JJ, Vincent TJ, Purchase IF: Br J Cancer 51:713, 1985.
10. Peto R, Roe FJC, Lee PN, Levy L, Clack J: Br J Cancer 32:411, 1975.
11. Parish SE: DPhil thesis, Oxford University, 1981.
12. Peto R, Parish SE, Gray R: "IARC Scientific Publication." Lyon: IARC, 1985.
13. Camner P, Philipson K, Friberg L: Arch Environ Hlth 24:82, 1972.
14. Pelkonen O, Nebert DW: Pharmacol Rev 34:189, 1982.
15. Suolinna EM, Vänttinen E, Aitio A: Toxicology 24:73, 1982.
16. Jett JR, Moses HL, Branum EL, Taylor WF, Fontana RS: Cancer 41:191, 1978.
17. Ayesh R, Idle JR, Ritchie JC, Crothers MJ, Hetzel MR: Nature 312:169, 1984.
18. Cartwright RA, Philip PA, Rogers HJ, Glashan RW: Carcinogenesis 5:1191, 1984.
19. Glowinski IB, Weber WW: J Biol Chem 257:1424, 1982.
20. Lower GM Jr, Bryan GT: Biochem Pharmacol 22:1581, 1973.
21. Cartwright A, Glashan RW, Rogers HJ, Ahmed RA, Barham-Hall D, Higgins E, Kahn MA: Lancet 2:842, 1982.
22. Rauscher FJ: In Mulvihill JJ, Miller RW, Fraumeni JF (eds): "Genetics of Human Cancer." New York: Raven Press, 1977, Foreword.
23. Shimizu H, Wu AH, Koo LC, Gao Y, Kolonel IN: JNCI (in press).
24. Epstein MA: Proc R Soc London Series B 221:1, 1984.
25. Armstrong RW, Armstrong MJ, Yu MC, Henderson BE: Cancer Res 43: 2967, 1983.
26. Englyst HN, Cummings JH: Analyst 109:937, 1984.
27. Bingham SA, Williams DRR, Cummings JH: Br J Cancer 52:399, 1985.
28. Hiatt RA, Friedman, GD, Bawol RD, Ury HK: JNCI 68:885, 1982.
29. Greenberg ER, Vessey MP, McPherson K, Doll R, Yeates D: Br J Cancer 51:691, 1985.

30. Moore JW, Clark MG, Takatani O, Wakabyashi Y, Hayward JL, Bulbrook RD: JNCI 71:749, 1983.
31. Stampfer MJ, Burring JE, Willett W, Rosner B, Eberlein K, Hennekens CH: Stat Med 4:111, 1985.
32. Stich HF, Stich W, Rosin MP, Vallejera MO: Int J Cancer 34:745, 1984.
33. Kvale G, Bjelke E, Gart JJ: Int J Cancer 31:397, 1983.
34. Willett WC, Polk F, Underwood BA, et al: N Engl J Med 310:430, 1984.
35. Beasley RP: Hepatology 2:215, 1982.
36. Umbenhauer D, Wild CP, Montesano R, Saffhill R, Boyle JM, Huh N, Kirstein U, Thomale J, Rajesnsky MF, Lu SH: (in press).
37. Garner C, Ryder R, Montesano R: Cancer Res 45:922, 1985.
38. Phizackerley PJR, Al-Dabbagh SA: Anal Biochem 131:242, 1983.
39. Forman D, Al-Dabbagh S, Doll R: Nature 313:620, 1985.
40. Al-Dabbagh S, Forman, D, Bryson D, Stratton I, Doll R: Br J Indust Med (in press).

Biochemical and Molecular Epidemiology of Cancer 127–134 (1986)

Genetic Oncodemes and Antioncogenes

Alfred G. Knudson, Jr.

Institute for Cancer Research, Fox Chase Cancer Center, Philadelphia, Pennsylvania 19111

The burden of cancer falls nonrandomly on a poulation. Some persons acquire cancer by chance alone. The somatic mutation hypothesis implies that background mutation rates would cause an irreducible burden of cancer in a population. A second group has a higher incidence of some cancer(s) because of exposure to environmental agents. A third group has a higher incidence as a result of genetic predisposition to environmental oncogenesis; xeroderma pigmentosum exemplifies this group. A fourth group is strongly predisposed to cancer because of inheritance of a mutation that constitutes one of the oncogenic steps. Each of these four groups can be called an *oncodeme,* a demographic unit with a peculiar susceptibility to a particular cancer.

The last group is of particular interest in that it has revealed a new class of "cancer genes" that is also important in the nonhereditary forms of the same cancers. Evidence has been assembled from the study of retinoblastoma (RB), Wilms tumor (WT), and neuroblastoma (NB) that two events are necessary in their causation. The first event is germinal in hereditary cases and somatic in nonhereditary cases, whereas the second event is somatic in both. The events are regarded as genetic (including mutation, deletion, and chromosome loss). The second event can arise de novo or by somatic recombination, in both cases leading to hemizygosity or homozygosity. Because the normal alleles of such genes are in effect antioncogenic, such loci have been calld *antioncogenes.* It was proposed that RB and WT would be the best models to test these hypotheses because constitutional deletion cases provide chromosomal localization of the relevant genes. Recent research of others has demonstrated that these mechanisms do operate and that such a group of cancer genes, different from oncogenes, exists.

Mutations in antioncogenes could provide the mechanism for oncogenesis in the common cancers. Each of the cancers includes a fourth oncodeme and each may be caused by two primary events, yet some cancers are apparently caused by primary changes in oncogenes or in their expression. Oncogenesis mediated by oncogene aberration may also involve two-hit kinetics and could, therefore, underlie the common cancers. Questions about these possibilities and about the interaction between oncogenes and antioncogenes remain to be answered.

Key words: oncodemes, hereditary cancer, cancer genes, oncogenes, antioncogenes

Received April 17, 1985.

© **1986 Alan R. Liss, Inc.**

To the extent that spontaneous somatic mutations can produce a cancer, there will always be some "background" incidence of that cancer, and we cannot anticipate eradication of the disease. Under conditions of an indefinite life span all individuals would ultimately contract some cancer. However, all indications are that this background incidence of cancer is a small part of the total and that much of human cancer occurs among persons who have a genetic susceptibility and/or oncogenic environmental exposure. We can begin by dividing a population into four subgroups, or *oncodemes* [1], with respect to the incidence of a particular cancer: (1) background oncodeme, in which the incidence is determined by random mutations in "normal" persons, (2) environmental oncodeme, in which the incidence is elevated by exposure to an oncogenic environmental agent, (3) environmental-genetic oncodeme, in which the incidence is determined by genetic susceptibility to an environmental agent, and (4) genetic oncodeme, in which genetic susceptibility is more important than either spontaneous or environmentally induced events. There could be more than one subgroup for each of the last three groups; for example, both smoking and asbestos are important agents in the etiology of lung cancer.

Very little is known about the third oncodeme. A well known but rare example is provided by skin carcinoma and melanoma in persons with xeroderma pigmentosum (XP). It appears that these cancers do not occur at increased frequency in XP subjects who are protected from sunlight. A basic defect in DNA repair leads to increased rates of mutation at all genetic loci following exposure to ultraviolet radiation, but the only mutations that seem to cause a problem are those that are oncogenic. It is almost certain that much of so-called environmental cancers occurs in this oncodeme, but there is still much to be learned.

The fourth oncodeme includes two classes of persons, those with enhanced rates of spontaneous occurrence of oncogenic events and those with a mutation that itself is one of the events on the path to cancer. The former may be exemplified by Bloom's syndrome, which has been reported to be associated with increased spontaneous mutation rates [2] and with increased rates of homologous chromosome exchange [3]. Such exchanges could in turn convert a cell that is heterozygous for a cancer mutation into one that is homozygous, thus revealing recessive cancer genes [4–6]. The second class of person harbors what can be called a *cancer mutation* and has revealed a new class of gene, which has been called *antioncogene* in order to distinguish it from the *oncogenes* originally associated with highly oncogenic retroviruses [7]. This is the class I wish to discuss here.

MATERIALS AND METHODS
Human Cases

There are at least 50 different known forms of hereditary cancer in man. In each form, susceptibility is transmissible to 50% of the offspring of affected persons. Penetrance of a given gene may be virtually 100% for these gene carriers. Familiar phenotypes of these mutations include heritable colon cancer (with or without polyps), breast cancer, skin cancer (nevoid basal cell carcinoma syndrome), pheochromocytoma, medullary carcinoma of the thyroid, and retinoblastoma. For purposes of analysis, attention was focused on the hereditary forms of three cancers observed in children: retinoblastoma, Wilms tumor, and neuroblastoma [8–10]. The advantages of studying the children's cancers are that the identification of affected persons is made early in life and that the hereditary cases constitute a significant fraction of all cases. The cases studied have been published previously [8–10], were seen at M.D. Anderson Hospital and Tumor Institute [8], or were seen at Children's Hospital of Philadelphia [11].

The data of interest were age of detection of tumor, bilaterality or unilaterality of tumor, number of tumors in some cases, associated phenotypic features, and karyotypes in a few cases.

Animal Cases

A putative animal model of dominantly heritable renal carcinoma in the rat has been reported by Eker and his colleagues [12,13]. We have recently begun a study of these animals with a principal objective of identifying homozygous offspring of matings between heterozygous rats. The heterozygous rat has a high penetrance for development of tumors by the age of 1 year, the mean number of tumors per animal being higher in the male than in the female. The studies include pathologic examination of the kidneys of heterozygous animals, the mating of heterozygous animals, and the examination of offspring, in some cases prenatally and in some cases postnatally.

RESULTS
Retinoblastoma, Wilms Tumor, and Neuroblastoma in Man

These studies demonstrated that the ages of detection of tumor are earlier for presumably heritable cases. Furthermore, the fraction of known cases yet undiagnosed by a given age declined in a semilog fashion for heritable cases, suggesting that tumor development required a single event in addition to the germinal mutation [8]. A similar plot for the ages of nonhereditary cases suggested that two events are necessary [8]. The results are contrasted in Figure 1.

From actual enumeration of tumors in the eyes of bilateral cases and from estimates of the relative frequencies of bilateral tumors, unilateral tumors, and absence of tumor, it was estimated that the numbers of tumors per heterozygous carrier of the mutant gene approximated a Poisson distribution, with $m \cong 3$ [8]. These data are summarized in Table I.

One interesting case of retinoblastoma was found to have a constitutional deletion of chromosome 13, extending from band q14 to band q22 [11].

Studies of Wilms tumor and neuroblastoma revealed similar differences in ages of onset between hereditary and nonhereditary cases [9,10]. Patients with aniridia showed the pattern of hereditary cases [9].

Hereditary Renal Carcinoma in the Rat

Some heterozygous animals can be identified by examination of the kidney following unilateral nephrectomy at the age of 5–6 months. Matings of heterozygous animals have resulted in litters of smaller (six to eight offspring) size than found for matings of heterozygous X normal matings (eight to 12 offspring). In two instances, hysterectomy was performed at 18 days of gestation and revealed a total of 22 placentas, 16 of which were normal and contained apparently normal fetuses and six of which were very small and contained no detectable fetus but rather masses of dead

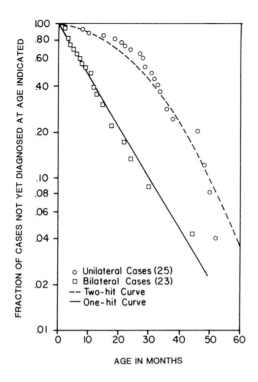

Fig. 1. Comparison of ages at diagnosis for hereditary (bilateral) and nonhereditary (unilateral) cases of retinoblastoma.

TABLE I. Frequency of Tumors in Heterozygotes for the Retinoblastoma Gene [8]

	Expected[a] (%)	Observed (%)
Tumors in one eye in bilateral cases		
1	43	53
2	33	26
3	17	14
4	6	6
5	1.8	1.5
Eyes affected per heterozygote		
0	5	1–10
1	35	25–40
2	60	60–75

[a]Assuming a Poisson distribution with m = 3.

or dying cells. Whether these cells are neoplastic is not yet known. Further studies are currently being conducted.

DISCUSSION

From the analysis of the ages of onset of retinoblastoma, Wilms tumor, and neuroblastoma, it was concluded that each of these tumors arose as a result of two events or "hits." The first event was regarded as a germinal mutation in hereditary cases and a somatic mutation in germinal cases.

Comparison of the deletion case of retinoblastoma to other deletion cases led to the conclusion that the critical chromosomal site was 13q14 [11], a conclusion that was corroborated in a case with a very small deletion entirely within this band [14]. The inclusion of the esterase D gene in these deletions and the existence of a population polymorphism for electrophoretic mobility of esterase D permitted a test of linkage in hereditary cases without deletion. From these data, it can be concluded that all hereditary cases resulted from mutation (or deletion) at the same locus [15,16].

Examination of nonhereditary cases has revealed deletion of this same site in the tumors of a few, although no deletion is found constitutionally [17–19]. This finding supports the original hypothesis that the first event affects the same site in all cases of retinoblastoma whether hereditary or nonhereditary.

Similar conclusions have been made for Wilms tumor. The aniridia cases were hypothesized to be deletions that include both a Wilms tumor locus and an aniridia locus [9]. The first report that supported this hypothesis described a translocation between chromosomes 8 and 11 and concluded that a portion of chromosome 8 was deleted [20]. Subsequent investigation revealed that the deletion was in chromosome 11 [21], in keeping with other deletion cases that had been reported in the meantime. The critical band is 11p13 [22]. As with retinoblastoma, some nonhereditary cases of Wilms tumor, without constitutional deletion, have been shown to have a deletion in tumor cells [23,24].

No constitutional deletion cases have been reported for neuroblastoma, nor has linkage with a known locus. However, many tumors reveal heterozygosity for a deletion in chromosome 1p, which might yet prove to be the locus of a neuroblastoma gene [25,26].

It was hypothesized that the second event in all three tumors was the development of homozygosity (or hemizygosity) and that these oncogenic mutations are recessive with respect to oncogenesis [4,27,28]. It was proposed that the second event could be a new one, such as submicroscopic mutation, deletion, or chromosomal loss by nondisjunction [4,28]. Six genotypes were proposed according to the six possible combinations of three aberrations, $13q^{rb}$ (submicroscopic mutation), $13q^-$ (deletion), or 13^- (chromosomal loss), although some genotypes would probably be lethal. It was also proposed that the second event might be mitotic recombination [4,28]. In fact, both classes of mechanism have been reported following the use of linked markers and karyotyping.

So, it appears that two human tumors, retinoblastoma and Wilms tumor, are attributable to recessive mutation (or loss) at a specific locus. Both tumors occur in two classes of individuals, one of "normal" phenotype and one heterozygous for germinal mutation at the relevant locus. Theoretically, there should be a third group of individuals who are homozygous for the mutation (Table II). In these hosts, no somatic event would be necessary, and every target cell in the susceptible tissue would become a tumor cell. Since all tissues are formed prenatally, such homozygous genotypes should prove lethal to the fetus [4]. In the rat model, in which heterozygotes are susceptible to a tumor in adult life, the homozygote dies prenatally. This finding supports the idea that homozygosity is both necessary and sufficient for oncogenesis in this system. No "third event" is necessary. These hereditary cancers of man and rat have revealed a new class of cancer gene, different from the oncogenes first

TABLE II. Tumors Caused by Recessive Genes in Hosts of Different Genotypes

	Genotype		
	Normal	Heterozygote	Abnormal
Host	$+/+$	$+/-$	$-/-$
Tumor	$-/-$	$-/-$	$-/-$
Somatic events	2	1	0
Tumor number	Rare	1	Many

discovered in certain retroviruses. Because the normal alleles of this new class of cancer gene are in effect antioncogenic, such genes have been called antioncogenes [1,7]. Oncogenes produce their effects via heightened or qualitatively aberrant expression, whereas antioncogenes do so through loss of expression.

How general might the mechanism of oncogenesis by mutation in antioncogenes be? Since nearly all cancers seem to contain the fourth oncodeme of hereditary form, it might be that most cancers, both in the hereditary and nonhereditary forms, can be caused by recessive mutations of antioncogenes. Using a mathematical model that relates cancer incidence to cellular events, Moolgavkar and Knudson [29] have shown that the age-specific incidences of the common cancers are consistent with two genetic events. The same events could, therefore, occur in the first oncodeme spontaneously and in the second and third oncodemes, accelerated by environmental agents, with or without genetic interaction with those agents.

The fourth oncodeme should never be large for common cancers, because genes with lethal behavior in homozygotes and occasional lethal behavior in heterozygotes will be maintained in a population only by recurrent mutation. If the survival value of the normal genotype is 1, of a lethal genotype 0, and of intermediate genotype $1-s$, and if the mutation rate is μ, then the frequency of heterozygotes is 2 (μ/s). If $\mu \leq 10^{-5}$ mutations per locus per generation and s ≥ 0.1, then the heterozygote frequency cannot exceed 2×10^{-4}. It is interesting that the two most frequent hereditary predispositions to cancer that have yet been defined, polyposis coli and neurofibromatosis, both have frequencies of this order of magnitude.

If common cancers can be caused by mutations in antioncogenes, how can we accommodate the evidence that at least some cancers, eg, Burkitt lymphoma, can be caused by primary change in the expression of an oncogene? The common form of Burkitt lymphoma in Africa is associated with EB virus infection and seems to belong to the second oncodeme, whereas EB-negative cases appear to belong to the first oncodeme. There is no evidence for a fourth oncodeme for this tumor. However, the underlying genetic defect, a translocation between chromosome 8 and chromosome 14, 2, or 22, is the same for both of the first two oncodemes, Translocations may be a common mechanism for oncogenesis via oncogenes in man. Just as with antioncogenes, such a mechanism might also involve two events. Can the common cancers of adults, which probably occur in all four oncodemes, be caused by either mechanism (Table III)? Are retinoblastoma and Burkitt lymphoma atypical extremes in their apparent causation by just one of these two mechanisms? These are questions to be answered in the future.

Finally, we can take note of the possibility that there is a final common pathway for oncogenesis via oncogenes and antioncogenes. Comings [30] proposed a model in which what are here called antioncogenes are regulators of oncogenes. Under such

TABLE III. Occurrence of Certain Cancers According to Oncodeme and Primary Mechanism

	Primary mechanism		
Oncodeme	Oncogene	Antioncogene	Unknown
I	BL	Rb, WT	S, C, Br, L
II	BL		S, C, Br, L
III			S, C(?), Br(?), L(?)
IV		Rb, WT	S, C, Br, L

Abbreviations used: BL, Burkitt lymphoma; Rb, retinoblastoma; WT, Wilms tumor; S, C, Br, L, carcinoma of skin, colon, breast, lung, respectively.

conditions cancer could result if the oncogene or one of its cis-acting elements was altered or if the product of an antioncogene was not formed. Another scenario is one in which antioncogenes code for differentiation products that operate at cell surfaces. Oncogenesis could result from loss of both normal copies of the antioncogenes or from insertion of an abnormal oncogene product into the cell surface. These possibilities likewise leave questions to be answered in the future.

ACKNOWLEDGMENTS

This study was supported in part by an appropriation from the Commonwealth of Pennsylvania and by Public Health Service grant CA06927 from the National Cancer Institute.

REFERENCES

1. Knudson AG: Cancer Res 45:1437, 1985.
2. Vijayalaxmi, Evans HJ, Ray JH, German J: Science 221:851, 1983.
3. Chaganti RSK, Schonberg S, German J: Proc Natl Acad Sci USA 71:4508, 1974.
4. Knudson AG: In: "Excerpta Medica International Congress Series no. 411, Proc Fifth Intl Cong Hum Genet." Amsterdam: Excerpta Medica, 1976, p 367.
5. Passarge E, Bartram CR: Birth Defects: Orig Art Ser XII, Number 1:177, 1976.
6. Festa RS, Meadows AT, Boshes RA: Cancer 44:1507, 1979.
7. Knudson AG: Prog Nucleic Acid Res Mol Biol 29:17, 1983.
8. Knudson AG: Proc Natl Acad Sci USA 68:820, 1971.
9. Knudson AG, Strong LC: J Natl Cancer Inst 48:313, 1972.
10. Knudson AG, Strong LC: Am J Hum Genet 24:514, 1972.
11. Knudson AG, Meadows AT, Nichols WW, Hill R: N Engl J Med 295:1120, 1976.
12. Eker R, Mossige J: Nature 189:858, 1961.
13. Eker R, Mossige J, Johannessen JV, Aars H: Diagn Histopathol 4:99, 1981.
14. Yunis JJ, Ramsay N: Am J Dis Child 132:161, 1978.
15. Sparkes RS, Murphree AL, Lingua RW, Sparkes MC, Field LL, Funderburk SJ, Benedict WF: Science 219:971, 1983.
16. Connolly MJ, Payne RH, Johnson G, Gallie BL, Allerdice PW, Marxhall WH, Lawton RD: Hum Genet 65:122, 1983.
17. Balaban G, Gilbert F, Nichols W, Meadows AT, Shields J: Cancer Genet Cytogenet 6:213, 1982.
18. Gardner HA, Gallie BL, Knight LA, Phillips RA: Cancer Genet Cytogenet 6:201, 1982.
19. Benedict WF, Banerjee A, Mark C, Murphree AL: Cancer Genet Cytogenet 10:311, 1983.
20. Ladda R, Atkins L, Littlefield J, Neurath P, Marimuthu KM: Science 185:784, 1974.
21. Francke U, Holmes LB, Atkins L, Riccardi VM: Cytogenet Cell Genet 24:185, 1979.
22. Riccardi VM, Hittner HM, Francke U, Yunis JJ, Ledbetter D, Borges W: Cancer Genet Cytogenet 2:131, 1980.
23. Kaneko Y, Egues MC, Rowley JD: Cancer Res 41:4577, 1981.

24. Slater RM, de Kraker J: Cancer Genet Cytogenet 5:237, 1982.
25. Brodeur G, Green AA, Hayes FA, Williams KJ, Williams DL, Tsiatis AA: Cancer Res 41:4678, 1981.
26. Gilbert F, Balaban G, Moorhead P, Bianchi D, Schlesinger H: Cancer Genet Cytogenet 7:33, 1982.
27. Knudson AG: Adv Cancer Res 17:317, 1973.
28. Knudson AG: Semin Oncol 5:57, 1978.
29. Moolgavkar SH, Knudson AG: J Natl Cancer Inst 66:1037, 1981.
30. Comings DE: Proc Natl Acad Sci USA 70:3324, 1973.

Biochemical and Molecular Epidemiology of Cancer 135–148 (1986)

Geographical Epidemiology and Migrant Studies

C.S. Muir and J. Staszewski

International Agency for Research on Cancer, 69372 Lyon Cedex 08, France

The differences in the patterns of cancer between regions, countries, and ethnic groups, and the changes in risk that occur when parts of a population migrate to another part of the world, constitute the most compelling evidence that the determinants of most human cancers are environmental in nature. On the basis of incidence, mortality, and relative frequency data, the world cancer burden has been estimated to be about 6 million new cases per year around 1975, the commonest cancers in males being in rank order lung, stomach, colon and rectum, mouth and pharynx, and prostate, and in females breast, cervix uteri, stomach, colon and rectum, and lung. Regional site patterns of cancer distribution are described. Following examination of intracountry variations, including the very large differences observed within the US, the changes in risk that occur on migration are discussed. Cancer levels in the host country of recent migrants can on occasion be used to estimate risks in the country of origin. The main significance of migrant studies lies in the fact that the relatively rapid and large changes that occur with increasing length of residence in the new homeland cannot be due to genetic factors. The results of recent migrant studies in the UK and Australia are discussed, and the suitability of migrant groups in transit from one set of exposures to another for the identification of risk factors and of their mode of action is reemphasized. The problems associated with migrant studies are examined.

Key words: cancer, incidence, mortality, migrants, geography, environment

Geographical descriptive epidemiology, of which migrant studies are but a part, is concerned mainly with the occurrence and pattern of diseases in general populations and with regional and ethnic variations. From such information stems the cardinal hypothesis underlying most of our work in cancer today, to wit, that the determinants of cancer are environmental, using that word in the broad sense of all that impinges on the human organism [1]. (This definition of environment includes not only discrete chemical carcinogens in air, food, and water and at work but also the less readily defined life-style factors such as dietary, social, and cultural habits.) The evidence for this statement is developed below, following a consideration of the likely global burden of cancer and of patterns of geographical distribution.

Received April 17, 1985.

© **1986 Alan R. Liss, Inc.**

SIZE OF THE CANCER BURDEN

Available incidence, mortality, and relative frequency data have recently been used to estimate the worldwide frequency of major cancer sites. Around 1975, when the world population was estimated to be 4,066 million persons, the five most frequent cancer sites (skin excluded) on a global basis in males were considered to be lung, stomach, colon and rectum, mouth and pharynx, and prostate; in females they were breast, cervix uteri, stomach, colon and rectum, and lung [2]. These sites alone comprised 53% and 60% of the 3.0 million and 2.9 million cancers estimated to occur in males and females, respectively. From a public health point of view, these estimates are of great value in drawing attention to the fact that for males at least 20% (lung and mouth and pharynx) of cancers are preventable with current knowledge (Table I).

International Variation

The world-wide pattern, by region of the world or by country, is far from uniform, however, and large international variation has been reported for most cancer sites. To characterize such regional incidence patterns, cancer incidence data around 1975 published in the most recent (fourth) volume of "Cancer Incidence in Five Continents" [3] are used unless otherwise stated. This approach has the advantage that the data are more accurate than those derived from Parkin et al [2], but they are much more restricted in global coverage, there being few incidence data for virtually all of Africa and most of Asia and large portions of Central and South America.

Stomach cancer incidence in Japan was some eight to ten times higher than among US whites, being intermediate in other countries—generally higher in southern American, eastern and central Europe, and Polynesia than in western and northern Europe, India, and Senegal.

Lung cancer was the commonest form of malignant disease in males of Western countries. The highest rates, recorded in US blacks, Polynesians, and UK and US whites, were two to four times as high as most of those recorded in South America, Israel, Norway, Sweden, or Spain, some five to ten times higher than in India, and 100 times greater than in Senegal (even a large degree of underreporting in Senegal can explain only a part of the difference). In females, the incidence of this cancer was over ten times higher in Polynesians and three to six times greater in US whites and blacks, in the UK, and in China than in India, France, or Spain.

Colon and rectum cancer incidence was highest in the developed, affluent countries, particularly in North America, lower in northern, central, and, particularly,

TABLE I. Estimated Global Number of New Cases of Cancer (in thousands) Around 1975, in Rank Order, by Site and Sex [2]

Rank	Males Site	No.	Females Site	No.
1	Lung	464	Breast	541
2	Stomach	422	Cervix uteri	459
3	Colon/rectum	251	Stomach	261
4	Mouth/pharynx	233	Colon/rectum	256
5	Prostate	198	Lung	127
	All	2,969	All	2,902

eastern Europe and Latin America, and lowest in India and Senegal, the rates there being one-fifth or less those of high-risk countries.

Cancer of the breast was the commonest malignancy in females of the Western countries, particularly in North American whites, being about three times as high as in China and India and over four times as great as in Japan and Senegal. The rates in western and northern Europeans and in Israeli Jews tended to be higher than in those from eastern and central Europe, Latin America, and Spain.

Cancer of the cervix uteri was particularly frequent in parts of Latin America, Asia, and eastern and central Europe, as well as among US blacks and Hispanics, the incidence being three to ten times as high as in Israel and Spain and two to five times greater than in US whites and Asians.

The incidence of prostate cancer was highest in US blacks, about twice that in US whites. The rates in US blacks were ten times as high as in India, China and Japan, or Senegal. The incidence decreased when passing from North American whites to northern and western Europe, with a lower incidence in Latin America and one still lower in eastern Europe and Israel.

Cancers of the buccal cavity and pharynx comprise an aggregation of sites with quite different epidemiological features. They include cancer of the lip (not rare in white males and particularly frequent in parts of Canada but rare in nonwhite populations), nasopharynx (very frequent in southern Chinese but rare in most other populations), salivary gland (rare almost everywhere), and the other parts of the mouth and pharynx (particularly frequent in India and among French males). Overall incidence for these sites combined was highest in French males, in Chinese and Indians, over six times as high in most of North American whites, Australia, Polynesia, Europe (Latin countries excluded), Israel, Senegal, or Japan.

Regional and National Site Patterns

Distinct site patterns are found for many countries and regions of the world [2,3]. In East Africa, for example, the most frequent cancer is that of the liver, whereas the incidence of cancer of the colon and rectum, as well as of the lung, appears to be lower than anywhere outside Africa. Cervix cancer appears to be twice as frequent as breast cancer, and esophageal cancer more frequent than stomach cancer. There is a high incidence of lymphoma, including Burkitt's lymphoma, in young East Africans.

Japan is characterized by a very high stomach cancer incidence, whereas the incidence of lung cancer, and particularly of breast, prostate, endometrial, and ovarian cancers and lymphatic leukemia, is very low compared to North America and western Europe. A similar, only somewhat less pronounced pattern (except for the relative absence of lymphatic leukemia), is found in Poland.

China has very high incidence rates for cancers of nasopharynx, esophagus, liver, penis, and uterine cervix and low rates for those cancers that are rare in Japan.

In India, there is a very high incidence of cancers of the mouth and pharynx and high levels of esophagus and uterine cervix cancers and a low incidence of cancer of the stomach, colon and rectum, liver, lung, breast, and prostate and the leukemias.

"Western" countries (North America, Australia, New Zealand, and western and northern Europe) are generally characterized by a high incidence of cancer of the lung, colon and rectum, breast, and prostate, but there are substantial differences between these countries even for these major sites. For further discussion of geographical patterns see Muir et al [4].

Intercountry Variation

Variation in cancer incidence and mortality within a country can also be large. Differences between US. whites and blacks have already been mentioned. Indeed, within the US there is a large spectrum of risk for many common cancers (Table II). A distinctive site pattern prevails in Utah—the state with a substantial Mormon population, which follows a life-style involving low tobacco and alcohol consumption. The incidence there of cancers of the mouth and pharynx, pancreas, larynx, lung, and urinary bladder (and also colon, rectum, breast, cervix, and kidney) was distinctly lower than in any other US white population, hence the inclusion of a special column for Utah in Table II.

Within the state of Utah, Mormons and non-Mormons also showed substantial differences in risk (Table III). Urban and rural Mormons tended to have similar risks, whereas among non-Mormons most sites showed an urban excess [5].

Within-country variation of cancer mortality has been studied more extensively because mortality data are available for a whole country much more often than are the incidence data. Cancer mortality atlases have been published recently for several

TABLE II. Variation in Cancer Incidence* Patterns Within the United States

Site (sex)	High	Low	Ratio H/L	Utah[b]
Lip (M)	Utah 10.3	Nonwhites < 1.0	> 10	
Nasopharynx (M)	Bay area Chinese 14.6	Connecticut, Iowa 0.5	ca 30	
Esophagus (M)	Atlanta black 19.3	Utah, Hawaii white 2.4	ca 8	
Stomach (M)	Hawaii Hawaiian 36.6	Atlanta white 5.7	ca 6	
Colon (M)	Connecticut 32.3	Hawaii Hawaiian 13.7	ca 2.5	20.3
Rectum (M)	LA[a] Japanese 21.7	Alameda black 6.7	ca 3	9.9
Liver (M)	Bay area Chinese 18.1	Utah 1.0	ca 18	
Gallbladder (F)	American Indian 22.2	Detroit black 1.1	ca 20	
Pancreas (M)	Bay area black 18.3	LA Japanese 4.7	ca 4	7.0
Lung (M)	New Orleans black 107.2	American Indian 8.1	ca 13	32.9
Malignant melanoma (M)	Hawaii white 11.8	LA black 0.7	> 10	
Breast (F)	Hawaii Hawaiian 87.5	American Indian 19.3	> 4	63.8
Cervix (F)	Atlanta black 26.4	Hawaii Japanese and Filipino 6.4	ca 4	7.5
Corpus (F)	Atlanta white 38.5	New Orleans and Alameda black 10.5	ca 3.5	
Ovary (F)	Bay area white 14.4	New Orleans black 5.5	< 3	
Prostate (M)	Alameda black 100.2	Bay area Japanese 12.7	ca 8	
Testis (M)	Hawaii white 5.0	Detroit black 0.8	ca 6	
Bladder (M)	New Orleans white 24.5	Hawaii Hawaiian 5.9	ca 4	16.5
Kidney (M)	Hawaii white 11.2	Chinese < 3.0	> 3	6.6
Thyroid (F)	Hawaii Hawaiian 17.6	New Orleans black 2.8	ca 6	
Multiple myeloma (M)	Bay area black 8.4	Chinese and Japanese ≤ 1.7	< 5	

*The average annual incidence rates [2] per 100,000 population are age-standardized to the world population. All rates given are based on more than ten cases.
[a]LA, Los Angeles.
[b]See text.

TABLE III. Standardized Incidence Rates* for Selected Sites in Utah (1969–1971) by Religion and Residence [5]

Site (sex)	Mormons		Non-mormons	
	Urban	Rural	Urban	Rural
All (M)	73	72	115	76
Tobacco-related (M)	44	43	106	59
Colon (M)	67	49	104	54
Lung (M)	37	39	96	54
Breast (F)	84	74	121	97
Cervix (F)	54	60	120	111

*Third National Cancer Survey Rate for all areas included = 100.

countries, including Belgium, Canada, China, England and Wales, the Federal Republic of Germany, Japan, The Netherlands, Poland, Switzerland, and the US. The US data by county have been the most extensively studied for elucidation of possible risk factors. Cancer incidence atlases have recently been published for Scotland and Norway.

Validity of Comparisons

The findings from geographical epidemiology discussed so far have several limitations. First, good-quality data on cancer occurrence are available for only a limited number of populations [3], and for many, especially those in developing countries, they are incomplete, doubtful, or nonexistent. (Indices of quality are discussed in [3].) Further, the variations detected between populations in cancer risks might be not true but artefactually produced by differences in cancer recognition associated with lack of medical infrastructure, willingness and ability to seek medical advice, etc. Finally, the interpretation of the etiological meaning of the differences in cancer risk is often difficult: Are they due to genetic or racial differences or to environmental factors?

Changes Over Time

If differences in cancer risk are genetic in origin, they should be relatively stable as a population changes its genetic composition very slowly, yet very large changes have been observed over the past 50 years in many countries in the risk of common cancers [6]. Such changes have been in both directions—cancer of the stomach falling nearly everywhere with the decline beginning at different times, cancer of the lung rising again at different rates and at different times, malignant melanoma rising in fair-skinned populations, etc. Such evidence does not exclude a role for genetic factors (for example, skin pigmentation for malignant melanoma), merely indicating that the environment is a major determinant of risk.

To summarize, geographical epidemiology provides information on the cancer burden of populations as well as on variation in cancer risk patterns by site over space and time. Incompleteness and inaccuracy of this information often limit its usefulness. Nonetheless the mere existence of differences in cancer pattern can give rise to hypotheses about cause. Conversely, if a hypothesis does not explain the observed distribution, it is incomplete or wrong [7].

CANCER IN MIGRANTS

Studies of cancer in migrants may help to resolve some of the problems raised above. First, they can provide proxy data on populations originating in countries where cancer is difficult to measure. Second, they demonstrate whether changes in the environment such as occur after migration are followed by changes in cancer risk and the time needed for such changes to appear. On occasion, etiology can be uncovered and mechanism of action suggested.

Surrogate Data

If data on the occurrence of cancer in a given population do not exist, or are of doubtful value, a proxy estimate can be obtained when such information is available for recent migrants originating from that population. For example, the low mortality from prostate cancer in Poland had been questioned because it is a disease of older ages for which statistical data from Poland had not been very reliable; a low mortality from this cancer, however, was also found in Polish-born Americans [8]. The elevation of nasopharyngeal cancer risk in Cantonese as compared to other Chinese had been demonstrated for Chinese migrants to Singapore long before reliable data from China became available [9,10]. Such estimates of incidence in the country of origin based on the incidence among migrants, however, are founded on the questionable assumptions that their cancer risk is representative for the total country and that there is no short-term change in risk associated with migration. As has been pointed out repeatedly [11,12], migrants are rarely a representative sample of the population of the country of origin and may exhibit a variety of biases including a healthy migrant effect, a skewed age distribution, and a variety of social class differences (see also below). The estimate is more credible if the incidence among migrants of the cancer in question differs considerably from that in the host population and also if it is of the same order in migrants from a given country in different countries of settlement, as for prostate cancer in Polish migrants to England and Wales and to Australia as well as in those moving to the US [12–14].

Differences in the completeness and accuracy of cancer recognition can be greater, and are much more difficult to assess, in between-country comparisons than when migrants from the countries in question are compared within a common host country where they presumably share largely similar diagnostic and reporting procedures. Hence migrant studies may help to determine whether the similarities or differences in cancer occurrence detected by geographical epidemiology studies are true. For example, a higher incidence of stomach cancer incidence in eastern Europe in comparison to that in western and southern Europe, and an even higher incidence in Japan, has been corroborated by the findings in migrants from these countries to the US [12,15,16].

Significance of Migrant Studies

The significance of changes in cancer risk after migration was recognized by Kennaway in 1944 [17], who stated: "the very high incidence of primary cancer of the liver found among negroes in Africa does not appear in negroes in the United States of America, and is therefore not of a purely racial character. Hence, the prevalence of this form of cancer in Africans may be due to some extrinsic factor, which could be identified," and again by Steiner in 1954 [18]. It was not until

Haenszel's papers of 1961 and 1968 [15,16] that the full significance of migrant studies became more widely appreciated, despite reports on cancer mortality among the foreign-born in Boston in 1929 [19], Smith's pioneering analysis of cancer mortality in Japanese in the US in 1956 [20], and the work of Eastcott in New Zealand and Dean in South Africa on lung cancer risk in British migrants published in 1954 and 1959, respectively [21,22].

Besides leading to the recognition of the importance of environmental factors in cancer etiology, migrant studies have helped to identify these factors and to elucidate their modes of action. It has been found repeatedly that identification of environmental cancer risk factors, especially of those related to life-style, is much easier in populations in transit, subject to sizeable changes in habits and exposures, than in populations with a stable and uniform way of life [23]. Migrants are just such populations in transit. It was thus possible, for example, to identify dietary risk factors for stomach cancer in Japanese migrants to the US, whereas these factors were so uniformly spread out in Japan that their detection there was virtually impossible [24].

The mode and time of action of environmental cancer risk factors can also be indicated by migrant studies. For example, results of the studies on cancer in migrants from such diverse countries as Japan and Poland to the US have indicated that events early in life, in childhood, determine the risk of stomach cancer, whereas the risk of colon cancer depends on factors acting in adulthood (Tables IV, V).

For breast cancer, the situation is more complicated. In Polish-born migrants to the US, the risk of breast cancer increased within their lifetimes to the high level of native American women, as did colon cancer risk. In Japanese migrants to the US, on the other hand, the risk remained low for breast cancer while it increased for colon cancer in a manner similar to that for Polish males. Colon cancer in Japanese females also increased but 10–15 years later than in males. The high incidence of breast cancer characteristic of native white American females was probably first reached by the third generation of American Japanese [25,26].

Migrant studies need not be limited to movements across international boundaries. The significance of changes in risk associated with intracountry migration have, however, seldom been studied. A major exception is the inquiry into lung cancer in

TABLE IV. Change in Mortality on Migration From Japan to the US [16]

Group	Stomach (M)	Colon (M)	Lung (M)	Breast (F)
Japan	100	100	100	100
Japan-born Americans	72	374	306	166
US whites	17	489	316	591

TABLE V. Change in Mortality Rate* on Migration From Poland to the US [12]

Group	Stomach (M)	Colon (M)	Lung (M)	Breast (F)
Poland (1959–1961)	38	3	17	6
Polish-born Americans (1950)	34	14	36	19
US native whites (1950)	10	13	31	22

*Age-standardized to the world population standard.

TABLE VI. Standardized Lung Cancer Mortality Ratios Adjusted for Smoking History by Selected Birth Place and Current Residence Categories (US white males 35 years of age and over) [27]

| | Birth place | |
Current residence	Same as current residence	Farm
Metropolitan counties		
500,000+	117	159
50,000–500,000	89	156
Rural, nonfarm	62	93
Farm	50	50

migrant and settled native populations of the US [27], which demonstrated the lowest risk for natives in rural areas and a higher risk for natives in urban areas, but the highest was recorded in migrants from rural to urban areas (see also below; Table VI).

Problems of Migrant Studies

Migrant studies have their own problems. Migrants are seldom a random sample of the population of the country of origin, but are as a rule a selected group, eg, landless farmers, members of the Armed Forces, skilled workers, members of an ethnic or religious minority, etc. They often originate mainly from some specific area(s) of the home country. As a result, the cancer risk pattern of the migrants may represent that of the country of birth inadequately. For example, the "old" Polish migration to the US, before World War II, consisted mainly of poor, landless farmers, and their colon cancer risk was presumably lower than that for Poland as a whole (in spite of this, colon cancer mortality among Polish-born Americans in 1950 was as high as in the native Americans in the high-risk areas where they had for the most part settled [12]). The cancer risk patterns of Jews in Poland may have differed widely from that of the other inhabitants.

Comparisons of migrants with the country of origin have usually been based on composite national data. This was often due to the lack of data on intracountry variation in cancer risk, to lack of knowledge on the place of origin within the country of birth of the migrants, or usually to lack of both these items of information. When the within-country variation in cancer risk is large, as in China, availability of that information becomes crucial for the assessment of change in risk and the interpretation of results. This point has been recently demonstrated in a study using Guangdong province rather than all-China data for comparison with US Chinese, a great majority of whom originated in Guangdong [28]. The magnitude of the differences in risk between the various Chinese dialect groups, all from the southern part of China, living in Singapore, emphasizes this point (Table VII) [10].

A further problem might be the fact that migrants differ in several aspects from the host population, settling mainly in some specific areas and occupations. Differences in the selection as well as in the patterns of settlement of migrants from different countries hamper the comparability of their cancer patterns. Polish-born Americans, for example, settled mainly in the cities of the northeastern states as industrial workers, Scandinavian-born Americans as farmers in the north-central states, and migrants from Japan as farm workers in Hawaii and California.

TABLE VII. Age-Standardized Cancer Incidence* per 100,000 per Annum in Principal Chinese Dialect Groups (Singapore 1968–1977, by sex) [10]

Group	Nasopharynx		Esophagus		Lung	
	M	F	M	F	M	F
Hokkien	15.2	5.3	27.5	6.7	73.2	14.6
Teochew	16.5	6.1	30.7	7.8	67.0	13.9
Cantonese	30.4	10.9	4.5	2.2	57.3	28.5
Hainanese	16.2	5.6	6.9	1.2	38.5	11.0
Hakka	12.8	4.8	8.4	2.8	43.1	11.9

*All rates are age-adjusted to the world standard population.

Migrants can be reluctant to use unfamiliar medical services or unable to afford to do so. The terminally ill may go "home" to die, thus remaining in the denominator but not appearing in the numerator of the rate.

Studies of Habits and Life-Style

The habits and life-style of the migrants can remain similar to those in their country of birth or change rapidly—usually to those of the host country—or remain unchanged in some aspects and changed (partly or completely) in others. To quote Steiner [18], "Factors such as climate, altitude, temperature, amount of solar and other types of irradiation and intercurrent disease may differ at once. . . . On the other hand, certain environmental factors some of which may be cultural change more slowly after migration. The choice of food and culinary practice, occupational exposures, sanitary habits, economic levels, and other factors may gradually change over a period of years. . . ." Such questions have seldom been studied (Japanese Americans being the notable exception), which is regrettable because these differences and changes are presumably the main causes of variation in cancer patterns of migrants from those of their countries of birth and of destination. If, as seems likely, much of the burden of breast, large bowel, and prostate cancer is in some way linked to diet [1] and given that dietary intake within a country may not vary sufficiently to be assessed readily by case-control methods, one might imagine that the advent of migrant groups, frequently at low risk for these cancers, would be quickly followed by appropriate studies. Yet such investigations are very few in number. There are several reasons for this. The governments of host countries may, for a variety of reasons, not wish to acknowledge the existence of migrants or to permit their identification, or the migrants themselves may be in the host country illegally and hence try to conceal their origin.

Recent Migrant Studies

It is not proposed to recapitulate the now classical findings of Haenszel [15] and Haenszel and Kurihara [16]. Migrant studies up to 1970 were well reviewed by Kmet [11]. Two large descriptive studies of cancer in migrants, however, were published recently.

"Immigrant Mortality in England and Wales 1970–78," published in 1984 [29], comprises the largest material on cancer in migrants since Haenszel's "Cancer Mortality in the Foreign-Born in the United States" [15] and covers also the other causes of death. Mortality from cancer by site and sex in immigrants from 17 countries is compared with mortality in England and Wales and also with mortality in the countries of birth when available (Table VIII). The authors conclude that "The size of the cancer differences, reflecting differences between countries, suggests that as yet there has been little adaptation of immigrants to the life-style of the new country (England and Wales) and/or the effects of exposure at home persist after migration. In contrast with American [ie, Haenszel's] observations, rates of cancer of the intestine, breast and prostate and other sites do not appear to have changed within first generation Asian and African immigrants and changed only partly in Poles."

The intriguing contrast with the American experience is perhaps due to the shorter residence of most immigrants in England and Wales, usually less than 20–30 years,* whereas in the US it was mainly greater than 25 years† and/or to a greater resistance to change in diet and life-style.

A different selection of migrants may also have played a role: Polish migrants to the UK were from higher socioeconomic classes and presumably at a lower risk of stomach cancer than the earlier migrants to the US originating mainly from poor rural farming areas.

The outstanding increase in lung and esophagus cancer risk, to a level much higher than that reported from either their country of origin or of adoption, observed for Polish-born Americans in 1950 and 1959–1961 mortality data (in the latter only for older ages) [12] and in the Buffalo case-control study [31], has not appeared in England and Wales, probably because of the same differences in migrant selection. A similar phenomenon was observed within the US for migrants from rural farming areas to urban areas: As was mentioned above, these migrants experienced higher

TABLE VIII. Standardized Mortality Ratios for Selected Common Cancers in Migrants to England and Wales: Comparison With Risk in Those Remaining in the Country of Origin [29]

	Ireland	Italy	Poland
Stomach cancer (M)			
SMR[a] of homeland	106	143	197
SMR of migrants	104	107	120
Colon cancer (M)			
SMR of homeland	116	84	43
SMR of migrants	118	27 (4)[b]	79
Rectum (M)			
SMR of homeland	85	72	61
SMR of migrants	112	59 (6)	71
Lung cancer (M)			
SMR of homeland	57	56	54
SMR of migrants	111	68	62
Breast cancer (F)			
SMR of homeland	88	67	45
SMR of migrants	88	85	97

[a]All comparisons based on England and Wales mortality experience with SMR of 100.
[b]Number in parentheses denotes number of deaths. All other SMRs based on more than ten deaths.

*Poles arrived mainly during 1940–1949, migrants from the U.S.S.R. in 1945–1949, and migrants from India, the Caribbean, and other Commonwealth countries mainly after 1960. By UN convention, the place of origin is determined by current political boundaries, not those at the time of migration [30].

†Most migrants arrived before 1924; mortality was analyzed for 1950.

lung cancer mortality than the lifelong city residents. As explanations, two hypotheses have been advanced. One proposes a lack of adaptation in persons born on farms, ". . . an abrupt imposition of additional particulate matter . . . from the urban atmosphere with no intervening period of gradual adaptation to an increasing load. This, when added to cigarette smoke, might overload and inhibit the action of the respiratory cilia in particle transport, and would thus permit longer contact of the particles, and any carcinogens adhering to their surfaces, with the epithelial cells." The other hypothesis postulates a better adaptation in the urban population rather than a lack of adaptation in the rural; exposure at birth, or even in utero, to small carcinogen doses might create some resistance, perhaps by preconditioning enzyme metabolism [27].

Whether the lack of change in the immigrants' cancer mortality was the effect of an insufficiently long period of residence in England and Wales could probably be assessed if the study was repeated with the new material available for the years around 1980, permitting in addition evaluation of time trends. Inclusion of information on the duration of residence in England and Wales would be particularly pertinent for immigrant groups arriving over a longer period of time (as most groups did) rather than within a limited period (eg, migrants from Poland or the USSR).

The second study, "Mortality From Cancer in Migrants to Australia, 1962–1971" [32], is based on smaller numbers and includes no information on mortality in the migrants' countries of birth. For some sites and immigrant groups, however, mortality is provided for three categories of duration of residence in Australia: 0–5 years (in this category the "healthy migrant" effect, reflected by a low mortality, is sometimes evident), 6–16 years, and 17+ years. The change in mortality towards the rates prevailing in Australia was usually most evident in immigrants residing in Australia for longer than 17 years (Table IX); this effect is well seen, for example, in breast cancer in Italian and Yugoslav migrants. Extension of the study for the next 10 years would be most interesting: Numbers of deaths would be increased, and time trends might become apparent. Inclusion of data on cancer mortality in the immigrants' countries of birth would be valuable as would, if possible, addition of one more category of duration of residence (say, 27+ years).

Age at Migration

Age at migration has seldom been taken into account, as in the study of cardiorespiratory disease mortality among British and Norwegian migrants to the US [33] (Table X). The observations are clear: Britons migrating at early ages to the US tended to have lower lung cancer risk than those migrating at age 15 years and over; for Norwegians the reverse obtained. Those migrating as adults seem to carry over the high (British) or low (Norwegians) risk of their country of birth, whereas those migrating as children appear to have acquired the intermediate risk of their host country.

That tabulations by age at migration can be of great value is indicated by a paper on melanoma in migrants to Australia: migrants arriving before the age of 10 years appeared to have a risk of superficial spreading melanoma similar to that of native-born Australians, whereas the estimated incidence in those arriving after the age of 15 years was approximately one-quarter the native-born rate, with arrival at later ages giving no additional advantage [34] (Table XI).

TABLE IX. Standardized Mortality Ratios* for Selected Common Cancers in Migrants to Australia by Length of Residence (1962–1971) [32]

Length of stay in Australia	Ireland	Italy	Poland	Greece	Yugoslavia
Stomach cancer (M)					
All periods	133	146	164	101	134
0–5 years	91 (6)[a]	165	128 (5)	—	—
6–16 years	166	165	188	—	—
17+ years	127	146	159	—	—
Colon cancer (M)					
All periods	110	62	98	64	72
0–5 years	—	20 (3)	—[b]	19 (2)	—
6–16 years	—	33	—	25 (3)	—
17+ years	—	79	—	86	—
Rectum cancer (M)					
All periods	130	82	96	57	90
0–5 years	—	35 (2)	—	0 (0)	—
6–16 years	—	51 (8)	—	0 (0)	—
17+ years	—	101	—	92	—
Lung cancer (M)					
All periods	143	102	129	103	166
0–5 years	171	68	185 (9)	—	153
6–16 years	228	72	113	—	189
17+ years	133	121	137	—	171
Breast cancer (F)					
All periods	124	73	84	74	45
0–5 years	76 (7)	43	—	—	18 (3)
6–16 years	80	60	—	—	39
17+ years	138	105	—	—	68 (9)

*All comparisons based on Australian mortality experience with SMR of 100.
[a]Numbers in parentheses denote numbers of deaths. All other SMRs based on more than ten deaths.
[b]Data not provided.

TABLE X. Effect of Age of Migration on Lung Cancer Mortality* Among British and Norwegian Male Migrants to the US by Age at Death [30]

Age at migration (years)	Age at death (years)	Mortality rate per 10,000	
		British	Norwegian
< 15	55–64	15	21
	65–74	34	21
15+	55–64	27	14
	65–74	38	16

*Mortality expressed per 10,000.

The use of SMRs in the recent studies, as well as in Haenszel's 1961 study, although legitimate, makes it impossible to compare the results of studies in the US, UK, and Australia directly. Addition of SMRs based on the mortality in the countries of birth (as in the 1968 paper on cancer in Japanese migrants to the US by Haenszel and Kurihara) could help in this respect, permitting statements like "in migrants from Poland, stomach cancer mortality decreased very little (from 100 to 96) towards the low (32) US mortality, and also towards (from 100 to 94) the somewhat higher (49) Australian mortality, while approximating (80) the still higher (78) mortality in England and Wales" (the numbers are fictitious). Direct standardization of the rates

TABLE XI. Relative Risk of Superficial Spreading of Melanoma by Age of Arrival in Australia [34]

Born in Australia	1.0
Age at arrival (years)	
0–4	1.2
5–9	1.4
10–14	0.7
15–19	0.3
20–24	0.3

to the "world" population as the standard would be better still when possible. However, numbers are often rather small.

Future Studies

Comparisons of shifts in cancer risks of migrants from the same country of birth to varying environments in different host countries such as in Indians to Natal and Singapore have been little exploited. Although data collection in the US, UK, and Australia should be continued and refined (as mentioned above, and also using cancer registration data on histological type, etc), the most useful information in this respect would be that from Argentina, Brazil, and, to a lesser extent, Canada (Europeans migrating to environments quite different from those of the US, UK, and Australia) [30]. Studies of changes in risk of Maghrebins to France would also be of great interest.

Analytical studies directed to relating the risk patterns of cancer and its precursors with information on life-style (smoking, alcohol consumption, diet, occupation, etc) have been carried out for US Japanese [24] and for migrants within Colombia [35,36]. Similar studies are required to explain the findings in other migrant populations. Increasing availability of mortality and incidence data on cancer in migrants covering relatively long time periods opens a new dimension in the studies; that of time trends.

In conclusion, despite their drawbacks, studies of changes in cancer risk in migrants still offer a means of identifying the determinants of cancer risk, in particular those aspects of diet likely to be most difficult to examine by case-control methods in native populations showing little background variation in food habits.

COMMENT

Geographical epidemiology provides data not only on the cancer burden of populations but also on variation in cancer risk patterns in space and time. Migrant studies take advantage of the great natural experiments that result when populations of a given genetic composition change environments. The ensuing alterations in site-specific cancer risk often permit easier identification of agents responsible for the changes observed and of the mode of action of these agents, including the influence of the age when exposures changed. Migrant studies are one of the most fascinating but least exploited fields in geographical epidemiology.

REFERENCES

1. Higginson J, Muir CS: J Natl Cancer Inst 63:1291, 1979.

2. Parkin DM, Stjernsward J, Muir CS: Bull WHO 62:163, 1984.
3. Waterhouse J, Muir CS, Shanmugaratnam K, Powell J (eds): "Cancer Incidence in Five Continents. Vol IV." Lyon: IARC (Scientific Publication No. 42), 1982.
4. Muir CS, Nectoux J: In Schottenfeld D, Fraumeni JF (eds): "Cancer Epidemiology and Prevention." Philadelphia: WB Saunders Co, 1982, pp 119–138.
5. Lyon JL, Gardner JW, West DW: In Cairns J, Lyon JL, Skolnick M (eds): "Cancer Incidence in Defined Populations, Banbury Report 4." Cold Spring Harbor NY: Cold Spring Harbor Laboratory, 1980, pp 3–28.
6. Magnus K (ed): "Trends in Cancer Incidence." Washington, DC: Hemisphere Publishing Corporation, 1982.
7. Muir CS: In Doll R, Vodopija I (eds): "Host Environment Interactions in the Etiology of Cancer in Man." Lyon: IARC (Scientific Publication No. 7), 1973, pp 1–13.
8. Staszewski J, Haenszel W: J Natl Cancer Inst 35:291, 1965.
9. Mekie DEC, Lawley M: Arch Surg 69:841, 1954.
10. Shanmugaratnam K, Lee HP, Day NE: "Cancer Incidence in Singapore 1968–1977." Lyon: IARC (Scientific Publication No. 47), 1983.
11. Kmet J: J Chronic Dis 23:305, 1970.
12. Staszewski J: "Epidemiology of Cancer of Selected Sites in Poland and Polish Migrants." Cambridge, MA: Ballinger Publishing Co., 1976.
13. Adelstein AM, Staszewski J, Muir CS: Br J Cancer 40:464, 1979.
14. Staszewski J, McCall M, Stenhouse NS: Br J Cancer 25:599, 1971.
15. Haenszel W: J Natl Cancer Inst 26:37, 1961.
16. Haenszel W, Kurihara M: J Natl Cancer Inst 40:43, 1968.
17. Kennaway EL: Cancer Res 4:571, 1944.
18. Steiner PE: Cancer: "Race and Geography." Baltimore: Williams and Wilkins, 1954.
19. Lombard HL, Doering CR: J Prev Med 3:343, 1929.
20. Smith RL: J Natl Cancer Inst 17:549, 1956.
21. Eastcott DF: Lancet 1:37, 1956.
22. Dean G: Br Med J 2:852, 1959.
23. Higginson J: J Natl Cancer Inst 37:527, 1966.
24. Haenszel W, Kurihara M, Segi M, Lee RKC: J Natl Cancer Inst 49:969, 1972.
25. Haenszel W: In Aoki K, Tominaga S, Hirayama T, Hirota Y (eds): "Cancer Prevention in Developing Countries." Nagoya: The University of Nagoya Press, 1982, pp 351–362.
26. Dunn JE: Natl Cancer Inst Monogr 47:157, 1977.
27. Haenszel W, Loveland DB, Sirken MG: J Natl Cancer Inst 28:947, 1962.
28. King H, Li J, Locke FB, Pollack ES, Tu J: Am J Public Health 75:237, 1985.
29. Marmot MG, Adelstein AM, Bubusu L: "Immigrant Mortality in England and Wales 1970–78." London: OPCS (Studies on Medical and Population Subjects No. 47), 1984.
30. Staszewski J, Muir CS, Slomska J, Jain K: J Chronic Dis 23:351, 1970.
31. Graham S, Levin ML, Lilienfeld AM, Sheehe P: Cancer 16:13, 1963.
32. Armstrong BK, Woodings TL, Stenhouse NS, McCall MG: "Mortality From Cancer in Migrants to Australia 1962–1971." Perth: The University of Western Australia, 1983.
33. Rogot E: Am J Epidemiol 108:181, 1978.
34. Holman CDAJ, Armstrong BK: JNCI 73:75, 1984.
35. Cuello C, Correa P, Haenszel W, Gordillo G, Brown C, Archer M, Tannenbaum S: J Natl Cancer Inst 57:1015, 1976.
36. Haenszel W, Correa P, Cuello C, Guzman N, Burbano LC, Lores H, Munoz J: J Natl Cancer Inst 57:1021, 1976.

DNA Methylation

Peter A. Jones, Lois Chandler, Timothy Kautiainen, Vincent Wilson, and Edith Flatau

USC Comprehensive Cancer Center, Los Angeles, California 90033

Several lines of evidence strongly suggest that the methylation of specific cytosine residues in the dinucleotide sequence CG in DNA is part of a potent gene silencing mechanism in vertebrate cells. First, methylation patterns are tissue specific and the hypomethylation of many genes is correlated with their active expression [1–6]. There have been some apparent exceptions to these generalizations, examples being the collagen and vitellogenin genes that can be expressed from heavily methylated sequences [7,8]. However, most of the evidence is still in line with the hypothesis that the undermethylation of specific sequences may be a necessary but not sufficient condition for gene activity.

Initially it was thought that the modification of single CG methylation sites would silence genes. However, recent results in several systems suggest that the methylation of domains within the 5′ or 3′ regions of genes may be more important than the modification of single sites. Examples of such domains include the albumin locus in rat hepatoma cell variants [9] and the promoter region of the human dihydrofolate reductase gene [10]. Domains of methylation in the 3′ region of a gene may also be important in gene control, and Wolf et al [11] have found a complete concordance between glucose-6-phosphate-dehydrogenase activity and hypomethylation of CG clusters, which may be important in X chromosome activation. Bird et al [12] have also recently found that about 30,000 islands of highly CG-rich sequences, which are deficient in methylation, are located throughout the mouse genome. These islands may well be associated with genes, and a similar conclusion was reached by Tykocinski and Max [13], who detected CG clusters in the major histocompatibility complex genes and in the 5′ region of other genes. Thus, domains of methylation, which may be localized to either the 5′ region, or 3′ region may be critical in the extinction of gene activity in differentiated cells, and the undermethylation of these sequences may be a necessary precondition for gene expression.

Vincent Wilson's present address is Laboratory of Human Carcinogenesis, National Cancer Institute, Building 37, Bethesda, MD 20205.

Edith Flatau's present address is Internal Medicine "B," Central Emek Hospital, Afula 18101, Israel.

Received May 7, 1985.

© **1986 Alan R. Liss, Inc.**

The second line of evidence that DNA methylation can control gene expression comes from experiments in which specific gene sequences are methylated before their introduction into recipient cells. For example, the methylation of the 5' region of the globin gene leads to its inactivity after transfection into recipient cells [14]. Similarly, the methylation of three CCGG sites in the promoter region of the E2A gene of adenovirus type II results in the inactivity of the sequence [15]. The methylation of retrovirus genomes by mammalian but not bacterial methylases renders the viruses noninfectious [16], and the genes can be reactivated by treatment with inhibitors of DNA methylation.

The third series of experiments that strongly implicates a role for cytosine methylation in eukaryotic gene control comes from studies using the nucleoside analogs 5-azacytidine (5-aza-CR) and 5-azadeoxycytidine (5-aza-CdR). These analogs are powerful inhibitors of the methylation of newly incorporated cytosine residues in DNA [17] and incorporation of the fraudulent bases often results in the activation of silent genetic information [18]. The large variety of systems that respond to 5-aza-CR [19] and the careful mapping of the demethylation induced provide strong corroborative evidence for a causative role for methylation in silencing genes.

If DNA methylation plays an important role in controlling gene expression in normal differentiated cell types, then it follows that abberations within this controlling mechanism may be implicated in the abnormal switching of genes that occurs during neoplastic transformation. Several studies have shown that DNA methylation patterns in naturally occurring human tumors are different from the tissues of origin [10–22]. Azacytidine can have strong effects on the stability of the transformed phenotype [23–26], suggesting that altered methylation patterns may play a role in neoplastic transformation and progression. We have therefore investigated the abilities of chemical carcinogens to interact with this DNA information coding system and have determined the levels of methylation in naturally occurring pediatric tumors. Aspects of methylation control, including levels of extractable methyltransferase activity in a variety of tumorigenic and nontumorigenic cell types, were also studied to determine whether changes in methylation capacity might play a role in the instability of the tumor phenotype.

INHIBITION OF DNA METHYLATION BY CHEMICAL CARCINOGENS

Many carcinogens are metabolized intracellularly to active electrophiles, which react to form adducts with guanine residues in DNA. Guanine residues are important for the enzymatic methylation of DNA since they occur both opposite and adjacent to potentially methylatable cytosine residues within DNA. The formation of adducts at methylation sites might therefore be expected to interfere with the normal inheritance of DNA methylation patterns. Carcinogens also induce DNA damage, including strand breaks, and some electrophiles can interact directly with the active sites of enzymes. We therefore determined whether ultimate chemical carcinogens would influence the ability of hemimethylated DNA substrates to accept methyl groups from S-adenosylmethionine in the presence of crude DNA methyltransferase preparations [27].

A range of ultimate chemical carcinogens, including MNNG, EMS, ENU, nitrogen mustard and benzo(a)pyrene diolepoxide, inhibited the transfer of methyl groups to hemimethylated DNA. The formation of alkali labile sites in the DNA substrate also lessened its ability to accept methyl groups in vitro but the substrate efficiency of the DNA was much less inhibited by the formation of thymine dimers or double-strand DNA breaks. The ultimate carcinogens also induced the formation of alkali labile lesions in DNA, but the degree of inhibition of DNA methyltransferase activity was greater than that which could be accounted for by this lesion alone. Thus the formation of adducts on guanine residues may also have played a role in inhibiting the DNA methyltransferase reaction. The experiments were not sufficiently refined to determine whether the inhibitory effect was due either to the formation of adducts at methyl acceptor sites or to general disruption of DNA secondary structure.

Certain of the carcinogens were also capable of reacting directly with the DNA methyltransferase enzyme, which apparently requires an active SH group for its function [28]. Thus, chemical carcinogens may be able to inhibit DNA methylation by at least three mechanisms, adduct formation, induction of strand breaks, and direct inhibition of the methyltransferase.

The genomic level of DNA 5-methylcytosine was also significantly diminished in Balb 3T3 cells treated with several aromatic hydrocarbons [29]. Benzo(a)pyrene-induced decreases in 5-methylcytosine levels were concentration dependent over the range of 0.1 to 1.0 mg/ml when determined 16 hr after the treatment period. All of the chemical carcinogens that were tested that were known to transform Balb 3T3 cells initiated significant reductions in 5-methylcytosine formation by 48 hr after exposure to the carcinogens. However, concentrations of some hydrocarbons that did not transform these cells, 5–50-fold above effective levels of oncogenic chemicals, also produced significant reduction in DNA methylation. We were not able to detect changes in genomic 5-methylcytosine levels in C3H 10T1/2 Cl 8 cells treated with aromatic hydrocarbons. Thus, while the inhibition of DNA methylation may be an important step in the initiation of transformation in certain mouse cells, decreases in the level of the modified base alone cannot account for the onset of this multistep process.

Overall, these experiments and those of several other investigators [30–33] demonstrated that carcinogenic agents may be able to cause heritable changes in the levels of DNA modification in certain cell types by a variety of mechanisms, including the formation of adducts, single-strand breaks, and direct inactivation of DNA methyltransferase enzymes. The net results of carcinogen treatment of cells may therefore be changes in gene expression that can be propagated in the absence of further carcinogen treatment. This is an important point, since theories of chemical carcinogenesis must accomodate the fact that the lesions induced by the carcinogens can be propagated without further exposure to carcinogens. In the next set of experiments, we examined 5-methylcytosine levels in a series of human tumor cell lines and naturally occurring human tumors to determine whether changes in DNA 5-methylcytosine levels may also be involved in naturally occurring cancers.

DNA METHYLATION IN HUMAN TUMOR CELL LINES AND FRESH PEDIATRIC TUMOR EXPLANTS

Several investigators have measured overall genomic levels of 5-methylcytosine in various tumor cell lines and animal tumors [34,35]. Results of these experiments have not been consistent, and decreased, increased, or unchanged levels of 5-methyl-cytosine have been reported in the various tumors examined. We therefore examined

the level of methylation in five human tumor cell lines, rhabdomyosarcoma, retinoblastoma, neuroblastoma, osteogenic sarcoma, and fibrosarcoma [36]. In general, the
DNA methylation level in these lines was not decreased when compared to human
fibroblasts. On the other hand, the methylation level in the HT1080 human fibrosarcoma cell line was decreased considerably from the value of 3.45% found in human
fibroblasts. Thus, some but not all oncogenically transformed cell lines have low
levels of DNA methylation.

We also examined the levels of DNA methylation in freshly explanted pediatric
tumors [36] to determine whether our failure to observe markedly decreased 5-
methylcytosine levels in cell lines was due to the selection pressures operational
during the establishment of cell lines in culture [37]. Methylation levels of approximately 3.4% of cytosines modified to 5-methylcytosine were found in one Wilms
tumor explant, two rhabdomyosarcomas, and one medullablastoma. These values
were similar to those of human fibroblasts. On the other hand, the methylation level
in two fresh explants of neuroblastoma were of the order of 2.7%, which were
decreased substantially from the values found in retinoblastoma tumors or fibroblasts.
These results indicate that generalized statements on the DNA methylation levels in
pediatric tumors probably cannot be made, although substantial variations may occur
between different tumor cell types. It may therefore be necessary to measure the
methylation status of specific genes within tumor cells before the potential role of
methylation in abberrant gene expression in tumors can be appreciated.

METHYLATION PATTERNS IN HUMAN TUMOR CELL LINES

DNA was extracted from human tumor lines, including osteogenic sarcoma,
rhabdomyosarcoma, and neuroblastoma cells, and analyzed for the methylation patterns of type I collagen and Ha *ras* genes. These experiments demonstrated considerable heterogeneity in the different tumor cell lines with regard to the methylation
status of the specific genes. The expression of the collagen gene was also examined,
but generalized statements about the methylation status of the gene and its expression
could not be made. The results showed considerable flexibility and heterogeneity in
the methylation status of these genes in different cell types, suggesting that tumors
are remarkably heterogeneous with respect to methylation patterns as originally
reported by Feinberg and Vogelstein [20,21] and Goelz et al [22].

METHYLATION CAPACITY OF HUMAN TUMOR CELLS

The results of these experiments with restriction endonucleases and specific
genes strongly suggested that abberations in DNA methylation control occur in cancer
cells. Additionally, there is evidence that the overall levels of methylation within
some but not all tumors and tumor cell lines may be changed from the levels in
normal cells. We have begun to investigate the levels of active DNA methyltransferase
enzymes within cells to determine whether these abnormal patterns and the level of
DNA modification may be due to changes in the methylation machinery.

The levels of DNA methyltransferase in tumorigenic and nontumorigenic cells
from four species were therefore examined by extracting methylase enzyme from
nuclei and assaying the activity of the extracted enzyme using hemimethylated DNA
substrates. These experiments have shown that the levels of extractable enzyme in the

tumorigenic cells were, in general, higher than in nontumorigenic cells. Furthermore, the levels of extractable enzyme did not correlate with the 5-methylcytosine content of the respective cell DNAs. For example, although the level of methylation in the tumorigenic cells was sometimes less than that in nontumorigenic varieties, the tumorigenic cells had increased levels of extractable enzyme. These results were unexpected and suggested that the overall 5-methylcytosine level is not determined solely by the level of active methylase. However, the increased level of enzyme may allow tumor cells greater flexibility in the establishment of new methylation patterns that might be responsible to some extent for the plasticity of the transformed phenotype.

SUMMARY

There is considerable evidence that the methylation of specific cytosine residues in DNA is part of a multilevel control system for gene expression in vertebrate cells. The evidence implicating methylation in the control of the activity of many genes is convincing and strongly supports the notion that methylation locks certain but not all genes in the "off" condition. Hypomethylation may therefore be a necessary but not sufficient condition for gene expression, and abberations in this controlling device may be implicated in faulty gene expression in cancer cells. Chemical carcinogens interfere with the process of DNA methylation in cells, and some tumors have decreased 5-methylcytosine levels and hypomethylation of specific sequences. Finally, an increased level of extractable methyltransferase exists in tumor cells, and this may allow greater flexibility contributing to the instability of the phenotype.

ACKNOWLEDGMENTS

This work was supported by grants CA39913 and CA40422 from the National Institutes of Health.

REFERENCES

1. Riggs AD: Cytogenet Cell Genet 14:9, 1975.
2. Holliday R, Pugh JE: Science 187:226, 1975.
3. Razin A, Riggs AD: Science 210:604, 1980.
4. Ehrlich M, Wang RY-H: Science 212:1350, 1981.
5. Doerfler W: Annu Rev Biochem 52:93, 1983.
6. Riggs AD, Jones PA: Adv Cancer Res 40:1, 1983.
7. McKeon C, Ohkubo H, Pastan I, deCrombruggle B: Cell 29:203, 1982.
8. Gerber-Huber S, May FEB, Westley BR, Felber BK, Hosbach HA, Andres A-C, Ryffel GU: Cell 33:43, 1983.
9. Orlofsky A, Chasin LA: Mol Cell Biol 5:214, 1985.
10. Shimada T, Nienhuis AW: J Biol Chem 260:2468, 1985.
11. Wolf SF, Dintzis S, Toniolo D, Persico G, Lunnen KD, Axelman J, Migeon BR: Nucleic Acids Res 12:9333, 1984.
12. Bird A, Taggart M, Frommer M, Miller OJ, Macleod D: Cell 40:91, 1985.
13. Tykocinski ML, Max EE: Nucleic Acids Res 12:4385, 1984.
14. Busslinger M, Hurst J, Flavell RA: Cell 34:197, 1983.
15. Langer K-D, Vardimon L, Renz D, Doerfler W: Proc Natl Acad Sci USA 81:2950, 1984.
16. Simon D, Stuhlman H, Jahner D, Wagner H, Werner E, Jaenisch R: Nature 304:275, 1983.
17. Jones PA, Taylor SM: Cell 20:85, 1980.

18. Jones PA: Cell 40:485, 1985.
19. Jones PA: Int Encyl Pharm Ther 28:17, 1985.
20. Feinberg AP, Vogelstein B: Nature 301:89, 1983.
21. Feinberg, AP, Vogelstein B: Biochem Biophys Res Commun 111:47, 1983.
22. Goelz SE, Vogelstein B, Hamilton SR, Feinberg AP: Science 228:187, 1985.
23. Frost P, Liteplo RG, Donaghue TP, Kerbel RS: J Exp Med 159:1491, 1984.
24. Kerbel RS, Frost P, Liteplo R, Carlow D, Elliot BE: J Cell Physiol Suppl 3:87, 1984.
25. Olsson L, Forchhammer J: Proc Natl Acad Sci USA 81:3389, 1984.
26. Olsson L, Due C, Diamont M: J Cell Biol 100:508, 1985.
27. Wilson VL, Jones PA: Cell 32:239, 1983.
28. Cox R: Cancer Res 40:61, 1980.
29. Wilson VL, Jones PA: Carcinogenesis 5:1027, 1984.
30. Lapeyre J-N, Becker FF: Biochem Biophys Res Commun 87:698, 1979.
31. Boehm TLJ, Drahovsky D: Carcinogenesis 2:39, 1981.
32. Lapeyre J-N, Walker MS, Becker FF: Carcinogenesis 2:873, 1981.
33. Pfohl-Leszkowicz A, Fuchs RPP, Keith G, Dirheimer G: J Cancer Res Clin Oncol 103:318, 1982.
34. Diala ES, Cheah MSC, Rowitch D, Hoffman RM: JNCI 71:755, 1983.
35. Gama-Sosa MA, Slagel VA, Trewyn RW, Oxenhandler R, Kuo K, Gehrke W, Ehrlich M: Nucleic Acids Res 11:6883, 1983.
36. Flatau E, Bogenmann E, Jones PA: Cancer Res 43:4901, 1983.
37. Wilson VL, Jones PA: Science 220:1055, 1983.

Biochemical and Molecular Epidemiology of Cancer 155–165 (1986)

Mechanism of Transformation by an Oncogene Coding for a Normal Growth Factor

Fernando Leal, Hisanaga Igarashi, Arnona Gazit, Lewis T. Williams, Vicente Notario, Steven R. Tronick, Keith C. Robbins, and Stuart A. Aaronson

Laboratory of Cellular and Molecular Biology, National Cancer Institute, Bethesda, Maryland 20205 (F.L., H.I., A.G., V.N., S.R.T., K.C.R., S.A.A.), and Howard Hughes Medical Institute, University of California, San Francisco, California 94143 (L.T.W.)

Recently, investigations of the genetic alterations that cause normal cells to become malignant have focused on a small set of cellular genes. Acute transforming retroviruses have substituted viral genes necessary for replication with these discrete segments of host genetic information [1,2]. When incorporated within the retroviral genome, these transduced cellular sequences, termed *onc* genes, acquire the ability to induce neoplastic transformation. The discovery that independent virus isolates have recombined with the same or closely related cellular protooncogenes implies that only a limited number of cellular genes are capable of acquiring transforming properties under these conditions.

The profound cellular alterations induced by the activated cellular transforming genes have some similarities to the growth-promoting actions of hormones and growth factors. Each exerts pleiotropic effects on cellular metabolism, including the induction of sustained cell replication. Interest in understanding the actions of *onc* genes has led to concerted efforts to isolate, amplify, and sequence such genes. The present report summarizes investigations that have linked one oncogene to a cellular gene encoding a normal growth factor.

PLATELET-DERIVED GROWTH FACTOR AND SIMIAN SARCOMA VIRUS

Simian sarcoma virus (SSV) was isolated from a fibrosarcoma of a woolly monkey and represents the only known sarcoma virus of primate origin [3]. The virus has been characterized in tissue culture [4], and its integrated DNA provirus has been cloned in infectious form [5]. Physical and biological characterization of its genome

Received June 25, 1985.

Published 1986 by Alan R. Liss, Inc.

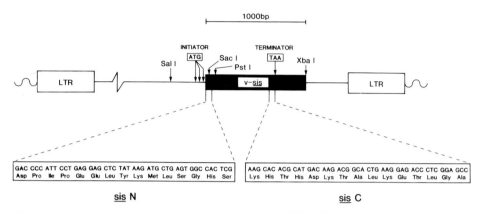

Fig. 1. Major structural features of simian sarcoma virus (SSV) DNA. The cell-derived sequence of SSV is indicated as a darkened rectangle. Signals for translation of the v-*sis*–coded protein are also indicated. The composition of *sis* N and *sis* C peptides was determined from the v-*sis* nucleotide sequence. LTR, long terminal repeat; bp, base pairs.

has localized its transforming gene to the cell-derived onc sequence, v-*sis* [6]. The SSV genome, including the v-*sis* region, has been sequenced [7]. Moreover, antibodies prepared against small peptides derived from the v-*sis* sequence have been used to identify the 28,000 dalton v-*sis* gene product, p28^{sis}, in SSV transformed cells [6,7]. Major structural features of the SSV genome as well as the location and composition of peptides used to generate anti-p28^{sis} sera are shown in Figure 1.

Platelet-derived growth factor (PDGF) is a heat-stable (100°C), cationic (pI, 9.8) protein [8]. It circulates in blood stored in the α granules of platelets and is released into serum during blood clotting [9]. It represents the major protein growth factor of human serum and is a potent mitogen for connective tissue and glial cells in culture [10–12]. Unreduced active PDGF exhibits multiple forms ranging in size from 28,000 to 35,000 daltons [8,13,14]. Reduction of PDGF produces inactive, smaller peptides ranging in size from 12,000 to 18,000 daltons [12,13].

Amino acid sequence analysis of the amino-terminal portions of both active human PDGF and its inactive, reduced peptides has revealed the presence of two homologous chains (PDGF-1 and PDGF-2) in active PDGF preparations [15]. These peptides are identical at eight of 19 positions near their amino termini, with no sequence gaps required for the homology alignment. Whether the active PDGF preparation is composed of a single protein formed by disulfide linkage of these two peptides or is composed of two proteins, each of which consists of a disulfide-linked dimer of one of the peptides, is not yet known.

PREDICTED AMINO ACID SEQUENCE HOMOLOGY BETWEEN p28^{sis} AND HUMAN PLATELET-DERIVED GROWTH FACTOR

The rapid proliferation of nucleotide sequence data (and thus predicted amino acid sequences for numerous proteins), in combination with the development of sequence data banks and computer programs for rapidly searching for similarities among these sequences [16], has recently led to a number of striking observations. One such discovery was that the amino acid sequence of one peptide chain of platelet-derived growth factor (PDGF), a potent human connective tissue cell mitogen, showed a high degree of match with a segment of the predicted v-*sis* sequence [17,18].

The predicted *sis* coding sequence, starting at residue 67, demonstrated an 84% match to PDGF-2 over this same stretch. Furthermore, in the total of 70 PDGF-2 residues identified, 87.1% corresponded to the p28^{sis} sequence. Taking into account the New World primate origin of v-*sis* [19], it was concluded that the v-*sis* transforming gene arose by recombination between the SSAV genome and a host cell gene for PDGF or a very highly related protein. The observed amino acid differences between human PDGF-2 and v-*sis* could be accounted for by the known degree of divergence between the genomes of humans and cebids [20]. In fact, a proteolytic cleavage signal (Lys-Arg) is present at residues 65–66 in the v-*sis* sequence, and the next residue commences the homology between v-*sis* and PDGF-2. Cleavage here would result in an approximately 20,000 dalton peptide corresponding closely in size to PDGF-2.

p28^{sis} IS STRUCTURALLY AND CONFORMATIONALLY RELATED TO PDGF

Efforts were undertaken to investigate the structural, immunological, and functional relationships of the v-*sis* gene product and human PDGF [21]. We utilized specific peptide antibodies to study the biosynthesis of the v-*sis*–coded transforming protein in SSV transformed cells. Marmoset cells infected with SSV were pulse-labeled with ^{35}S-methionine for various times, extracted, and then immunoprecipitated with the appropriate antisera. The immunoprecipitates were then analyzed on SDS-gels in the presence or absence of reducing agent (Fig. 2A).

The following events in the biogenesis and posttranslational modification of the SSV transforming protein were shown to occur. First, a 28,000 dalton single peptide chain is synthesized and rapidly undergoes disulfide bond-mediated dimerization to a 56,000 dalton specifies. The 56 K dimer is then cleaved at its amino terminal end. The products of these proteolytic events detected under reducing conditions are single chains of 11 K (amino terminal) and 20 K (C terminal) peptides (designated p11^{sis} and p20^{sis}, respectively).

Other steps involved in the processing of p28^{sis} were uncovered by studies utilizing anti-PDGF serum. Under nonreducing conditions, the same sized species recognized by the anti-*sis* C-terminal serum were detected (Fig. 2B). In addition, the PDGF antiserum detected a 24 K protein that was not recognized by the *sis* N terminal- or *sis* C terminal-specific antisera. This species appeared to be the most stable processed form of the *sis* gene product. These results demonstrated that the v-*sis* gene product assumed a conformational structure similar to that of a PDGF-2 dimer and established an immunological cross-reactivity between this transforming gene product and human PDGF.

THE v-*sis* GENE PRODUCT IS FUNCTIONALLY EQUIVALENT TO PDGF

Studies of the biosynthesis of the v-*sis* protein have shown that the polypeptide is associated with cell membranes [22]. Utilizing SSV transformed cell membranes as the source of v-*sis*–coded protein, we devised a means of functionally characterizing cell-associated molecules that could be unequivocally identified as products of the v-*sis* gene. As shown in Table I, it was possible to demonstrate that v-*sis* translational products synthesized by and associated with SSV transformed cells specifically induce

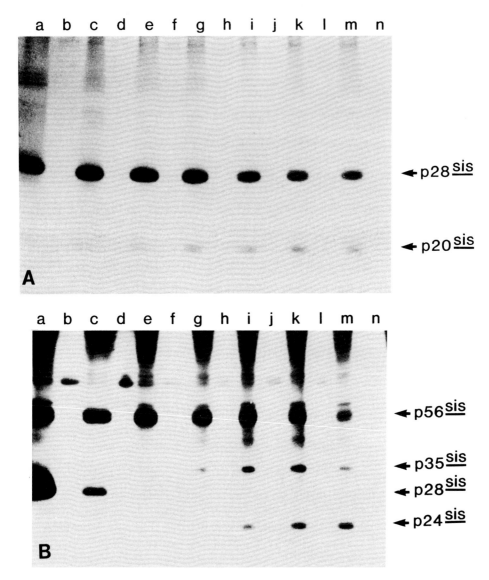

Fig. 2.   Pulse-chase analysis of the v-*sis* translational product. HF/SSV cells were pulse-labeled for 15 min with ^{35}S-cysteine and methionine and chased for periods of 0 (lanes a and b), 15 (lanes c and d), 30 (lanes e and f), 45 (lanes g and h), 60 (lanes i and j), 75 (lanes k and l), and 90 (lanes m and n) min. Cell lysates were incubated with anti-*sis* C (A, lanes a, c, e, g, i, k, and m), anti-PDGF (A, lanes a, c, e, g, i, k, and m) or nonimmune rabbit (lanes b, d, f, h, j, l, and n) serum. Immunoprecipitates were analyzed by polyacrylamide gel electrophoresis in reducing (A) or nonreducing (B) conditions.

DNA synthesis in quiescent fibroblasts. Moreover, v-*sis*–coded proteins possessed the capacity to bind PDGF receptors and to induce tyrosine phosphorylation of PDGF receptors. In each case, it was possible to establish the v-*sis*–coded nature of these activities by specific inhibition with antibodies directed against different regions of the v-*sis* gene product [23]. These findings demonstrated that the SSV transforming protein is functionally equivalent to PDGF.

TABLE I. SSV Transforming Gene Product Possesses Fibroblast-Specific Mitogenic Activity

Mitogen	Protein added (μg)	Inhibiting peptide antibody[a]	^{3}H-Thymidine incorporation[b]	
			BALB/MK	NIH/3T3
SSV transformed	—	*sis*-N	NT	29,125
cell membrane	—	*sis*-N	NT	27,555
protein	—	—	2,840	26,641
	20	—	2,976	497,111
	20	*sis*-N	2,676	244,023
	20	*sis* N[c]	2,702	484,275
	20	*sis*-C	2,462	110,260
	20	*sis* C[c]	2,814	486,970
Uninfected cell membrane protein	20	—	2,898	28,868
PDGF	0.003	—	2,485	255,621
EGF	0.001	—	195,320	362,514

[a]The amount of antibody required to precipitate all of the *sis* gene product recognized in membrane preparations was determined in parallel immunoprecipitation experiments using ^{35}S-labeled HF/SSV cells as the source of membrane protein. The antibody concentration utilized was in twofold excess.
[b]BALB/MK or NIH/3T3 cells were plated in 96 well culture dishes and grown to confluence without media changing. Sixteen hours after test samples were added, medium was supplemented with 2 μCi ^{3}H-thymidine (New England Nuclear; specific activity 20 Ci/mmol) per well and incubated an additional 5 hr. Trichloroacetic acid-insoluble material was measured by scintillation counting. EGF and PDGF receptor grades were purchased from Collaborative Research. Raw counts without substraction of background are shown. NT, not tested.
[c]Antibodies were incubated with homologous peptide prior to inhibition study.

The ability of different anti-*sis* peptide sera to recognize various processed dimer forms of the v-*sis* translational product in SSV transformed cells made it possible to determine which forms possessed PDGF-like functions. Several processed forms, as well as the unprocessed p56^{sis} dimer itself exhibited these activities. In addition to the precursors p28^{sis}, p56^{sis}, and p42^{sis}, which are recognized by anti-*sis* N serum, anti-*sis* C serum which also detects p35^{sis}, a homodimer species representing from 5 to 10% of the total v-*sis* gene product. By comparing the residual PDGF-like activity following treatment by *sis* N and *sis* C antisera, we estimate that p35^{sis} may be severalfold more active in receptor competition or mitogenesis assays than less processed forms. All of these studies established that processing at amino and carboxy termini of this the p56^{sis} dimer is not required for its PDGF-like functions, although it appears that more mature forms may possess higher specific activities [23].

EVIDENCE THAT SSV TRANSFORMING ACTIVITY IS MEDIATED BY THE PDGF RECEPTOR

As summarized above, v-*sis* translational products possess the known functional activities of PDGF, including the ability to bind PDGF receptors, stimulate PDGF receptor authophosphorylation, and induce DNA synthesis of quiescent fibroblasts. If transformation by SSV were directly mediated by the interaction of v-*sis* products with cellular PDGF receptors, one would expect to observe a strict correlation between target cells susceptible to SSV transformation and cell types possessing

PDGF receptors. To address this question, we investigated the ability of SSV to transform a variety of cells in culture. We analyzed those cell types shown to possess PDGF receptors, including fibroblasts and smooth muscle cells, as well as cultures derived from epithelial or endothelial tissues, which lacked PDGF receptors. As a control, we compared the transforming activity of SSV with that of another acute transforming retrovirus, Kirsten-MSV, rescued by the same helper virus.

As shown in Table II, Kirsten-MSV efficiently transformed each of the target cells analyzed. In contrast, SSV showed a more restricted pattern. We observed high titered SSV transforming activity for fibroblasts and smooth muscle cells. However, there was no discernible morphological or detectable growth alteration of either epithelial or endothelial cells in response to SSV infection. The complete correlation between those assay cells susceptible to SSV transformation and those possessing PDGF receptors strongly implies that SSV transforming activity is mediated by the obligatory interaction of its *sis* gene product with the PDGF receptor.

MECHANISM OF v-*sis* TRANSFORMATION

The discovery that v-*sis* encodes a protein closely related in its predicted sequence [17,18] to human PDGF provided early experimental evidence that transforming genes act to perturb normal cellular pathways by which growth factors and their receptors induce cellular proliferation. More recently, close homology between the predicted v-*erb*-B product and the EGF receptor [24], as well as possible links between other oncogene products and growth factor/hormone receptors that share tyrosine kinase activity, have been discovered. Demonstrations that v-*sis* translational products synthesized by and associated with SSV transformed cells specifically bind PDGF receptors, stimulate tyrosine phosphorylation of the PDGF receptor, and induce DNA synthesis in quiescent fibroblasts have provided direct experimental evidence for this concept.

After synthesis on membrane-bound ribosomes, the $p28^{sis}$ monomer rapidly forms a homodimer in the endoplasmic reticulum and travels through the Golgi apparatus toward the cell periphery where it is further processed at both termini [22]. Recent evidence indicates that the LDL receptor travels along a similar intracellular

TABLE II. Susceptibility of Cell Types That Possess or Lack PDGF Receptors to SSV Transformation*

Tissue cell line	Presence of surface PDGF receptors	Transforming activity	
		SSV	Ki-MSV
Fibroblast			
Mouse (NIH/3T3)	+	+	+
Human skin	+	+	+
Smooth muscle			
Bovine	+	+	+
Endothelial			
Bovine aorta	−	−	+
Epithelial			
Mink (MvlLu)	−	−	+

*Biological activity of rescued transforming virus was determined by direct focus [40] or soft agar colony-forming [41] assays. Foci or colonies were scored at 14–21 days following infection.

pathway [25–27]. Moreover, sequence analysis of the EGF receptor predicts a protein whose receptor domain is translocated across the ER with its kinase domain occupying a cytoplasmic orientation [28]. If the PDGF receptor were processed in an analogous manner, its receptor domain might very well proceed along the same intracellular route as newly synthesized *sis*/PDGF-2–like dimers. If so, it is possible that the SSV transforming protein binds its PDGF-receptor target within the confines of the transformed cell.

PDGF provides a proliferative stimulus only to those cells that possess specific surface receptors for the growth factor. We observed a strict correlation between those cell types possessing PDGF receptors and those susceptible to transformation by SSV. Although there are undoubtedly other differences between fibroblasts as compared to endothelial or epithelial cells in addition to their PDGF receptor status, our findings strongly suggest that the v-*sis* gene product must interact with the PDGF receptor to manifest its transforming activity. Thus, it appears that the PDGF-like activities of v-*sis* translational products are those functions responsible for its ability to alter normal cellular growth control, leading suitable target cells along the pathway to malignancy.

THE HUMAN *sis* PROTOONCOGENE IS THE STRUCTURAL GENE FOR PDGF POLYPEPTIDE CHAIN 2

In view of the striking structural and functional similarities between human PDGF and the viral *sis* oncogene product, we have explored, at the molecular level, the role of the human *sis* protooncogene in human malignancies. To characterize the human *sis*/PDGF-2 locus, we isolated v-*sis*–related sequences from a bacteriophage library of normal human DNA [29]. These clones represented a continuous stretch of approximately 30 kbp. By Southern blotting analysis and hybridization with a v-*sis* probe, five v-*sis*–homologous restriction fragments were identified that could be localized within a 15 kbp region. Nucleotide sequence analysis of the v-*sis*–related regions demonstrated that an open reading frame was contained within the first five c-*sis* (human) exons. However, the 5′-most exon lacked a translation initiation codon [29,30]. Thus, c-*sis* coding sequences are incompletely represented in SSV. This conclusion is further supported by the observation that a 4.2 kbp *sis*-related transcript is present in human cells [31]. When the predicted c-*sis* (human) coding sequence was compared with that of the polypeptides representing PDGF-2, there was essentially complete homology [29,32,33]. These findings demonstrated that the c-*sis* (human) locus is the structural gene for PDGF-2.

EXPRESSION OF THE NORMAL CODING SEQUENCE FOR HUMAN *sis*/PDGF-2 INDUCES CELLULAR TRANSFORMATION

The transcription of c-*sis* (human) was studied by using probes derived from introns and exons of the PDGF-2 gene. A 4.2 kb mRNA in the A2781 human tumor cell line was detected by a v-*sis* probe and by c-*sis* probes representing each of the c-*sis* exons (unpublished observations). The only other probe that hybridized to the same sized message was derived from a region 10 kbp upstream of the 5′-most v-*sis*–related exon of human c-*sis*. This probe (pc-*sis*1) did not detect v-*sis* RNA and thus might represent a non-*sis*-related exon of the c-*sis* transcriptional unit. Nucleotide sequence analysis of pc-*sis*1 was performed and revealed the presence of three open reading frames each of which was initiated by a methionine codon. Donor splice sites were found at positions within pc-*sis*1 that would allow for in-phase translation when spliced to the acceptor splice site in the first v-*sis*–related exon [34].

The DNA of a c-*sis* (human) phage clone, λ-c-*sis* clone 8, that contained all of the PDGF-2 coding sequences [29] was introduced into NIH/3T3 cells via transfection to study the structural requirements for c-*sis* gene expression. The sequences contained within the λ-c-*sis* clone 8 were incapable of transforming cells and they did not synthesize transcripts as determined by cotransfection experiments using a selectable marker gene (pSV2-gpt). Moreover, positioning a retroviral LTR upstream of the λ-c-*sis* clone 8 coding regions failed to confer transforming activity [34].

Since the putative upstream exon of c-*sis* (human) contained a potential amino terminal sequence for a PDGF/*sis* precursor, but not identifiable promoter signals, this segment was ligated in the proper orientation between the retroviral LTR and first exon of c-*sis* (human) clone 8. As shown in Figure 3, by transfection of NIH/3T3 cells with this molecular construct, transforming activity comparable to that of SSV DNA was observed (10^5 ffu/pmol) [34]. Thus, our findings provide direct evidence for a model in which the constitutive expression of the human gene for a normal growth factor in a cell susceptible to its growth-promoting actions can result in cell transformation.

Transformants induced by the activated human *sis*/PDGF-2 coding sequence contained two major *sis*/PDGF-2–related protein species of 52,000 and 35,000 daltons, which were detected using anti-*sis* peptide serum and nonreducing assay conditions. In contrast, a 26,000 dalton species, presumed to be the primary translational

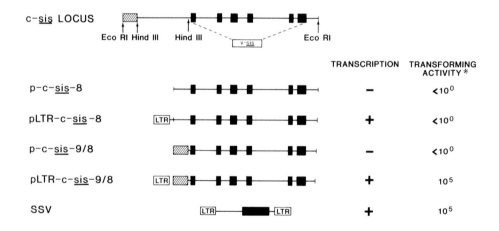

*Focus-forming units per pmol of PDGF-2 coding sequences

Fig. 3. Expression of the normal PDGF-2 coding sequence in mouse fibroblasts induces morphological transformation. Genomic DNA molecules cooled in plasmid vectors were transfected onto NIH/3T3 cells and tested for transcriptional activation and transforming activity. A filled box indicates a c-*sis*/PDGF-2 exon related to v-*sis*; a hatched box indicates the upstream c-*sis*/PDGF-2 exon not related to v-*sis*. LTR, retrovirus long terminal repeat.

product, was observed under reducing conditions. These findings imply that the putative upstream exon sequences served to initiate translation of a PDGF-2 precursor molecule, which underwent dimer formation and subsequent processing. In light of our knowledge that the human *sis* gene codes for PDGF-2 and our findings of highly efficient transforming activity by the construct, we conclude that normal human PDGF-2 expressed in NIH/3T3 cells is sufficient to induce transformation.

These studies have potentially important implications concerning the role of normal genes coding for growth-regulatory molecules in the neoplastic process. A number of growth-promoting molecules have been shown to be released by a variety of tumor cells [35–38]. In some cases, such molecules have been postulated to play a role in the neoplastic state of these cells. However, the alternative possibility exists that the expression of such factors is a secondary result of the genetic instability and dedifferentiated state known to exist in tumor cells.

Our present findings establish that derepression of the coding sequence for a normal human growth factor can cause it to acquire transforming properties in an appropriate target cell. Moreover, when incorporated by a retrovirus, the v-*sis*/ PDGF-2 transforming gene has been shown to induce fibrosarcomas and glioblastomas [39; our unpublished observations]. Many human glioblastomas and fibrosarcomas express *sis*/PDGF-2 transcripts [31], whereas normal fibroblasts and glial cells so far analyzed do not [31; our unpublished observations]. Thus, transcriptional activation of this gene could be involved in the induction of naturally occurring tumors of connective tissue origin. If so, it will be important to gain more detailed knowledge of the regulation of the human *sis* protooncogene to determine what mechanisms may lead to its transcriptional activation.

REFERENCES

1. Bishop JM: Cellular oncogenes and retroviruses. In Snell EE, Boyer PD, Meister A, Richardson CC (eds): "Annual Review of Biochemistry." Palo Alto: Academic Press, Vol 52, 1983, pp 301–354.
2. Weiss RA, Teich N, Varmus H, Coffin RJ: "Molecular Biology of Tumor Viruses, RNA Tumor Viruses," 2nd ed. New York: Cold Spring Harbor, 1982.
3. Theilen GH, Gould D, Fowler M, Dungworth DL: C-type virus in tumor tissue of a woolly monkey (*Lagothrix spp.*) with fibrosarcoma. JNCI 47:881, 1971.
4. Aaronson SA: Biologic characterization of mammalian cells transformed by a primate sarcoma virus. Virology 52:562, 1973.
5. Robbins KC, Devare SG, Aaronson SA: Molecular cloning of integrated simian sarcoma virus: Genome organization of infectious DNA clones. Proc Natl Acad Sci USA 78:2918, 1981.
6. Robbins KC, Devare SG, Reddy EP, Aaronson SA: *In vivo* identification of the transforming gene product of simian sarcoma virus. Science 218:1131, 1982a.
7. Devare SG, Reddy EP, Law JD, Robbins KC, Aaronson SA: Nucleotide sequence of the simian sarcoma virus genome: Demonstration that its acquired cellular sequences encode the transforming gene product, p28*sis*. Proc Natl Acad Sci USA 80:731, 1983.
8. Antoniades HN, Scher CD, Stiles CD: Purification of human platelet-derived growth factor. Proc Natl Acad Sci USA 76:1809, 1979.
9. Kaplan DR, Chao FC, Stiles CD, Antoniades HN, Sher CD: Platelet alpha-granules contain a growth factor for fibroblasts. Blood 53:1043, 1979.
10. Rosse R, Glomset J, Kariya B, Harker L: A platelet-dependent serum factor that stimulates the proliferation of arterial smooth muscle cells in vitro. Proc Natl Acad Sci USA 71:1207, 1974.
11. Scher CD, Shepard RC, Antoniades HN, Stiles CD: Platelet-derived growth factor and the regulation of the mammalian fibroblast cell cycle. Biochim Biophys Acta 560:217, 1979.
12. Heldin CH, Westermark B, Wasteson A: Platelet-derived growth factor: Purification and partial characterization. Proc Natl Acad Sci USA 76:3722, 1979.

13. Heldin CH, Westermark B, Wasteson A: Demonstration of antibody against platelet-derived growth factor. Exp Cell Res 136:255, 1981.

14. Deuel TF, Huang JS, Proffit RT, Baenziger JU, Chang D, Kennedy BB: Human platelet-derived growth factor. Purification and resolution into two active protein fractions. J Biol Chem 256:8896, 1981.

15. Antoniades HN, Hunkapiller MW: Human platelet-derived growth factor (PDGF): Amino terminal amino acid sequence. Science 220:963, 1983.

16. Wilbur WJ, Lipman DJ: Rapid similarity searches of nucleic acid and protein data banks. Proc Natl Acad Sci USA 80:726, 1983.

17. Doolittle RF, Hunkapiller MW, Hood LE, Devare SG, Robbins KC, Aaronson SA, Antoniades HN: Simian sarcoma virus *onc* gene, v-*sis*, is derived from the gene (or genes) encoding a platelet-derived growth factor. Science 221:275, 1983.

18. Waterfield MD, Scrace GT, Whittle N, Stroobant P, Johnsson A, Wasteson A, Westermark B, Heldin CH, Huang JS, Deuel TF: Platelet-derived growth factor is structurally related to the putative transforming protein p28*sis* of simian sarcoma virus. Nature 304:35, 1983.

19. Robbins KC, Hill RL, Aaronson SA: Primate origin of the cell-derived sequences of simian sarcoma virus. J Virol 41:721, 1982.

20. Wilson AC, Carlson SS, White TJ: Biochemical evolution. Annu Rev Biochem 46:573, 1977.

21. Robbins KC, Antoniades HN, Devare SG, Hunkapiller MW, Aaronson SA: Structural and immunological similarities between simian sarcoma virus gene product(s) and human platelet-derived growth factor. Nature 305:605, 1983.

22. Robbins KC, Leal F, Pierce JH, Aaronson SA: The v-*sis*/PDGF-2 transforming gene product localizes to cell membranes but is not a secretory protein. EMBO J 4:1783–1792, 1985.

23. Leal F, Williams LT, Robbins KC, Aaronson SA: Evidence that the v-*sis* gene product transforms by interaction with the receptor for platelet-derived growth factor. Science 230:327–330, 1985.

24. Downward J, Yarden Y, Mayes E, Scrace E, Totty N, Stockwell P, Ullrich A, Schlessinger J, Waterfield MD: Close similarity of epidermal growth factor receptor and v-*erb*-B oncogene protein sequences. Nature 307:521, 1984.

25. Schneider WJ, Beisiegel U, Goldstein JL, Brown MS: Purification of the low density lipoprotein receptor, an acidic glycoprotein of 164,000 molecular weight. J Biol Chem 257:2664, 1982.

26. Tolleshaug H, Hobgood KK, Brown MS, Goldstein JL: The LDL receptor locus in familial hypercholesterolemia: Multiple mutations disrupt transport and processing of a membrane receptor. Cell 32:941, 1983.

27. Gething M-J, Sambrook J: Construction of influenza haemagglutinin genes that code for intracellular and secreted forms of the protein. Nature 300:598, 1982.

28. Ullrich A, Coussens L, Hayflick JS, Dull TJ, Gray A, Tam AW, Lee J, Yarden Y, Libermann TA, Schlessinger J, Downward J, Mayes ELV, Whittle N, Waterfield MD, Seeburg PH: Human epidermal growth factor receptor cDNA sequence and aberrant expression of the amplified gene in A431 epidermal carcinoma cells. Nature 309:418, 1984.

29. Chiu I-M, Reddy EP, Givol D, Robbins KC, Tronick SR, Aaronson SA: Nucleotide sequence analysis identifies the human c-*sis* proto-oncogene as a structural gene for platelet-derived growth factor. Cell 37:123, 1984.

30. Josephs SF, Dalla Favera R, Gelmann EP, Gallo RC, Wong-Staal F: 5' viral and human cellular sequences corresponding to the transforming gene of simian sarcoma virus. Science 219:503, 1984.

31. Eva A, Robbins KC, Andersen PR, Srinivasan A, Tronick SR, Reddy EP, Ellmore NW, Galen AT, Lautenberger JA, Papas TS, Westin EH, Wong-Staal F, Gallo RC, Aaronson SA: Cellular genes analogous to retroviral *onc* genes are transcribed in human tumor cells. Nature 295:116, 1982.

32. Johnsson A, Heldin C-H, Wasteson A, Westermark B, Devel TF, Huang JS, Seeburg PH, Gray A, Ullrich A, Scrace G, Stroobant P, Waterfield MD: The c-*sis* gene encodes a precursor of the B chain of platelet-derived growth factor. EMBO J 3:921, 1984.

33. Josephs SF, Guo C, Ratner L, Wong-Staal F: Human proto-oncogene nucleotide sequence corresponding to the transforming region of simian sarcoma virus. Science 223:487, 1984.

34. Gazit A, Igarashi H, Chiu I-M, Srinivasan A, Yaniv A, Tronick SR, Robbins KC, Aaronson SA: Expression of the normal human *sis*/PDGF-2 coding sequence induces cellular transformation. Cell 39:89, 1984.

35. DeLarco JE, Todaro GJ: Growth factors from murine sarcoma virus transformed cells. Proc Natl Acad Sci USA 75:4001, 1978.

36. Heldin CH, Westermark B, Wateson A: Chemical and biological properties of a growth factor from human-cultured osteosarcoma cells: Resemblance with platelet derived growth factor. J Cell Physiol 105:235, 1980.

37. Nister M, Heldin CH, Wateson A, Westermark B: A platelet-derived growth factor analog produced by a human clonal glioma cell line. Ann NY Acad Sci 397:25, 1982.

38. Graves DT, Owen AJ, Antoniades HN: Evidence that a human osteosarcoma cell line which secretes a mitogen similar to platelet-derived growth factor requires growth factors present in platelet-poor plasma. Cancer Res 43:83, 1983.

39. Wolfe LG, Deinhardt F, Theilen GJ, Rabin H, Kawakami T, Bustad LK: Induction of tumors in marmoset monkeys by simian sarcoma virus, type 1 (*lagothrix*): A preliminary report. JNCI 47:1115, 1971.

40. Aaronson SA, Rowe WP: Nonproducer clones of murine sarcoma virus transformed BALB/3T3 cells. Virology 43:9, 1970.

41. Shin S, Freedman VH, Risser R, Pollack R: Tumorigenicity of virus-transformed cells in nude mice is correlated specifically with anchorage independent growth in vitro. Proc Natl Acad Sci USA 72:4435, 1975.

Biochemical and Molecular Epidemiology of Cancer 167–176 (1986)

The Role of Active Oxygen in Tumor Promotion

Peter A. Cerutti

Department of Carcinogenesis, Swiss Institute for Experimental Cancer Research, 1066 Epalinges/Lausanne, Switzerland

PARADIGMS IN MULTISTEP CHEMICAL CARCINOGENESIS

Tumor promoters modulate gene expression resulting in the proliferation rather than differentiation of initiated cells. Selection and clonal expansion of promoted initiated cells is facilitated when promoters speed up the terminal differentiation of surrounding noninitiated cells and when they are particularly toxic to them. Only an "ideal" promoter may possess all the above qualities, and the importance of the different activities may vary for different organ systems. Promotion results mostly in benign neoplasms and only rarely in carcinomas. Many of the benign neoplasms regress, but some of them spontaneously progress to malignant tumors. Progression is usually associated with karyotypic changes [1–6].

For many years, the paradigm has been 1) that promoters in contrast to initiators do not cause DNA damage and DNA sequence changes, 2) that their effects are reversible (at least in early stages), and 3) that they are only effective when applied repeatedly *after* initiator treatment. There exists no endogenous or xenobiotic promoter that rigorously complies with all these rules and important "exceptions" to the above paradigms have been discovered that have to be taken seriously. For example, most promoters that induce a cellular prooxidant state induce DNA damage by indirect action [7], and even the membrane-active phorbolester promoter phorbol-12-myristate-13-acetate (PMA) has been shown to cause DNA single-strand breakage, sister chromatid exchanges (SCE), and chromosomal aberrations in leukocytes [8,9], cultured mouse epidermal cells [10], and basal cells of mouse epidermis in vivo [11]. (The notion that even epithelial and endothelial cells can establish prooxidant states has recently received experimental support: 1) It was found that PMA induces chemiluminescence in mouse epidermal cells [12] and 2) that active oxygen is formed following treatment with the D,T-diaphorase inhibitor menadione could be directly demonstrated in endothelial cells by epr-spectroscopy [13].)

Received May 17, 1985.

© **1986 Alan R. Liss, Inc.**

The second paradigm has been challenged by the finding that a single application of PMA to dimethylbenz(a)anthracene (DMBA)-initiated skin of NMRI mice is remembered for many weeks (half-life ~ 10 weeks) after which time promotion can be completed by the application of the second stage promoter RPA [14]. In analogous experiments in SENCAR mice, the treatment with PMA had no effect when it was followed 8 weeks later by the second-stage promoter mezerein [15]. Although the observation that PMA alone can induce a small number of tumors [16,17] might indicate the presence of some spontaneously initiated cells, the successful and efficient induction of tumors by a reversed regimen, ie, PMA application first, then DMBA after a delay of several weeks, then second-stage promoter RPA [18], is in direct violation of paradigm 3. According to formal terminology, PMA acted as initiator and DMBA as first-stage promoter in this experiment. This interpretation adheres to the initial premise of multistep, chemical carcinogenesis, namely that it is possible to distinguish clearly classes of agents with nonoverlapping biological properties. However, ideal representatives for these classes are exceptions among xenobiotics and may not exist. We have previously suggested considering quality gradients [19]. Within the frame of a four-step carcinogenesis model, ie, initiation, first-stage promotion, second-stage promotion, progression, such quality gradients could be complex. For example, a given compound could be a strong initiator and first-stage promoter, another a strong initiator and progressor, etc. There are six permutations for the simple mixing of two strong qualities. Recent evidence suggests that certain qualities are related, however. Hennings et al [20] reported that agents usually considered to be strong initiators (4-nitro-quinoline-N-oxide; N-methyl-N'-nitro-N-nitroso-guanidine; urethane) were particularly active as progressors for mouse skin papillomas. A relationship between the quality of promoters and progressors is indicated by the finding of T. Slaga and collaborators (personal communication) that benzoylperoxide is a particularly potent progressor on the other hand. These considerations suggest that cyclic rather than sequential regimen, eg; initiator, promoter, initiator, promoter, etc, or initiation on the background of chronic promotion, might be particularly efficient and relevant to the in vivo situation.

In this discussion, we have not questioned the usefulness of the concept of multistep carcinogenesis nor of the distinction of initiation, promotion, progression as mechanistically different stages involving multiple genes. Rather, major difficulties in present research are seen in the lack of carcinogens with highly selective properties and in the definition on a molecular level of a unique sequence of events a cell has to pass through on the pathway to malignancy. Work with endogenous promoters such as hormones and growth factors might circumvent some of these difficulties.

SIGNAL TRANSDUCTION BY PROMOTERS THAT BIND TO SPECIFIC MEMBRANE RECEPTORS

The primary site for early action of many mouse skin promoters is the plasma membrane. The interaction occurs with specific receptors in the case of the phorbolester promoters, teleocidin, lyngbyatoxin, mezerein [2,21], and endogenous peptide hormones. As a consequence, protein kinase C is activated. For peptide hormones the stimulation is mediated by diacylgylcerol, which is produced from phosphatidyl-inositol by the action of a phosphodiesterase [22,23]. The simultaneous release of inositol-triphosphate is likely to act as signal for Ca^{2+} mobilization from the endoplasmic reticulum [24]. These events quickly result in an increase in the cytoplasmic pH by an unknown mechanism involving the Na^+/H^+ antiporter. It has been noted that several oncogene products appear to act at different stages of the same signal transduction pathway [24,25]. The phorbolester promoters directly stimulate protein kinase C, which serves as its membrane receptor, and do not cause any immediate large changes in intracellular Ca^{2+} distribution. Nevertheless, PMA induces an increase in cytoplasmic pH comparable to that observed for peptide hormones in quiescent mouse thymocytes and Swiss 3T3 fibroblasts [26]. Evidently, sufficient Ca^{2+} is available for the activation of the Ca^{2+}-dependent protein kinase C.

EARLY EFFECTS OF PROOXIDANT PROMOTERS THAT DO NOT BIND TO SPECIFIC MEMBRANE RECEPTORS

For many promoters, there is no evidence that they bind to membrane receptors, although some of them may affect membrane structure in a less specific manner. Examples for mouse skin are anthralin, cantharidin, phenols, benzo(e)pyrene, 7-bromomethylbenz(a)anthracene, iodoacetic acid, a number of peroxy-compounds, and the Ca^{2+} ionophore A-23187. Organic peroxides and hydrogenperoxide are complete promoters or stage I promoters for SENCAR mice [25], and various oxidizing agents induce the capacity for anchorage-independent growth and tumorigenicity in cultured Balb/C epidermal cells $JB6P^+$ [18,29]. Indeed, superoxide produced extracellularly by xanthine/xanthine oxidase or by human neutrophils promotes and transformes cultured mouse embryo fibroblasts C3H10T1/2 to focus formation and tumorigenicity [30,31]. An early effect of prooxidant promoters appears to be the mobilization of mitochondrial Ca^{2+} [32]. We have found that arachidonic acid-hydroperoxide specifically induces Ca^{2+} release in a sequence of reactions involving the degradation of the peroxide by glutathione peroxidase, an increase in mitochondrial NAD^+, and ADP-ribosylation of the $Ca^{2+}/2H^+$ antiporter. However, the corresponding hydroxyl-arachidonic acid derivative and free arachidonic acid also elicited Ca^{2+} release, albeit with diminished efficiency (C. Richter and P. Cerutti, unpublished). Mitochondrial Ca^{2+} mobilization might trigger a cascade of events similar to that induced by peptide hormone promoters. It is interesting to note that PMA accelerates hydrolysis of ATP in rat liver mitochondria [33]. Figure 1 presents a heuristic scheme of the interrelated pathways of signal transduction of polypeptide hormones, phorbol-ester-type promoters, and prooxidant promoters.

PARACRINE AND CLASTOGENIC ACTION OF INFLAMMATORY CELLS IN TUMOR PROMOTION

Inflammation is necessary but not sufficient for promotion in mouse skin [34]. An early event following the application of PMA and many other promoters is the infiltration of polymorphonuclear cells (PMN) and later macrophages in response to chemotactic signals. These phagocytic cells react to the exposure with PMA and other membrane-active compounds with an oxidative burst and the release of a complex mixture of phospholipids, free arachidonic acid (AA), and AA metabolites. It was suggested by Goldstein et al [35] that the active oxygen released by inflammatory cells might exert a promotional effect on initiated epidermal cells in neighboring tissue. This model has been elaborated on by several laboratories [11,31,36,37], and

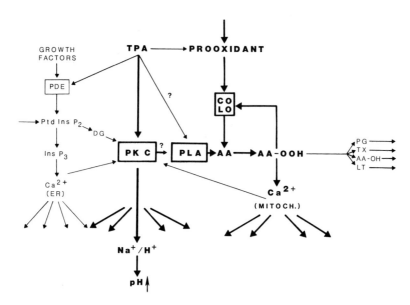

Fig. 1. Pathways of signal transduction of polypeptide hormones, phorbol-ester-type promoters, and prooxidant promoters.

there is convincing evidence that PMA can induce DNA and chromosomal damage in leukocytes and that leukocytes release a diffusible clastogenic factor (CF) [38]. The formation of DNA strand breakage, ring-saturated thymine, and SCE in response to PMA was demonstrated in cocultures of PMN or macrophages with fibroblasts [7,39,40] and mouse epidermal cells [11]. As was mentioned above, PMA stimulation of PMN induced the transformation of cocultured C3H10T1/2 cells [31]. The PMA-induced CF from human monocytes has been biochemically characterized. It consists of H_2O_2, reduced iron, AA-hydroperoxides and other lipids, and free AA [7,41]. This mixture of lipids and phospholipids undergoes radical chain reactions that may initiate autooxidation reactions, disturb the Ca^{2+} and pH homeostasis in the target cell, and ultimately induce DNA and chromosomal damage.

The hydroxy-AA metabolites contained in the chromatographed monocyte CF derive from the corresponding hydroperoxy precursors, ie, 5- and 11- and 15-HETE from 5- and 11- and 15-HPETE, thromboxane B_2 and prostaglandin E_2 from prostaglandin G_2, and 15-hydroperoxy prostaglandin E_2. In the tissue and the metastable CF preparations, these hydroperoxy metabolites are of sufficient stability to reach neighboring epithelial and mesenchymal cells. Indeed, we have demonstrated by alkaline elution analysis that exogenous 15-hydroperoxy-AA efficiently breaks DNA in mouse fibroblasts (T. Ochi and P. Cerutti, unpublished).

The role of DNA damage and chromosomal aberrations induced by prooxidant promoters remains unclear. As was discussed above, the formation of relatively large numbers of random DNA breaks could be involved in the modulation of gene expression [42,43], and rare chromosomal rearrangements might play a role in late steps of tumorigenesis. If CF was more toxic to noninitiated than initiated cells, it might also facilitate selection and clonal expansion of the latter. In addition to its clastogenicity, the "paracrine" action of the complex mixture of active phospholipid and AA derivatives which are released by PMA-stimulated leukocytes may contribute to the role of inflammation in promotion and progression. For example, the CF mixture contains prostaglandin $F_2\alpha$, which mobilizes intracellular Ca^{2+} [25] and enhances PMA promotion of DMBA-initiated mouse skin [44]. Topical application of various chemically stable AA metabolites on initiated mouse skin did not produce striking results [44], but endoperoxide analogs of prostaglandins were active promoters [45]. Monocytes also release complement components, monokines, and mononuclear cell-conditioned factor. These mediators of inflammation may contribute to the role of phagocytes in promotion/progression [46].

Immediate effects of promoters observed in a large portion of a cell population can hardly be the consequence of rare mutations or chromosomal aberrations. However, because of their potent clastogenic activities, prooxidant promoters could play a role in protooncogene activation by gene rearrangement or gene amplification (without the induction of gross chromosomal changes). For the same reason, they may also represent potent progressors, as suggested by the results of T. Slaga (personal communication) mentioned above. The contention that initiators induce all the genetic changes necessary for neoplastic growth involving promoter-induced selection and clonal expansion [15] can only be ascertained when initiated, nonpromoted cells are available for genetic analysis.

MODULATION OF GENE EXPRESSION BY PROMOTERS

In contrast to viral carinogens, chemicals do not introduce new genetic information into the target cell. Rather, they modulate the expression of cellular genes. Therefore, the finding of Balmain et al [47] that the level of rasH transcripts was increased in individual and pooled papillomas from DMBA-initiated and PMA-promoted SENCAR mice was of particular interest. However, in similar work by Toftgard et al [48] and T. Slaga (personal communication), no significant changes in the expression of rasH, rasK, fos, myc, and raf protooncogenes could be detected in pooled papillomas with the exception that abl-RNA was decreased below constitutive levels. It should also be mentioned that the two cloned pro-genes of JB6 P^+ mouse epidermal cells have no resemblance to 12 retroviral oncogenes to which they have been compared [49]. In contrast, an increase in the expression of rasH and mos protooncogenes was discovered in primary mouse hepatomas that may be in an early stage of promotion [50].

It appears likely that promoter action is more complex than the direct activation of retroviral-type protooncogenes. A case in point is the observation that PMA treatment strongly enhanced the transformation of mouse embryo fibroblasts C3H10T1/2 with the cloned human bladder cancer cellular rasH gene [51]. These results suggest that tumor promoters modulate the expression of cellular genes that complement or enhance the function of activated oncogenes. Prooxidant stress genes and certain genes under hormonal control might be regulated by promoters. For example, the proviral gene of mouse mammary tumor virus (MMTV) can be induced to transcribe in virally infected cells both by the glucocorticoid hormone dexamethasone (DEX) and the tumor promoter PMA. Previous studies have shown that there are specific DNA sequences in the MMTV long terminal repeat (LTR) necessary for the induction of transcription by DEX [52]. To determine whether transcriptional changes in gene expression induced by PMA also involve specific DNA sequences, we used mouse L cells transfected with chimeric MMTV plasmids. Thymidine kinase-deficient (tk⁻) Ltk⁻aprt⁻ cells were transformed to tk+ with a plasmid construction containing various deletion fragments of the MMTV LTR joined to the herpes simplex tk gene. Cells successfully transfected were selected in HAT medium and propagated. Cytoplasmic RNA was isolated from cultures that had been treated with either DEX or PMA. The constructions and experimental procedures have been described previously [52]. The RNA was analyzed for transcriptional activity of the plasmid by RNA blot hybridization. As is shown in Table I, both PMA and dexamethasone require a region between −105 and −204 base pairs from the cap site for transcription (Gruenert, Buetti, Diggelmann, and Cerutti, unpublished). The fact that the induction of complete viral sequences was more efficient than all the constructions containing only LTR sequences suggests that there exist additional recognition sequences outside the LTR.

When cDNA libraries from a murine thymic leukemia T-cell line were screened for PMA-inducible sequences, the most abundant species were related to MMTV. MMTV-related RNA was also induced by PMA in normal spleen cells from Balb/c and C57BL/6 mice. Sequence analysis revealed that MMTV-related cDNA clones included part of the env gene and the right LTR of MMTV [53]. In a different system, the same specific 5′ sequences of the rat prolactin gene were recognized for the induction of the transcription of downstream sequences in response to EGF and PMA in human A431 cells [54]. Important insights about the mechanism of modulation of gene expression are also obtained from studies of induction of EBV by PMA [55].

PROMOTER-INDUCED POSTTRANSLATIONAL MODIFICATIONS OF PROTEINS

The spectrum of proteins being phosphorylated in response to PMA by protein kinace C and other kinases is presently being characterized in several laboratories. Among others, the EGF [56], insulin [57], and somatomedin C [58] receptors, 80-kD heat shock protein [59], two 28-kD "stress" proteins [60], and the histones H2B and H4 [61] serve as acceptors. We have recently discovered that PMA induces a second type of posttranslational protein modification, namely poly-ADP ribosylation [62–64]. This modification is of particular interest in that it specifically involves chromosomal proteins and might, therefore, play a role in promoter-induced modulation of gene expression.

TABLE I. Inducibility by PMA of Transcription of Constructs Containing Various Deletions in MMTV-LTR

L cells containing	DEX[a]	PMA[a]	DEX/PMA
Total virus	7.9	7.7	1.0
Construct with complete LTR	4.4	2.1	2.1
Construct with LTR sequences from capsite to −600	6.9	4.6	1.5
Construct with LTR sequences from capsite to −204	4.4	2.2	2.0
Construct with LTR sequences from capsite to −105	ND	ND	—

[a]Treatment of transformed mouse L cells with either 10^{-6} M DEX or 20 ng/ml PMA for 24 hr. Densitometer readings of dot blots are listed.

As was mentioned above, many promoters induce a cellular prooxidant state, and antioxidants have antipromotional activity [7,65]. Poly-ADP ribosylation of chromosomal proteins might play a role in the mechanism of action of prooxidant promoters; it is intimately related to the redox state of the cell, DNA strand breakage, and chromatin conformation. Evidence for the participation of poly-ADP ribosylation in DNA repair, cell differentiation [66,67], and malignant transformation [68–70] has been obtained. Our recent finding that PMA and superoxide cause an increase in poly-ADP ribosylation of nuclear proteins in mouse fibroblasts C3H10T1/2, and human skin fibroblasts is intriguing. In contrast to poly-ADP ribosylation by the methylating agent N-methyl-N'-nitro-N-nitrosoguanidine, de novo RNA and protein synthesis are required [62–64]. Multiple nuclear proteins serve as poly-ADPR acceptors in response to PMA treatment in 10T1/2 cells. Preliminary results suggest that histones H2B and H2A are poly-ADP ribosylated. However, according to Western blot analysis, the major acceptor is ADP ribosyl transferase itself. In the PMA-treated samples, major bands correspond to proteolytic fragments of the transferase. The reaction is inhibited by the antioxidant enzyme catalase and the protease inhibitor antipain. Fragmentation of the enzyme could represent a response to PMA-induced cellular stress. Indeed, similar transferase fragmentation is induced in permeabilized human lymphocytes by the alarmon Ap4A [71].

ACKNOWLEDGMENTS

The original work reported in this article was supported by grants from the Swiss National Science Foundation and the Swiss Association of Cigarette Manufacturers.

REFERENCES

 1. Pitot H: Contributions to our understanding of the natural history of neoplastic development in lower animals to the cause and control of human cancer. Cancer Surv 2:519–537, 1983.
 2. Weinstein IB, Gattoni-Celli S, Kirschmeier P, Lambert M, Hsiao W, Backer J, Jeffrey A: Multistage carcinogenesis involves multiple genes and multiple mechanisms. Cancer Cells 1:229–237, 1984.
 3. Schulte-Hermann R, Timmermann-Trosiener I, Schuppler J: Response of liver foci in rats to hepatic tumor promoters. Toxicol Pathol 10:63–70, 1982.
 4. Yuspa SH: Mechanisms of initiation and promotion in mouse epidermis. In: "The Role of Cocarcinogens and Promoters in Human and Experimental Carcinogenesis." Lyon: IARC (in press).
 5. Hicks RM: Pathological and biochemical aspects of tumor promotion. Carcinogenesis 4:1209–1214, 1983.
 6. Slaga TJ (ed): "Mechanisms of Tumor Promotion, Vol III. Tumor Promotion and Carcinogenesis In Vitro." Boca Raton, FL: CRC Press, 1983.
 7. Cerutti P: Prooxidant states and tumor promotion. Science 227:375–381, 1985.
 8. Emerit I, Cerutti P: Tumor promoter phorbol-12-myristate-13-acetate induces chromosomal damage via indirect action. Nature 293:144–146, 1981.
 9. Birnboim H: DNA strand breakage in human leukocytes exposed to a tumor promoter, phorbol-myristate-acetate. Science 215:1247–1249, 1982.
10. Dzarlieva R, Fusenig N: Tumor promoter 12-0-tetradecanoyl-phorbol-13-acetate enhances sister chromatid exchanges and numerical and structural chromosome aberrations in primary mouse epidermal cultures. Cancer Lett 16:7–17, 1982.
11. Dutton DR, Bowden GT: Indirect Induction of a clastogenic effect in epidermal cells by a tumor promoter. Personal communication, 1985.
12. Fischer S, Adams L: Inhibition of tumor promoters stimulated chemiluminescence in mouse epidermal cells by inhibition of arachidonic acid metabolism. AACR Proc 25:82, 1984.

13. Rosen G, Freeman B: Detection of superoxide generated by endothelial cells. Proc Natl Acad Sci USA 81:7269–7273, 1984.

14. Fürstenberger G, Sorg B, Marks F: Tumor promotion by phorbol esters in skin: Evidence for memory effect. Science 220:89–91, 1983.

15. Hennings H, Yuspa S: Two-stage promotion in mouse skin: an alternative explanation. JNCI (in press).

16. Burns F, Albert R, Altschuler B, Morris E: Environ Health Perspect 50:309, (1983).

17. Astrup E, Iversen O, Elgjo K: The tumorigenic and carcinogenic effect of TPA when applied to the skin of Balb/cA mice. Virchows Arch B Cell Pathol 33:303, 1980.

18. Marks F, Fürstenberger G, Kinzel V: J Cancer Res Clin Oncol 109:A16, 1985.

19. Ide M, Kaneko M, Cerutti P: Benzo(a)pyrene and ascorbate-CuSO$_4$ induce DNA damage in human cells by direct action. In McBrien PCH, Slater TF (eds): "Protective Agents in Cancer." New York: Academic Press, 1983, pp 125–140.

20. Hennings H, Shores R, Wenk M, Spengler E, Tarone R, Yuspa S: Malignant conversion of mouse skin tumours increased by tumour initiators and unaffected by tumour promoters. Nature 304:67–69, 1983.

21. Weinstein I, Gattoni-Celli S, Kirschmeier P, Lambert M, Hsiao W, Backer J, Jeffrey A: Multistage carcinogenesis involves multiple genes and multiple mechanisms. Cancer Cell 1:229–237, 1984.

22. Kikkawa U, Kaibuchi K, Castagna M, Yamanishi J, Sano K, Tanaka Y, Miyake R, Takai Y, Nishizuka Y: In Greengard P (ed): "Advances in Cyclic Nucleotide and Protein Phosphorylation Research." New York: Raven Press, 1984, pp 437–442.

23. Nishizuka Y: The role of protein kinase C in cell surface signal transduction and tumour promotion. Nature 308:693–698, 1984.

24. Berridge M, Irvine R: Inositol triphosphate, a novel second messenger in cellular signal transduction. Nature 312:315–321, 1984.

25. Hesketh T, Moore J, Morris J, Taylor M, Rogers J, Smith G, Metcalfe J: A common sequence of calcium and pH signals in the mitogenic stimulation of eukaryotic cells. Nature 313:481–484, 1985.

26. Sporn M, Roberts A: Autocrine growth factors and cancer. Nature 313:745–747, 1985.

27. Slaga T, Klein-Szanto A, Triplet L, Yotti L, Trosko J: Skin Tumor promoting activity of benzoylperoxide, a widely used free radical generating compound. Science 213:1023–1025, 1981.

28. Gindhart T, Srinivas L, Colburn N: Benzoylperoxide promotion of transformation of JB6 mouse epidermal cells: Inhibition by ganglioside GT but not retinoic acid. Carcinogenesis 6, 1985.

29. Nakamura Y, Colburn N, Gindhart T: Role of reactive oxygen in tumor promotion: Implication of superoxide anion in promotion of neoplastic transformation in JB-6 cells by TPA. Carcinogenesis 6, 1985.

30. Zimmerman R, Cerutti P: Active oxygen acts as a promoter of transformation in mouse C3H/10T1/2/C18 fibroblasts. Proc Natl Acad Sci USA 81:2085–2087, 1984.

31. Weitzman S, Weitberg A, Clark E, Stossel T: Phagocytes as carcinogens: Malignant transformation produced by human neutrophils. Science 227:1231–1233, 1985.

32. Lötscher H, Winterhalter K, Carafoli E, Richter C: Hydroperoxides can modulate the redox state of pyridine nucleotides and the calcium balance in rat liver mitochondria. Proc Natl Acad Sci USA 76:4340–4344, 1979.

33. Backer J, Weinstein I: A phorbolester tumor promoter accelerates hydrolysis of ATP by isolated rat liver mitochondria. Proc Am Assoc Cancer Res 24:109, 1983.

34. Slaga T, Fischer S, Weeks C, Klein-Szanto A: Cellular and biochemical mechanisms of mouse skin tumor promoters. In Hodgson E, Bend J, Philpot R (eds): "Reviews in Biochemical Toxicology." New York: Elsevier-North Holland, Vol III, 1981.

35. Goldstein B, Witz G, Amoruso M, Troll W: Protease inhibitors antagonize the activation of polymorphonuclear leukocyte oxygen consumptions. Biochem Biophys Res Commun 88:854–860, 1979.

36. Cerutti P, Amstad P, Emerit I: Tumor promoter phorbolmyristate-acetate induces membrane-mediated chromosomal damage. In Nygaard O, Simic M (eds): "Radioprotectors and Anticarcinogens." New York: Academic Press, 1983, pp 527–538.

37. Birnboim H: Importance of DNA strand breakage in tumor promotion. In Nygaard O, Simic M (eds): "Radioprotectors and Anticarcinogens." New York: Academic Press, 1983, pp 539–556.

38. Emerit I, Cerutti P: Tumor promoter phorbol-12-myristate-13-acetate induces a clastogenic factor in human lymphocytes. Proc Natl Acad Sci USA 79:7509–7573, 1982.

39. Weitberg A, Weitzman M, Destrempes M, Latt S, Stossel N: Stimulated human phagocytes produce cytogenetic changes in cultured mammalian cells. N Engl J Med 308:26–30, 1983.

40. Lewis J, Adams D: Induction of 5,6-ring-saturated thymine bases in NIH-3T3 cells by phorbol-ester-stimulated macrophages: Role of reactive oxygen intermediates. Cancer Res 45:1270–1276, 1985.

41. Kozumbo W, Muhlematter D, Jorg A, Emerit I, Cerutti P: unpublished.

42. Scher W, Friend C: Breakage of DNA and alterations in folded genomes by inducers of differentiation in Friend erythroleukemic cells. Cancer Res 38:841–849, 1978.

43. Johnstone A, Williams G: Role of DNA breaks and ADP-ribosyl transferase activity in eukaryotic differentiation in human lymphocytes. Nature 300:368–370, 1982.

44. Fischer S, Gleason G, Hardin L, Bohrmann J, Slaga T: Prostaglandin modulation of phorbol ester skin tumor promotion. Carcinogenesis 1:245–248, 1980.

45. Lupulescu A: Tumorigenic potential of endoperoxide analogs. Experientia 40:209, 1984.

46. Whiteley P, Needleman P: Mechanism of enhanced fibroblast arachidonic acid metabolism by mononuclear cell factor. J Clin Invest 74:2249–2253, 1984.

47. Balmain A, Ramsden M, Bowden G, Smith J: Activation of the mouse cellular Harvey-ras gene in chemically induced benign skin papillomas. Nature 307:658–660, 1984.

48. Toftgard R, Roop D, Yuspa S: Proto-oncogene expression during two stage carcinogenesis in mouse skin. Carcinogenesis 6:655–657, 1985.

49. Gindhart T, Nakamura Y, Stevens L, Hegameyer G, West M, Smith B, Colburn N: Genes and signal transduction in tumor promotion: Conclusions from studies with promoter resistant variants of JB-6 mouse epidermal cells. In Mass M, Kaufman D, Siegfried J, Steele V, Nesnow S (eds): "Carcinogenesis—A Comprehensive Survey Vol 8. Cancer of the Respiratory Tract: Predisposing Factors." New York: Raven Press, 1985, pp 341–368.

50. Pitot H, Grosso L, Dunn T: The role of the cellular genome in the stages of carcinogenesis. In Bishop J, Rowley J, Greaves M (eds): "Genes and Cancer." New York: Alan R. Liss, Inc., 1984, pp 81–98.

51. Hsiao W, Gattoni-Celli S, Weinstein I: Oncogene-induced transformation of C3H10T1/2 cells is enhanced by tumor promoters. Science 226:552–555, 1984.

52. Buetti E, Diggelmann H: Glucocorticoid regulation of mouse mammary tumore virus: Identification of short essential DNA region. EMBO J 1423–1429, 1983.

53. Kwon B, Weissman S: Mouse mammary tumor virus-related sequences in mouse lymphocytes are inducible by 12-O-tetradecanoyl phorbol-13-acetate. J Virol 52:1000–1004, 1984.

54. Supowit S, Potter E, Evans R, Rosenfeld M: Polypeptide hormone regulation of gene transcription: Specific 5′-genomic sequences are required for epidermal growth factor and phorbol ester regulation of prolactin gene expression. Proc Natl Acad Sci USA 81:2975–2979, 1984.

55. Zur Hausen H, Bornkamm G, Freese U, Hecker E: Persisting oncogenic herpes virus induced by tumor promoter TPA. Nature 272:373–375, 1978.

56. Iwashita S, Fox C: Epidermal growth factor and potent phorbol tumor promoters induce epidermal growth factor receptor phosphorylation in a similar but distinctively different manner in human epidermoid carcinoma A431 cells. J Biol Chem 259:2559–2567, 1984.

57. Takayama S, White M, Lauris V, Kuhn C: Phorbolesters modulate insulin receptor phosphorylation and insulin action in cultured hepatoma cells. Proc Natl Acad Sci USA 81:7797–7801, 1984.

58. Jacobs S, Sayyoun N, Saltiel A, Cuataracas P: Phorbol-esters stimulate the phosphorylation of receptors for insulin and somatomedin C. Proc Natl Acad Sci 80:6211–6213, 1983.

59. Gindhart T, Stevens L, Copley M: Transformation and tumor promoter sensitive phosphoproteins in JB6 mouse epidermal cells: One is also sensitive to heat stress. Carcinogenesis 5:1115–1121, 1984.

60. Welch W: Phorbolester, Calcium Ionophore or serum added to quiescent rat embryo fibroblast cells all result in elevated phosphorylation of two 28,000-Dalton mammalian stress proteins. J Biol Chem 260:3058–3062, 1985.

61. Patskan G, Baxter CS: Specific stimulation by phorbol-esters of the phosphorylation of histones H2B and H4 in murine lymphocytes. Cancer Res 45:667–672, 1985.

62. Singh N, Poirier G, Cerutti P: Tumor promoter phorbol-12-myristate-13-acetate induces poly ADP-ribosylation in human monocytes. Biochem Biophys Res Commun 126:1208–1214, 1985.

63. Singh N, Poirier G, Cerutti P: Tumor promoter phorbol-myristate-acetate induces a prooxidant state which causes the accumulation of poly ADP-ribose in fibroblasts. In "Proc 7th Int. Symp. ADP-Ribosylation Reactions." New York: Springer Verlag, 1985, pp 298–302.

64. Singh N, Poirier G, Cerutti P: Tumor promoter phorbol-12-myristate-13-acetate induces poly ADP-ribosylation in fibroblasts. EMBO J 4:1491–1494, 1985.
65. Kensler T, Trush M: Role of reactive oxygen radicals in tumor promotion. Environ Mutagen 6:593–616, 1984.
66. Hayaishi O, Ueda K (eds): "ADP-Ribosylation Reactions: Biology and Medicine." New York: Academic Press, 1982.
67. Miwa M, Hayaishi O, Shall S, Smulson M, Sugimura T (eds): "ADP-Ribosylation, DNA repair and Cancer." Tokyo: Scientific Societies Press, 1983.
68. Sugimura T, Miwa N: Poly ADP-ribose and cancer research. Carcinogenesis 4:1503–1506, 1983.
69. Kun E, Kirsten E, Milo G, Kurian P, Kumari H: Cell cycle dependent intervention and in vitro poly (ADP-ribosyl)ation of nuclear proteins in human fibroblasts. Proc Natl Acad Sci USA 80:7219–7223, 1984.
70. Borek C, Morgan W, Ong A, Cleaver J: Inhibition of malignant transformation in vitro by inhibitors of poly ADP-ribose synthesis. Proc Natl Acad Sci USA 81:243–247, 1984.
71. Surowy C, Berger N: Diadenosine 5′,5‴-P′-P⁴-tetraphosphate stimulates processing of ADP-ribosylated poly (ADP-ribose) polymerase. J Biol Chem 258:579–583, 1983.

Biochemical and Molecular Epidemiology of Cancer 177–190 (1986)

Toward the Decline of Lung Cancer

Marc T. Goodman and Ernst L. Wynder

Cancer Research Center of Hawaii, University of Hawaii at Manoa, Honolulu, Hawaii 96813 (M.T.G.) and Division of Epidemiology, Mahoney Institute for Health Maintenance, American Health Foundation, New York, New York 10017 (E.L.W.)

Recent declines in the rate of lung cancer among young adults in the United States and Europe cannot be explained completely by reductions in the prevalence of current smoking. The effect of other factors on trends in lung cancer incidence and mortality are discussed, including the role of smoking cessation, alterations in the tar and nicotine content of cigarettes, occupational exposure, air pollution, and nutrition.

Key words: lung cancer decline, smoking cessation, low-tar yield cigarettes, occupational exposures, air pollution, nutrition

During the past four decades there has been a dramatic increase in the incidence of lung cancer in men throughout much of the world. Lung cancer is the leading cause of cancer death in men in most countries, and in 1985 it will be the leading cause of cancer mortality in women in the United States [1]. An examination of sex-specific incidence rates in this country demonstrates a steady increase in the number of new cases of disease, especially among the older cohorts. The rate of increase is declining among younger men, while among women the incidence rates are still climbing rather sharply.

Data from the National Center for Health Statistics show a drop in age-specific mortality among men born after 1930 and possibly among women born after 1940 [2] (see Figs. 1, 2). Among white males, decreases in the incidence rates for cohorts aged 25–34 years were found in both the Third National Cancer Survey [3] and in the more recent Surveillance, Epidemiology End Results (SEER) data [4]. Increases in lung cancer incidence for white men aged 35–44 did not peak until about 1970, when the Third National Cancer Institute data were collected, declining somewhat by the end of the 1970s. Mortality rates among this group decreased from 15 to 12 per 100,000 per year between 1969 and 1979 [5]. While mortality rates among white males between 35 and 44 years of age were stable during the 1970s, increases were still being recorded among the older age cohorts. Incidence and mortality data indicate that rates may also be declining among women under 35 years of age, although sample sizes are too small to be certain [5].

Received May 28, 1985.

© **1986 Alan R. Liss, Inc.**

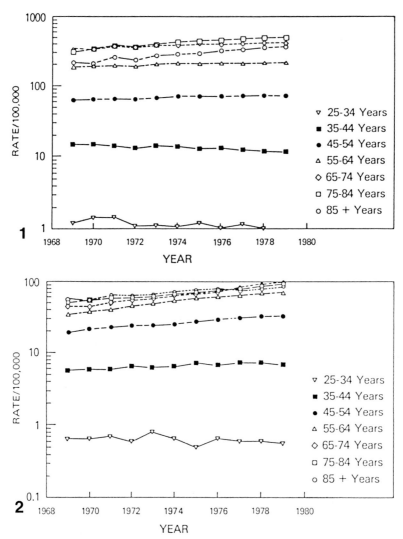

Fig. 1.   Age-specific US lung cancer mortality trends among white males. Reprinted from Devesa et al, with permission [5].

Fig. 2.   Age-specific US lung cancer mortality trends among white females. Reprinted from Devesa et al, with permission [5].

The purpose of this communication is to review possible reasons for secular trends in the incidence and mortality for lung cancer. The extent to which changing patterns of tobacco consumption in the United States and the rest of the world have contributed to these trends will be considered in addition to the role of smoking cessation, alterations in the tar and nicotine content of cigarettes, occupational factors, air pollution, and diet. It is hoped that this epidemiological exercise will add to the understanding of factors that may affect the downward trend of lung cancer incidence in younger, United States' male cohorts.

RESULTS

Tobacco Consumption

Smoking habits, especially in the United States, have undergone significant change during the past few decades. In 1955, over one half (54%) of the adult ($\geqslant 20$ years) male population and 27% of adult females were present smokers of cigarettes [6]. Adult cigarette smoking decreased among men by 1965 to 49% and increased among women to 32%. By 1980, it was estimated that these percentages had declined to 38% of adult men and 30% of adult women. Among men, this decline was greatest among the youngest and oldest age groups, with a 33% decline among 20–24 year-olds and a 37% decline among men over the age of 65 (Table I).

The decrease in the proportion of cigarette smokers between 1965 and 1980 was not as great among women. There were 22% fewer smokers among women aged 20–24 and an increase of 75% among women over the age of 65, from 10% in 1965 to 17% in 1980.

Consistent with these changes in smoking patterns, the proportion of never-smokers by age cohort has also changed [2] (Fig. 3). The percentage of never-smokers in the population increased for all men less than 45 years of age and for women less than 35 years old. Almost one-half of the men below the age of 25 had never smoked cigarettes in 1980 compared to less than one-third in this age group in 1965. Among women below 25 years of age, 50.8% claimed to be never-smokers in 1965 versus 56.3% in 1980. Thus, by 1980, young adult men and women were smoking to about the same extent.

What effect will this change in smoking habits have on lung cancer rates? It has been established that trends in mortality rates from lung cancer closely parallel changes in per capita cigarette consumption after a sufficient lag period has elapsed. Thus, the increased smoking prevalence in men born between 1910 and 1930 and in women born between 1920 and 1950 in the United States no doubt led to the "epidemic" of lung cancer occurring in the 1970s and 1980s [2]. This displays the strong coherence of the association of smoking behavior by birth cohort and subsequent mortality experience. In England and Wales, where per capita cigarette smoking plateaued earlier than it did in the United States, there has been a steady decline in the number of deaths from lung cancer, especially among younger male cohorts,

TABLE I. Percentage Change in the Proportion of Present and Former Smokers Among Adults in the United States by Sex, 1965 vs 1980

| Age group (years) | Percent change in proportion | | | |
| | Present smoker[a] | | Former smokers[b] | |
	Male	Female	Male	Female
20–24	−33	−22	+34	+51
25–34	−29	−28	+40	+45
35–44	−27	−40	+34	+97
45–64	−21	−4	+53	+99
$\geqslant 65$	−37	+75	+69	+215
All ages $\geqslant 65$	−27	−13	+50	−91

[a]Present smoker has smoked at least 100 cigarettes and non smokers include occasional smokers.
[b]Former smokers stopped smoking at least 1 year prior to interview.
From the Surgeon General, 1982 [2].

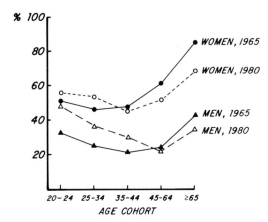

Fig. 3.   Percentage distribution of those who have never smoked cigarettes in the United States by age and sex, 1965 vs 1980. From the Surgeon General, 1982 [2].

presumably as the relative proportion of smokers in the younger generations diminishes.

To illustrate this point, a comparison of mortality data from different time periods is informative [7] (Table II). In investigating the trend of decreasing mortality from lung cancer among the younger cohorts of men, the 50% decline in death rates cannot be adequately explained by the 20% decline in smoking prevalence [8]. Similarly, an analysis of prospective data of 10,000 males has shown that only 55% of the difference in lung cancer incidence between geographic areas in Finland and Norway between 1953 and 1962 could be predicted by variations in smoking habits [9]. A second analysis of these data, using risk indices for 1975–1979, displayed a slightly better fit (64%) when plotted against the original smoking indices for 1962, but still left over one third of the variation unexplained [10].

Smoking Cessation

There is no doubt that the cessation of tobacco smoking stops the increase in excess risk associated with continued use of tobacco products [11–15]. In a case-control study conducted by our group [16], we found that among subjects who had smoked for 20 years or more, cessation of cigarette smoking did not alter the risk of lung cancer for about 3 years, followed by a gradual decline in risk approaching that for a nonsmoker after 10 to 15 years. The speed of the decline was dependent on the history of the amount and duration of smoking. The lag period for the reduction in risk associated with smoking cessation is affected in part by selection bias. For instance, smokers with symptomatic conditions will often quit smoking because of discomfort or their physician's advice. This effect diminishes with time, because of selective mortality, since people in poor health will die more rapidly than people in good health.

US trends in smoking cessation correspond inversely to secular patterns in the proportion of current smokers. Between 1965 and 1980, the proportion of ex-smokers among adults in the United States increased from 20 to 30% among men and 8 to 16% among women (see Table I). Increases in the relative proportion of ex-smokers in the population were greater with increasing age for both sexes. Also, the increased

TABLE II. Decreases in Lung Cancer, Comparing 1978 Data With Data for the Worst-Affected Generations of Men in England and Wales and in the United States

Age (years)	England and Wales				United States			
	Worst-affected generation (born ca 1910–1911)[a]		Rates for 1978 compared with those for worst-affected generation		Worst-affected generation (born ca 1910–1911)[a]		Rates for 1978 compared with those for worst-affected generation	
	Mortality/ million men	Period of observation	Mortality/ million men in 1978	Decrease (%/year)[b]	Mortality/ million men	Period of observation	Mortality/ million men in 1978	Decrease (%/year)[b]
30–34	40	1941–45	17	58/35	24	1958–62	17	30/18
35–39	98	1946–50	63	36/30	73	1963–67	62	15/13
40–44	253	1951–55	138	45/25	219	1968–72	192	12/8
45–49	597	1956–60	385	36/20	502	1973–77	480	4/3
50–54	1,234[c]	1961–65	1,047	15/15	?	1980	1,021	—[e]
55–59	2,219[d]	1966–70	1,912	14/10	?	1985	1,647	—[f]
60–64	3,577[d]	1971–75	3,315	7/5	?	1990	2,625	—[g]
65–69	5,018	1978	5,018	—	?	1995	3,557	—[g]

[a]These are the generations with the highest death rates at ages 35–44, when substantial effects of smoking first became evident. However, if in the future the number of cigarettes smoked per individual will decrease, or the effective dose of noxious chemicals per cigarette will decrease, the benefits at some particular attained age to these two worst-affected generations may be greater than to the immediately previous generations. The maximum American lung cancer rates in old age may therefore be seen, at around the turn of the century, in the generation born in the few years before this "worst-affected" generation.

[b]Percentage decrease, comparing age-specific mortality in 1978 with that for the worst-affected generation (born 1910–11 in England and Wales, born 1927–28 in the United States).

[c]Might have been materially larger but for changes in cigarette composition.

[d]Would have been materially larger but for changes in cigarette composition.

[e]US mortality at ages 50–54 years should reach a maximum by ca 1980.

[f]US mortality at ages 55–59 years is still rising.

[g]US mortality at ages 60–64 and 65–69 years is still rising rapidly.

Reprinted from Doll and Peto [7], with permission.

percentage of former smokers during the 15-year period was larger among women than among men within each age category. This may be accounted for, in part, by the much larger percentages of ever-smokers and former smokers among men. For instance, 28% of men over the age of 64 were categorized as former smokers in 1965 compared to 4% of women. These percentages increased to 47% of men in 1980 (representing a 69% increase) and 14% of women (representing a 215% increase).

To what extent has smoking cessation contributed to the apparent reversal in the spiralling rate of lung cancer deaths? It was noted earlier that cigarette smoking cessation would not immediately produce a reduction in risk of lung cancer for smokers, but would certainly prevent large increases in risk similar to those experienced by continuing smokers. While it is difficult to assess fully the effects of tobacco smoking cessation on recent trends in lung cancer mortality, several prospective studies present evidence that smokers who quit do indeed reduce their risk of lung cancer. Data from 20 years of observation on male British doctors showed that mortality decreased with the duration of cigarette smoke cessation, although at the end of 15 years it was still two times that of never-smokers [12]. Two other prospective studies, the Multiple Risk Factor Intervention Trial (MRFIT) [17] in the United States and the Whitehall Study of London Civil Servants in England [18] have examined the relationship of smoking cessation to lung cancer risk. The MRFIT Study, including 12,866 high risk (heavy cigarette consumption, high blood pressure, high serum cholesterol) men, showed 81 deaths from lung cancer in the intervention group compared to 69 deaths among the usual care group after 7 years of follow-up. The difference between these mortality rates was not significant. Smoking intervention, including basic behavioral modification techniques and hypnosis, reduced the proportion of ever cigarette smokers in the study group from 63.8 to 32.3% after 72 months. The proportion of ever-smokers among the usual care group was reduced from 63.5% to 45.6% after 72 months. This study might be used to support the contention that smoking cessation does nothing to reduce the risk of lung cancer. One needs to ask, however, whether a reduction in mortality should have been expected. Participants in the MRFIT program were selected specifically because they were considered at high risk of coronary heart disease. They were generally all heavy smokers at the outset of the trial. American Cancer Society data on smoking cessation show that long-term smokers (20 or more years) of a pack or more of cigarettes per day had much less substantive risk reduction than did people smoking less than a pack per day before quitting [19,20] (Table III). When mortality ratios for ex-cigarette smokers compared to never-smokers were analyzed by years of smoking cessation, quitters for 10 years or more had mortality ratios of 1.08 among light smokers in contrast to 1.50 among heavy smokers. Thus, substantial reductions in mortality were not as apparent in previously heavy smokers. The MRFIT participants were not only

TABLE III. Mortality Ratio of Current Cigarette Smokers and Ex-smokers*

No. of cigarettes smoked per day	Current cigarette smokers	Stopped (years)		
		1	1–10	10+
<20	1.61	2.04	1.30	1.08
20+	2.02	2.69	1.82	1.50

*The mortality ratio of men who never smoked was set at 1.00.
Reprinted from Hammond and Horn [19], with permission.

heavy, long-term smokers, but the follow-up data reported were only for a 7-year period—perhaps too short to demonstrate a significant change.

A report of 10 years of observation in the Whitehall study, a randomized trial of smoking cessation in 1,445 male smokers aged 40–59 years who were at high risk of cardiorespiratory disease, showed a small, significant difference in mortality between the intervention group (I) and normal care group (NC) [18]. The I group, consisting of 714 smoking men, were given advice on smoking cessation, while the NC group of 731 men were left alone. Lung cancer death rates were reduced to a similar extent in participants of both groups who gave up smoking. Overall, lung cancer mortality was 23% lower in the I group (calculated as the estimated proportionate reduction in 10 year risk), although this reduction was not significant. Two reasons for the absence of an effect may have been that 1) the one third of smokers who gave up cigarettes in the I group continued to smoke pipes and cigars, and 2) while a decline in lung cancer risk among heavy smokers may be expected by the end of 9 years, differences in the number of cigarettes smoked per day in the I and NC groups were small, averaging three or four cigarettes by the final postal inquiry.

Tar and Nicotine Yields

The dose-response relationship found between the risk of lung cancer and the number of cigarettes smoked per day prompted the belief that lower tar in cigarettes would lead to a diminution in the risk of lung cancer. Reports in the literature have been ambiguous regarding the effects on mortality of these reductions in tar yield [21–33], although there now appears to be a clearer picture of possible benefits [23]. Peto and Doll [34] have proposed that much of the decreasing rate of lung cancer in British men before the age of 50 years may have resulted from the introduction of the filter-tipped cigarette. The British data show that the younger cohorts smoke 20% fewer cigarettes than the older cohorts—a difference that does not alone account for reductions in the rate of lung cancer found among men under the age of 45 years (see Table II). This finding conforms with expectations, since individuals who are less than 50 years will have been smoking cigarettes on average since the middle 1950s when substantial tar reductions in cigarettes were taking place. Changes in mortality rates that have occurred in cohorts older than 50 years are difficult to assess, since the majority of these patients began smoking with nonfilter cigarettes. Thus, studies of trends in mortality for this age group will include a large number of people who smoked low-tar cigarettes for only a fraction of their smoking lives (Goodman and Wynder, unpublished data, 1985) (Figs. 4, 5). Other problems such as smoking compensation, changes in cigarettes smoked per day, and tobacco smoke inhalation may also affect these findings. For instance, between 1965 and 1980, the percentage of male adult (≥ 20 years) smokers who smoked at least 25 cigarettes per day rose from 25 to 34%, while the proportion of individuals smoking less than 15 cigarettes per day fell from 28 to 23% [6] (Fig. 6). Among women, these percentages were even more divergent, rising from 14 to 24% of individuals smoking more than 24 cigarettes per day and falling from 44 to 34% of women smoking less than 15 cigarettes per day.

The tar yield of both filter-tipped and nonfilter cigarettes in the United States and in most other industrialized societies has declined sharply over the past few decades (Fig. 7). Smokers who do not compensate in full for the reduction in nicotine by smoking more cigarettes, puffing more frequently or with greater volume, or by

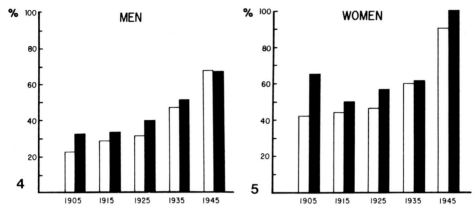

Fig. 4.   Filter cigarette usage as a percentage of lifetime smoking experience by birth cohort. Open bars, cases (N = 969). Closed bars, controls (N = 1,938).

Fig. 5.   Filter cigarette usage as a percentage of lifetime smoking experience by birth cohort. Open bars, cases (N = 375). Closed bars, controls (N = 749).

inhaling more deeply can expect to decrease their risk of lung cancer somewhat. Such a decrease would occur primarily among long-term smokers of low-yield cigarettes (ie, < 10 mg tar). An assessment of the effect of these changes in smoking habits is difficult because, to date, relatively few smokers have smoked low-yield cigarettes for more than 10 years: about 2% of our male and 4% of our female controls. As suggested in a recent report [33] and in accordance with our data, it is probable that the risk of lung cancer may be measured in direct proportion to the tar yield of the preferred brand of cigarettes smoked, once appropriate adjustment has been made for duration and amount.

Occupational Factors and Air Pollution

Although there is a large attributable risk of smoking to lung cancer, there is no doubt that lung cancer is a multifactorial disease. A number of occupational exposures have been established as risk factors for lung cancer, including exposure to arsenic, asbestos, bischloromethyl ether, chromium, ionizing radiation, mustard gas, nickel, and polycyclic hydrocarbons in soot, tar, and oil [35]. Furthermore, these substances may not be representative of the full spectrum of potential carcinogens. Weak risk factors to which a large proportion of the population is exposed may produce substantial changes in the background of lung cancer deaths. Since many of the substances listed above have been in use for less than the average induction period for lung cancer, it is probable that current mortality reflects early stages in what may be an upward trend in rates. Doll and Peto [7] have criticized the Occupational Safety and Health Administration estimates [36] of the proportion of all cancers attributable to occupation (20% or more) on the basis of what they deem to be severe overestimation of the number of individuals in the United States who are heavily exposed to occupational carcinogens.

It is difficult to separate the effects of smoking and socioeconomic status from occupational and other factors [37] (Fig. 8). For instance, there is a strong interaction

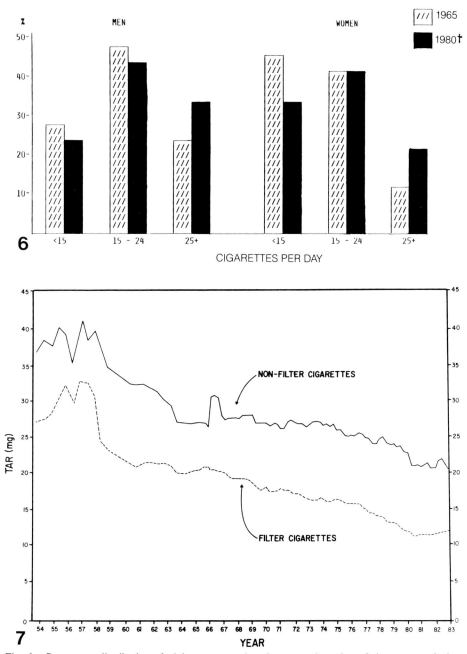

Fig. 6.   Percentage distribution of adult current smokers by grouped number of cigarettes smoked per day and sex, 1965 vs 1980. A current smoker has smoked at least 100 cigarettes and now smokes (includes occasional smokers). The 1980 data are for the last 6 months of 1980. From the Surgeon General, 1983 [6].

Fig. 7.   Sales-weighted average tar deliveries, 1954–1983.

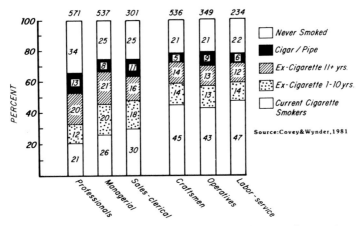

Fig. 8.   Age-standardized smoking rates by occupational level of white male controls aged 41 through 70 years. Reprinted from Covey and Wynder [37], with permission.

between smoking and asbestos on the risk of lung cancer. The importance of testing for synergy between smoking (and socioeconomic status?) and these occupational exposures seems particularly important in view of the fact that there appears to have been no increase in the proportion of never-smokers developing lung cancer over the past 35 years [2,6]. Doll and Peto [7] attributed approximately 11,000 lung cancers to occupational factors in the United States, comprising 15% of male and 5% of female lung cancers. They recommend, and we concur, that there is a strong need for a case-control study based on a representative sample of US cases to clarify the relationship between smoking and occupation and the rate of lung cancer.

Air pollution has been investigated quite extensively in association with the risk of lung cancer because of the direct route of exposure and urban/rural differences in the rate of lung cancer unexplained by variations in tobacco consumption [38]. A large number of pollutants have been identified as carcinogens based on animal and occupational evidence [39,40], which has led to speculation of a causal relationship. The low rate of lung cancer in nonsmoking Seventh-Day Adventists living in Los Angeles or Greeks and Japanese living in heavily polluted Athens and Yokohama suggests that if there is an effect of air pollution on lung cancer risk it is small at best.

Nutrition

Another consideration is whether improvements in the dietary status of young adults may have added to the current trends in the decline of lung cancer incidence in the United States among this group. The role of dietary fat, fruits and vegetables, vitamin A, retinoids, and other micronutrients in the etiology of lung cancer has been the subject of a great number of recent investigations. Examinations of nutritional factors in the induction of lung cancer are difficult not only because of the overwhelming affect of tobacco smoke on risk but also as a result of the problems inherent in obtaining reliable dietary information. These problems have been reviewed by us in some detail in an earlier article [41]. As a result of these and other research obstacles, it is premature to come to any conclusions regarding the effect of nutritional excesses, deficiencies, or imbalances on the incidence of lung cancer. In spite of these reservations, two prospective studies with sample sizes large enough for appropriate statistical analysis provide suggestive evidence that daily consumption of green-yellow vegetables reduces the risk of lung cancer [42,43]. The relatively low incidence of lung cancer in Japan compared to that in the United States while caused, in large part, by differences in smoking patterns, may also be influenced by dietary differences [43]. Although the comparatively low consumption of fruits and green and yellow vegetables in Japan in the past would be inconsistent with the hypothesized protective effect of β-carotene, the intake of dietary fats, which may also enhance lung carcinogenesis, is also lower.

Doll and Peto [7] have posited that a reduction of US lung cancer deaths by 20% may be brought about by dietary means. We regard this issue as open. Investigations of macro- and micronutrients, especially of carotinoids on lung cancer risk are indicated. Case-control studies of lung cancer and nutrition must be conducted in a manner allowing for appropriate adjustment for smoking habits and socioeconomic status. Furthermore, we need to recognize that it may not be possible to obtain reliable dietary histories from cancer patients. Prospective studies with large-scale blood collection and storage for later analysis should be initiated to resolve the issue [44].

DISCUSSION

When the link between tobacco smoking and the risk of lung cancer was established in the early 1950s, it was apparent that the incidence of lung cancer would soon become the leading cause of cancer death among men and, perhaps in the future, among women. This prediction has unfortunately been realized.

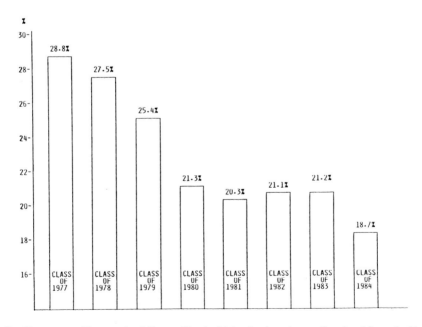

Fig. 9. Teenage smoking trends: daily smoking by high school graduates. Reprinted from the National Institute on Drug Abuse [47], with permission.

Following the release of the first Surgeon General's Report in 1964 [45] there have been gradual changes in smoking habits in the United States in addition to overall reductions in the tar yields of cigarettes. First, there was a sharp increase in males who quit smoking, especially among the middle-aged, upper-income groups. This was followed by a rise in the proportion of never-smokers among young men. These trends have led to an approximate 50% reduction in the percentage of male smokers compared to rates 30 years ago.

Women have also begun to stop smoking in increasing numbers, although not to the same extent as men. The overall percentage of female smokers, however, has doubled since 1950. Hence, the rate of new lung cancer cases continues to climb, and it is expected that the rate of this incline will not fall off for years to come.

Superimposed on these changes in the prevalence of cigarette smoking is the fact that the tar yield of American-manufactured cigarettes is about one half of what it was in 1950. Since most smokers are unlikely to compensate completely for this decline in tar yield, it is likely that smokers of low-tar yield cigarettes will reduce their risk of lung cancer significantly, an effect mostly to be seen among young cohorts. Efforts to reduce further the tar yields of cigarettes on the market should continue. The average tar yield of cigarettes should not exceed 10 mg.

Obviously, occupational carcinogens need to be controlled to the greatest extent possible. Air pollution, though unlikely to affect the risk of lung cancer, should be monitored and reduced for other public health reasons such as general hygiene. At this time, no specific dietary advice can be given for the possible prevention of lung cancer.

Those of us who have been involved in etiological research on tobacco-related cancers may derive some satisfaction from the turnaround in the lung cancer rates in most of the developed world. Anti-smoking campaigns have been obviously successful and should now focus on high risk groups such as women and lower income smokers. Young people should be admonished not to start smoking or, if they have already done so, to quit. That these preventive efforts have been fruitful is evidenced by a recent report released by the National Institute on Drug Abuse showing that the prevalence of teenage smoking continues to decline [46] (Fig. 9). The reduction in the risk of lung cancer in individuals who quit offers a special incentive to those in public health whose goal is the elimination of a preventive disease. We who have expended a great deal of energy toward the reduction of lung cancer and the tobacco-related diseases can now see light at the end of the tunnel.

ACKNOWLEDGMENTS

The authors thank Ms. Sheila Petty and Ms. Roz Fieland for their editorial assistance in the preparation of this manuscript. This study was supported by Public Health Service grant CA-17613 from the National Cancer Institute.

REFERENCES

1. American Cancer Society: "Cancer Facts and Figures—1984." New York: American Cancer Society, 1983.
2. United States Public Health Service: "The Health Consequences of Smoking—Cancer." Rockville, MD: DHS Pub No (PHS) 82-50179, 1982.

3. Cutler SJ, Young JL (eds): Natl Cancer Inst Monogr 41:1–454, 1975.
4. Young JL, Percy CL, Asire AJ (eds): Natl Cancer Inst Monogr 57:1–1082, 1981.
5. Devesa SS, Horm JW, Connelly RR: In Mizell M, Correa P (eds): "Lung Cancer: Causes and Prevention." New Orleans, LA: Verlag Chemie International, 1984.
6. United States Public Health Service: "The Health Consequences of Smoking—Cardiovascular Disease." Rockville, MD:DHHS Pub No (PHS) 84-50204, 1984.
7. Doll R, Peto R: J Natl Cancer Inst 66:1191, 1981.
8. Doll R: "Prospects for Prevention." London: Royal College of Physicians, 1982.
9. Pederson E, Magnus K, Mork T, et al: Acta Pathol Microbiol Scand: Suppl 199, 1969.
10. Teppo L: In Mizell M, Correa P (eds): "Lung Cancer: Causes and Prevention." New Orleans, LA: Verlag Chemie International, 1984.
11. Rogot E, Murray JL: Public Health Rep 95:213, 1980.
12. Doll R, Peto R: Br Med J 2(6051):1525, 1976.
13. Hammond EC: Am J Public Health 55:682, 1965.
14. Hammond EC: Natl Cancer Inst Monogr 19:127, 1966.
15. Hirayama T: "Smoking in Relation to the Death Rates of 265,118 Men in Tokyo." Tokyo: National Cancer Center Research Institute, 1967.
16. Wynder EL, Stellman SD: Cancer Res 37:4608, 1977.
17. Multiple Risk Factor Intervention Trial Research Group: JAMA 248:1465, 1982.
18. Rose G, Hamilton PJS, Colwell L, Shipley MJ: J Epidemiol Commun Health 36:102, 1982.
19. Hammond EC, Horn D: JAMA 166:1159, 1958.
20. Hammond EC, Horn D: JAMA 166:1294, 1958.
21. Wynder EL, Stellman SD: J Natl Cancer Inst 62:471, 1979.
22. Garfinkel L: In "Banbury Report No 3." Cold Spring Harbor, NY: Cold Spring Harbor Laboratory, 1980, p 19.
23. Lee N, Garfinkel L: J Epidemiol Commun Health 35:16, 1981.
24. Bross IJ, Gibson R: Am J Public Health 58:1396, 1968.
25. Hammond EL, Garfinkel L, Seidman H, et al: In Hiatt HH, Winsten JA (eds): "Origins of Human Cancer—Book A." Cold Spring Harbor, NY: Cold Spring Harbor Laboratory, 1977, p 101.
26. Kunze M, Vutuc C: In "Banbury Report No 3." Cold Spring Harbor, NY: Cold Spring Harbor Laboratory, 1980, p 29.
27. Hammond EC, Garfinkel L, Seidman H, et al: Environ Res 12:263, 1976.
28. Hawthorne VM, Fry JS: J Epidemiol Commun Health 32:260, 1978.
29. Reid DD: Natl Cancer Inst Monogr 19:287, 1966.
30. Dean G, Lee PN, Todd GF, et al: "Tobacco Research Council Research Paper No 14." London: Tobacco Research Council, 1977.
31. Wynder EL, Mabuchi K, Beattie EJ: JAMA 213:2221, 1970.
32. Wynder EL, Mushinski M, Stellman S: "Proceedings of the Third World Conference on Smoking and Health." New York, Vol 1, 1975.
33. Lubin J, Blot WJ, Berrino F: Int J Cancer 33:569, 1984.
34. Peto R, Doll R: In Mizell M, Correa P (eds): "Lung Cancer: Causes and Prevention." New Orleans, LA: Verlag Chemie International, 1984.
35. Blot WJ: In Mizell M, Correa P (eds): "Lung Cancer: Causes and Prevention." New Orleans, LA: Verlag Chemie International, 1984.
36. Bridbord K, Decoufle P, Fraumeni JF, et al: "Estimates of the Fraction of Cancer in the United States Related to Occupational Factors." Bethesda, MD: National Cancer Institute, National Institute of Environmental Health Services, and National Institute for Occupational Safety and Health, 1978.
37. Covey LS, Wynder EL: J Occup Med 23:537, 1981.
38. Wynder EL, Hoffmann D: Proc Natl Conf Air Pollution 1143, 1963.
39. Hoffmann D, Wynder EL: In Stern AC (ed): "Air Pollution." New York: Academic Press, 1977, p 361.
40. U.S. Environmental Protection Agency: "Health Assessment Document for Polycyclic Organic Matter." Washington, DC: Office of Research and Development, 1978.
41. Wynder EL, Goodman MT: Epidemiol Rev 5:177, 1983.

42. MacLennan R, Da Costa J, Day NE, et al: Int J Cancer 20:854, 1977.

43. Hirayama T: Nutr Cancer 1:67, 1979.

44. Wald N, Idle M, Boreham J, Bailey A: Lancet 2:813, 1980.

45. United States Public Health Service: "Smoking in Health: Report of the Advisory Committee of the Surgeon General of the Public Health Service." Rockville, MD: PHS Publ No 1103, 1964.

46. "Smoking and Health Reporter." Bloomington, IN: National Interagency Council on Smoking and Health, Vol 2, 1985.

Biochemical and Molecular Epidemiology of Cancer 191–204 (1986)

Tumorigenic Agents in Tobacco Products and Their Uptake by Chewers, Smokers, and Nonsmokers

Dietrich Hoffmann, Stephen S. Hecht, Assieh A. Melikian, Nancy J. Haley, Klaus D. Brunnemann, John D. Adams, and Ernst L. Wynder

American Health Foundation, Valhalla, New York 10595

We discuss the fact that nicotine contributes significantly to the carcinogenic potential of tobacco and tobacco smoke by giving rise to relatively high concentrations of N′-nitrosonornicotine and 4-(methylnitrosamino)-1-(3-pyridyl)-1-butanone (NNK). These tobacco-specific nitrosamines are metabolically activated by α-hydroxylation. In the case of NNK, the α-hydroxylation leads to an unstable intermediate which is capable of methylating DNA to 7-methylguanine and the promutagenic O^6-methylguanine. Catechol is the major known cocarcinogen in tobacco smoke. The coadministration to mouse skin of benzo(a)pyrene (BaP) and catechol leads to a decrease in the levels of glucuronide and sulfate conjugates of BaP metabolites and to increased formation of 3-hydroxyBaP and of *trans*-7,8-dihydroxy-7,8-dihydroBaP, which, in turn, increases formation of *trans*-7,8-dihydroxy-*anti*-9,10-epoxy-7,8,9,10-tetrahydroBaP adducts with DNA.

We also review the findings that have demonstrated that smokers of low-yield cigarettes will at least partially compensate for the low nicotine delivery by increasing their smoking and inhalation intensity. Furthermore, we discuss the relative risk assessment of environmental tobacco smoke exposure, showing that nonsmokers absorb only a small percentage of the smoke inhaled by active smokers. Uptake of environmental tobacco smoke by infants of smoking mothers, however, can be significant. The ongoing elucidation of endogenous formation of carcinogens as a consequence of inhalation of smoke or ingestion of tobacco juices is also discussed.

Key words: nicotine, tobacco-specific nitrosamines, catechol, cocarcinogenesis, smokers' compensation, environmental tobacco smoke, endogenous formation of carcinogens

It has been recognized for more than three decades that tobacco smoking is causatively associated with several types of cancer. It is less well known that also

Abbreviations used: BaP, benzo(a)pyrene; BPDE, BaP-7,8-diol-9,10-epoxide; NAB, nitrosoanabasine; NAT, nitrosoanatabine; NDELA, nitrosodiethanolamine; NDMA, nitrosomethylamine; NNAL, 4-(methylnitrosamino)-1-(3-pyridyl)-1-butan-1-ol; NNK, 4-(methylnitrosamino)-1-(3-pyridyl)-1-butanone; NNN, N′-nitrosonornicotine; NPYR, N-nitrosopyrrolidine; VNA, volatile nitrosamines; "Passive Smoking" is a commonly used term for Environmental Tobacco Smoke (ETS) Exposure.

Received April 17, 1985.

© **1986 Alan R. Liss, Inc.**

tobacco chewers and snuff dippers face an increased risk for cancer, namely, cancer of the oral cavity and, possibly, cancers of other sites, caused by the action of organ-specific carcinogens present in tobacco. More recently, the question of an increased risk for lung cancer caused by (passive) environmental tobacco smoke exposure has surfaced [1–3].

In the past, our tobacco research program has been directed toward the isolation and identification of tumor initiators, tumor promoters, cocarcinogens, and organ-specific carcinogens [4]. More recently, however, we have focused on three specific areas in tobacco carcinogenesis, namely, the contribution of nicotine to the carcinogenic potential of tobacco products [5], the cocarcinogenic effect of catechol [6], and the uptake of toxic agents and their fate in chewers, smokers, and nonsmokers [7,8].

NICOTINE-DERIVED N-NITROSAMINES

Occurrence

Although it has been known for a long time that nicotine is the major determinant for tobacco habituation [9], only the research efforts in the past decade have revealed the importance of this major tobacco alkaloid in tobacco carcinogenesis [10]. During aging, curing, and fermentation as well as during smoking, nicotine gives rise to N′-nitrosonornicotine (NNN) and 4-(methylnitrosamino)-1-(3-pyridyl)-1-butanone (NNK). The minor tobacco alkaloids nornicotine, anatabine, and anabasine also form the corresponding nitrosamines (Fig. 1). In cigarette smoke, 25–45% of NNN and NNK originate by transfer from the tobacco, and the remainder is pyrosynthesized [11,12].

Levels of tobacco-specific nitrosamines in US tobacco products and in mainstream and sidestream smoke are listed in Table I. These quantitative data represent the highest concentrations of carcinogenic nitrosamines reported in any consumer products and respiratory environments, perhaps with the exception of a few rare occupational environments. The high exposure of tobacco consumers to nitrosamines is especially apparent in a comparison of the estimated exposure of US residents to nitrosamines from various sources (Table II) [10,13].

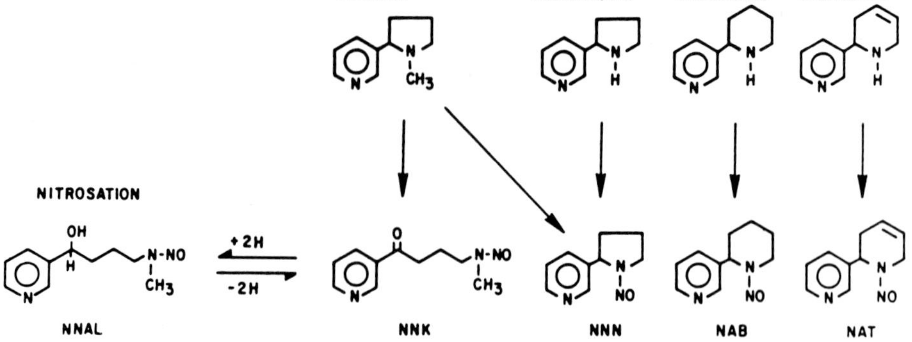

Fig. 1.   Formation of tobacco-specific N-nitrosamines.

TABLE I. Tobacco-Specific Nitrosamines in Commercial US Tobacco Products

Tobacco product[a]	NNN	NNK	NAT + NAB[b]
Smokeless tobacco			
Chewing tobacco (ppb)	3,500–8,200	100–3,000	500–7,000
Snuff (ppb)	800–89,000	200–8,300	200–4,000
Mainstream smoke			
Cigarettes-NF (ng/cig.)	120–950	80–770	140–990
Cigarettes-F (ng/cig.)	50–310	30–150	60–370
Little cigar-F (ng/cigar)	5,500	4,200	1,700
Cigar (ng/cigar)	3,200	1,900	1,900
Sidestream smoke			
Cigarettes-NF (ng/cig.)	1,700	410	270
Cigarettes-F (ng/cig.)	150	190	150

[a]NF, cigarette without filter tip; F, cigarette with filter tip.
[b]NAT, nitrosoanatabine; NAB, nitrosoanabasine.
Reprinted from Hoffmann and Hecht [10], with permission.

TABLE II. Estimated Exposure of US Residents to Nitrosamines

Source of exposure	Nitrosamines	Primary exposure route	Daily intake (μg/person)	
Beer	NDMA	Ingestion	0.34	
Cosmetics	NDELA	Dermal absorption	0.41	
Cured meat; cooked bacon	NPYR	Ingestion	0.17	
Scotch whiskey	NDMA	Ingestion	0.03	
Cigarette smoking	VNA	Inhalation	0.3	
	NDELA	Inhalation	0.5	
	NNN	Inhalation	6.1	
	NNK	Inhalation	2.9	16.2
	NAT+NAB	Inhalation	7.2	
Snuff dipping	VNA	Ingestion	3.1	
	NDELA	Ingestion	6.6	
	NNN	Ingestion	75.0	
	NNK	Ingestion	16.1	164.5
	NAT+NAB	Ingestion	73.4	

Reprinted from Hoffmann and Hecht [10], with permission.

Carcinogenicity

The significance of these exposure data is heightened by the carcinogenic potency of NNN and NNK in mice, rats, and Syrian golden hamsters (Table III) [10]. A single dose of 0.005 mmol of NNK (1 mg) induced tumors of the respiratory tract in 50% of the hamsters [14]. NNK, given to rats at a dose of approximately 0.1 mmol, induced tumors of the liver (4/29 rats), of the nasal cavity (6/29), and of the lung (12/29). The same molar dose of N-nitrosodimethylamine (NDMA) induced only liver tumors (5/26) and one nasal cavity tumor (1/26) [10].

In addition to the high carcinogenic potency of NNN and NNK, it is intriguing that, at three dose levels, NNK induced significantly more lung tumors in male rats than in females, while such difference in response was not seen with regard to tumors of the nasal cavity and of the liver (Table IV) [15]. The induction of lung cancer in rats by NNK represents the first known system that would lend itself to a study of the

TABLE III. Carcinogenicity of Tobacco-Specific Nitrosamines

Nitros-amine	Species and strains	Route of application	Principal target organs	Dose (mmol)
NNN	A/J mouse	ip	Lung	0.12 (mouse)
	F344 rat	sc	Nasal cavity, esophagus	0.2–3.4 (rat)
		po	Esophagus, nasal cavity	1.0–3.6 (rat)
	Sprague-Dawley rat	po	Nasal cavity	8.8 (rat)
	Syrian golden hamster	sc	Trachea, nasal cavity	0.9–2.1 (hamster)
NNK	A/J mouse	ip	Lung	0.12 (mouse)
	F344 rat	sc	Nasal cavity, lung, liver	0.2–2.8 (rat)
	Syrian golden hamster	sc	Trachea, lung	0.9 (hamster)
			Nasal cavity	0.005 (hamster)
NAT	F344 rat	sc	None	0.2–2.8 (rat)
NAB	F344 rat	po	Esophagus	3–12 (rat)
	Syrian golden hamster	sc	None	2 (hamster)
NNA	A/J mouse	ip	None	0.12 (mouse)

Reprinted from Hoffmann and Hecht [10], with permission.

TABLE IV. Induction of Tumors in F344 Rats

NNK Group	Effective No. of rats (sex)	Percent rats with tumors		
		Lung[a]	Nasal cavity[b]	Liver[c]
I. 9.0 mmol/kg	15 M	93	93	40
	15 F	60*	93	33
II. 3.0 mmol/kg	15 M	87	87	27
	15 F	47*	80	27
III. 1.0 mmol/kg	27 M	85	74	11
	27 F	30*	37*	15
IV. Solvent control	26 M	0	0	12
	26 F	4	0	4

[a]Total of squamous cell carcinoma, adenoma, and adenocarcinoma (control, adenoma only).
[b]Benign and malignant tumors.
[c]Benign and malignant tumors (control, adenoma only).
*Difference between males and females $p < 0.05$.
Reprinted from Hoffmann et al [15], with permission.

differences in lung cancer susceptibility between males and females [16]. There is some suggestive evidence from epidemiological studies that women may indeed have decreased susceptibility toward lung cancer [16].

Metabolic Activation and DNA-Binding

N-Nitrosamines are enzymatically converted to unstable intermediates that can react with nucleophilic centers in cellular macromolecules. Although the structures of these electrophilic, unstable intermediates have not been unambiguously character-ized, evidence suggests that the reactive species are diazohydroxides [17]. Figure 2 shows a scheme of the generally accepted route of metabolic activation of NDMA; it begins with α-hydroxylation and leads to N-methyl-N-hydroxymethylnitrosamine,

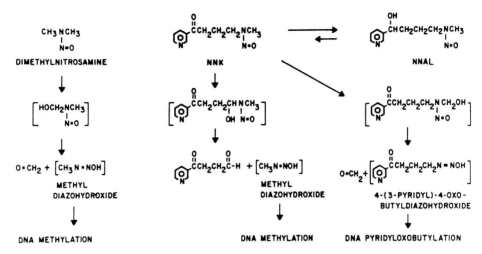

Fig. 2. Metabolic activation of *N*-nitrosodimethylamine and NNK. Structures in brackets are likely intermediates that have not been isolated.

which has a half-life of approximately 10 sec at pH 7 [18]. This intermediate decomposes to a methylating species, most likely methyldiazohydroxide. In vitro and in vivo studies have shown that, upon activation, NDMA reacts with DNA, yielding upon hydrolysis 7-methylguanine, O^6-methylguanine, 3-methyladenine, and several other products [19]. Extensive studies have documented that O^6-methylguanine is important in regard to tumor initiation [19].

Figure 2 depicts the α-hydroxylation of NNK, which occurs on the methylene group and the methyl group. As in the case of NDMA, the α-hydroxylation of the methylene group leads to methyldiazohydroxide.

In explants of human buccal mucosa, trachea, esophagus, bronchus, peripheral lung, and urinary bladder, NNN and NNK are metabolically activated by α-hydroxylation similar to these reactions in laboratory animals, but to a lesser extent [20].

Recently, our group has shown that the treatment of rats with NNK leads to the formation of 7-methylguanine and O^6-methylguanine in DNA of the lung, the liver, and the nasal mucosa [21]. The development of a biotin-avidin enzyme-linked immunosorbent assay for O^6-methylguanosine now opens the possibility for measuring DNA-methylation by NNK in tissues of animals and possibly also of tobacco consumers [22].

In summary, during tobacco processing and smoking, nicotine gives rise to the highly carcinogenic NNK. Upon metabolic activation, this nitrosamine can form the promutagenic DNA adduct O^6-methylguanine (Fig. 3) [10].

COCARCINOGENIC EFFECT OF CATECHOL ON MOUSE SKIN

Mouse skin bioassays have been widely used for the identification of tumor initiators, tumor promoters, and cocarcinogens in tobacco "tar" [4]. Fractionation studies in conjunction with bioassays have delineated that the tumor initiators reside primarily in those neutral subfractions that contain the polynuclear aromatic hydrocarbons and that the major cocarcinogens reside in the weakly acidic portion (Fig. 4)

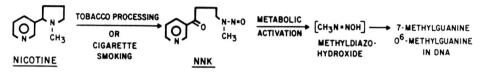

Fig. 3.   Scheme linking nicotine to formation of the promutagenic DNA adduct O^6-methylguanine. Reprinted from Cancer Research, with permission.

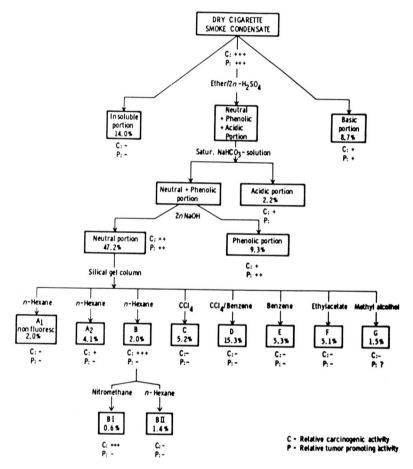

Fig. 4.   Fractionation of cigarette smoke condensate and test results of the end fractions for tumorigenic activities in mouse skin. C, relative carcinogenic activity; P, relative tumor promoting activity.

[23,24]. The neutral subfractions B and BI do not induce tumors by themselves, but, in combination with the weakly acidic portion, they possess most of the tumorigenic potency of the total "tar" [4]. Catechols were shown to be major cocarcinogens in the weakly acidic portion and, thus, in the total "tar" [24,29,30]. The delineation of mechanism(s) involved in the cocarcinogenic effect of catechol is currently being attempted by examining the effects of catechol on the metabolic activation of benzo(a)pyrene (BaP) in mouse skin and on the binding of BaP-metabolites to DNA

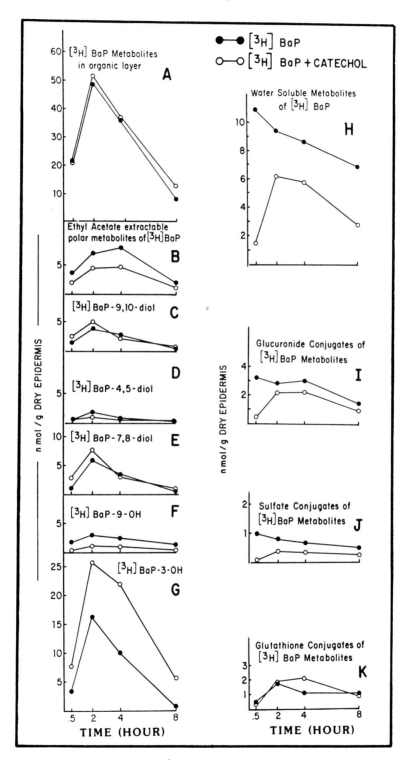

Fig. 5. Levels of various metabolites of [³H]BaP in mouse skin in the absence (●) and presence (○) of catechol.

and protein at various time intervals. This involves concurrent application to mouse skin of 15 μg of [^{3}H]BaP and 500 μg of catechol [25]. Catechol shows little effect on the total amount of BaP metabolized in mouse skin, but it does affect the relative proportions of BaP metabolites. Figure 5 summarizes our findings to date. While catechol decreased the proportions of ethyl acetate-soluble polar metabolites (Fig. 5B) and quinones and of water-soluble polar metabolites (Fig. 5H), it caused a twofold increase in the levels of unconjugated 3-hydroxy-BaP (Fig. 5G). Catechol also increased the levels of unconjugated *trans*-7,8-dihydroxy-7,8-dihydroBaP (Fig. 5E) and of *trans*-9,10-dihydroxy-9,10-dihydroBaP (Fig. 5C) 30 min after treatment. However, subsequently the levels of these two BaP-dihydrodiols in the treated mice decreased to the levels of those in the control animals.

Catechol increased the binding of *trans*-7,8-dihydroxy-9,10-epoxy-7,8,9,10-tetrahydroBaP (BPDE) to DNA about 2.3-fold 8 hr after treatment. The ratio of *anti*- to *syn*-BPDE adducts was elevated 1.6-fold 2 hr after treatment and about 2.9-fold 8 hr post treatment (Fig. 6). This was due to the fact that only the *anti* form was increased and not the *syn* form. The increased formation of *anti*-BPDE-DNA adducts in the presence of catechol may be one factor for its cocarcinogenicity on mouse skin. We are also intrigued by the twofold increased rate of formation of 3-hydroxyBaP in the presence of catechol. We study these aspects in depth because of the importance of mechanisms of cocarcinogenesis for environmental carcinogenesis *per se.*

UPTAKE OF SMOKE CONSTITUENTS
Low-Nicotine Cigarettes

The observation of a clear dose-response relationship of cigarette smoking and cancer risk has led to a demand for and to the development of cigarettes with low smoke yields, since it was unrealistic to expect full compliance with smoking cessation efforts. However, the smokers of low-yield cigarettes responded to the diminished yield of nicotine by changing their smoking patterns, ie, they increased the intensity of smoking and the depth of inhalation [1,7,25].

This phenomenon has been observed by several investigators in as many different countries [1,7,25]. We have studied some aspects of this smoking behavior in two groups of six smokers each who were given filter cigarettes with stabile draw resistance and tar yields but with incremental variations in nicotine delivery (as measured by standardized machine smoking).

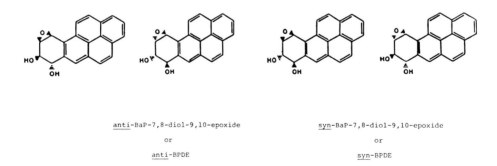

anti-BaP-7,8-diol-9,10-epoxide   syn-BaP-7,8-diol-9,10-epoxide

or   or

anti-BPDE   syn-BPDE

Fig. 6.   Structures of *anti*-BaP-7,8-diol-9,10-epoxides and *syn*-BaP-7,8-diol-9,10-epoxides.

In group 1, six smokers whose customary brand yielded 0.73 ± 0.39 mg of nicotine per cigarette in machine-generated mainstream smoke were given cigarettes with ultra-low-yield (0.06 mg), low-yield (0.4 mg), medium-yield (0.7 and 0.9 mg), and high-yield (1.3 mg) nicotine, respectively, for a period of 1 week. Their uptake of nicotine was determined immediately after smoking the first cigarette of the new brand and after 1 week of smoking the new brand. The overall assessment of smoke uptake was made by radioimmunoassays for nicotine and its major metabolite, cotinine, in the serum of smokers as well as by carboxyhemoglobin measurements and by determining thiocyanate, the hepatic detoxification product of the gaseous smoke constituent hydrogen cyanide [25].

As shown in Figure 7, the smoker who shifts from the customary medium-yield cigarette to one with ultra-low-nicotine yield reflects this by serum nicotine reductions of 80–90%, while switching to the low-yield cigarette brings about a serum nicotine reduction of only ≈20%. Smoking of the cigarette with high-nicotine yield leads at first to elevated serum nicotine but, after 1 week, when the smoker is acclimatized to the new brand, the serum nicotine level is no higher than that measured after smoking the customary brand. Figure 8 demonstrates similar findings for smokers who switched to a high-nicotine cigarette and were then gradually titrated to medium-, low-, and ultra-low yields. Again, significant decreases in serum nicotine occurred only with ultra-low-yield cigarettes. In all other cases there was compensation. Generally, the trend of the cotinine data was comparable to that for nicotine. Carboxyhemoglobin and thiocyanate levels in the blood were not significantly altered, since compensation through smoking behavior need not markedly affect the mainstream smoke delivery of carbon monoxide and hydrogen cyanide. Thus, we conclude that the nicotine delivery in the smoke is a major factor for the smoker's compensation, which is observed by switching to low-yield cigarettes. Smoke yields measured with machine-

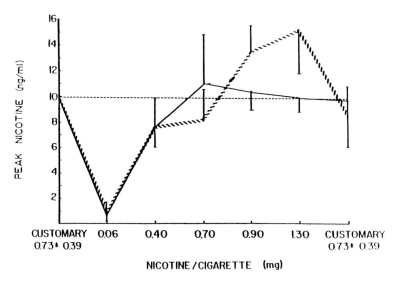

Fig. 7.   Plasma nicotine levels in smokers who received cigarettes with incrementally increasing nicotine content as determined under standard smoking conditions. The line set at 10 ng/ml represents the levels noted with the customary brand of cigarette. All values are means ± S.E.

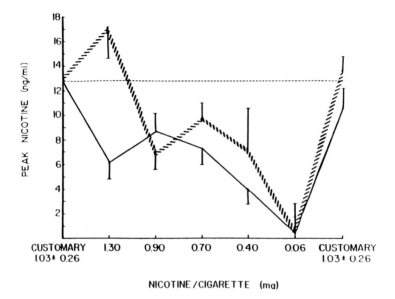

Fig. 8. Plasma nicotine levels in smokers who received cigarettes with incrementally decreasing nicotine content as determined under standard smoking conditions. The dotted horizontal line represents the levels noted with the customary brand of cigarette. All values are means ± S.E.

smoking procedures are not representative of the smoke yields obtained with various smoking behaviors of the consumers.

Environmental Tobacco Smoke

Since 1981, several epidemiological studies have inferred that the nonsmoking wives of cigarette smokers have a somewhat greater risk for lung cancer than the nonsmoking wives of nonsmokers [1,3]. On the other hand, at least one prospective study and three case control studies failed to observe a significantly higher lung cancer rate for "passive smokers" compared to nonsmokers. Furthermore, it is rather difficult in these epidemiological studies to adjust for all confounders for lung cancer. Therefore, there was a need for risk assessment by actually measuring smoke uptake after environmental exposure and to compare such measurements with those from active smokers.

We created a laboratory setting that enabled us to expose nonsmokers under controlled conditions to cigarette smoke-polluted environments. Exposure was twice daily for 5 days, and blood, saliva, and urine samples were taken from the volunteers in this study before exposure in the morning and immediately after the second 80 min exposure in the late afternoon. Nicotine and cotinine were determined in the physiological fluids by radioimmunoassays.

Figure 9 demonstrates that nicotine levels in the morning did not exceed a few nanograms per milliliter of saliva, but they showed a dramatic increase to 1.9 µg/ml after the second exposure.

Cotinine levels rise gradually up to 30 ng/ml and recede only slowly after the second exposure. Cotinine appears in the saliva following uptake of nicotine and persists in physiological fluids longer than nicotine as a result of the gradual detoxification that occurs in the liver. Cotinine levels also remain elevated for longer

ENVIRONMENTAL SMOKE UPTAKE

SALIVA

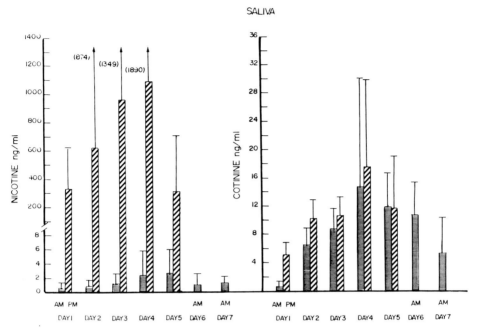

Fig. 9. Left (AM) columns: before entering the "smoke room" in the morning. Right (PM) columns: directly after the second 80 min smoke exposure during the same day.

periods because of its half-life of 18–20 hr in contrast to the half-life of nicotine, which is about 20 min. Figure 10 presents nicotine and cotinine concentrations in the urine after passive smoke exposure. Nicotine levels decrease more slowly in urine than in saliva but remain relatively high even 2 days after exposure (100 μg/mg creatinine). Nicotine and cotinine levels in the saliva and urine of environmentally exposed persons have never amounted to more than a few percent of the corresponding levels found in smokers who consumed 20 cigarettes per day.

However, the effects of environmental smoke exposure are not the same for all individuals. With special consideration for the susceptibility to respiratory infections and other ailments of infants during the first year of life, we measured the degree of uptake of tobacco-specific markers of exposure in the urine of infants whose mothers were smokers yet were not breastfeeding these children.

Figure 11 shows the relatively high urinary cotinine levels in some of the exposed infants and indicates a dose response between the cigarette consumption of the mother or primary caretaker and the urinary cotinine level of the exposed infants. We find this observation most important and plan to initiate a larger study on infants in cooperation with Dr. R. Greenberg of the University of North Carolina in Chapel Hill [26].

Endogenous Formation of Nitrosamines

Tobacco carcinogenesis has largely been concerned with the study of exogenous formation of carcinogens and their inhibition and with an assessment of the biological properties of various smoke constituents. More recent developments in research techniques have enabled us to consider also the fate of inhaled or ingested tobacco

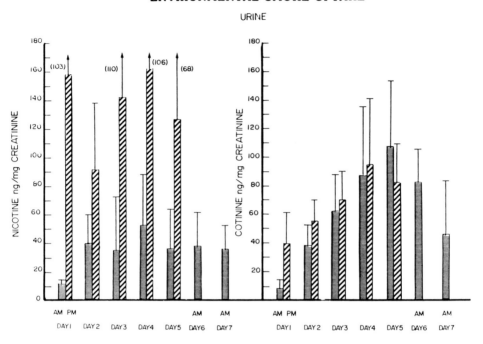

Fig. 10.   Left (AM) columns: before entering the "smoke room" in the morning. Right (PM) columns: immediately after the second 80 min smoke exposure during the same day.

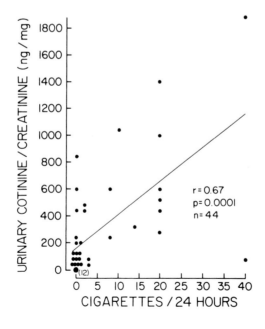

Fig. 11.   Relationship between the number of cigarettes smoked by mothers in the previous 24 hr and cotinine in urine of their infants.

TABLE V. Endogenous Formation of N-Nitrosoproline (NPRO) in Humans

Group	Protocol	μg NPRO/24 hr urine in nonsmokers	N	μg NPRO/24 hr urine in nonsmokers	N	P
1	Control diet	3.6	13	5.9	13	0.047
2	Diet + proline	3.6	14	11.8	14	0.031
3	Diet + proline + vitamin C	4.7	13	4.6	13	0.46

Reprinted from Hoffmann and Brunnemann [8], with permission.

components in vivo. The endogenous nitrosation of amino compounds was of special concern since the smoke of a cigarette contains up to 600 μg of nitrogen oxides and since nicotine and other tobacco-alkaloids are readily available precursors for the formation of carcinogenic nitrosamines. Moreover, hydrogen cyanide, one of the gaseous smoke constituents, is upon inhalation and detoxification in the liver converted to thiocyanate, which is a powerful catalyst for nitrosation reactions as was shown by in vitro and in vivo studies [27,28]. Therefore, we compared the urinary excretion of nitrosoproline (NPRO) in 15 cigarette smokers and 15 nonsmokers after standardizing the dietary proline intake and after giving proline supplements. Monitoring endogenous nitrosation through the use of proline is especially suitable for several reasons. First, proline is a naturally occurring amino acid. Second, its nitrosation product, N-nitrosoproline, is almost quantitatively excreted in urine without further metabolism [8]. Third, NPRO is nontoxic and noncarcinogenic.

Our findings in smokers and nonsmokers, presented in Table V, indicate that the smokers excrete significantly more NPRO in urine than do nonsmokers. Addition of 300 mg of proline per day to the diet elevated NPRO excretion by the smokers even further while no such increase of NPRO was observed in the nonsmokers' urine. Last, ascorbic acid supplements were effective inhibitors of NPRO formation even in the smokers who had received dietary supplements of proline. Thus, the role of tobacco smoke inhalation in facilitating endogenous nitrosation reactions is apparent and we can assume that endogenous nitrosation of nicotine and other tobacco amines may likewise occur. The detection of these reaction products would be indistinguishable from the uptake of exogenous tobacco-specific nitrosamines and many of their metabolism products would be the same as those derived from nicotine itself.

Therefore, we are currently probing methods that will allow us to determine without ambiguity whether tobacco-specific nitrosamines and other carcinogenic nitrosamines are in fact formed as a result of endogenous nitrosation reactions.

ACKNOWLEDGMENTS

These studies are supported by grants CA-17613 and 2PO1-CA-29580 from the National Cancer Institute and grant ES 03278 from the National Institutes of Environmental Health Sciences, Department of Health and Human Services, respectively.

We thank Bertha Stadler and Ilse Hoffmann for their editorial assistance.

REFERENCES

1. U.S. Surgeon General: "The Health Consequences of Smoking—Cancer." DHHS Publ No (PHS) 82-50179, 1982, p 332.

2. International Agency for Research on Cancer: "Betel Quid and Tobacco Chewing, Snuff Dipping and Some Nitroso Compounds." IARC Monograph, Vol 37, 1985 (in press).
3. International Agency for Research on Cancer: "Tobacco Smoking." IARC Monograph, Vol 38, 1985 (in press).
4. Hoffmann D, Wynder EL, Rivenson A, LaVoie EJ, Hecht SS: Progr Exp Tumor Res 26:43, 1983.
5. Hoffmann D, LaVoie EJ, Hecht SS: Cancer Lett 26:67, 1985.
6. Melikian AA, Leszcynska JM, Hecht SS, Hoffmann D: Carcinogenesis 7:9, 1986.
7. Haley NJ, Axelrad CM, Tilton KA: Am J Public Health 73:1050, 1983.
8. Hoffmann D, Brunnemann KD: Cancer Res 43:5570, 1983.
9. Johnston LM: Lancet 2:742, 1942.
10. Hoffmann D, Hecht SS: Cancer Res 45:935, 1985.
11. Hoffmann D, Dong M, Hecht SS: JNCI 58:1841, 1977.
12. Adams JD, Lee SJ, Vinchkoski N, Castonguay A, Hoffmann D: Cancer Lett 17:339, 1983.
13. National Research Council: "The Health Effects of Nitrate, Nitrite, and N-Nitroso Compounds." Washington, DC: National Academy Press, 1981, p 529.
14. Hecht SS, Adams JD, Numoto S, Hoffmann D: Carcinogenesis 4:1287, 1983.
15. Hoffmann D, Rivenson A, Amin S, Hecht SS: J Cancer Res Clin Oncol 108:81, 1984.
16. U.S. Surgeon General: "The Health Consequences of Smoking for Women." Washington, DC: U.S. Department of Health and Human Services, 1980, p 385.
17. Michejda CJ, Kroeger-Koepke MB, Koepke SR, Sieh DH: Am Chem Soc Symp Ser 174:3, 1981.
18. Mochizuki M, Anjo T, Okada M: Tetrahedron Lett 21:3693, 1980.
19. Pegg OE: Rev Biochem Toxicol 5:83, 1983.
20. Castonguay A, Stoner GD, Schut HA, Hecht SS: Proc Natl Acad Sci 80:6694, 1983.
21. Castonguay A, Tharp R, Hecht SS: IARC Sci Publ 57: 805, 1984.
22. Foiles PG, Trushin N, Castonguay A: Carcinogenesis 6:989, 1985.
23. Hoffmann D, Wynder EL: Cancer 27:848, 1971.
24. Hecht SS, Carmella S, Mori H, Hoffmann D: JNCI 66:163, 1981.
25. Haley NJ, Sepkovic DW, Hoffmann D, Wynder EL: J Clin Pharmacol Ther 38:164, 1985.
26. Greenberg RA, Haley NJ, Etzel RA, Loda FA: N Engl J Med 310:1075, 1984.
27. Boyland E, Walker SE: Nature 248:601, 1974.
28. Ohshima H, Bereziat H: Carcinogenesis 3:115, 1982.
29. Van Duuren BL, Katz C, Goldschmidt BM: JNCI 51:703, 1973.
30. Van Duuren BL, Goldschmidt BM: JNCI 56:1237, 1976.

Biochemical and Molecular Epidemiology of Cancer 205–211 (1986)

Human Cytochrome P-450 Isozymes: Polymorphism and Potential Relevance in Chemical Carcinogenesis

F. Peter Guengerich, Tsutomu Shimada, Linda M. Distlerath, Paul E.B. Reilly, Diane R. Umbenhauer, and Martha V. Martin

Department of Biochemistry and Center in Molecular Toxicology, Vanderbilt University School of Medicine, Nashville, Tennessee 37232

Many chemical carcinogens are oxidized to their reactive forms by cytochrome P-450 (P-450) enzymes, and variation in these P-450s may contribute to host factors in carcinogenesis. Polymorphisms have been reported for several P-450–mediated activities, and we report the purification of P-450 isozymes involved in four of these: debrisoquine 4-hydroxylase, phenacetin O-deethylase, mephenytoin 4-hydroxylase, and nifedipine oxidase. The purified proteins differ in apparent monomeric molecular weight, amino acid composition, immunochemical properties, and substrate specificity. Antibody and DNA probes for these P-450s have been prepared and may ultimately be of use in human risk assessment.

Key words: chemical carcinogenesis, genetic polymorphism, cytochrome P-450, debrisoquine 4-hydroxylation

Many chemicals are not carcinogenic themselves but exert their effects only after biotransformation to electrophiles which react with DNA [1]. A common enzymatic step in such bioactivation is mixed-function oxidation by cytochrome P-450 (P-450) [2]. The isozymic composition of P-450 in experimental animals is known to vary as a function of age, sex, and induction regimen [3], and the activation and detoxication of carcinogens can be influenced by these changes.

Questions then arise about the interindividual variation of P-450s in humans and the potential contribution to cancer risk. Genetic polymorphisms have been identified in the oxidation of drugs in humans [4–8] (Table I). The possibility exists that a P-450 isozyme involved in oxidation of one of these drugs might also be involved in the bioactivation or detoxication of a carcinogen. Thus, individuals with either unusually high or low rates of oxidation of the drug might be at special risk from a given carcinogen. In this regard Idle and his associates [12,13] have suggested that individuals with unusually high debrisoquine 4-hydroxylase activity may be more prone to

Received June 6, 1985.

© **1986 Alan R. Liss, Inc.**

TABLE I. Human P-450s Involved in Polymorphisms

P-450	Polymorphism	Homologous rat enzyme	References
P-450$_{DB}$	Debrisoquine, sparteine, etc	P-450$_{UT-H}$	9–11
P-450$_{PA}$	Phenacetin	P-450$_{ISF-G}$	11[a]
P-450$_{MP}$	Mephenytoin	P-450$_{UT-I}$	4, 21
P-450$_{NF}$	Nifedipine	P-450$_{PCN-E}$	4, 22

[a]Dannan et al, manuscript in preparation.

lung tumors related to cigarette smoking and possibly to liver tumors caused by aflatoxin B$_1$.

To understand better these polymorphisms and their relevance to carcinogenesis we have begun to characterize the enzymes in detail. To date we have purified and raised antibodies to the four P-450s listed in Table I, which all appear to be involved in polymorphisms of drug oxidation.

MATERIALS AND METHODS

Sources of Human Liver Microsomes

Liver samples were obtained from individuals who met accidental deaths and donated other tissues for transplant. Arrangements were handled through the Nashville Regional Organ Procurement Agency. Tissues were perfused and chilled within 15–30 min of death and frozen ($-70°C$) in small pieces as described elsewhere [14].

Purification of P-450s

Microsomes were solubilized with sodium cholate and fractionated to obtain electrophoretically homogeneous P-450$_{DB}$, P-450$_{PA}$, P-450$_{MP}$, and P-450$_{NF}$ using combinations of n-octylamino Sepharose, DEAE-cellulose, hydroxylapatite, and CM-cellulose chromatography. The methods are described in detail elsewhere [11,21–22]. Purity was established using sodium dodecyl sulfate-polyacrylamide gel electrophoresis, prosthetic group analysis, and various immunohistochemical criteria [4,11,21,22].

Reconstitution of Catalytic Activities

Purified P-450s were reconstituted with rabbit or rat NADPH-P-450 reductase and L-α-1,2-dilauroyl-sn-glycero-3-phosphocholine as described elsewhere [15]. In some cases purified human liver cytochrome b_5 was added after other components were mixed.

Immunochemical Studies

Antibodies were raised to purified P-450s in rabbits as described elsewhere [16]. Specificity of antisera and estimates of concentrations of individual P-450s in microsomal samples were made using immunoblotting methods [15]. Immunoinhibition studies were done using immunoglobulin G fractions and human liver microsomes as previously described [3,11,16,17].

RESULTS

Human liver P-450$_{DB}$, P-450$_{PA}$, P-450$_{MP}$, and P-450$_{NF}$ were purified to electrophoretic homogeneity using chromatographic methods. Further evidence supportive of the high purity of these preparations was obtained by prosthetic group analysis and immunochemical methods [11]. The apparent monomeric molecular weights all differ, and difference indices for the determined amino acid compositions also indicate dissimilarity of the four P-450s. In the case of P-450$_{MP}$, two molecular weight variants (P-450$_{MP-1}$ and P-450$_{MP-2}$) were isolated and found to be indistinguishable from each other by a number of criteria, including N-terminal amino acid sequences; however, the two forms are apparently coded for by distinct mRNAs, as shown by in vitro translation studies with liver samples. The N-terminal sequence of P-450$_{MP}$ is compared to those of other human, rat, and rabbit P-450s in Figure 1.

Antibodies were raised to each of the four purified P-450s and were shown to be specific as judged by double immunodiffusion and immunoblotting analysis [4,11]. Each antibody inhibited the catalytic activity of its homologous antigen in human liver microsomes, consonant with the view that it is the major enzyme involved in each of the polymorphisms. Antibodies were also used to make comparisons of structural similarity with rat liver P-450s (Table I). Considerable homology was observed in some cases (which is not really related to the N-terminal sequence alone [Fig. 1]). However, this gross structural structure homology does not always carry over to similarity of function. P-450$_{UT-I}$ does not catalyze mephenytoin 4-hydroxylation, but P-450$_{PCN-E}$ does. Both P-450$_{UT-A}$ and P-450$_{PCN-E}$ catalyze nifedipine oxidation.

All of the purified P-450s expressed their individual catalytic activities when reconstituted in the usual manner. However, when rough calculations are made using the immunochemically determined estimates of P-450 concentration and the catalytic activity in microsomal preparations, the turnover numbers of the purified enzymes are somewhat less than expected. In the case of P-450$_{MP}$ and P-450$_{NF}$, the addition of purified human liver cytochrome b_5 stimulated catalytic activity (and anticytochrome b_5 inhibited these activities in microsomal preparations).

The substrate specificities of the four P-450s were assessed using both reconstitution assays and immunoinhibition assays with microsomal fractions. The conclusions of our studies to date are presented in Table II. Others have found that 2-acetylaminofluorene metabolism is not catalyzed by P-450$_{DB}$ [20]. In further considerations of substrate specificity, we have tried to correlate the different polymorphic activities in various human liver samples. The results support our conclusions (Table II) that debrisoquine 4-hydroxylation and bufuralol 1′-hydroxylation are catalyzed by the same enzyme [4,11]. In other cases some correlation is found but other studies (*vide supra*) do not support the view that the same enzyme is involved in both activities [11].

We have also quantified each of the four P-450s in liver microsomes using the antibodies. In the of case P-450$_{NF}$ a significant correlation ($r = 0.78$, $n = 32$, $p < 0.005$) between nifedipine oxidase activity and immunodetectable protein was observed when samples from various patients were examined. The correlation was almost as good when a monoclonal antibody was used to repeat the study ($r = 0.65$, $n = 39$, $p < 0.005$). However, with the other three P-450s (P-450$_{DB}$, P-450$_{PA}$, and P-450$_{NF}$) we did not see a significant correlation between catalytic activity and immunodetectable protein.

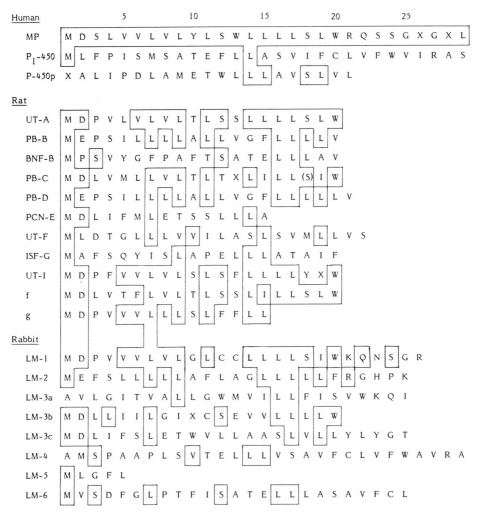

Fig. 1. N-Terminal sequences of human P-450s. Sequences for P-450$_{MP}$ [21], P-450p (Guzelian and Wrighton, personal communication), P$_1$-450 [18], and the rat and rabbit P-450s [19] are derived from the indicated references.

DISCUSSION

We have started to purify and characterize the human P-450s to ascertain their roles in chemical carcinogenesis and drug toxicity in humans. Known polymorphisms of drug metabolism in humans provide a link between in vitro catalytic activities and patients that can facilitate further studies. The partial characterization of the enzymes shown to be involved in four polymorphisms is described here. Purification of the P-450s is important in the development of immunochemical and DNA probes that can be used for further assessment of the enzymes' role.

Immunochemical inhibition of catalytic activity has been the major tool used in establishing substrate specificity of the individual P-450s (Table II). Enzyme reconsti-

TABLE II. Apparent Substrate Specificity of Human P-450s

P-450	Activities	Activities shown not to be associated with each P-450
P-450$_{DB}$ [17]	Debrisoquine 4-hydroxylation Sparteine Δ^5-oxidation Bufuralol 1'-hydroxylation Encainide O-demethylation Propranolol 4-hydroxylation Lasiocarpine oxidation Monocrotaline oxidation	S-Mephenytoin 4-hydroxylation Nifedipine oxidation Phenacetin O-deethylation 7-Ethoxycoumarin O-deethylation Acetanilide 4-hydroxylation Aniline 4-hydroxylation Diazepam N-demethylation Benzo(a)pyrene hydroxylation Benzo(a)pyrene-7,8-dihydrodiol 9,10-epoxidation N,N-Dimethylnitrosamine N-demethylation Trichloroethylene oxidation Vinylidene chloride oxidation Aflatoxin B$_1$ 2,3-epoxidation Aflatoxin B$_1$ 8-hydroxylation Ethylmorphine N-demethylation Morphine N-demethylation d-Benzphetamine N-demethylation Aminopyrine N-demethylation 1-Naphthylamine 2-hydroxylation 2-Naphthylamine N-hydroxylation 2-Naphthylamine 1-hydroxylation 2-Naphthylamine 6-hydroxylation 2-Aminofluorene N-hydroxylation 2-Aminofluorene 5-hydroxylation Azoprocarbazine N-oxidation
P-450$_{PA}$	Phenacetin O-deethylation	Debrisoquine 4-hydroxylation S-Mephenytoin 4-hydroxylation Nifedipine oxidation
P-450$_{MP}$	S-Mephenytoin 4-hydroxylation S-Mephenytoin N-demethylation S-Nirvanol 4-hydroxylation Diphenylhydantoin 4-hydroxylation	R-Mephenytoin 4-hydroxylation R-Mephenytoin N-demethylation R-Nirvanol 4-hydroxylation N-Methyl diphenylhydantoin 4-hydroxylation Diazepam N-demethylation Nifedipine oxidation d-Benzphetamine N-demethylation 4-Nitroanisole O-demethylation Benzo(a)pyrene hydroxylation Bufuralol 1'-hydroxylation Phenacetin O-deethylation
P-450$_{NF}$	Nifedipine oxidation Testosterone 6β-hydroxylation Aldrin epoxidation 17β Estradiol 2-hydroxylation 17β Estradiol 4-hydroxylation	S-Mephenytoin 4-hydroxylation Phenacetin O-deethylation Bufuralol 1-hydroxylation

TABLE III. Correlation of Polymorphic Activities in Human Liver Microsomes

	Correlation coefficient $(r)^a$			
	Bufuralol 1'-hydroxylation	Phenacetin O-deethylation	S-Mephenytoin 4-hydroxylation	Nifedipine oxidation
Debrisoquine 4-hydroxylation	0.86 (16)*	0.62 (43)*	0.24 (20)	0.04 (22)
(±)Bufuralol 1'-hydroxylation		0.68 (9)*	−0.08 (10)	0.11 (8)
Phenacetin O-deethylation			0.11 (20)	0.27 (13)
S-Mephenytoin 4-hydroxylation				−0.06 (21)

$^a n$ in parentheses (n being the number of liver samples from individual humans).
*Statistically significant at least at the $p < 0.025$ confidence level.

tution and correlation studies (Table III) have been used to complement these findings. The work to date suggests that enzymes are reasonably specific and that many carcinogens are not oxidized by the particular enzymes studied here. The results agree that any correlation between debrisoquine 4-hydroxylation and aflatoxin B_1-induced liver tumors [12] does not have a metabolic basis. The complexity of cigarette smoke does not permit definite conclusions related to the case of the lung cancer study [13], although benzo(a)pyrene metabolism does not appear to be involved.

The question of the basis of the polymorphisms arises. The lack of correlation between catalytic activity and immunochemically detectable protein in the cases of P-450$_{DB}$, P-450$_{PA}$, and P-450$_{MP}$ suggests that polymorphism may occur in the structural genes for each enzyme. (The two forms P-450$_{MP-1}$ and P-450$_{MP-2}$ have similar catalytic activities, and the presence of the two forms does not explain the polymorphism.) In the case of P-450$_{NF}$, regulation may be at the transcriptional level. The levels of P-450$_{DB}$ and P-450$_{PA}$ appear to be very low (a few percent of the P-450 pool), while P-450$_{MP}$ and P-450$_{NF}$ appear to account for something on the order of an average of 20% of the P-450 pool. Fetal livers are consistently devoid of P-450$_{MP}$ but not P-450$_{NF}$. P-450$_{NF}$ may be inducible by certain drugs such as dexamethasone. P-450$_{NF}$ appears to have important physiological substrates (Table II).

In addition to the approach of using antibodies to elucidate the substrate specificities of these P-450s toward other drugs and carcinogens, we are also applying recombinant DNA methods to better understand the polymorphisms. Human liver mRNA was reverse transcribed to form cDNA, which was inserted into bacteriophage λgt11 to prepare an expression library of 10^7 members. Screening with antibodies and subsequent plaque purification produced clones corresponding to P-450$_{DB}$, P-450$_{PA}$, P-450$_{MP}$, P-450$_{NF}$, and human cytochrome b_5. These cDNAs are being developed further to generate useful probes that can be used to isolate full-length clones for sequencing, to measure mRNA levels, to find and identify any alterations in structural genes, and ultimately to develop further that can be used for screening patients' samples for polymorphisms.

ACKNOWLEDGMENTS

These studies were supported by NIH grants CA 30907 and ES 00267. We thank Dr. G.R. Wilkinson for providing drug standards.

REFERENCES

1. Miller EC, Miller JR: Cancer 47:2337, 1981.
2. Wislocki PG, Miwa GT, Lu AYH: Enzym Basis Detox 1:135, 1980.
3. Waxman DJ, Dannan GA, Guengerich FP: Biochemistry 24:4409, 1985.
4. Guengerich FP, Distlerath LM, Reilly PEB, Wolff T, Shimada T, Umbenhauer DR, Martin MV: Xenobiotica (in press).
5. Küpfer A, Preisig R: Semin Liver Dis 3:341, 1983.
6. Sloan TP, Mahgoub A, Lancaster R, Idle JR, Smith RL: Br Med J 2:655, 1978.
7. Kalow W, Otton SV, Kadar D, Endrenyl L, Inaba T: Can J Physiol Pharmacol 58:1142, 1980.
8. Boobis AR, Murray S, Kahn GC, Robertz G-M, Davies DS: Mol Pharmacol 23:474, 1983.
9. Larrey D, Distlerath LM, Dannan GA, Wilkinson GR, Guengerich FP: Biochemistry 23:2787, 1984.
10. Distlerath LM, Guengerich FP: Proc Natl Acad Sci USA 81:7348, 1984.
11. Distlerath LM, Reilly PEB, Martin MV, Davis GG, Wilkinson GR, Guengerich FP: J Biol Chem 260:9057, 1985.
12. Ritchie JR, Idle JR: In Bartsch A, Armstrong B (eds): "Host Factors in Human Carcinogenesis." Lyon: International Agency for Research in Cancer, 1982, pp 381–384.
13. Ayesh R, Idle JR, Ritchie JC, Crothers MJ, Hetzel MR: Nature 312:169, 1984.
14. Wang PP, Beaune P, Kaminsky LS, Dannan GA, Kadlubar FF, Larrey D, Guengerich FP: Biochemistry 22:5375, 1983.
15. Guengerich FP, Dannan GA, Wright ST, Martin MV, Kaminsky LS: Biochemistry 21:6019, 1982.
16. Kaminsky LS, Fasco MJ, Guengerich FP: Methods Enzymol 74:262, 1981.
17. Wolff T, Distlerath LM, Worthington MW, Groopman JD, Hammons GJ, Kadlubar FF, Prough RA, Martin MV, Guengerich FP: Cancer Res 45:2116, 1985.
18. Jaiswal AK, Gonzalez FJ, Nebert DW: Science 228:80, 1985.
19. Black SD, Coon MJ: In Ortiz de Montellano PR (ed): "Cytochromes P-450." Plenum Press: New York (in press).
20. McManus ME, Boobis AR, Michin RF, Schwartz DM, Murray S, Davies D, Thorgeirsson SS: Cancer Res 44:5692, 1984.
21. Shimada T, Misono KS, Guengerich FP: J Biol Chem 261:909, 1986.
22. Guengerich FP, Martin MV, Beaune PH, Kremers P, Wolff T, Waxman DJ: J Biol Chem (in press).

Biochemical and Molecular Epidemiology of Cancer 213–226 (1986)

Growth, Differentiation, and Neoplastic Transformation of Human Bronchial Epithelial Cells

Curtis C. Harris, George H. Yoakum, John F. Lechner, James C. Willey
Brenda Gerwin, Susan Banks-Schlegel, Tohru Masui, and George Mark

Laboratory of Human Carcinogenesis, Division of Cancer Etiology, National Cancer Institute, Bethesda, Maryland 20205

Pathways of growth and differentiation have been studied in normal human bronchial epithelial cells cultured in serum-free medium. Diminished responsiveness to inducers of terminal squamous differentiation, for example, TGF-β and/or autocrine production of growth factors (eg, gastrin-releasing factors), may provide lung carcinoma cells with a selective clonal expansion advantage. Human bronchial epithelial cells have also been employed to investigate the role of specific oncogenes in carcinogenesis and tumor progression. Using the protoplast fusion method for high frequency gene transfection, the v-Ha-*ras* oncogene initiates a cascade of events in the normal human bronchial cells leading to their apparent immortality, aneuploidy, and tumorigenicity with metastasis in athymic nude mice. These results suggest that oncogenes may play an important role in human carcinogenesis.

Key words: human, epithelial cells, growth, differentiation, transformation

We are investigating the molecular and cellular mechanisms controlling growth and differentiation of human bronchial epithelial cells and the dysregulation of these controls during the multistage process of carcinogenesis. The general strategy employed in these studies is shown in Figure 1. After developing conditions for the replicative culture of normal human lung epithelial cells, the effects of carcinogens and tumor promoters on their growth properties, differentiation programs, and tumorigenic potential are investigated. Epidemiological studies, clinical observations, and investigations in animal models provide clues to which carcinogens to utilize in

Abbreviations used: TGF-β, type β transforming growth factor; GRP, gastrin-releasing factor; NRK, normal rat kidney; DAG, diacylglycerol; NHBE, normal human bronchial epithelial; PA, plasminogen activator; Epi, epinephrine; CLE, cross-linked envelope; BDS, whole blood-derived serum; HCG, human chorionic gonadotropin; TPA, 12-O-tetradecanoylphorbol-13-acetate; GTP, guanine triphosphate; LTR, long terminal repeat.

Received August 7, 1985.

© **1986 Alan R. Liss, Inc.**

these in vitro model systems. Cultured human cells can also be used to test genetic hypotheses, including the role of specific oncogenes in the multistage carcinogenic process.

CONTROL OF GROWTH AND TERMINAL DIFFERENTIATION IN HUMAN BRONCHIAL EPITHELIAL CELLS

Pathways of growth and terminal differentiation are highly regulated in the normal bronchial epithelium (Fig. 2). We are currently investigating the regulation of

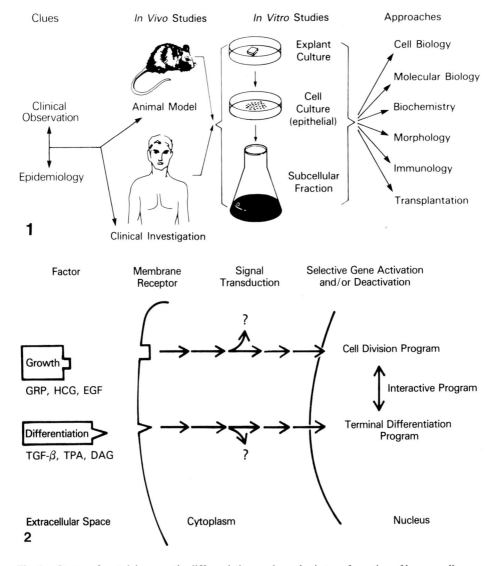

Fig. 1.   Strategy for studying growth, differentiation, and neoplastic transformation of human cells.

Fig. 2.   Growth and differentiation pathways in human bronchial epithelial cells.

these pathways using bronchial epithelial cells cultured in a serum-free, chemically defined culture medium [1]. In a search for specific growth factors, we tested whether or not "ectopic" hormones produced by lung carcinomas might be autocrine growth factors. For example, gastrin-releasing peptide (bombesin) is frequently found in small cell carcinomas [2,3], and human chorionic gonadotropin is detected in many nonsmall cell carcinomas [4]. These hormones significantly enhance the growth of normal bronchial epithelial cells in vitro (Figs. 3, 4) by binding to specific membrane receptors, leading to the transduction of a signal to the nucleus and subsequent activation of the genes essential for cellular replication. For example, normal bronchial epithelial cells have about 7,000 high affinity receptors for gastrin-releasing factor that can be blocked with chemical analogs such as spantide (Willey et al, unpublished results).

The pathway for terminal squamous differentiation in human bronchial epithelial cells can also be initiated by ligands binding to specific membrane receptors. Type β transforming growth factor (TGF-β) (also known as *epithelial inhibitor*), is an example of such a polypeptide [5]. TGF-β was first characterized by its ability to induce reversible phenotypic transformation of normal rat kidney (NRK) cells in the presence of epidermal growth factor (EGF) [6,7]. More recently, it has been shown to inhibit the growth of some cell types [8,9]. Our study shows that TGF-β inhibits the growth of normal human bronchial epithelial (NHBE) cells and, in addition, is a potent inducer of squamous differentiation in this system. TGF-β induced the following terminal differentiation markers of NHBE cells: 1) clonal growth inhibition [10,11]; 2) irreversible inhibition of DNA synthesis; 3) an increase in extracellular plasminogen activator (PA) activity [12,13]; 4) an increase in Ca ionophore-induced, cross-linked envelope (CLE) formation [14,15]; and 5) an increase in cell area [10,16]. Whole blood-derived serum (BDS) also induced terminal differentiation markers of NHBE cells [10,17]. Anti-TGF-β antibody was able to neutralize the inhibition of DNA synthesis by either TGF-β or BDS in a dose-dependent fashion. These findings clearly demonstrate that TGF-β is the primary serum factor that induces terminal squamous differentiation of NHBE cells.

It has been reported that NRK cells and murine AKR-2B cells have specific receptors for TGF-β with Kd 25–30 and Kd 33 pM and 17,000 and 10,500 binding sites per cell, respectively [18,19]. TGF-β receptors on NHBE cells have a higher affinity, with Kd 13 $\pm$ 3 pM and 10,000 $\pm$ 3,000 binding sites per cell. The 50% inhibitory dose for TGF-β on DNA synthesis of NHBE cells was about 0.4 pM. Thus, as shown for NRK cells, the effect of TGF-β on NHBE cells may be mediated by specific receptors for TGF-β and only a small fraction of these receptors need be occupied for TGF-β to inhibit the growth of NHBE cells.

In addition to endogenous molecules, there are exogenous agents that can induce terminal squamous differentiation of normal bronchial epithelial cells in vitro (Fig. 5). These agents appear to mediate their effects by activating protein kinase C and/or by increasing intracellular calcium ion concentration. These effects may be due to direct interaction (eg, 12-O-tetradecanoylphorbol-13-acetate [TPA] by activation of protein kinase C) and/or to indirect mechanisms mediated by membrane lipid peroxidation and generation of active oxygen species that modify mitochondrial membranes leading to release of calcium ions into the cytosol [20]. In addition, exogenous aldehydes, including those found in tobacco smoke (ie, formaldehyde, acrolein, and acetaldehyde), and peroxides may produce the same effects.

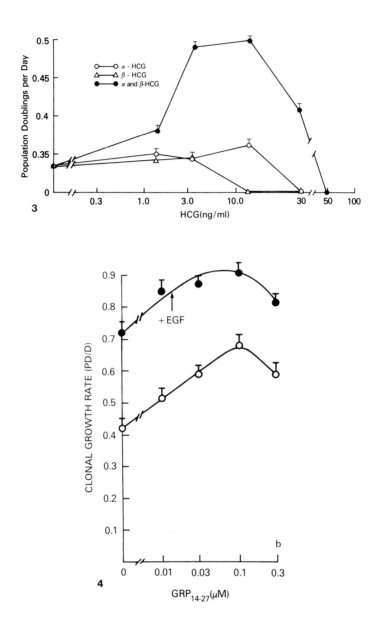

Fig. 3.   Effect of α and β human chorionic gonadotropin on clonal growth rate of human bronchial epithelial cells.

Fig. 4.   Effect of gastrin-releasing peptide on clonal growth rate of human bronchial epithelial cells. Five thousand cells in 1 ml of dissolved in LHC medium) plastic culture dishes containing 3 ml of LHC medium with or without EGF. Twenty-four hours later, the media were removed and replaced with media containing varying concentrations of GRP$_{14\text{-}27}$. Cells were incubated for a total of 7 days, with a medium change after 4 days. Dose-response experiments were with GRP$_{14\text{-}27}$. $\bigcirc$, EGF absent; $\bullet$, EGF present.

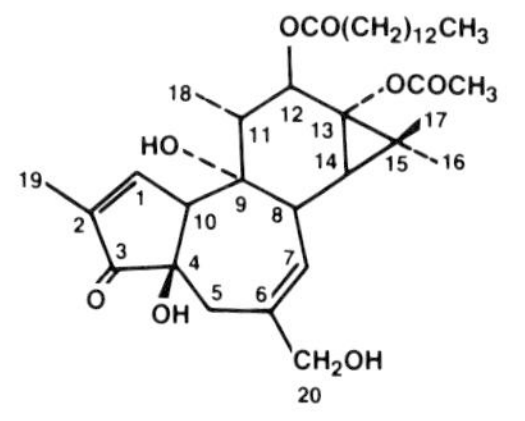

12-0-Tetradecanoyl-phorbol-13-acetate

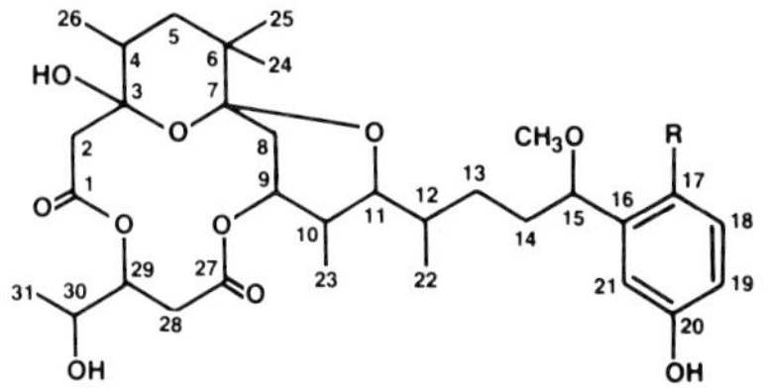

Aplysiatoxin, R = Br
Debromoaplysiatoxin, R = H

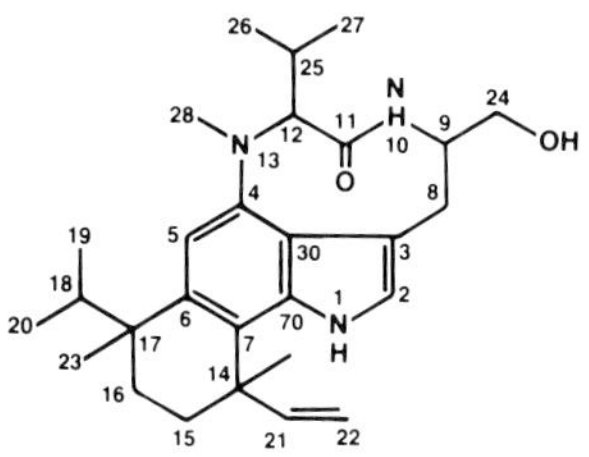

Teleocidin B

$CH_2 = O$
Formaldehyde

$CH_2 = CH - CH = O$
Acrolein

$CH_3 - CH = O$
Acetaldehyde

H_2O_2
Hydrogen Peroxide

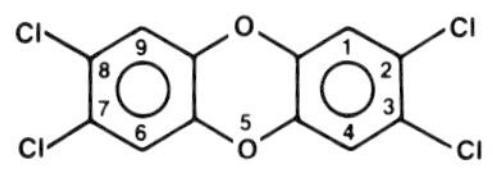

2,3,7,8-Tetrachlorodibenzo-*p*-dioxin

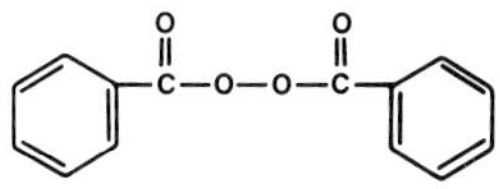

Benzoyl Peroxide

Fig. 5. Tumor promoters, aldehydes, peroxides, and a dioxin are inducers of terminal squamous differentiation of human bronchial epithelial cells.

Several studies have shown that lung carcinoma cell lines exhibit diminished responsiveness to differentiation inducers [10,21,22]. We do not as yet understand why malignant cells are relatively insensitive to agents that induce the terminal differentiation of their normal counterparts. To study this phenomenon, a controlled cell culture system is indispensible. Using a serum-free culture system for NHBE cells, we have shown that BDS, specifically the platelet fraction, induced terminal squamous differentiation of NHBE cells, while malignant human lung carcinomas did not respond to this differentiation-inducing effect of BDS [10,17]. Moreover, BDS enhances growth of malignant cells in a dose-dependent manner. We found that TGF-β, one of the defined factors found in human platelets, is a potent growth inhibitor and an inducer of squamous differentiation for NHBE cells but not lung carcinoma cells cultured in monolayer under serum-free conditions. Therefore, BDS contains both growth factors and inducers of terminal squamous differentiation, and the specificity of response to these agents resides at the cellular level (Fig. 6). Fibroblasts respond primarily to growth factors, for example, platelet-derived growth factor. In contrast, NHBE cells respond primarily to inducers of differentiation (ie, TGF-β), whereas carcinoma cells are generally unresponsive to TGF-β and are stimulated to divide by as yet unidentified growth factors in BDS. In conclusion, an imbalance between the pathways of growth and differentiation could lead to a selective clonal expansion advantage of preneoplastic and neoplastic cells, while normal epithelial cells respond by terminal differentiation.

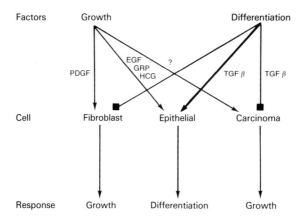

Fig. 6. Blood-derived serum contains both growth factors (eg, platelet-derived growth factor [PDGF], epiderminal growth factor [EGF], gastrin-releasing peptide [GRP] and human chorionic gonadotropin [HCG]) and differentiation inducers (eg, transforming growth factor β in epithelial cells).

Recently, there have been many reports linking the *ras* p21 oncogene products with the guanosine triphosphate (GTP)-binding protein system that controls adenylate cyclase activity [23–28]. We recently showed that epinephrine antagonized the action of the differentiation-inducing factor TGF-β (Masui et al, unpublished results). Moreover, NHBE cells transfected by v-Ha-*ras* oncogene are insensitive to differentiation-inducing stimuli, such as TPA, BDS, and TGF-β [29; Masui et al, unpublished data]. Thus, the abilities of either epinephrine or p21 *ras* to block differentiation may be linked to activation of the stimulatory GTP-binding protein pathways. This hypothesis could provide a feasible role for the *ras* oncogene during epithelial carcinogenesis.

MALIGNANT TRANSFORMATION OF HUMAN BRONCHIAL EPITHELIAL CELLS BY TRANSFECTED HARVEY RAS ONCOGENE

Three families of oncogenes, *ras*, *raf*, and *myc*, have so far been associated with human lung cancer (Fig. 7). Approximately 10% of the carcinoma cell lines have yielded *ras*-mutated protooncogene sequences when their DNA were transfected into mouse NIH-3T3 cells [for review, see 30]. The *myc* family of protooncogenes has been found to be activated by amplification in many cell lines established from small cell carcinoma of the lung [31].

Minna [31] recently described a third member of this family, L-*myc*, which has a highly conserved region of nucleotide sequence homology in the second exon with c-*myc* and N-*myc*. The third family, *raf*, is also found to be overexpressed in small carcinomas (Mark et al, unpublished results) by an as yet undiscovered mechanism probably related to the gene rearrangements caused by the deletion in the short arm of chromosome 3 (p14-23) near the site of one of the *raf* protooncogenes (p25) [32]. Mark et al [33] recently identified a *raf*-related putative protooncogene (c-*pks*) on chromosome X. Analysis of DNA and amino acid sequence data suggests that the members of the *raf* oncogene family are receptors with serine/threonine kinase activity and may have functional similarities to protein kinase C.

Because the above-mentioned associations are not proof that these protooncogenes actually play an intrinsic role in human lung carcinogenesis and/or the mainte-

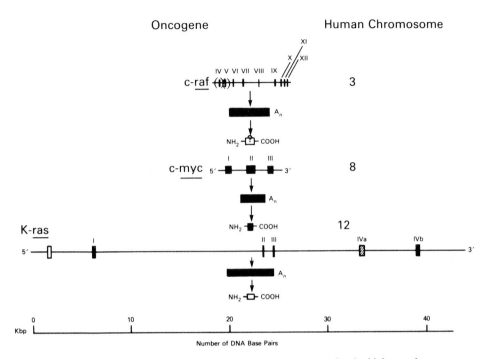

Fig. 7. Three families of oncogenes (*ras*, *raf*, and *myc*) have been associated with human lung cancer.

TABLE I. Strategy for Studying Neoplastic Transformation of Human Bronchial Epithelial Cells by Transfected Oncogenes

A. Select oncogenes associated with lung cancer
B. Use progenitor epithelial cells of bronchogenic carcinoma
C. Develop and use high frequency gene transfection method
D. Develop and use conditions to select preneoplastic and neoplastic cells
E. Establish criteria to identify preneoplastic and neoplastic cells

nance of the malignant phenotype, we considered it important to determine the phenotypic alterations caused by these sequences following their transfection into NHBE cells in vitro.

Our strategy for these investigations is outlined in Table I. NHBE cells were chosen for these studies because they are the progenitor cells of bronchogenic carcinoma. We had previously developed serum-free media to culture the cells and had shown that they replicate for 20 to 40 cell generations, retain a diploid karyotype, and are responsive to both exogenous and endogenous inducers of terminal squamous differentiation [6,10,13,17,21,22].

The calcium-phosphate method of Graham and van der Eb [34] has become the standard method for gene transfer into rodent fibroblasts. However, knowing that high concentrations of calcium ions are cytotoxic to human epithelial cells and that a moderate concentration (ie, a few micromoles) enhances pathways of terminal squamous differentiation [10], we developed an alternative method [35] which is illustrated in Figure 8. A plasmid is constructed to contain the oncogene(s) and may also contain a positive selectable marker gene (eg, *gpt* or *neo*). The number of plasmids per host

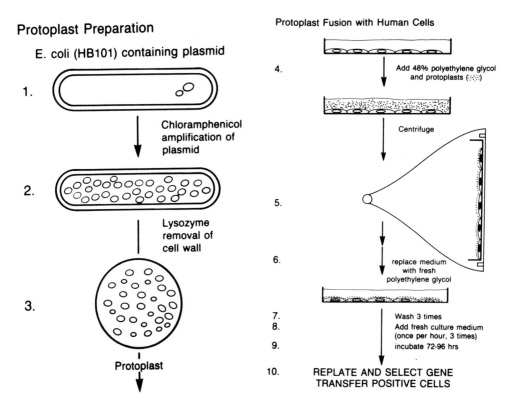

Fig. 8.   Schematic diagram of the protoplast fusion method of gene transfection.

bacteria is amplified 20- to 100-fold by chloramphenicol treatment. Protoplasts are then formed by enzymatically removing the bacterial cell wall with lysozyme. The protoplasts are sedimented onto the surface of the epithelial cells by centrifugation and, in the presence of purified polyethylene glycol, the membranes of the protoplasts and epithelial cells fuse, permitting access of plasmids to the interior of the human cells. The frequency of stable integration of genes transfected in human epithelial cells by this method is as high as that achieved by the calcium-phosphate method in rodent fibroblasts (ie, approximately 1 to 5 × 10^{-3}).

Selection pressures to isolate presumptive neoplastic cells were based on the hypothesis that such cells have a defect in their differentiation pathways. Whereas the normal cells are responsive to these inducers of differentiation, human carcinoma cell lines are relatively resistant and continue to grow in the presence of TPA, an exogenous inducer or BDS, which contains TGF-β, an endogenous inducer of terminal squamous differentiation [5]. Maintenance of the normal cells either at confluence or in suspension causes terminal differentiation. These observations formed the foundation for our experimental design.

We chose the *ras* family of oncogenes to initiate our investigations [29] because of 1) their frequent association with human carcinomas, including those of the lung [36–38]; 2) their genetic dominance in the transformation of murine cells; and 3) the well-defined point mutations in the structural gene. The native form of v-Ha-*ras* was selected because of its small size, its strong Moloney long terminal repeat (LTR) transcriptional promoter, and its readily identifiable phosphorylated protein, p21 [39–41]. We consider the introduction of v-Ha-*ras* to be a direct genetic test of the transforming potential of Ha-*ras* p21 in human bronchial epithelial cells.

The experimental design of these studies is based on the use of inducers of terminal squamous differentiation for isolating abnormal cells. NHBE cells were grown in serum-free LHC-4 medium, as previously described [1], and were passaged at 200,000 cells per 50 mm tissue culture dish. When the cells were 70 to 80% confluent, they were transfected by protoplast fusion using an *Escherichia coli* strain (HB 101) carrying plasmid H1, which contains v-Ha-*ras* on a 5.4 kbp Eco R1 fragment [42]. Selection of differentiation-resistant transfected NHBE cells was initiated by growth in LHC-4 medium containing 2% BDS, which induces terminal squamous differentiation in the NHBE cells within 7 to 10 days. This selection yielded v-Ha-*ras* transfectants at a frequency of approximately 10^{-3}. When the transfected cells became 80% confluent, the cells were subcultured by dissociation and reseeding at one-third cell density to test for their capacity for indefinite growth. The cells were maintained at confluence as a second selective pressure, and after 2 months, four multilayered cellular foci (TBE-1, -2, -3, and -4) appeared. These four foci were subcultured as individual cultures and have continued to grow indefinitely (ie, > 120 cell generations). One of these cell lines (TBE-1) has been extensively studied [29].

The phenotypic properties of the NHBE cells, TBE-1 cells, TBE-1SA (anchorage-independent TBE-1 cells), and TBE-1SAT (cells isolated from tumors formed by TBE-1SA cells injected into irradiated athymic nude mice) are listed in Table II. The v-Ha-*ras*-transfected cells are not induced to differentiate terminally by either 2% BDS or 100 nM TPA. TBE-1 cells are presumed to produce a growth factor because the growth rate of the cells at clonal density increases by a factor of 5 when autogenously conditioned medium is used as a supplement. TBE-1 cells also rarely grow in semisolid medium. When they are xenotransplanted into athymic nude mice, TBE-1 cells initially produce small, regressing tumors, and after 7 to 10 months tumors reappeared in only a few mice. In contrast, cells isolated from colonies of TBE-1 cells growing in agar (ie, TBE-1SA) have a higher activity of type IV collagenase and produce progressively growing tumors with a latency period of approximately 2 months. These tumor cells (ie, TBE-1SAT) have been shown to be of human origin on the basis of their isoenzyme patterns and the chromosomal analysis of the cultured cells. When TBE-1SAT cells are injected into athymic nude mice, they again display their tumorigenic properties. When analyzed by immunoperoxidase staining, these anaplastic tumors contain small amounts of keratin (the presence of which has been confirmed by immunoprecipitation using antiserum to total keratin purified from human stratum corneum) (Fig. 9); they also produce β human chorionic gonadotropin. Determining whether the growth factor activity found in conditioned media from these cells is β human chorionic gonadotropin will require additional investigations.

The TBE cells have a high metastatic potential (Table II). Metastasis to liver, lung, spleen, and kidney has been frequently observed from TBE cells growing at subcutaneous sites in the athymic nude mouse. Therefore, they may prove to be useful in model studies of metastases and their prevention. It is of interest that murine NIH/3T3 cells transfected with human tumor DNA containing activated *ras* oncogenes express the metastatic phenotype in athymic nude mice [43]. Preliminary results indicate that discrete genomic sequences may be involved [44].

TABLE II. Summary of the Phenotypic Properties of Normal Human Bronchial Epithelial Cells (NHBE) and v-Ha-*ras*-Transfected HBE Cells (TBE-1 and TBE-1SA) and TBE-1SAT Cells Isolated From Tumor Tissue*

Cell name	Differentiation response		Conditioned medium response		Anchorage indepen-dence	Tumorigenicity in athymic nude mice (subcutaneous)		Type IV collagenase activity
	2% BDS	TPA	NRK M-104	ACRM M-104		Frequency	Metastasis	
NHBE	+	−	ND	ND	−	−	−	+
TBE-1	−	−	−	+	+	+ (2/16)[b]	+	+ +
TBE-1SA[a]	−	−	ND	+	+	+ (13/14)	+ +	+ + +
TBE-1SAT	−	−	ND	+	+	+ (9/10)[c]	+ +	ND

*Phenotypic characteristics associated with the neoplastic properties of carcinoma cells, transformed cells grown in cell culture that were tested for v-Ha-*ras*–transfected normal human bronchial epithelial cells (TBE-1 and TBE-1SA) and the parent cell type. Column 2 indicates the differentiation response of NHBE grown in LHC-4 medium supplemented with 2% blood-derived serum (BDS) or 100 nM 12-O-tetradecanoylphorbol-13-acetate (TPA); the resistance of v-Ha-*ras*–transfected cells to in vitro stimuli for squamous differentiation is indicated by the capacity for growth in LHC-4 medium containing these agents. The v-Ha-*ras*–transfected cells do not produce a tumor cell growth factor capable of supporting the anchorage-independent growth of normal rat kidney (NRK) cells. However, clonal growth of TBE-1 cells requires 10 to 50% MCDB-104, LHC-4, or RPMI 1640 medium conditioned by 3 days of growth with 50% confluent TBE-1 cultures. This finding indicates that TBE-1 cells elaborate an autogenous factor required for the growth of TBE-1 cells resulting in an autogenous conditioned medium response for (ACMR) TBE-1 cells. The ability to form colonies during growth in soft agar was used to isolate TBE-1 derivatives capable of anchorage-independent growth (TBE-1SA). Early passage TBE-1 cells did not form colonies during growth in soft agar when seeded at 10^6 cells/60 mm dish. The relationship of anchorage independence to tumorigenicity is indicated by the relative increase in tumorigenicity observed for TBE-1SA cells. ND, not done.
[a]The anchorage-independent population isolated after soft agar growth of TBE-1 was named TBE-1SA.
[b]After 14 days the nodules regressed when 10^6 or 2×10^7 TBE-1 cells were injected subcutaneously in irradiated athymic nude mice. After 7 months, tumors reappeared in a few animals at 9 to 12 months.
[c]The TBE-1SAT cells isolated from tumors are now > 1.0 cm after transplant and are continuing to grow. It remains to be determined if the TBE-1SAT cells are more tumorigenic.

The transfected v-Ha-*ras* oncogene apparently caused NHBE cells to become immortal and malignant as judged by their continued growth, aneuploidy, and tumor-igenicity in athymic nude mice. The mechanism by which the v-Ha-*ras* p21 initiates this multistage process is unknown. The possibility was tested that a secondary alteration causing increased expression of a non-*ras* oncogene might have occurred. Total cell RNA was extracted from TBE-1, TBE-1SA, and TBE-1SAT cells. This RNA was screened by "dot-blot" hybridization with probes specific for H-*ras*, N-*myc*, c-*myc*, and *raf*. In no case was increased expression observed relative to a normal human bronchial epithelial cell control.

Because aneuploidy was an early observation we propose that the mutant p21 causes biochemical changes that interfere with mitosis and cause chromosomal rear-rangements, including loss of specific chromosomes containing cancer-suppressor genes that allow the emergence of the malignant cells from the population of less malignant cells in response to the selective pressures provided by BDS, high-density cell cultures, and growth in semisolid medium (Fig. 10). Constant stimulation of the G-protein system caused by activated *ras* p21 may be responsible for extending the life span of the cells. These selection pressures are potent inducers of terminal squamous differentiation of NHBE cells, but human lung carcinoma cell lines are

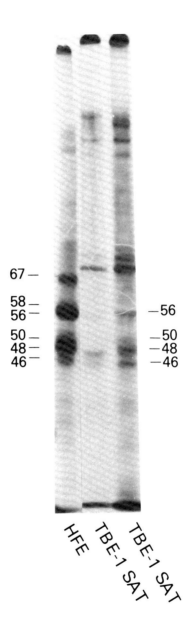

Fig. 9.   Presence of keratin in tumors formed following injection of TBE-1SA cells into athymic nude mice. Keratins from ^{35}S-methionine–labeled cell extracts of tumors (designated TBE-1SAT) derived from TBE-1SA cells were immunoprecipitated selectively with antiserum to total keratin purified from human stratum corneum and resolved electrophoretically on an 8.5% polyacrylamide gel. In addition to a 56 kd keratin band, TBE-1SAT cells containing predominantly small-sized keratins (46, 48 and 50 kd) are shown; HFE designates proteins from human foreskin epithelial cells.

TABLE III. Hypothetical Imbalance Between Control of Growth and Terminal Differentiation in Preneoplastic and Neoplastic Cells

A. Extracellular
    1. Increase in quantity and/or potency of growth factor
    2. Decrease in quantity and/or potency of differentiation factor
B. Membrane receptor
    1. Qualitative change, eg, truncated growth factor receptor not requiring ligand for activation of signal transduction
    2. Quantitative increase of normal growth factor receptors
    3. Qualitative change in differentiation factor receptor, eg, binding of ligand to it does not transduce signal
    4. Quantitative decrease of normal differentiation factor receptors
C. Signal transduction
    1. Activation of growth signal transduction unrelated to receptor
    2. Inactivation of differentiation signal transduction
D. Selective gene activation and/or major deactivation
    1. Stimulation of cell division program
    2. Inhibition of terminal differentiation program

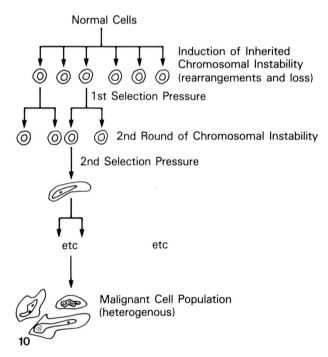

Fig. 10.   A simple model of selection of preneoplastic and neoplastic cells during random chromosomal rearrangements and losses caused by an inherited induction of chromosomal instability.

relatively resistant and continue to grow [10,21] (Fig. 11). It is of interest that although TPA was not used as a selective pressure in their isolation, the transformed cells nonetheless acquired a resistance to induction of differentiation by TPA. This observation implies a more generalized defect in the differentiation program of these transformed cells.

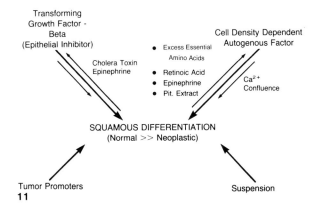

Fig. 11. Inducers of terminal squamous differentiation in normal human bronchial epithelial cells. Neoplastic transformmed cells are relatively unresponsive.

The data noted above are consistent with the hypothesis that preneoplastic and neoplastic human bronchial epithelial cells have an imbalance in their growth and differentiation programs (Table III). Such an imbalance would provide these cells with a selective growth expansion advantage over the normal epithelial cells. *In vitro* carcinogenesis studies using cells from experimental animals have also provided data supporting this hypothesis. Defects in control of cellular differentiation have been associated with the initiation phase of carcinogenesis in mouse epidermal cells [45] and 3T3 T proadipocytes [46].

REFERENCES

1. Lechner JF, Haugen A, McClendon IA, Pettis EW: In Vitro 18:633, 1982.
2. Moody TW, Pert CB, Gazdar AF, Carney DN, Minna JD: Science 214:1246, 1981.
3. Roth KA, Evans CJ, Weher E, Barchas JD, Bostwick DG, Bensch KG: Cancer Res 43:5411, 1983.
4. Trump BF, Wilson T, Harris CC: In Ishikawa S, Hayata Y, Suemasu K (eds): "Lung Cancer 1982." Amsterdam: Excerpta Medica, 1982, pp 101–124.
5. Masui T, Wakefield LM, Lechner JF, LaVeck MA, Sporn MB, Harris CC: Proc Natl Acad Sci USA (in press).
6. Roberts RF, AB, Anzano MA, Lamb LC, Smith JM, Sporn MB: Proc Natl Acad Sci USA 78:5339, 1981.
7. Roberts AB, Anzano MA, Lamb LC, Smith JM, Frolik CA, Marquardt H, Todaro GJ, Sporn MB: Nature 295:417, 1982.
8. Tucker RF, Shipley GD, Moses HL, Holley RW: Science 226:705, 1984.
9. Roberts AB, Anzano MA, Wakefield LM, Roche NS, Stern DF, Sporn MB: Proc Natl Acad Sci USA 82:119, 1985.
10. Lechner JF, McClendon IA, LaVeck MA, Shamsuddin AM, Harris CC: Cancer Res 43:5915, 1983.
11. Wille JJ Jr, Pittelkow MR, Shipley GD, Scott RE: J Cell Physiol 121:31, 1984.
12. Isseroff RR, Fusenig NE, Rifkin DB: J Invest Dermatol 80:217, 1983.
13. Willey JC, Saladino AJ, Ozanne C, Lechner JF, Harris CC: Carcinogenesis 5:209, 1984.
14. Sun T-T, Green H: Cell 9:511, 1976.
15. Rice RH, Green H: Cell 18:681, 1979.
16. Green H: Cell 11:405, 1977.
17. Lechner JF, Haugen A, McClendon IA, Shamsuddin AM: Differentiation 25:229, 1984.
18. Tucker RF, Branum EL, Shipley GD, Ryan BJ, Moses HL: Proc Natl Acad Sci USA 81:6757, 1984.

19. Frolik CA, Wakefield LM, Smith DM, Sporn MB: J Biol Chem 259:10995, 1984.
20. Cerutti P: In Harris C (ed): "Biochemical and Molecular Epidemiology of Cancer." New York: Alan R. Liss, Inc., 1986, pp 167, (this volume).
21. Willey JC, Moser CE Jr, Lechner JF, Harris CC: Cancer Res 44:5124, 1984.
22. Willey JC, Moser CE Jr, Harris CC: Cell Biol Toxicol 1:145, 1984.
23. Gilman AG: Cell 36:577, 1984.
24. Kataoka T, Powers S, Cameron S, Fasano O, Goldfarb M, Broach J, Wigler M: Cell 40:19, 1985.
25. Toda T, Uno I, Ishikawa T, Powers S. Kataoka T, Broek D, Cameron S, Broack J, Matsumoto K, Wigler M: Cell 40:27, 1985.
26. McGrath JP, Capon DJ, Goeddel DV, Levinson AD: Nature 310:644, 1984.
27. Hurley JB, Simon MI, Teplow DB, Robishaw JD, Gilman AG: Science 226:860, 1984.
28. Manne V, Bekesi E, Kung H-F: Proc Natl Acad Sci USA 82:376, 1985.
29. Yoakum GH, Lechner JF, Gabrielson EW, Korba BE, Malan-Shibley L, Willey JC, Valerio MG, Shamsuddin AM, Trump BF, Harris CC: Science 227:1174, 1985.
30. Land H, Parada LF, Weinberg RA: Science 222:771, 1983.
31. Minna J: Paper presented at UCLA Symposium on Biochemical and Molecular Epidemiology of Cancer.
32. Bonner TI, O'Brien SJ, Nash WG, Rapp UR, Morton CC, Leder P: Science 223:71, 1984.
33. Mark GE, Seeley TW, Shows TB, Mountz JD: Submitted for publication.
34. Graham FL, van der Eb AJ: Virology 52:456, 1973.
35. Yoakum GH, Korba BE, Lechner JF, Tokiwa T, Gazdar AF, Seeley T, Siegel M, Leeman L, Autrup H, Harris CC: Science 222:385, 1983.
36. Nakano H, Yamamoto F, Neville C, Evans D, Mizuno T, Perucho M: Proc Natl Acad Sci USA 81:71, 1984.
37. Perucho M, Goldfarb M, Shimiza K, Lama C, Fogh J, Wigler M: Cell 27:467, 1981.
38. Yuasa Y, Srivastana SK, Dunn CY, Rhim JS, Reddy EP, Aaronson SA: Nature 303:775, 1983.
39. Spandidos DA, Wilkie NM: Nature 310:469, 1984.
40. Shih TY, Papageorge AG, Stokes PE, Weeks MO, Scolnick EM: Nature 287:686, 1980.
41. Furth ME, Davis LJ, Fleurdelys B, Scolnick EM: Virology 43:294, 1982.
42. Ellis RW, DeFeo D, Maryak JM, Young HA, Shih TY, Chang EM, Lowy DR, Scolnick EM: J Virol 36:408, 1980.
43. Thorgeirsson UP, Turpeenniemi-Hujanen T, Williams JE, Westin EH, Heilman CA, Talmadge JE, Liotta LA: Mol Cell Biol 5:259, 1985.
44. Bernstein SC, Weinberg RA: Proc Natl Acad Sci USA 82:1726, 1985.
45. Kawamura H, Strickland JE, Yuspa SH: Cancer Res 45:2748, 1985.
46. Scott RE, Maercklein PB: Proc Natl Acad Sci USA 82:2995, 1985.

Biochemical and Molecular Epidemiology of Cancer 227–231 (1986)

Epidemiology of Primary Liver Cancer

Richard H. Decker and Mary C. Kuhns

Hepatitis Research, Diagnostics Division, Abbott Laboratories, North Chicago, Illinois 60064

Cancer of the liver is the seventh most common cancer worldwide, with an incidence somewhat less than one-half that of esophageal and lung cancer. However, in certain parts of the world it is the most common cancer. A major focus of attention on the etiology of primary hepatocellular carcinoma (HCC) has been directed to the relationship of chronic hepatitis B to HCC because of a convincing body of epidemiologic evidence that connects the two diseases. It should be pointed out that there is evidence that other environmental factors and probably host factors play a part in HCC, particularly in those areas of the world that have low endemicity of HBV, but it is clear that the majority of cases of HCC worldwide have some association with HBV.

It was first postulated in the 1950s that viral hepatitis could be the cause of HCC [1,2], but until the late 1960s it was not possible to test the hypothesis directly. Upon the discovery of the hepatitis B antigen and the development of better tests for it and other markers of HBV [3], numerous studies were initiated that have provided strong evidence of a causal association of HBV and liver cancer. Epidemiologic data have supported two additional lines of evidence for chronic HBV as a risk factor for liver cancer: 1) the evidence that similar hepadnaviruses cause both chronic hepatitis and HCC in at least two animals, the woodchuck (WHV) and the Peking duck (DHBV) [4]; and 2) biochemical evidence that hepatitis B viral DNA or parts of it at least are integrated into cellular genes of tumor cells and hepatocytes far more often in HBV carrier patients with HCC than in other control groups [5–8].

This discussion will deal only with the key epidemiologic data of HCC. There are three types of epidemiologic studies dealing with HBV and HCC: geographical data, case-control studies, and prospective studies.

GEOGRAPHICAL DATA

The estimate of there being around 200 million HBV carriers worldwide is generally accepted [9]. This is about 5% of the world's population. Approximately

Received July 15, 1985.

© **1986 Alan R. Liss, Inc.**

40% of the chronic carriers are infected at birth, when it has been shown that 90% of infected newborns become chronic carriers [10–13]. The incidence of virus carriership was illustrated by Szmuness [14], with the highest incidence of chronic HBV in Africa and Southeast Asia. These population centers also represent the population centers with the highest incidence rates of HCC. Alternately, the lowest rates of chronic hepatitis B worldwide are in the United States and western Europe, where there are low incidence rates of HCC. This correlation holds for areas with intermediate frequency of HBV carriers and intermediate incidence of HCC. There are exceptions to this geographical approach that need further exploration, but in general the overall correlation of incidence of HBV and incidence of HCC is good [15–17]. Sub-Saharan Africa and southeast Asia, with carrier rates exceeding 10%, also have the highest incidences of HCC, eg 99.3/100,000 males in Mozambique [18]. In areas with intermediate carrier rates of 2–5% such as north Africa, the Middle East, and southern Europe or low carrier rates (0.2–0.5%) such as the United States and northern Europe, the incidence is intermediate and low, respectively. A low incidence is 0.9/100,000 males [19].

CASE-CONTROL STUDIES

Numerous case control studies have been generated over the past 12 years [14,15,17,18,20–22], and data are not consistent even in the same areas and following similar protocols. One explanation is apparent: Methods for testing HBV markers in the serum have been changing during this time. The aim of the case-control study is to compare the frequency of HBV carriers among liver cancer patients with frequency of carriers in appropriate control groups, and from these data to determine relative risks of carriers to acquire HCC. In the data presented in Table I, summarized from data from Szmuness [14], the incidence of chronic hepatitis B carriers among liver cancer patients from several regions of the world are compared with the incidence of carriers among controls in that area. The carrier incidence among cancer patients is higher than in control groups for all regions and generally correlates with occurrence of disease. Great Britain is an obvious exception, and the incidence of chronic hepatitis B in US patients with liver cancer is also lower than in other regions. Since these are also regions of low risk for chronic HBV, it could be theorized that HCC caused by alternate factors will emerge when the most prominent risk factor is less common in a region.

TABLE I. Frequency of HBsAg in HCC Patients and Controls*

	Percent positive for HBsAg	
Country	HCC	Controls
Greece	66.6	5.0
Great Britain	16.0	—
United States	26.0	0.0
Mozambique	62.0	14.7
Uganda	47.0	6.0
Senegal	64.1	13.0
Taiwan	90.0	15–20
Vietnam	82.0	8–20

*This table represents a summary of RIA data from Szmuness [14].

From these data, Szmuness calculated the relative risk of HB carriers for acquiring liver cancer, and from more complete data Munoz and Linsell [18] recently updated these figures. The estimated relative risk for carriers in high incidence regions of the world was found to be 10 or above, while the relative risks (RR) in areas like the United States and western Europe were as high as 68. RR values greater than 10 are taken to mean that the factor under consideration is probably a casual factor. For a point of comparison, cigarette smoking carries an RR of 20 for lung cancer. Not only is the association of chronic hepatitis B and HCC strong, but it is also specific. HBV has not been causally linked to any other cancers. It could be that HCC is the result of cirrhosis rather than chronic infection, because cirrhosis is often found in HCC-affected liver specimens at autopsy. However, patients with cirrhosis from causes other than HBV do not have a high risk of HCC, while patients with HBV-related HCC have a much higher risk [10,22–25]. Additionally, the association of HBV and liver cancer does not reflect a subsequent infection or particular susceptibility to HBV in patients who have liver cancer. We have previously noted that nearly half of HBV carriers acquire their infection at birth. This was followed up relative to subsequent HCC by Larouse et al [26], who investigated the etiology of HCC in 23 patients in Senegal, Africa. In Senegal hepatitis B is endemic and patients acquired HCC at a unusually early mean age of 32 years. Larouse et al tested the hepatitis B carrier status of the mothers of these patients and found that 71% were chronic carriers, compared to 14% of mothers of 28 matched control subjects of the same age groups and communities. These data are consistent with the premise that the patients acquired their HBV infection from their mothers at birth and that their HCC *followed* these infections.

Most of the case-control studies have made the epidemiologic correlation between HCC and the hepatitis B carrier state (eg, chronic serum HBsAg) rather than with acute hepatitis B infection followed by recovery, and most findings suggest that the presence of antibodies to HBV, indicative of prior exposure and recovery, do not carry a significant RR, even though integration of the viral genome into hepatocyte DNA can occur in acute hepatitis B with recovery. Recently, however, Brechot et al [27] tested liver specimens of 20 HBsAg-negative patients with HCC for the presence of HBV DNA by blot hybridization and reported the presence of HBV DNA sequences in all 20 of the patient specimens.

PROSPECTIVE STUDIES

Perhaps the most persuasive epidemologic studies relative to chronic HBV and HCC are the prospective studies, which are very time consuming but are now beginning to bear fruit. Studies with Eskimos in Alaska, Chinese in Hong Kong and Singapore, Japanese in Tokyo, and Chinese in Taiwan and Peoples Republic of China have been initiated or have been ongoing for up to 10 years. Two such studies illustrate the data derived. Lu et al have studied a population in Qidong County, China, where the incidence of HCC is $50/10^5$/year, as reported by Sun and Chu [28]. Of a population of 14,694 enrolled, 17.4% were found to be carriers. Up to 5.5 years into the study there were 41 cases of HCC, with 33 of them among the carrier population, giving an incidence rate of $234.4/10^5$/year, compared to an incidence rate of 13.5 for the noncarrier group. Thus, the carrier incidence was 17.5 times the control group. The Taiwan data of Beasley and Hwang [24,25] represent the most completed prospective study with even stronger correlation results. This study, begun 10 years ago, enrolled nearly 23,000 government employees and has had a 95% follow-up. Data on 8 years of this study were recently described. This population, like the Qidong study, had a high HBV carrier incidence (15%) at recruitment, and the rate of development of HCC among the carriers was $526/10^5$/year, compared to only $2/10^5$/year among the control group. The risk of developing HCC among carriers in this study was a remarkable 220 times that among the control group.

Beasley and Hwang also calculated death by cause between carrier and control groups from the data of this study, and they found that in 8 years, over 50% of deaths in the carrier group were liver disease related and that one third the deaths were from HCC. From this, it can be expected that the cause of death by HCC in the carrier population would approach a rate of 50% before the subjects live long enough to begin to die of other age-related causes.

CONCLUSION

To date, the prospective studies have all dealt with populations endemic for HBV carriers and it remains to be determined if the correlations hold true for populations at lower risk for both hepatitis B and HCC. As the denominator (chronic hepatitis B) decreases, it is possible that the numerator (HCC) will contain proportionately more cases of non-B-related liver cancer, such that alternate or multifactoral relationships will emerge. It has already been found that geographical distribution of HCC and possible environmental exposure to aflatoxin appear to correlate more closely than do HBV and HCC [18, 28]. However, better data dealing with actual exposure to such potential carcinogens is difficult to acquire; efforts to generate methods for these data was reported by Dr. Sun and Dr. Groopman at the Proceedings meeting. Prince has used case-control data to calculate the incidences of HBV-related HCC and suggests that it may not be necessary to include environmental factors other than HBV to explain HCC [29]. Unfortunately, macroepidemiology is dependent data often outside of one or two investigators' control and includes variables that are quite intolerable to the laboratory scientist. Despite these limitations the epidemiologists have provided us with a great deal of knowledge of the etiology of liver cancer, in what must be considered among the classics of cancer epidemiology.

REFERENCES

1. Payet M, Camain R, Pene P: Rev Int Hepatol 4:1, 1956.
2. Steiner PE, Davies JN: Br J Cancer 11:523, 1957.
3. Blumberg BS, Gerstley BJ, Hungerford DA, London WT, Sutnick AI: Ann Intern Med 66:924, 1967.
4. Summers J: Hepatology 1:179, 1981.
5. Edman JC, Gray P, Valenzuela P, Rall LB, Rutter WJ: Nature 286:535, 1980.
6. Brechot C, Pourcel C, Louise A, Rain B, Tiollais P: Nature 286:533, 1980.
7. Chakraborty PR, Ruiz-Opazo N, Shouval D, Shafritz DA: Nature 286:531, 1980.
8. Marion PL, Salazar FH, Alexander JJ, Robinson WS: J Virol 33:795, 1980.
9. Arthur MJP, Hall AJ, Wright R: Lancet i: 607, 1984.
10. Beasley RP: Hepatology 2:21S, 1982.
11. Okada K, Kamiyama I, Inomata M, et al: N Engl J Med 294:746, 1976.
12. Beasley RP, Trepo C, Stevens CE, et al: Am J Epidemiol 105:94, 1977.
13. Beasley RP, Hwang LY, Stevens CE, et al: Hepatology 3:135, 1983.

14. Szmuness W: Prog Med Virol 24:40, 1978.
15. Beasley RP, Hwang LY: In Vyas GN, Dienstag JL, Hoofnagle JH (eds):"Viral Hepatitis and Liver Disease." Orlando FL: Grune and Stratton, 1984, pp 209–224.
16. Beasley RP, Lin CC, Chien CS, et al: Hepatology 2:553, 1982.
17. Beasley RP, Blumberg B, Popper H, et al: In Okuda K, MacKay I (eds):"Hepatocellular Carcinoma." Geneva: UICC Report Vol 17, 1982, p 60.
18. Munoz N, Linsell A: In Correa P, Haenszel W (eds):"Epidemiology of Cancer of the Digestive Tract." The Hague: Martinus Nijhoff, 1982 pp 161–165.
19. Doll R, Payne P, Waterhouse J (eds): "Cancer Incidence in Five Continents." Berlin: Springer, 1966.
20. Prince AM, Szmuness W, Michon J, et al: Int J Cancer 16:376, 1975.
21. Tong MJ, Sun SCM, Schaefer BT, et al: Ann Intern Med 75:687, 1971.
22. Tabor E, Gerety RJ, Voegel CL, et al: JNCI 58:1197, 1977.
23. Obata H, Hayashi N, Motoike Y, et al: Int J Cancer 25:741, 1980.
24. Beasley RP, Hwang LY, Lin CC: Lancet 2:1129, 1981.
25. Beasley RP, Hwang LY: Semin Liver Dis 4:113, 1984.
26. Larouze B, London WT, Saimot G, Werner B, Lustbadere ED, Payet M, Blumberg BS: Lancet 2:534, 1976.
27. Brechot C, Nalpas B, Courouce AM, et al: N Engl J Med 306:1384, 1982.
28. Sun T, Chu Y: J Cell Physiol (Suppl) 3:39, 1984.
29. Prince AM: In Vyas GN, Cohen S, Schmid R (eds): "Viral Hepatitis." Philadelphia: Franklin Institute Press, 1978, p 460.

Biochemical and Molecular Epidemiology of Cancer 233–256 (1986)

Aflatoxins as Risk Factors for Liver Cancer: An Application of Monoclonal Antibodies to Monitor Human Exposure

John D. Groopman, William F. Busby, Jr., Paul R. Donahue, and Gerald N. Wogan

Boston University School of Public Health, Environmental Health Section, Boston, Massachusetts 02118 (J.D.G.) and Massachusetts Institute of Technology, Department of Applied Biological Sciences, Cambridge, Massachusetts 02139 (W.F.B., P.R.D., G.N.W.)

Aflatoxins belong to a class of compounds known as mycotoxins, which are a group of chemically diverse secondary fungal metabolites that induce a variety of toxic responses in humans and animals when foods or feeds containing these compounds are ingested. Well over 100 structurally characterized mycotoxins are currently known, with newly identified compounds being added to this list at a rapid rate [1–3]. Most of these mycotoxins have not been implicated in any toxic syndromes in animals or people. Others, such as aflatoxin B_1 (AFB_1) and certain trichothecenes, have been implicated in highly lethal episodic outbreaks of mold poisoning in exposed human and animal populations. Several other mycotoxins have been directly identified in the human food supply [4], and many more toxins have been identified in laboratory cultures of molds, which had, in turn, been isolated from human foods from various parts of the world [1]. These mycotoxins have recently been comprehensively reviewed by Busby and Wogan [5].

Since the discovery of the aflatoxins in 1960, there has been an increasing concern about the possible health hazards engendered by the introduction of toxic, and possibly carcinogenic, compounds into foods by toxigenic molds. There is an enormous literature pertaining to various aspects of the aflatoxins that reflects upon their significant impact on human and animal health and the associated economic consequences. AFB_1 occupies a unique position among other chemical carcinogens. Its extreme potency as an animal toxin and hepatocarcinogen, its wide distribution in the human food supply, and its implication as a liver carcinogen in man have combined to stimulate a great deal of productive inquiry into its metabolism, its biochemical mode of action, and the procedures for monitoring human exposure. Comparable amounts of integrated information exist for few other carcinogens. Thus, results obtained in studies with AFB_1 have served not only as a guidepost for investigations

Received July 8, 1985.

© **1986 Alan R. Liss, Inc.**

with other environmental chemical carcinogens but also as a basis for fuller under-standing of the mechanisms underlying the phenomena associated with chemical carcinogens *per se*.

The aflatoxins were first discovered as a consequence of an epizootic outbreak in 1960 of a disease that resulted in the deaths of many thousands of young turkeys, ducks, and pheasants in eastern and southern England [6]. This disease, known as *turkey X disease*, was characterized by lethargy and loss of appetite, resulting in death within a week. Postmortem examination revealed extensive hepatic necrosis and hemorrhage, with frequent engorgement of the kidneys. Microscopic examination of the liver showed parenchymal degeneration and bile duct proliferation. A similar extensive outbreak of the disease occurred almost simultaneously in ducklings in Kenya and Uganda. Later, in 1960, pigs and calves were also affected [7].

Thorough veterinary examinations failed to uncover evidence of biological transmission of the disease in turkeys, and a microbiological or viral etiology was ruled out [6]. Attention was therefore turned to possible chemical contamination of the feed, although no significant amounts of any known toxin were detected. Because of the fact that over 80% of the reported cases occurred within 100 miles of London, it was soon established that affected flocks of birds had been fed meal produced by only a single mill from among a number of mills owned by the same company. The contaminant was further traced to a shipment of Brazilian peanut meal, when feed produced by a second mill of the company was suddenly implicated in additional cases of the disease. This meal, called *Rossetti* meal because of the name of the ship in which it was imported, proved to be highly toxic to chicks and ducklings [8–10] and eventually carcinogenic to rats [11]. Sargeant et al [9], although unsuccessful in isolating fungi from the sterile Rossetti meal, did isolate the common fungus *Aspergillus flavus* from a highly toxic sample of Ugandan peanuts. The cultured fungus produced a toxin that was eventually designated *aflatoxin* from the contraction of *A flavus toxin*.

The following areas will be briefly discussed in this review: 1) the occurrence of aflatoxins as natural food contaminants and their role in human liver cancer and acute aflatoxicosis; 2) the carcinogenicity of AFB_1 to experimental animals, with particular emphasis on primates; 3) aflatoxin chemistry and metabolism, including metabolic activation and DNA adduct formation; and 4) current methodologies using monoclonal antibodies to detect and quantitate aflatoxins and their metabolites, including DNA adducts, in human and animal samples.

HUMAN DISEASE AND AFLATOXIN EXPOSURE
Occurrence of Aflatoxins in Human Foods

Human populations can be exposed to aflatoxins by the consumption of com-modities that have been directly contaminated by toxigenic strains of *A flavus* and *A parasiticus* during growth, harvest, or storage. Secondary exposure may occur by the consumption of products such as meat and other edible tissues, milk and dairy products, and eggs derived from animals that have consumed aflatoxin-contaminated feeds.

In addition to factors that control or influence the growth of *A flavus* or *a parasiticus*, other variables can affect aflatoxin production in contaminated human foods. These include strain of the invading fungus, genetic susceptibility of the host plant (in the case of field contamination) and harvested commodity (in the case of storage contamination), chemical composition of the commodity, and stress factors (eg, drought conditions and insect damage) that increase the probability of fungal infections [12]. Thus virtually limitless possibilities exist for interaction between the various parameters affecting growth and aflatoxin production.

Since the requirements for aflatoxin production are relatively nonspecific, the molds can produce toxins on almost any foodstuff that will support growth. This is exemplified by the diverse types of commodities that become contaminated with aflatoxin. Nearly all agricultural commodities are potentially subject to contamination with aflatoxins when appropriate conditions are present during growth, harvest, or storage. It is important to note that obvious contamination of a commodity with *A flavus* or *A parasiticus* does not necessarily indicate the presence of aflatoxins, and the appearance of a sound, uninfected sample of commodity does not preclude the existence of significant quantities of aflatoxins.

Current guidelines for aflatoxin contamination of agricultural commodities in the United States is 20 μg total aflatoxins/kg (20 ppb), except for raw, shelled peanuts, which may contain 25 μg/kg [13]. The rationale for the higher limits set for raw peanuts was based on both the expectancy of a reduction in aflatoxin content following roasting and sorting (at which point the 20 μg/kg limit would be in effect) and a compromise reached to ensure the voluntary cooperation by peanut shellers. Although a tolerance level of 15 μg/kg for consumer peanut products in the United States has been proposed, no final action has yet been taken. The US Food and Drug Administration (FDA) has also set a practical action guideline of 0.5 μg AFB_1/liter (0.5 ppb) for fluid milk.

The regulatory control of aflatoxin in human foods and animal feeds in other countries as of 1976 has been summarized by Stoloff [14]. At that time, 18 countries regulated aflatoxin levels with the emphasis on peanuts and peanut products. Generally, acceptance limits for human foods ranged from the limits of analytical sensitivity up to 50 μg AFB_1/kg (50 ppb AFB_1).

Human Liver Cancer

Aflatoxins are among the few chemically identified and widely disseminated environmental carcinogens for which quantitative estimates of human exposure have been systematically sought. Despite the fact that significant differences in responsiveness are known to exist among animal species [5], it is reasonable to assume that man might respond to either acute or chronic effects of the toxins whenever exposure takes place through contamination of dietary components. It also seems reasonable to assume that the character and intensity of the human response might vary depending on factors such as age, sex, nutritional status, concurrent exposure to other agents (eg, viral hepatitis or parasitic infestation), as well as the level and duration of exposure to aflatoxins.

As information has accumulated on various aspects of the aflatoxin problem, it has become apparent that the risk of exposure to aflatoxins is much less in technologically developed countries than in developing ones. Reduced exposure is attributable to the combined effects of several factors contributing to the prevention of contamination of foods or food-raw materials, such as rapid postharvest drying of crops and controlled storage conditions. Although data on the occurrence of aflatoxins in foods have indicated the widespread geographic nature of the problem, little quantitative information on human exposure has been obtained because the samples were randomly collected and few actual intake studies were performed.

Primary liver cancer is not a prevalent form of cancer in Western countries; however, there are certain geographical areas of the world where the incidence is significantly elevated, namely, Southeast Asia, China, southern India, and Sub-Saharan Africa [15,16]. These regions correspond for the most part to climates where temperature and humidity would favor mold contamination of human foodstuffs. This correlation is not perfect, since other tropical regions, such as parts of South America, for example, are not characterized by high rates of liver cancer.

Several epidemiological studies were designed to obtain information on the relationship of estimated dietary intake of aflatoxin to the incidence of primary human liver cancer in different parts of the world. Information is now available from Uganda [17,18], the Philippines [19], Swaziland [20], Kenya [21], Thailand [22,23], and Mozambique [24], which had the highest incidence of human liver cancer in the world at the time of these studies and an estimated daily per capita consumption several times greater than the next highest intake regions in Thailand and Swaziland [16].

Summary data from four of these studies are presented in Table I, which contains information on aflatoxin ingestion and liver cancer incidence arranged in order of incresing value for each parameter. It can be seen that aflatoxin ingestion varied over a range of values from 3 to 222 ng/kg body weight per day. Estimated liver cancer incidence values extended from a minimum of 2.0 to a maximum of 35.0 cases/100,000 population per year. There was a positive association between the two parameters in that high intakes of aflatoxin were consistently associated with high incidence rates. The association was most apparent in connection with incidence rates

TABLE I. Aflatoxin Ingestion and Liver Cancer Incidence in Humans*

	Dietary aflatoxin intake (ng/kg of body weight/d)	Cases of liver cancer in adults (> 15 years old)			
		Men		Women	
Population		No./100,000 population/year	Incidence	No./100,000 population/year	Incidence
Kenya					
High altitude	3–5	1	3.1	0	0
Medium altitude	6–8	13	10.8	6	3.3
Low altitude	10–15	16	12.9	9	5.4
Swaziland					
Highveld	5–9	9	7.0	2	1.4
Middleveld	9–14	24	14.8	5	2.2
Lebombo	15–20	4	18.7	0	0
Lowveld	43–53	35	26.7	7	5.6
Thailand[a]					
Songkhala	5–8	—	—	—	—
Ratburi	45–77	—	—	—	—
Mozambique[b]	222	—	35.0	—	15.7

*Data were compiled for 1 year in Thailand, 3 years in Mozambique, and 4 years in Kenya and Swaziland.
[a]Statistics for the total population were cases per 100,000 population with an incidence of 6.0. In Ratburi, Thailand, statistics for the total population were two cases per 100,000 population per year with an incidence of 2.0
[b]Incidence for the total population was 25.4 cases per 100,000 population per year.

for adult men, for which large numbers of cases were involved, consequently yielding more precise estimates of disease incidence. The incidence of liver cancer in these studies was a linear function of the log of dietary aflatoxin intake [25,26].

Taken together, these data provide strong circumstantial evidence of a putative causal relationship between aflatoxin ingestion and liver cancer incidence in humans. Although this evidence does not constitute proof that aflatoxins are the cause of liver cell carcinoma in man, these data, together with the extensive animal data on aflatoxin carcinogenicity, are sufficient to indicate that exposure to the carcinogen is associated with elevated risk of this form of cancer and therefore warrants continued investigations into effective means for monitoring and control of aflatoxin occurrence as food contaminants.

More detailed information on the possible role of aflatoxins in human liver carcinogenesis may be found in the reviews by Wogan [27], van Rensburg [28], and Shank [15,25].

Within the past 10 years a very strong correlation has also been established between human primary liver cancer and hepatitis B virus (HBV) infection. Areas of high prevalence of HBV in Africa and Asia also coincide with areas where aflatoxin contamination of the human food supply is also elevated. Thus two plausible, perhaps interactive, etiologic factors for induction of liver cancer in humans have been identified.

Several lines of evidence have converged to indicate that liver cancer (hepatocellular carcinoma [HCC]) and active or chronic HBV infection are causally related [29–30], although there is no association between HCC and previous HBV infection [30]. The presence of antibodies to the hepatitis B surface antigen (HBsAg) in serum was used to establish geographic and regional relationships between HCC and HBV in Southeast Asia and China, India and Sub-Saharan Africa [30,31]. Exceptions to the association exist, however, in that HCC is uncommon and HBV prevalent in Egypt and Greenland [30], although the quality of the Greenland data has been questioned [32].

Lines of evidence to support the putative causal link between HCC and HBV can be summarized as follows: 1) the demonstration of family clusters of HCC and HBV where there is strong indication that HBV is vertically transmitted to the offspring from a maternal carrier in an infectious state [29,32]; 2) the demonstration of HBV marker proteins in the nontumorous portion of the liver in HCC patients [29–31]; 3) putative precancerous changes (liver cell dysplasia) in patients with chronic HBV infection [30]; and 4) the demonstrated integration of HBV DNA into liver cell DNA from patients with HCC [33–36].

Complete elucidation of the pathogenesis of human HCC must, however, take into account several points [30]. First, chronic HBV infection is not the sole etiologic factor in HCC, since some cases are not related to HBV. Second, chronic HBV infection is, by itself, not sufficient to cause HCC, since only a fraction of the individuals infected ever go on to develop HCC. Thus, other factors including individual susceptibility, general health, immunologic competence, and aflatoxin exposure are possibly important determinants in the developments of HCC. Clearly these developments have indicated the need for additional investigations into the interrelationships of aflatoxin, HBV infections, and HCC.

Acute Aflatoxicosis

Data confirming clinical indications of acute aflatoxicosis in humans have been sparse, although there is substantial evidence for aflatoxin consumption by selected populations [15,25]. For example, Campbell et al [37] detected aflatoxin M_1 (AFM_1), a hydroxylated metabolite of AFB_1, in the urine of Filipinos ingesting peanut butter heavily contaminated with approximately 500 μg AFB_1/kg. It was estimated that 1–4% of the ingested aflatoxin was excreted as this metabolite.

Suggestive evidence of acute aflatoxicosis has been reported from Taiwan and Uganda [15,25]. The syndrome was characterized by vomiting, abdominal pain, pulmonary edema, and fatty infiltration and necrosis of the liver. More extensive documentation of an outbreak of putative aflatoxin poisoning was provided from western India in 1974 [15,28]. Unseasonal rains and scarcity of food prompted the consumption of heavily molded corn (five specimens analyzed contained 6–16 mg aflatoxin/kg corn) by people in over 200 villages. Of the nearly 400 patients examined there were over 100 fatalities, with death in most instances caused by gastrointestinal hemorrhage. The illness was not infectious and occurred only in households where the contaminated corn was consumed. Histopathology of liver specimens revealed extensive bile duct proliferation, a lesion often noted in experimental animals after acute aflatoxin exposure. However, the possibility of the concurrent presence of other mycotoxins was not evaluated; therefore, multiple etiology cannot be ruled out.

There is strong evidence that a disease of children in Thailand, with symptoms identical to those of Reye syndrome, was associated with aflatoxicosis [15,25]. The disease was characterized by vomiting, convulsions, coma, and death, with cerebral edema and fatty involvement of the liver, kidney, and heart noted at autopsy. Aflatoxin poisoning was suggested as a possible cause since the symptoms of Reye syndrome in humans closely approximated those observed with acute aflatoxicosis in monkeys. In one case, consumption of aflatoxin-contaminated rice in a Thai household was apparently associated with a Reye syndrome fatality. Later studies showed that this rice sample was also contaminated with other toxigenic *Aspergillus* species, one of which (*A clavatus*) produced the edema-inducing toxin cytochalasin E and two tremorgens. In subsequent investigations Shank et al [38] demonstrated AFB_1 in the liver, brain, kidney, bile, and gastrointestinal tract contents of 22 out of 23 Thai fatalities. In seven of these cases AFB_1 content was substantially elevated relative to the low levels of AFB_1 detected in 10 out of 15 patients dying from other causes.

It should be noted that aflatoxin residues have not been associated with incidences of Reye syndrome in the United States, where a viral etiology is suspected [25]. Despite an initial report in which AFB_1 was detected at the parts per trillion level in the blood and/or liver of seven Reye syndrome patients in the southern United States [39], a follow-up study from the same laboratory showed that AFB_1 also occurred in the serum and urine from control subjects not suffering from the disease [40]. Therefore, no significant difference was observed between the two populations. However, since aflatoxin was detectable in over 20% of the samples, recent ingestion of contaminated food was indicated. Food preference questionnaires suggested a link between consumption of cornmeal and corn break and the appearance of aflatoxin in the subjects.

CARCINOGENESIS IN EXPERIMENTAL ANIMALS

AFB_1 has been shown to be a potent carcinogen in many species of animals, including rodents, nonhuman primates, and fish [5]. Generally, the liver was the primary target organ affected, where the toxin induced a high incidence of hepatocellular carcinomas and lower incidences of other tumor types. Under appropriate circumstances, dependent on such variables as animal species and strain, dose, route of administration, and dietary factors, significant incidences of tumors have been induced at sites other than the liver.

Most of the published information on AFB_1 carcinogenicity has been obtained from studies in rats, which are highly susceptible to the toxin. There has, however, been an increasing literature in recent years dealing with the carcinogenic responses of the rainbow trout (an even more sensitive species than the rat) and the monkey (possibly a more appropriate model for human risk estimation). Such experiments have often examined dose-response characteristics and the influences of such parameters as route of administration, size and frequency of dose, and the sex, age, and strain of the test animal. Effects of various modifying factors on carcinogenic responses have been evaluated, including diet, hormonal status, liver injury, microsomal enzyme activity, and concurrent exposure to other carcinogens. Several studies have examined the potency and structure-activity relationships of aflatoxin congeners, structural analogs, and metabolites as inducers of liver tumors.

AFB_1 has been demonstrated to induce liver tumors in two species of lower primates fed a diet containing 2 mg AFB_1/kg: the tree shrew (*Tupaia glis*) [41] and the marmoset (*Saguinus oedipomidas*) [42]. All liver tumors of the tree shrew were classified as hepatocellular carcinomas and developed in a manner similar to those of the rat [41,43]. Liver tumor incidence was 100% in surviving females (six of six) and 50% (three of six) in males [41]. Unlike the case with rats, in the marmoset histologic observation revealed the association of cirrhotic changes with liver tumor development [42].

Rhesus monkeys have also proven to be susceptible to AFB_1 carcinogenicity. In three reports on single animals, two cases of hepatocellular carcinoma [44,45] and one of cholangiocarcinoma [46] were observed in animals treated with AFB_1 for 5.5 to 6 years by an oral or a mixed oral and intramuscular dosing regimen. More recent data on 47 monkeys, representing three species (rhesus, cynomolgus, and African green) that had received AFB_1 by ip and/or po routes for periods greater than 2 months, have been published [47]. Primary liver tumor incidence was 19% (5/26) in animals surviving for longer than 6 months, and total tumor incidence in these animals was 50% (13/26). The five primary liver tumors included two hepatocellular carcinomas and three hemangioendothelial sarcomas. There were also six gall bladder or bile duct carcinomas, which in five cases extended to the liver parenchyma.

Extensive biological data indicate the high potency of AFB_1 as a toxin and carcinogen for a wide variety of animals species [5]. This information has provided the impetus for studies on metabolism and DNA adduct formation reactions of AFB_1 aimed at understanding the underlying molecular mechanisms of how this compound initiates these processes.

CHEMISTRY, METABOLISM, AND DNA ADDUCT FORMATION

The aflatoxins are highly substituted coumarins containing a fuse dihydrofurofuran moiety. The toxic principles were extracted and isolated from *A flavus* cultures by investigative groups in the United Kingdom and The Netherlands [48–50] and structurally identified by a group in the United States [51–53]. Four major aflatoxins were produced. Aflatoxins B_1 and B_2 (AFB_1 and AFB_2) were so designated because of their strong blue fluorescence under ultraviolet light, whereas aflatoxins G_1 and G_2 (AFG$_1$ and AFG$_2$) fluoresced greenish-yellow. As shown by the chemical structures in Figure 1, the B toxins were characterized by the fusion of a cyclopentenone ring to the lactone ring of the coumarin structure; the G toxins contained an additional fused lactone ring. AFB$_1$ and, to a lesser extent, AFG$_1$ were responsible for the biological potency of aflatoxin-contaminated meals and crude fractions derived from toxigenic *A flavus* cultures. These two toxins possessed an unsaturated bond at the 2,3 position (the 8,9 position according to the IUPAC nomenclature) on the terminal furan ring. The essentially inactive AFB$_2$ and AFG$_2$ were saturated at this position.

The aflatoxins are soluble in methanol, chloroform, and other organic solvents but are only sparingly soluble in water (10–30 μg/ml). The toxins strongly absorb ultraviolet light (362 nm), with extinction coefficients in methanol or ethanol varying from 17,100 for AFG$_2$ to 24,000 for AFB$_2$. Fluorescence emission occurs at 425 nm for AFB$_1$ and AFB$_2$ and at 450 nm for AFG$_1$ and AFG$_2$. Though aflatoxins are quite stable in foods and feeds, they are rapidly deactivated by extremes of pH (less than 3 or more than 10), oxidizing agents, or exposure to ultraviolet light in the presence of oxygen [14].

The aflatoxins are primarily metabolized in animals by the microsomal mixed function oxygenase system, a complex organization of cytochrome-coupled, O_2- and NADPH-dependent enzymes localized mainly on the endoplasmic reticulum of liver cells but also present in kidney, lungs, skin, and other organs. These enzymes catalyze the oxidative metabolism of AFB$_1$, resulting in the formation of various hydroxylated derivatives, as well as an unstable, highly reactive expoxide metabolite. Detoxification of AFB$_1$ is accomplished by enzymatic conjugation of the hydroxylated metabolites with sulfate or glucuronic acid to form water-soluble sulfate or glucuronide esters that are excreted in urine or bile. An alternative route for removal of AFB$_1$ from the organism involves the enzyme-catalyzed reaction of the epoxide metabolite with glutathione and its subsequent excretion in the bile. The known detoxification pathways of AFB$_1$ metabolism have been summarized in Figure 2.

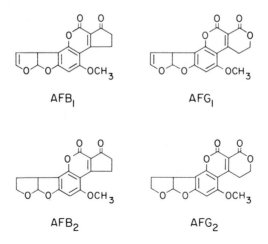

Fig. 1.   Structures of aflatoxins.

During the course of AFB_1 metabolism, the reactive electrophilic epoxide can covalently react with various nucleophilic centers in cellular macromolecules such as DNA, RNA, and protein. The consequences of this "activation" reaction may be opposite to those of detoxification and potentially pose a biological hazard to the cell or organism and constitute a putative mechanism by which many compounds, including AFB_1, exert toxic, carcinogenic, and genotoxic effects [54,55]. The pathways by which AFB_1 is metabolized into macromolecular-binding species have also been depicted in Figure 2. Comprehensive reviews of aflatoxin metabolism have been published by Busby and Wogan [5], Campbell and Hayes [56], and Shank [57], to which the reader is referred for further details.

The first AFB_1-DNA adduct was identified by Essigmann et al, [58] as 2,3-dihydro-2-(N^7-guanyl)-3-hydroxy-AFB_1 (AFB_1-N^7-Gua) (Fig. 3), the major product liberated from DNA modified in vitro with AFB_1 and a rat liver microsomal activation system. Its presence was subsequently confirmed in vivo [59,60]. The binding of AFB_1 residues to DNA in vivo was essentially a linear function of dose at a given time after treatment [59,61]. A modification level of 125–1,100 AFB_1 residues per 10^7 nucleotides was observed in rat liver 2 hr after ip dosing with 0.125–1.0 mg AFB_1/kg [59]. Similarly, rainbow trout embryo DNA was modified at much lower levels (one to six residues per 10^7 nucleotides) in direct proportion to AFB_1 concentration following incubation for 1 hr with 0.25–1.0 mg/liter AFB_1 [62]. Initial binding levels in DNA have been observed to drop rapidly within hours after AFB_1 treatment [63–65]. For example, maximum modification of rat liver DNA (1,250 residues per 10^7 nucleotides) was noted no later than 30 min after a 1 mg AFB_1/kg dose but declined to a level of 160 residues per 10^7 nucleotides 36 hr after treatment, giving an apparent half-life of AFB_1 binding to DNA of approximately 12 hr [61].

A number of other components, in addition to AFB_1 dihydrodiol (Fig. 3), were isolated from nucleic acid hydrolysates activated in vivo and in vitro with AFB_1. These adducts, designated I and IV by Lin et al [60], were apparently related to AFB_1-N^7-Gua by a precursor-product relationship. Thus, when AFB_1-N^7-Gua was treated under mildly alkaline conditions (pH 9.6), it was converted to these two other adducts. Furthermore, when both I and IV were subjected to additional acid hydrolysis, AFB_1 dihydrodiol was formed as the major product, along with small amounts of AFB_1-N^7-Gua. Low levels of I were detected when IV was hydrolyzed, and vice versa. On the basis of these results and spectral data, I was presumptively identified as 2,3-dihydro-2-(N^5-formyl-2,5,6-triamino-4-oxopyrimidin-N^5-yl)-3-hydroxy AFB_1 (AFB_1-FAPyr) (Fig. 3), a formamidopyrimidine derivative of AFB_1-N^7-Gua that contained an opened imidazole ring [60,66]. This proposed structure has recently been verified [66]. A ring-closed structure, 2,3-dihydro-2-(8,9-dihydro-8-hydroxy-guan-^{7}-yl)-3-hydroxy-AFB_1, was suggested for IV, although structural confirmation was not obtained [60]. Hertzog et al [66] have disputed this structure, proposing instead that IV is a ring-opened isomer of I (AFB_1-FAPyr).

At the present time, it appears that between 95 and 98% of the aflatoxin residues bound to DNA have been accounted for by chemical structure analysis. This work provides the chemical basis for producing monoclonal antibodies that recognize these DNA adducts so that the antibodies may be employed as highly specific probes for quantifying the occurrence of adducts as well as other products of AFB_1 metabolism in biological samples.

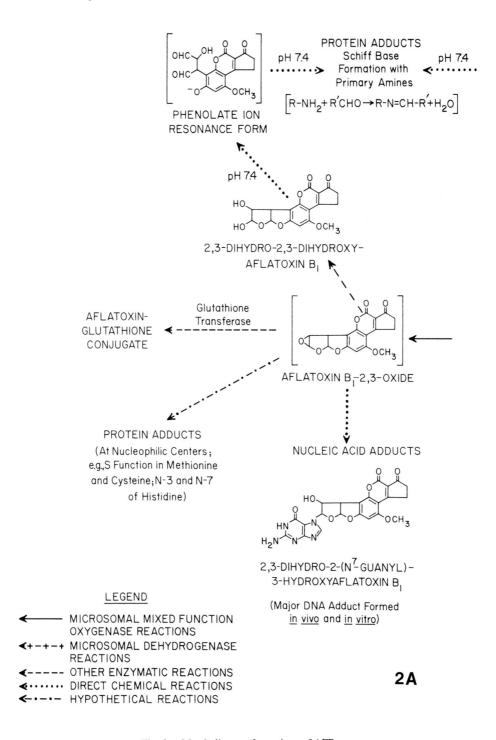

Fig. 2.   Metabolic transformations of AFB₁.

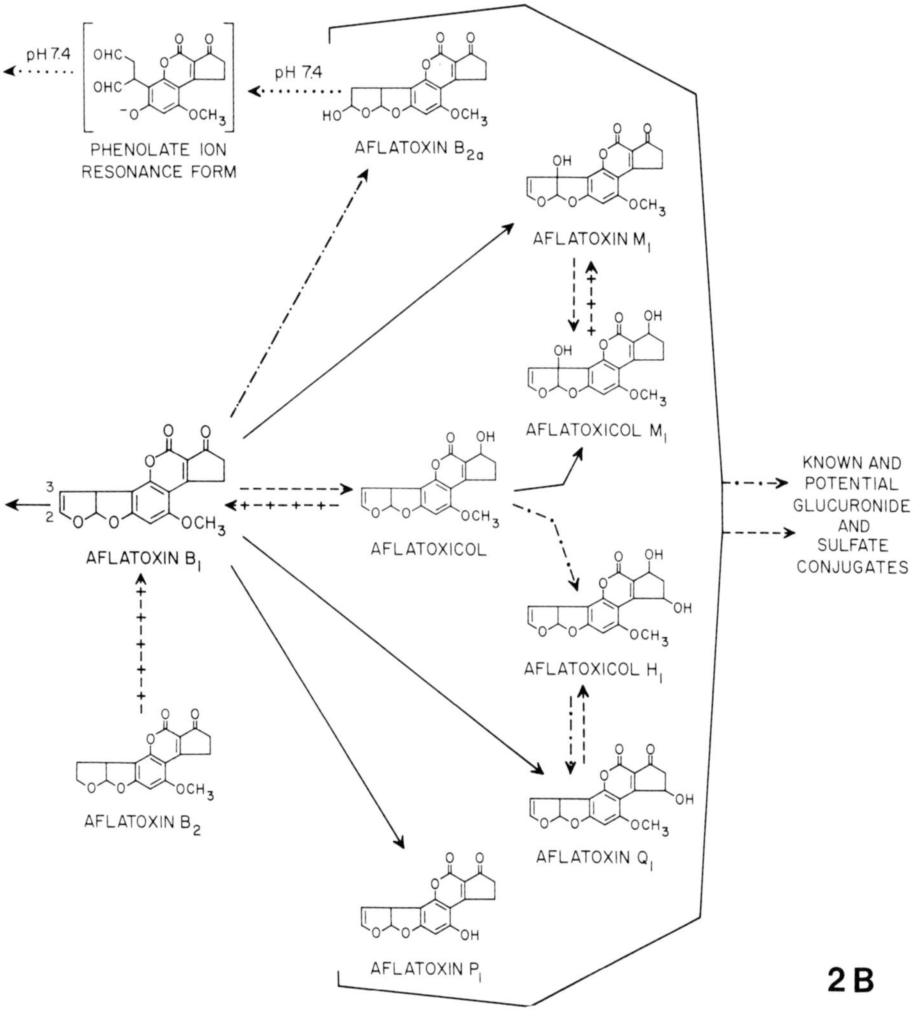

PHENOLATE ION
RESONANCE FORM

AFLATOXIN B$_{2a}$

AFLATOXIN M$_1$

AFLATOXICOL M$_1$

AFLATOXIN B$_1$

AFLATOXICOL

AFLATOXICOL H$_1$

KNOWN AND
POTENTIAL
GLUCURONIDE
AND
SULFATE
CONJUGATES

AFLATOXIN B$_2$

AFLATOXIN Q$_1$

AFLATOXIN P$_1$

2 B

IMMUNOLOGICAL DETECTION

Monoclonal Antibodies That Recognize Aflatoxins

Over the last 6 years we have produced various monoclonal antibodies that recognize aflatoxins, using antigens ranging from aflatoxin-modified DNA to afla-toxin-adducted proteins. These antibodies are being used in conjunction with such chemical analytic techniques as noninvasive screening methodologies to monitor human exposure to these environmentally occurring mycotoxins. These methods depend on the ability to quantify aflatoxin and its metabolites, including DNA adducts, in readily accessible compartments, such as serum and urine.

Earlier, we reported a chemical protocol to quantify AFB$_1$-N^7-Gua in urine [67] based on the isolation of AFB$_1$-DNA adducts from human urine by preparative and analytical liquid chromatography. A radiometric labeling technique using ^{3}H-dimethyl sulfate was used to tag the AFB$_1$-N^7-Gua at the 7 position of the guanine moiety. This

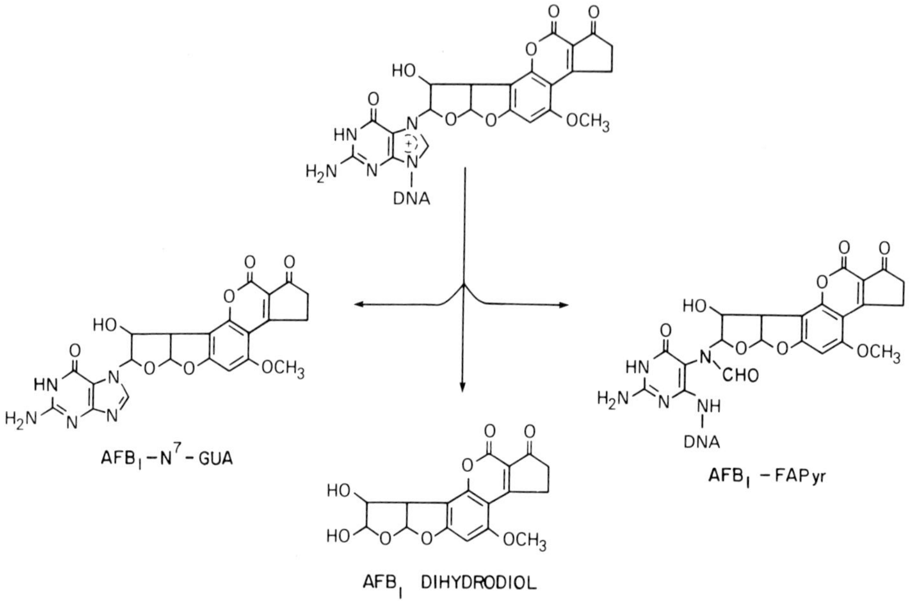

Fig. 3.   AFB$_1$-DNA adducts.

postlabeling technique is specific for the AFB$_1$-N^7-Gua adduct, and in vitro we obtained a limit of detectability in spiked samples of 1 pg AFB$_1$-N^7-Gua/ml urine. However, when we attempted to apply these methods to in vivo urine samples, nonspecific interfering materials often prevented the attainment of this level of sensitivity. Therefore, we have combined chemical analytic and radiometric procedures with a monoclonal antibody-affinity chromatography column both to purify the aflatoxin adducts and metabolites from urine and to confirm their identity.

The goal of developing a reusable monoclonal antibody-affinity chromatographic column for rapid isolation of aflatoxin metabolites and their adducts from human urine and serum samples required the production of high affinity monoclonal antibodies that recognize aflatoxins. The initial endeavors to produce aflatoxin-specific monoclonal antibodies culminated in the production of five antibodies, which were obtained after fusion of mouse P3 × 63 myeloma cells with spleen cells isolated from BALB/c mice that had been immunized with AFB$_1$-adducted DNA complexed with methylated bovine serum albumin. Selected hybridomas were found to produce monoclonal antibodies specific for modified DNA containing both AFB$_1$-N^7-Gua and AFB$_1$-FAPyr, suggesting that these DNA adducts share a common antigenic determinant. These antibodies recognized AFB$_1$-adducted DNA in a competitive ELISA (using USERIA methodology) with a limit of detectability as low as one AFB$_1$ residue per 1,355,000 nucleotides [68,69].

Monoclonal antibody 1-A-2 from these initial hybridomas is two to three times more sensitive than 1-B-2 in detecting AFB$_1$-DNA adducts. The USERIA with 1-A-2 is eightfold more sensitive at 50% inhibition than ELISA (250 fmol vs 2,000 fmol AFB$_1$ bound to DNA) compared with 1-B-2 (Figs. 4, 5). Antibodies 1-D-2, 1-E-2,

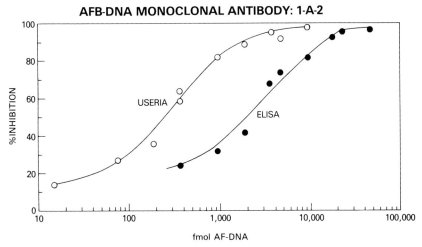

Fig. 4. Competitive inhibition curves for Mab 1-A-2.

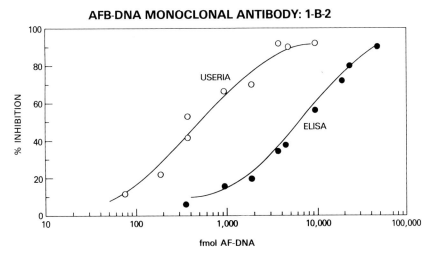

Fig. 5. Competitive inhibition curves for Mab 1-B-2.

and 1-F-2 were tested only with ELISA and were found to have 50% inhibition values similar to 1-B-2 (range 5,000–12,000 fmol AFB_1 adducted to DNA).

Monoclonal antibodies 1-A-2 and 1-B-2 were further characterized for isotype and antigen specificity. Both 1-A-2 and 1-B-2 were determined to be of mouse IgG1 isotype. Experiments were perfomred to ascertain if they were specific for the major AFB_1-guanine adducts AFB_1-N^7-Gua and AFB_1-FAPyr and to measure their cross-reactivity to other aflatoxin congeners and oxidative metabolites of AFB_1. These monoclonal antibodies apparently recognize only AFB_1 bound to DNA, since the following concentrations of compounds resulted in less than 2% inhibition in a competitive ELISA: 11,000 pmol AFB_1; 530 pmol AFB_2; 32,000 pmol aflatoxin $P_1(AFP_1)$; 5,100 pmol aflatoxin M_1 (AFM_1); 10,000 pmol aflatoxin B_{2a} (AFB_{2a}); 260 pmol aflatoxin G_1 (AFG_1); 2,000 pmol AFB_1 dihydrodiol (AF-Diol); 2,100 pmol

AFB$_1$-N^7-Gua; and 2,100 pmol AFB$_1$-FAPyr. Finally, it was determined that neither 1-A-2 nor 1-B-2 recognized 5.5 pmol of benzo[a]pyrene metabolite bound to DNA at a level of 1.24 adducts per 100 nucleotides. These data support the hypothesis that these monoclonal antibodies have an epitope for an altered conformation in DNA resulting only from the covalent binding of AFB$_1$.

Antibodies 1-A-2 and 1-B-2 were used for the quantification of rat liver DNA modified with AFB$_1$ in vivo. ^{3}H-AFB, was administered to rats at dosages ranging from 0.01 to 1.0 mg AFB$_1$/kg to represent subacute exposure levels [5] and the adducted DNA was isolated from liver 2 hr later. The AFB$_1$ residue per 35,000, 251,000, and 1,355,000 nucleotides and HPLC analysis of these nucleic acids revealed that 75–80% of the adducts bound were chromatographically identical to the AFB$_1$-N^7-Gua adduct. The nucleic acids were treated with 0.1 N KOH (at 37°C for 10 min) to convert quantitatively the AFB$_1$-N^7-Gua adducts to the AFB$_1$-FAPyr derivative. Representative results of inhibition experiments using the USERIA and monoclonal antibody 1-A-2 are shown in Figure 6. The 50% inhibition level using in vivo-modified DNA was 350 fmol AFB$_1$ bound to DNA compared with 250 fmol AFB$_1$ bound for in vitro-modified DNA. This discrepancy is attributed to the necessity of applying 3–90 μg of in vivo-modified DNA to the microwells compared with 5 ng of in vitro-adducted DNA for these competition analyses. Therefore, monoclonal antibodies directed toward AFB$_1$-modified DNA can be used to quantitate AFB$_1$ bound in vivo in rat liver to DNA at levels as low as one AFB$_1$ residue per 1,355,000 nucleotides. A major disadvantage of these initial antibodies was the lack of cross-reactivity with other aflatoxin congeners and metabolites also expected to be found in environmental samples.

Since the initial antibodies produced from animals immunized with AFB$_1$-modified DNA did not cross react with other aflatoxin derivatives, attempts to produce high affinity monoclonal antibodies with the desired range of reactivity were continued. Female BALB/By CJ mice were immunized with AFB$_1$-adducted bovine γ globulin (BGG) in complete Freund's adjuvant [70]. Seven of the 10 mice injected were found to produce significant anti-AFB$_1$ serum titers as measured by noncompetitive ELISA. Spleen cells from five of these mice were fused with SP-2 myeloma cells, and a number of monoclonal antibodies, grown as ascites fluid, were obtained.

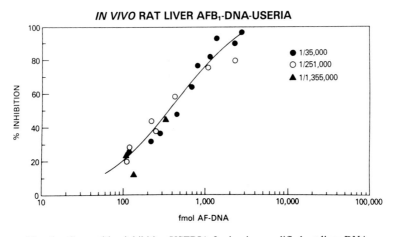

Fig. 6.   Competitive inhibition USERIA for in vivo-modified rat liver DNA.

One of these antibodies (2B11) proved to be a high affinity IgM (2B11) with many of the desired properties.

A value for the affinity constant of 2B11 determined from data obtained by competitive RIA was 1×10^9 liters/mole, using the method described by Muller [71]. The specificities of 2B11 in the competitive RIA for AFB_1 and its metabolites, including the major aflatoxin B_1-DNA adducts(AFB_1-N^7-Gua and AFB_1-FAPyr), are depicted in Figures 7 and 8. The 50% inhibition levels for AFB_1, AFB_2, and AFM_1 were found to be 3.0 pmol (1 ng), whereas those for AFG_1, AFG_2, and aflatoxin Q^1 (AFQ_1) were 60.0, 84.0, and 275.0 pmol, respectively. These data clearly indicate that the epitope for 2B11 recognition of aflatoxin lies in the coumarin ring and the cyclopentenone ring of the aflatoxin molecule.

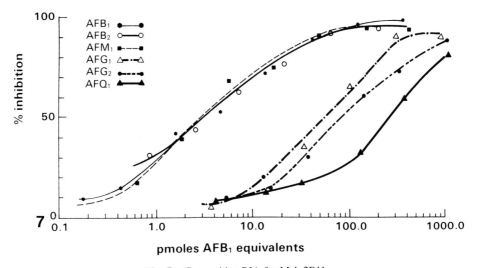

Fig. 7. Competitive RIA for Mab 2B11.

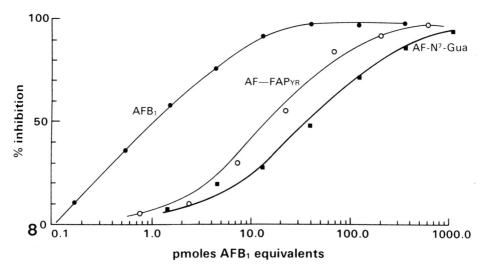

Fig. 8. Competitive RIA for Mab 2B11 and DNA adducts.

Figure 8 depicts the specificity and 50% inhibition values in the competitive RIA of 2B11 for AFB_1 (3.0 pmol) and the two major aflatoxin-DNA adducts AFB_1-FAPyr (24.0 pmol) and AFB_1-N^7-Gua (89.0 pmol). Based on the data in Figure 7, high recognition by the antibody was expected for the two aflatoxin-DNA adducts. In addition, data in Figure 8 indicate that the antibody is about four times more sensitive in detecting the AFB_1-FAByr adduct than the AFB_1-N^7-Gua adduct (24.0 pmol versus 89.0 pmol). This finding was unanticipated, since the aflatoxin moiety is identical in these adducts and the parent molecule. These observations suggest that the epitope for the antibody may be partially obstructed in adducts because of the stereochemistry of covalent binding of aflatoxin to guanine. Experiments (data not shown) using AFB_1-modified DNA and BSA in the competitive RIA determined that the 50% inhibition levels for these macromolecularly-bound aflatoxins were 10.0 and 12.0 pmol in a 300 μl assay, respectively. The similarity of these results with AFB_1 bound to either DNA or protein tend to support the suggestion that the epitope recongized by the monoclonal antibody may become sterically hindered when AFB_1 is coupled to a larger molecule.

Solid Phase Chromatography Using IgM Monoclonal Antibody 2B11

Efforts were initiated to produce a preparative monoclonal antibody affinity column to isolate aflatoxins from complex biological fluids. Ascites fluid containing antibody 2B11 was initially fractionated by precipitation with saturated ammonium sulfate followed by dialysis against PBS. The antibody was further purified by HPLC in a steric exclusion (molecular weight separation) chromatographic mode, which was employed to take advantage of the high molecular weight (MW 900,000) of the IgM in purification of the antibody. The purified antibody, having been assayed for activity by noncompetitive RIA, was bound to a solid phase matrix of Sepharose 4B. The columns made for these experiments contained 1 mg of antibody per millimeter of column volume.

Initial experiments were performed to determine the ability of the antibody column to bind ^{3}H-AFB_1. In these studies the concentration of ^{3}H-AFB_1 was 1 ng (3 pmol) in 10 ml phosphate-buffered saline (PBS), pH 7.4. A level that would approximate concentrations expected in body fluids of people exposed to contaminated foods. When the sample containing the ^{3}H-AFB_1 was applied to the column, about 10% of the radioactivity washed through in the loading and PBS wash phase. This loss was attributable to tritium exchange and was independently verified by other analytic procedure. The column was then washed with 2 M potassium thiocyanate, a commonly used elution buffer for antibody affinity chromatography, and less than 2% of the applied ^{3}H-AFB_1 was eluted. Sequential washes with phosphate buffer, pH 3.0; diethanolamine buffer, pH 9.9; and phosphate buffer, pH 2.0, removed less than 1% of the applied ^{3}H-AFB_1. However, quantitative elution of the bound ^{3}H-AFB_1 was achieved using 50% dimethylsulfoxide (DMSO) in phosphate buffer, pH 7.4 (50% DMSO buffer). The antibody column was regenerated by washing the column with PBS, pH 7.4, and to date we have used and regenerated this column more than 150 times with no apparent loss of activity.

To determine the optimal DMSO concentration for elution of AFB_1, the affinity column, prewashed as indicated, was eluted sequentially with 1, 5, 10, 20, 30, and

40% DMSO-PBS. A total loss of less than 4% of the applied AFB_1 was eluted by these DMSO solutions, and quantitative recovery was obtained only with 50% DMSO. Similar results were also obtained with solutions of dimethylformamide (DMF) in PBS. These properties emphasize the potential of this column for use as a preparative tool in recovery of aflatoxins from complex biological mixtures.

The capacity of the antibody affinity column to bind AFB_1 was determined by radiometric and absorbance techniques and was found to bind 1–1.3 μg of AFB_1 from 10 ml of PBS per 1 ml of column bed volume.

Isolation of AFB_1 previously added to human urine, serum, and milk was performed to test the applicability of the column to biological samples. Freshly collected human urine (10 ml) was centrifuged or filtered through a 0.45 μm filter and spiked with 1 ng ^{3}H-AFB_1. When urine was applied directly to the affinity column, 60% of the applied AFB_1 failed to bind to the column. However, by employing the protocol outlined in Figure 9, we were able to obtain quantitative binding of the ^{3}H-AFB_1 to the column and recovery in the 50% DMSO buffer. Thus, interfering materials in urine can be effectively removed by employing a preparative C18-Sep-Pak (Waters Associates, Milford, MA) stage in the isolation procedure. In previous studies, we have consistently found that 90–95% of aflatoxins applied to C18-Sep-Paks can be recovered [67].

Human serum (10 ml) or human milk (10 ml) spiked with ^{3}H-AFB_1 (1 ng) was also applied directly to the antibody column without prior treatment, and quantitative binding and recovery into 50% DMSO were observed in both instances. Unlike urine samples, a preparative step using the C18-Sep-Pak was not required for the quantitative recovery of the carcinogen from serum or milk.

Experiments were also performed to determine the recovery of ^{3}H-AFB_1-N^7-Gua (10 ng) spiked into PBS. In these experiments we found that quantitative recovery of the AFB_1-DNA adduct could also be achieved without any preparative clean-up step. Further studies are underway to determine the ability to recover these adducts from human serum and urine.

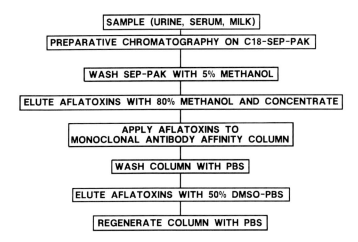

Fig. 9. Outline of aflatoxin isolation scheme.

Affinity Chromatography and HPLC Analysis of AFB$_1$-Treated Rat Urine

Urine samples from rats treated with ^{14}C-AFB$_1$ fractioned on the 2B11 monoclonal antibody affinity column were analyzed by competitive RIA, and the results were compared with the amount of aflatoxin determined from the radioactivity data. A precise correspondence (data not shown) was obtained, indicating that the majority of the aflatoxin derivatives in the rat urine would be recognized by the monoclonal antibody. These data also demonstrate that the competitive RIA has the requisite sensitivity to determine aflatoxin content in biological samples.

Two adult male Fisher 344 rats were each injected with 1 mg ^{14}C-AFB$_1$ per kilogram body weight and their urine collected for 20 hr, by which time 10–12% of the radiolabel had been excreted into the urine. Aliquots (100 μl) of each urine sample, containing 290 and 310 ng of ^{14}C-AFB$_1$ equivalents, respectively, were diluted with 1.9 ml of PBS and applied to the antibody affinity column, and 65% of the applied ^{14}C became bound to the affinity matrix. The eluate containing the initially unretained aflatoxin moieties was recycled back through the column, but this second passage failed to result in further binding. These data indicate that the unretained aflatoxins are not immunologically recognized by the antibody and thus are consistent with the specificity reported for this monoclonal antibody. The retained aflatoxins were eluted from the column with 50% DMSO-PBS and analyzed by analytic reversed-phase HPLC (Fig. 10) [72].

Representative HPLC chromatograms of the UV and the radioactivity aflatoxin profiles in the rat urine are found in Figures 11 and 12, respectively. The predominant metabolite was AFM$_1$, accounting for between 41 and 50% of the recovered ^{14}C. AFP$_1$ and AFB$_1$ were also detected but together account for less than 10% of the radioactivity and/or UV absorbance. The AFB$_1$-N^7-Gua adduct was a major metabolite and comprised 16% of the applied radioactivity. The level of AFB$_1$-N^7-Gua in the urine corresponded to the amount calculated from the pharmacokinetic data of Bennett et al [73]. The overall recovery of the radioactive aflatoxins applied to the HPLC column was greater than 95%. The unretained material from the affinity column (PBS washes) was analyzed by preparative HPLC procedures. All of the radiolabeled aflatoxin from this fraction chromatographed as unretained polar derivatives of AFB$_1$. These data show that the major metabolites isolated from urine of rats treated with AFB$_1$ are AFM$_1$, AFP$_1$, and AFB$_1$-N^7-Gua. It appears highly probable that by using other monoclonal antibodies with different specificities, the entire component of urinary aflatoxin derivatives, including the oxidative conjugates, could be quantitated.

Analysis of Human Urine from Individuals Exposed to AFB$_1$

People who had been exposed to AFB$_1$ from dietary sources were identified for a pilot study by collaborators of ours at the Institute of Health in Beijing, China [72]. Urine samples from those exposed were used to gain preliminary evidence of the applicability of the monoclonal antibody affinity column and HPLC analysis procedures for monitoring individuals for aflatoxin exposure. For this study, 20 individuals were selected, and the intake of AFB$_1$ from the diet on the previous day was calculated to be from 13.4 to 87.5 μg. Competitive RIA of the samples eluted from the monoclonal antibody column showed that the aflatoxin concentration in the collected urine was in the 0.1 to 10 ng/ml range. These data were calculated using a linear extrapolation of the RIA data. Further experiments need to be performed to verify

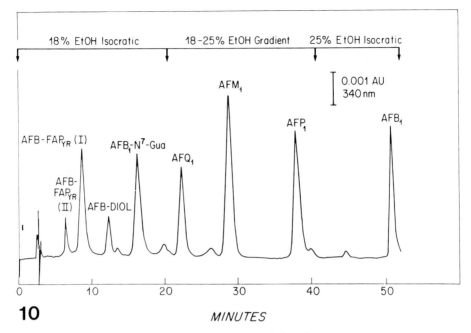

Fig. 10.   HPLC separation of aflatoxins.

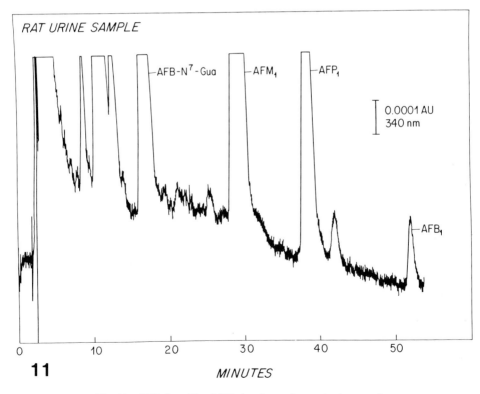

Fig. 11.   HPLC profile of UV absorbance from rat urine sample.

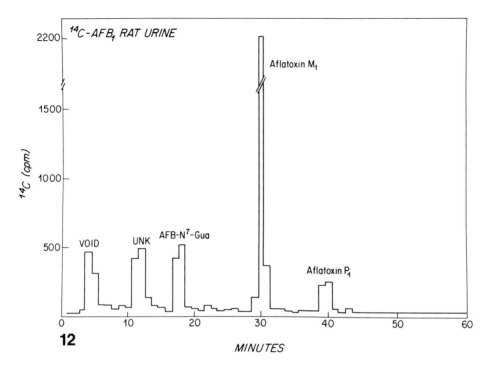

Fig. 12.   HPLC profile of radioactivity from rat urine sample.

that linear extrapolation is consistent with the pharmacokinetics of urinary aflatoxin excretion in humans. Therefore, these results should be interpreted as representing the range of aflatoxin content in these samples.

Urine samples from individuals who had been exposed to the highest dose (87.5 μg) the previous day were run on the antibody affinity column and then analyzed by analytic HPLC. An HPLC profile from one such sample is depicted in Figure 13, demonstrating the presence of the major AFB_1-DNA adduct AFB_1-N^7-Gua at levels representing between 7 and 10 ng of the adduct. These data indicate that the monoclonal antibody columns, coupled with HPLC, can quantify aflatoxin-DNA adducts in human urine samples obtained from environmentally exposed people in less than 1 hr.

Summary of Aflatoxin Monoclonal Antibody Research

We have been using monoclonal antibody technology to produce antibodies that recognize aflatoxins to develop noninvasive methodologies in conjunction with other chemical analytic techniques to monitor human exposure to environmentally occurring carcinogens. These methods require the ability to quantify aflatoxin and their metabolites, including DNA adducts, in readily accessible compartments such as serum and urine and to permit efficient analysis of many samples in a relatively short period of time.

Earlier literature reports have described techniques such as thin layer chromatography, high performance liquid chromatography, and immunological assays to prepare and analyze aflatoxin-containing samples for aflatoxin metabolites, including

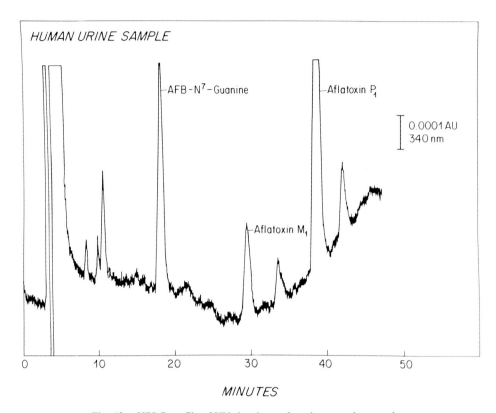

Fig. 13.   HPLC profile of UV absorbance from human urine sample.

DNA adducts. These methods have sufficient sensitivity to allow the measurement of AFM$_1$ and aflatoxin-DNA adducts in human urine [37,74]. However, the fundamental disadvantage of many of these procedures is the lengthy preparation time required before the sample can be submitted to analytic analysis. The new methods we have reported here are rapid enough (less than 1 hr) to be applied to large-scale epidemiologic studies for measurement of aflatoxin exposure in populations. Furthermore, these procedures permit the resolution and quantitation of individual aflatoxin congeners and metabolites. An example of this approach, discussed earlier, used a preparative monoclonal antibody affinity column in conjunction with HPLC to achieve the accurate and sensitive measurement of AFB$_1$-N^7-Gua in urine without nonspecific interference from other materials present in the sample that were found using a radiometric postlabeling technique [72].

The development of a reusable monoclonal antibody affinity chromatographic column first required the production of high affinity monoclonal antibodies that recognize aflatoxins, a task that culminated in the production of an antibody specific for AFB$_1$-adducted DNA. A competitive ELISA showed a limit of detectability of one AFB$_1$ residue per 1,355,000 nucleotides [68,69]. Since these antibodies did not cross react with the aflatoxin derivatives expected to be found in human urine and serum samples, attempts were continued to develop high affinity monoclonal antibodies with a wider range of selectivity. One antibody, an IgM (2B11), was found to have a particularly high affinity toward aflatoxins [70]. In the competitive RIA a 50% inhibition value of about 3 pmol is routinely obtained with this antibody, and there is a lower limit of detectability of approximately 300 fmol for AFB_1, AFB_2, and AFM_1. When this antibody is bound to a solid phase matrix, a reusable column can be prepared that selectively isolates aflatoxins from complex mixtures, such as urine, serum, and milk. These techniques have also been applied to experimental models and human samples, and data from these studies indicate the applicability of these procedures to population-based studies. Isolates from this column chromatographed by HPLC show very little contamination by nonaflatoxin derivatives. We have also recently produced monoclonal antibodies specific for AFM_1 and AFQ_1 and are in the process of producing a monoclonal antibody with higher affinity for the AFB_1-N^7-Gua adduct. By using these new antibodies, we hope to develop further the monoclonal antibody affinity chromatography procedures and subsequent immunologic analysis for quantifying these metabolites in human samples.

REFERENCES

1. Busby WF Jr., Wogan GN: In Riemann H, Bryan FL (eds): "Food-Borne Infections and Intoxications," 2nd ed. New York: Academic Press, 1979, pp 519–610.
2. Rodricks JV, Hesseltine CW, Mehlman MA (eds): "Mycotoxins in Human and Animal Health." Park Forest South, IL: Pathotox, 1977.
3. Shank RC (ed): "Mycotoxins and N-Nitroso Compounds: Environmental Risks." Boca Raton, FL: CRC, 1981, Vol 2.
4. Ciegler A, Burmeister HR, Vesonder RF, Hesseltine CW: In Shank RC (ed): "Mycotoxins and N-Nitroso Compounds: Environmental Risks." Boca Raton, FL: CRC, 1981, Vol 1, pp 1–50.
5. Busby WF, Wogan GN: In Searle CE (ed): "Aflatoxins in Chemical Carcinogens," 2nd ed. Washington, DC: American Chemical Society, 1985, pp 945–1136.
6. Goldblatt LA: In Goldblatt LA (ed): "Aflatoxin." New York: Academic Press, 1969, pp 1–11.
7. Allcroft R: In Goldblatt LA (ed): "Aflatoxin." New York: Academic Press, 1969, pp 237–264.
8. Asplin FD, Carnaghan RBA: Vet Rec 73:1215–1219, 1961.
9. Sargeant K, Sheridan A, O'Kelly J: Nature 192:1095–1096, 1969.
10. Sargeant K, Carnaghan RBA, Allcroft R: Chem Industry 53–55, 1963.
11. Lancaster MC, Jenkins FP, Philp J: Nature 192:1095–1096, 1961.
12. Ciegler A: Mycopathologia 65:5–11, 1978.
13. Stoloff L: J Assoc Off Anal Chem 63:1067–1073, 1980.
14. Stoloff L: In Rodricks JV, Hesseltine CW, Mehlman MA (eds): "Mycotoxins in Human and Animal Health." Park Forest South IL: Pathotox, 1977, pp 7–28.
15. Shank RC (ed): "Mycotoxins and N-Nitroso Compounds: Environmental Risks." Boca Raton, FL: CRC, 1981, pp 107–140.
16. Szmuness W: Prog Med Virol 24:40–69, 1978.
17. Alpert ME, Hutt MSR, Wogan GN, Davidson CS: Cancer 28:253–260, 1971.
18. Alpert ME, Hutt MSR, Davidson CS: The Lancet 1:1265–1267, 1968.
19. Campbell TC, Salamat L: In Purchase IFH (ed): "Mycotoxins in Human Health." New York, MacMillan, 1971, pp 271–280.
20. Peers FG, Gilman GA, Linsell CA: Int J Cancer 17:167–176, 1976.
21. Peers FG, Linsell CA, Br J Cancer 27:473–484, 1973.
22. Shank RC, Wogan GN, Gibson JB, Nondasuta A: Food Cosmet Toxicol 10:61–69, 1972.
23. Shank RC, Gordon JE, Wogan GN, Nondasuta A, Subhamani B: Food Cosmet Toxicol 10:71–84, 1972.
24. van Rensburg SJ, van der Watt JJ, Purchase IFH, Coutinho LP, Markham R: S Afr Med J 48: 2508a–2508d.
25. Shank RC: In Kraybill HF, Mehlman MA (eds): "Environmental Cancer." New York: John Wiley and Sons, 1977, pp 291–318.
26. Linsell CA, Peers FG: Trans R Soc Trop Med Hyg 71:471–473, 1977.
27. Wogan GN: Cancer Res 35:3499–3502, 1975.

28. van Reinsburg SJ: In Rodricks JV, Hesseltine CW, Mehlman MA (eds): "Mycotoxins in Human and Animal Health." Park Forest South, IL: Pathotex, 1977, pp 699–711.

29. Blumberg BS: Public Health Rep 95:427–435, 1980.

30. Hadziyannis SJ: Spriain nger Semin Immunopathol 3:473–485, 1981.

31. Popper H, Gerber MA, Thung SN: Hepatology 2:1S–9S.

32. Beasley RP: Hepatology 2:21S–26S, 1982.

33. Shafritz DA, Kew MC: Hepatology 1:1–8, 1981.

34. Shafritz DA: Hepatology 2:35S–41S, 1982.

35. Shafritz DA, Shouval D, Sherman HI, Hadziyannis SJ, Kew MC: N Engl J Med 305:1067–1073, 1981.

36. Brechst C, Pourcel C, Louise A, Rain B, Toillais P: Nature 286:533–535, 1980.

37. Campbell TC, Caedo JP, Bulatao-Jayme J, Salamut L, Engel RW: Nature 227:403–404, 1970.

38. Shank RC, Bourgois CH, Keschamras N, Chandavimol P: Food Cosmet Toxicol 9:501–507, 1971.

39. Ryan NJ, Hogan GR, Hayes AW, Unger PD, Siraj MY: Pediatrics 64:71–75, 1979.

40. Nelson DB, Kimbrough R, Landrigan PS, Hayes AW, Yang GC, Benanides J: Pediatrics 66:865–869, 1980.

41. Reddy JK, Svoboda DJ, Rao MS: Cancer Res 36:151–160, 1976.

42. Lin JJ, Liu C, Svoboda DJ: Lab Invest 30:267–278, 1974.

43. Newberne PM, Rogers AE: In Shank RC (ed): "Mycotoxins and N-Nitroso Compounds: Environmental Risks." Boca Raton, FL: CRC, 1981, pp 51–106.

44. Gopalan C, Tulpule PG, Krishnamurthi D: Food Cosmet Toxicol 10:519–521, 1972.

45. Adamson RH, Correa P, Dalgard DW: JNCI 50:549–553, 1973.

46. Tilak TBG: Food Cosmet Toxicol 13:247–249, 1975.

47. Sieber SM, Correa P, Dalgard DW, Adamson RH: Cancer Res 39:4545–4554, 1979.

48. van der Zijden ASM, Blanche Koelensmid WAA, Boldingh J, Barrett CB, Ord WO, Philp J: Nature 195:1060–1062, 1962.

49. Nesbitt BF, O'Kelly J, Sargeant K, Sheridan A, Nature 195:1062–1063, 1962.

50. Hartley RD, Nesbitt BF, O'Kelly J: Nature 198:1056–1058, 1963.

51. Asao T, Buchi G, Abdel-Kader MM, Chang SB, Wick EL, Wogan GN: J Am Chem Soc 85:1706–1707, 1963.

52. Asao T, Buchi G, Abdel-Kader MM, Chang SB, Wick EL, Wogan GN: J Am Chem Soc 87:882–886, 1965.

53. Chang SB, Abdel-Kader MM, Wick EL, Wogan GN: Science 142:1191–1192, 1963.

54. Miller JA: Cancer Res 38:559–576, 1970.

55. Miller EC: Cancer Res 38:1479–1496, 1978.

56. Campbell TC, Hayes JR: Toxicol Appl. Pharmacol 35:199–222, 1976.

57. Shank RC: J Toxicol Environ Health 2:1229–1244, 1977.

58. Essigmann JM, Croy RG, Nadzan AM, Busby WF Jr., Reinhold VN, Buchi G, Wogan GN: Proc Natl Acad Sci USA 74:1870–1874, 1977.

59. Croy RG, Essigmann JM, Reinhold VN, Wagon GN, Proc Natl Acad Sci USA 75:1745–1749, 1978.

60. Lin JK, Miller JA, Miller EC: Cancer Res 37:4430–4438, 1977.

61. Groopman JD, Busby WF Jr., Wogan GN: Cancer Res 40:4343–4351, 1980.

62. Croy RG, Nixon JE, Sinnhuber RO, Wogan GN: Carcinogenesis 1:903–909, 1980.

63. Garner RC, Wright CM: Chem Biol Interact 11:123–131, 1975.

64. Garner RC, Martin CN, Lindsay Smith JR, Coles BF, Tolson MR: Chem Biol Interact 26:57–73, 1979.

65. Hertzog PJ, Lindsay Smith JR, Garner RC: Carcinogenesis 1:787–793, 1980.

66. Hertzog PJ, Lindsay Smith JR, Garner RC: Carcinogenesis 1:723–725, 1982.

67. Donahue PR, Essigmann JM, Wogan GN: "Banbury Report 13: Indicators of Genotoxic Exposure." Cold Spring Harbor, NY: Cold Spring Harbor Laboratory, 1982, pp 221–229.

68. Haugen A, Groopman JD, Hsu IC, Goodrich GR, Wogan GN, Harris CC: Proc Natl Acad Sci USA 78:4124–4127, 1981.

69. Groopman JD, Haugen A, Goodrich GR, Harris CC: Cancer Res 42:3120–3124, 1982.

70. Groopman JD, Trudel LJ, Donahue PR, Rothstein A, Wogan GN: Proc Natl Acad Sci USA 81:7728–7731, 1984.
71. Muller R: J Immunol Methods 34:345–352, 1980.
72. Groopman JD, Donahue PR, Zhu J, Chen J, Wogan GN: Proc Natl Acad Sci USA 82 (in press), 1985.
73. Bennett RA, Essigmann JM, Wogan GN: Cancer Res 41:650–654, 1982.
74. Autrup H, Bradley K, Shamsuddin A, Wakhisi J, Wasunna A: Carcinogenesis 4:1193–1195, 1983.

Biochemical and Molecular Epidemiology of Cancer 257–270 (1986)

HBV DNA Replication State and Disease Activity During Persistent Infection and Hepatic Oncogenesis

David A. Shafritz

Albert Einstein College of Medicine, Marion Bessin Liver Research Center, Bronx, New York 10461

The use of molecular hybridization technology has enabled the scientific community to study hepatitis B virus (HBV)-related diseases through the detection of specific HBV DNA sequences in human tissues. Using cloned HBV DNA probes of high specific activity and Southern blot techniques, HBV DNA has been found in hepatocellular carcinoma (HCC) from HBsAg carriers in all areas of the world [1–7]. Provided that tissue preservation and DNA extraction are satisfactory, integration of HBV DNA into one or a discrete number of sites has been reported in most tumors in which viral DNA sequences have been found. Each tumor shows a unique banding pattern of integrated HBV DNA molecules, although bands of similar size have been found in many tumors [2]. In regions of liver adjacent to the tumor, integration of HBV DNA has also been found with the same, a partially related, or a totally different pattern of integrated HBV DNA [3–6,8]. HBV DNA integration into the liver genome of HBV carriers in the absence of HCC has also been reported [3–5,8]. However, detailed events concerning the integration process and precisely how this relates to development of hepatic malignancy has not yet been elucidated.

Molecular hybridization techniques have also been used to detect HBV DNA in human serum either by extracting total nucleic acids [8–12] or by directly spotting serum onto a nitrocellulose filter and hybridizing the filter with purified, cloned HBV DNA [13,14]. Using hybridization techniques in conjunction with immunologic detection of HBV marker proteins and traditional histologic analysis, we have studied virus replication, serum hepatitis B e antigen (HBeAg)/antihepatitis B e (anti-HBe) status, underlying liver disease activity, and the integration state of HBV DNA in selected HBV carriers. The present report summarizes our published findings [14,15] in three groups of patients: 1) individuals with chronic HBV-related states ranging from chronic carriers without histologic evidence of liver disease to carriers with chronic persistent hepatitis, chronic active hepatitis, or cirrhosis; 2) patients on chronic

Received August 7, 1985.

© **1986 Alan R. Liss, Inc.**

hemodialysis therapy; and 3) hepatitis B surface antigen (HBsAg) carriers with HCC.

MATERIALS AND METHODS
Patient Populations and Serologic Studies

Sera from several groups of patients, stored at $-20°C$, were studied. Group I was composed of 35 Greek patients all with serum containing HBsAg by conventional radioimmunoassay (RIA) (see below). This group represented a wide variety of chronic HBV-related states, including chronic carriers with normal liver by routine histology, patients with chronic persistent or chronic active hepatitis, carriers with cirrhosis, and several patients with cirrhosis and HCC. Antihepatitis B surface antigen (anti-HBs), HBeAg, anti-HBe, and anti-HBc were also evaluated. Group II consisted of 15 chronic hemodialysis and/or renal transplant patients and other persons working in a hospital environment, all of whom were serologically HBsAg positive. Five of these patients had undergone immunosuppressive therapy and two had received bilateral nephrectomies. Group III was composed of 10 HBsAg carriers undergoing initial evaluation of liver disease by a hepatologist. Negative controls (serum from healthy subjects negative for HBV markers) and positive controls (purified HBV DNA or serum from patients with known high titers of HBV) were included in each analysis.

Serologic studies of HBV markers (HBsAg, anti-HBs, anti-HBc, HBeAg, and anti-HBe) were performed with RIAs using commercially available (Abbott, N. Chicago, IL) reagent kits (AUSRIA II for HBsAg, AUSAB for anti-HBs, and CORAB for anti-HBc and HBeAg/anti-HBe). Histologic analysis of liver and tumor specimens was performed by routine staining (Masson trichome and hematoxylin and eosin) after fixation of tissue in neutral formalin and embedding in paraffin.

Immunologic Analysis of Liver for HBsAg, HBcAg, and δ Antigen

Liver biopsy specimens, needle or surgical, were snap frozen and cut in a cryostat. Unfixed air-dried sections, 5 μm thick, were examined by direct immunofluorescence (IF) or immunoperoxidase (IP) for HBsAg, hepatitis B core antigen (HBcAg), and δ antigen (δ-Ag) by methods previously described in detail [18,19]. In brief, fluorescein-conjugated antibodies to HBsAg, HBcAg, and δ-Ag (the latter kindly donated by Dr. M. Rizzetto) were applied to carefully washed sections and incubated for 30 min at 37°C. They were then washed twice in PBS for 10 min and examined under a fluorescent microscope (Vanox, Olympus, Lake Success, NY).

In each experiment, one positive and one negative control liver section was included for HBsAg, HBcAg, and δ-Ag detection. The specificity of HBsAg, HBcAg, and δ-Ag fluorescence was checked by absorption and blocking tests. All antisera used were also tested for nonspecific staining of control liver specimens obtained from HBsAg-negative persons. Moreover, cryostat sections from each specimen were reexamined for HBsAg, HBcAg, and δ-Ag by the direct IP technique using peroxidase-conjugated antibodies to HBsAg and HBcAg and to δ-Ag, kindly donated by Drs. L. Overby and M. Rizzetto, respectively. All histochemical studies were performed without knowledge of the serologic results of HBV DNA detection.

Hybridization of Serum and Liver DNA Extracts for HBV DNA Sequences

Human serum was analyzed for HBV DNA sequences using molecular hybridization techniques as previously reported [2,4,14,15]. In brief, 10–15 μl of serum was applied directly to a 0.45 U pore size nitrocellulose filter sheet (Schleicher and Schuell, Keene, NH), spotting 5 μl for each application and drying the paper between applications. Known positive and negative control samples were included in each analysis. The paper was treated with 0.5 N NaOH, neutralized with 1 M Tris-HCl, pH 7.4, and 0.5 M NaCl, treated with proteinase K (Boehringer/Mannheim) at 200 μg/ml for 1 hr at 37°C, washed twice with 2× SCC (0.30 M NaCl and 0.03 M Na citrate), baked *in vacuum* at 80° for 2 hr, prehybridized, and hybridized at 68°C for 24–36 hr in a solution containing Denhardt's solution (0.1% bovine serum albumin, 0.1% Ficoll, and 0.1% polyvinyl pyrollidone), 6× SSC (0.9 M NaCl and 0.09 M Na citrate), 0.1% sodium dodecyl sulfate (SDS), 0.025 M sodium phosphate buffer, pH 6.5, 200 μg/ml denatured calf thymus DNA, and $1^{-2} \times 10^7$ cpm of repurified, recombinant cloned HBV DNA labeled with ^{32}P to a specific activity of 2–4×10^8 cpm/μg DNA. Subsequent to hybridization, the nitrocellulose filter was washed, dried, and autoradiographed as described [2,4,14,15].

For hybridization analysis of liver tissue, total DNA was extracted from small portions of frozen percutaneous or surgical biopsy specimens, digested in 20 to 30 μg aliquots with restriction endonuclease Hind III, electrophoresed through an 0.8% agarose slab gel, transferred to a nitrocellulose filter, and hybridized with [^{32}P]HBV DNA also as previously reported [2,4]. Use of a purified HBV DNA probe ($\sim 3,250$ base pairs), separated and reisolated from the plasmid cloning vehicle (pA01, approximately 8,700 base pairs) and the stringency of the hybridization and washing conditions employed ensured that hybridization would detect only sequences complementary to HBV DNA [2,4,14,15].

RESULTS
Sensitivity and Scoring of HBV DNA Spot Hybridization Test

The sensitivity of the spot hybridization method by applying progressively decreasing amounts of purified HBV DNA to a nitrocellulose filter and detecting sequences complementary to [^{32}P]HBV DNA is shown in Figure 1. After 24 hr of autoradiography, 0.2–0.5 pg of HBV DNA sequences was detected and after 5 days, and 0.05–0.1 pg HBV DNA was visualized as a circular spot where DNA was applied to the filter (the last positive spot for each time of autoradiogram exposure reproduced poorly on the photograph). The spots were cut out and counted by liquid scintillation, confirming the high sensitivity of the autoradiographic method. A simple qualitative scoring system was developed on the basis of intensity of hybridization from trace to 4^+ (noted at the bottom of Fig. 1).

Detection of HBV DNA in the Serum of HBsAg Carriers

Serum HBV DNA analysis in HBsAg-positive persons, excluding those with HCC, are shown in Table I. Three groups of patients were studied: long-term surface antigen carriers (HBsAg$^+$) from Greece, patients undergoing initial evaluation of chronic liver disease in the United States, and patients from a renal analysis-transplant service. All HBsAg$^+$/HBeAg$^+$ carriers (28 of 28) showed HBV DNA in the serum. To our surprise, half (16 of 32) of the HBsAg$^+$/anti-HBe$^+$ carriers also showed HBV DNA in the serum. This result was found in all three population groups and was strikingly different from previous scattered reports of HBV DNA in the serum of a few HBsAg$^+$/anti-HBe$^+$ patients [8,10–12]. HBV DNA was also detected in the

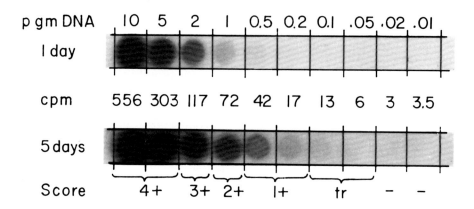

Fig. 1.   Spot hybridization test for detection of HBV DNA sequences. Recombinant cloned, repurified HBV DNA in serial dilution was spotted in 3 μl aliquots onto a nitrocellulose filter and hybridized with denatured ^{32}P-labeled HBV DNA of specific activity 3.5 × 10^8 cpm/μg. Details concerning the hybridization conditions are given in the text and by Lieberman et al [14]. The spot with 0.05 pg HBV was clearly visible on the original autoradiogram after 5 days of exposure but did not reproduce on the photograph. Reprinted from Lieberman et al [14], with permission.

TABLE I. Detection of HBV DNA in Serum Compared to HBeAg/Anti-HBe Status in HBsAg Carriers*

Carrier status	Serum HBV DNA (positive/total)
HBsAg$^+$/HBeAg$^+$	28/28
HBsAg$^+$/anti-HBe$^+$	16/32
HBsAg$^-$/anti-HBe$^+$	3/6

*Patients positive or negative for both HBeAg and anti-HBe are not included.

serum of three of six patients who were negative for HBsAg but positive for anti-HBc and anti-HBe (one was also positive for anti-HBs). In 85% of our positive cases, HBV DNA was detected in 10 μl of serum applied directly to a nitrocellulose filter. All trace positive and negative results were confirmed by extracting nucleic acids from 200–300 μl of serum and applying the entire extract to the nitrocellulose filter.

An example of the utility and simplicity of the serum HBV DNA spot hybridization test is illustrated in Figure 2. In each case, 10 μl of serum was applied directly to the filter. Samples 1 (4$^+$), 3 (4$^+$), and 7 (1$^+$) are from HBsAg/HBeAg carriers from the renal dialysis-transplant unit and patients 1 and 3 were implicated epidemiologically in transmission of hepatitis B infection to other persons. Sample 12 (4$^+$) is a carrier in the dialysis unit whose serum was HBsAg$^+$/anti-HBe$^+$. Hybridization with this specimen was as strong as any other we have observed during the last 3 years. For comparison, sample 9 (3$^+$–4$^+$) is from a patient with acute hepatitis B infection who became negative for serum HBV DNA after clinical infection cleared (spot 10). This suggests that some hepatitis B carriers have serum HBV DNA levels in the range observed during acute HBV infection and such carriers may be HBeAg$^+$ or anti-HBe$^+$. Together with the data in Table I, these results indicate further that we can no longer rely simply on seroimmunologic testing to determine whether hepatitis B virus is present or absent in the bloodstream.

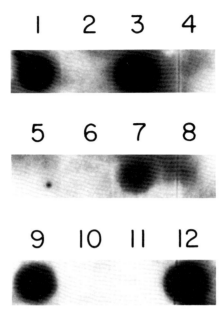

Fig. 2. HBV DNA spot hybridization test with selected serum specimens from HBsAg carriers and control patients. Spots 1, 3, and 7: HBsAg$^+$/HBeAg$^+$ carriers from renal dialysis unit; spot 12: HBsAg$^+$/anti-HBe$^+$ carrier from renal dialysis unit; spot 9: a patient acutely infected with HBV; spot 10: the same patient as spot 9 after resolution of infection; spots 2, 4, 5, 6, 8, and 11: negative controls or patients with anti-HBs following hepatitis B exposure or after infection had cleared. Reprinted from Lieberman et al [14], with permission.

TABLE II. Serum HBV DNA, HBeAg/Anti-HBe Status, HBcAg, and Liver Histology in Long-Term HBsAg Carriers* From Greece

Serum status	No. of patients	Liver HBcAg	Active liver disease
HBeAg$^+$/HBV DNA$^+$	7	7	7
Anti-HBe$^+$/HBV DNA$^+$	12	9	12
Anti-HBe$^+$/HBV DNA$^-$	10	1	3

*Chronic persistent hepatitis, chronic active hepatitis, or chronic active hepatitis with cirrhosis.

Molecular Forms of HBV DNA in the Liver in Relation to Virus Replication, Liver Disease Activity, and Serologic HBV Marker Status

To investigate further the pathophysiologic significance of HBV DNA in the serum of HBsAg$^+$/anti-HBe$^+$ carriers, a comparison was made between serum HBV DNA, HBeAg/anti-HBe status, HBcAg in hepatocyte nuclei (another index of virus replication), and histologic assessment of liver disease activity (Table II). Three groups of long-term carriers from Greece were studied: HBeAg$^+$/HBV DNA$^+$, anti-HBe$^+$/HBV DNA$^+$, and anti-HBe$^+$/HBV DNA$^-$. All seven HBeAg$^+$/HBV DNA$^+$

patients had chronic liver disease (chronic persistent hepatitis, chronic active hepatitis, or chronic active hepatitis with cirrhosis). HBcAg was detected in hepatocyte nuclei in all seven HBeAg[+]/HBV DNA[+] patients. Twelve out of 12 patients who were anti-HBe[+]/HBV DNA[+] also had active chronic liver disease and nine were positive for HBcAg in hepatocyte nuclei. In contrast, only three of 10 anti-HBe[+]/HBV DNA[−] patients had active liver disease and only one had hepatocyte nuclear core antigen. Six HBsAg carriers with normal liver histology were serum anti-HBe[+]/HBV DNA[−] and negative for hepatocyte nuclear core antigen. The major point of Table II is that all serum HBV DNA positive patients had active chronic liver disease, regardless of whether they were HBeAg or anti-HBe positive. Most of these patients also were positive for core antigen in hepatocyte nuclei, whereas only one serum HBV DNA negative patient showed hepatocyte nuclear core antigen. In addition, all of the patients with normal liver histology (ie, normal except for the presence of "ground-glass" hepatocytes) were serum HBV DNA negative. These results clearly demonstrate a correlation between serum HBV DNA, virus replication in liver, and continued activity of chronic liver disease, independent of the HBeAg/anti-HBe status.

To explore further the meaning of these observations, HBV DNA hybridization was performed with DNA extracts from percutaneous liver biopsies obtained from 17 of these patients. Total cellular DNA was digested with restriction enzyme Hind III, electrophoresed through an agarose gel, transferred to a nitrocellulose filter, and hybridized with repurified [^{32}P]-labeled cloned HBV DNA (Fig. 3). The major question here was in what molecular form would HBV DNA be found and under what circumstances was it integrated into the host liver cell genome? In five HBsAg[+]/HBeAg[+] patients analyzed (data from three are shown in Fig. 3, lanes 1–3), abundant free virion and lower molecular weight replicating forms of HBV DNA were found. In three HBsAg[+]/anti-HBe[+] patients with "normal" liver histology, discrete bands containing HBV DNA sequences of unique size greater than HBV genome length were present (see Fig. 3, lanes 4 and 6). No hybridization was obtained with other liver DNA extracts applied to the gel and analyzed simultaneously (for example, see Fig. 3, lane 5). This ruled out the possibility of nonspecific hybridization or trapping of the [^{32}P]HBV DNA probe by cellular DNA. These findings are consistent with integration of HBV DNA into the liver cell genome and the clonal propagation of hepatocytes containing these integrated HBV DNA sequences. However, since limited material was available, we could not rule out the possibility that some or all of these high molecular weight DNA molecules containing HBV sequences might represent concatomers, "superforms," or other extrachromosomal oligomers of HBV DNA [18], although these have not been reported in man. In these specimens, there was little or no free viral DNA in the liver (Fig. 3, lanes 4 and 6), nuclear HBcAg was not present, and serum HBV DNA was negative.

In serologically HBsAg[+]/anti-HBe[+]/HBV DNA[−] carriers from Greece with no histologic evidence of active liver disease, there was one additional interesting observation. These patients often showed a "ground-glass" appearance in the cytoplasm of many hepatocytes [19,20]. These so-called ground-glass hepatocytes contain abundant HBsAg and often appear in focal accumulations or clusters (Fig. 4). This is readily demonstrated by immunofluorescent staining of cryostat sections of liver for HBsAg (Fig. 5). In approximately 50% of these patients, we have found HBV DNA sequences in discrete bands of high molecular weight DNA. Therefore, it is possible that focal or nodular accumulations of hepatocytes containing cytoplasmic HBsAg

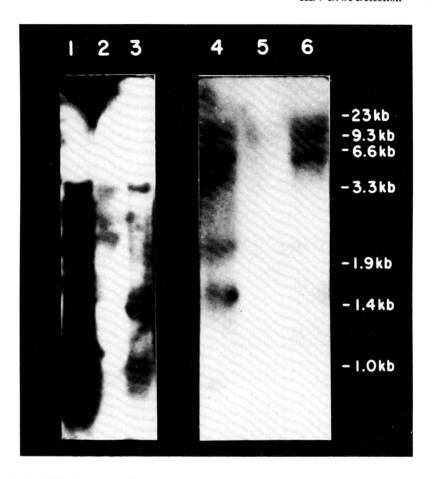

Fig. 3. Hybridization analysis for HBV DNA sequences in total DNA extracts from percutaneous liver biopsy specimens from serologically HBsAg$^+$/HBeAg$^+$/HBV DNA$^+$ and HBsAg$^+$/anti-HBe$^+$/HBV DNA$^-$ carriers. Serologically HBsAg$^+$/HBeAg$^+$/HBV DNA$^+$ carriers: lanes 1, 2, and 3; serologically HBsAg$^+$/anti-HBe$^+$/HBV DNA$^-$ carriers: lanes 4 and 6; negative control liver: lane 5. Reprinted from Hadziyannis et al [15], with permission.

represent clones of cells derived from single hepatocytes containing integrated HBV DNA that have been stimulated to divide. These patients generally show little or no free or replicating forms of HBV DNA in the liver, no hepatocyte nuclear core antigen, and no HBV DNA in the serum. This provides additional support to the concept that HBsAg production in these patients is derived from integrated HBV DNA sequences. Absence of virion production as part of a nonreplicating cycle of virus infection could also explain the tendency to accumulate HBsAg in these cells.

In patients actively replicating virus (HBsAg$^+$/HBeAg$^+$/HBV DNA$^+$ in serum), focal or nodular accumulations of HBsAg$^+$ hepatocytes and integrated HBV DNA sequences in unique banding patterns are not usually found. These patients show both HBsAg (cytoplasmic) and HBcAg (nuclear) distributed randomly throughout the hepatic parenchyma (Fig. 6). However, both focal or nodular and random distributions of HBsAg can be found in separate areas of liver in some patients at postmortem examination. These persons are usually anti-HBe$^+$ but still have active liver disease,

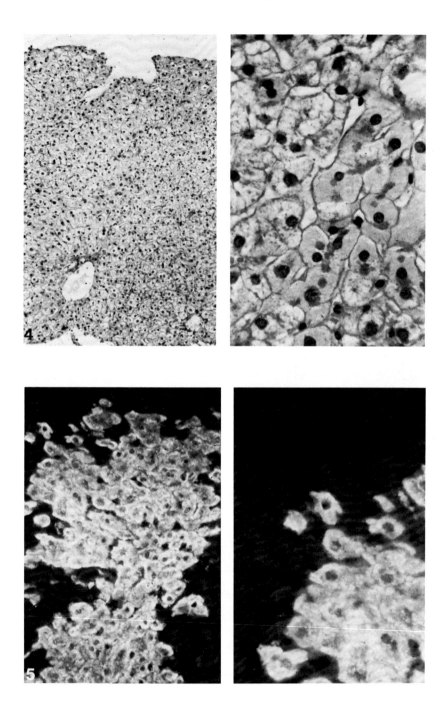

Fig. 4. Histologic evaluation of hepatic parenchyma in serologically HBsAg$^+$/anti-HBe$^+$/HBV DNA$^-$ carrier from Greece. There is no evidence of inflammatory liver disease, acute or chronic, and many hepatocytes have a "ground-glass" appearance as is shown on the left. This is illustrated at higher magnification on the right.

Fig. 5. Direct immunofluorescence for HBsAg in cryostat section of liver from a serologically HBsAg$^+$/anti-HBe$^+$/HBV DNA$^-$ carrier from Greece. Accumulations of HBsAg in the cytoplasm of many hepatocytes in groups or clusters is shown on the left. The cytoplasmic distribution of this HBsAg is shown at higher magnification on the right. HBcAg was not present in replicate sections of this liver.

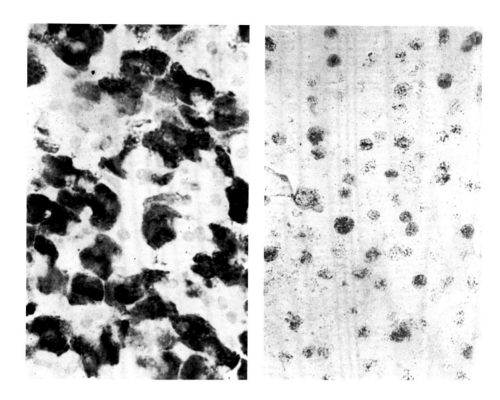

Fig. 6.   Distribution of HBsAg and HBcAg in the liver of a serologically HBsAg$^+$/HBeAg$^+$/HBV DNA$^+$ carrier with chronic active hepatitis. This patient showed IP-positive material for HBsAg (left) and HBcAg (right) in many hepatocytes in a random distribution.

HBcAg in hepatocyte nuclei, and HBV DNA in serum (Shafritz and Hadziyannis, unpublished observations). They constitute a third category of mixed infection (replicating and nonreplicating HBV in different regions of the liver).

HBV DNA in Hepatocellular Carcinoma Tissue From HBsAg Carriers

The vast majority of studies report integration of HBV DNA sequences into the host genome in hepatocellular carcinoma tissue of HBsAg carriers. This was demonstrated initially with the PLC/PRF/5 cell line [21,22]. Our subsequent studies with primary tumors from this same population [2,4] (Fig. 7), as well as those of others [5,6], established that the integrated HBV DNA molecules are present as unique bands on gel electrophoresis and hybridization analysis (Southern blot). This indicates that the site(s) of viral DNA integration is the same in a large proportion of the cells comprising the tumor. The presence of a single or fixed number of discrete bands in the hybridization analysis indicates monoclonality or oligoclonality of the tumor cell population. Since integration of HBV DNA into the nontumorous liver of tumor patients and into the liver of carriers without HCC has been reported, this clearly indicates that integration of HBV DNA precedes development of HCC. Generally, the genomic organization of integrated HBV DNA in tumors is more complex than that of the free virus, often containing deletions, inversions, and duplications of viral

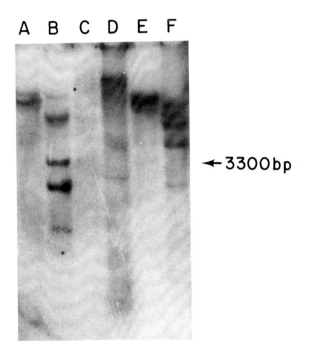

Fig. 7. Hybridization pattern of integrated HBV DNA sequences in hepatocellular carcinoma specimens from six South African black male HBsAg carriers. Restriction enzyme digestion was with Hind III. No free HBV genomes or virus replication intermediates were identified in these specimens. Reprinted from Shafritz and Kew [2], with permission.

sequences, as well as deletions of cellular sequences [23]. However, these findings are not always observed (Hino and Rogler, unpublished observations).

DISCUSSION

From various studies, it appears that DNA extracts from liver biopsies of HBsAg carriers show integrated HBV DNA [15,16,18]. Precisely when integration occurs, however, has not been elucidated. If only small amounts of HBV DNA are integrated, or if early in the course of disease integration sites are spread throughout the host genome, this will be difficult to determine. During progression of the carrier state, it is possible that hepatocytes expressing all viral components are continuously being removed or selectively destroyed by viral cytopathic effects or host immunological responses. Therefore, hepatocytes containing integrated HBV DNA, but which are not expressing full virions, may be preferentially retained. This could lead to an increased proportion of integrated HBV DNA in longer term carriers and would correlate with an increased ability to detect integrated HBV DNA in HBsAg carriers who are anti-HBe rather than HBeAg positive. This could lead to two stages in the integration process—early nonspecific integration, in which HBV DNA is diffusely distributed throughout the host genome, and later specific integration, in which cells containing integrated HBV DNA in unique sites have been selected for survival and/ or multiplication by host or other factors related to immune resistance or increased cell division rates. A similar selection mechanism for hepatocytes containing integrated HBV DNA could occur during antiviral therapy of carriers with Ara-A and/or interferon [24]. This could explain continued HBsAg expression in most patients in whom viral replication has been permanently inhibited by these agents [25] and could render these patients at increased risk to develop hepatocellular carcinoma [24].

Integration of HBV DNA in Relation to Potential Oncogenicity

All published studies are consistent with the interpretation that integration of HBV DNA into the hepatocyte genome precedes the development of hepatocellular carcinoma by months or years. The exact time at which integration occurs, the relationship between integration and HBV serum markers (as well as their progression), and the frequency with which integration leads to development of hepatocellular carcinoma require further study. From epidemiologic evidence [26,27], it would appear that 10 years of the HBV carrier state, and more often 20–30 years, is usually required to develop hepatocellular carcinoma. Therefore, individuals developing the carrier state in the first few years of life may be at greatest risk to develop hepatocellular carcinoma.

The finding of integrated HBV DNA in many hepatocellular carcinomas and in all hepatocellular carcinomas in which viral sequences are present suggests strongly that HBV is oncogenic or stimulates oncogenesis. In various animal models and tissue culture systems infected with "tumor" viruses, the presence of integrated viral DNA (proviral DNA in the case of RNA tumor viruses) often correlates with the ability of these viruses to transform cells [28,29]. Cells that are transformed and contain integrated viral genomes are generally "nonpermissive" for viral replication, as found for the PLC/PRF/5 cell line. In contrast, when cells permissive for replication are infected with the same virus, the virus does not become integrated and the cells are not transformed. Therefore, whether HBV persistence and integration lead to cellular transformation needs to be explored. Clearly, the presence of a unique or specific HBV DNA integration pattern in gross liver and tumor specimens (regardless of whether these patterns are the same or different) suggests that the bulk of cells in these specimens are derived from single progenitor cells that contain integrated HBV DNA and that have been stimulated to divide. In some instances, the histologic appearance of these abnormal cells may be difficult to distinguish from normal hepatocytes or cells within regenerating liver nodules. Whether the integrated HBV DNA acts as a mutagen, activates or enhances expression of a cellular oncogene or oncogenes, or in some other way alters cellular gene expression or growth properties remains to be determined. At present, it does not appear that HBV is a directly transforming virus, but even this is not certain, since no system has yet been established to study the properties of HBV in cell culture.

Proposed Events During Integration of HBV DNA, Transformation of Hepatocytes, and Development of Hepatocellular Carcinoma

A schematic model of events leading to transformation of hepatocytes during HBV infection is presented in Figure 8. At the extremes of persistent viral infection, there appears to be two types of HBV carriers, those who continue to replicate the virus and demonstrate continued liver disease activity (shown on the right) and those who do not replicate the virus and show little or no liver disease activity (shown on the left). In the former patients, the bulk of HBV DNA in liver is in free virions or

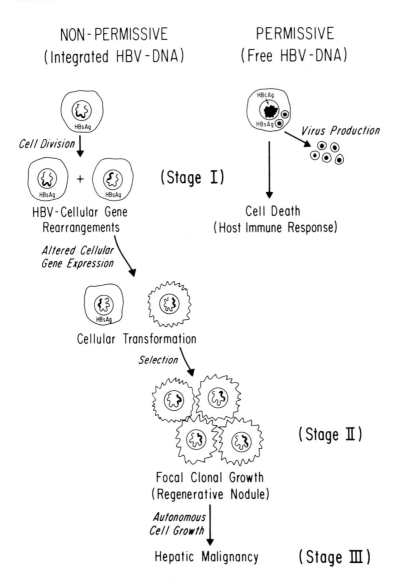

NON-PERMISSIVE
(Integrated HBV-DNA)

PERMISSIVE
(Free HBV-DNA)

Fig. 8.   Conceptual model illustrating possible events following HBV infection and integration of HBV DNA into the liver cell genome that might ultimately lead to the development of HCC. On the right are shown HBV carriers who continue to replicate the virus and demonstrate continued liver disease; on the left are shown HBV carriers who do not replicate the virus and show little or no liver disease activity. Reprinted from Shafritz and Rogler [23], with permission.

replicating forms and integration into unique sites in the host genome is not observed. In the latter cases, only integrated HBV DNA is present and virions are not produced. A mixed type of persistent infection may also occur in which features of active liver disease (virus replication) and focal accumulations of HBsAg with no evidence of active liver disease (virus nonreplication) are found in different regions of liver.

In patients in whom HBV is present but is no longer replicating, it may be more difficult for host immune responses to rid the liver of infected hepatocytes than in patients with active virus replication. Under this "negative" selection pressure, there may be accumulation of hepatocytes containing integrated HBV DNA as compared to hepatocytes that are actively producing virus (stage I). Under a variety of circumstances and conditions that stimulate hepatocyte cell division over many years (host responses, humoral or hormonal factors, contact with hepatotoxins, ethanol ingestion, chemical carcinogens such as aflatoxin, superinfection with other viruses, and so forth), a series of rearrangements of HBV DNA and/or cellular sequences in the host genome may occur and lead to production of hepatocytes with abnormal phenotypic properties (cellular transformation). Tumor promoting or DNA modifying agents could also contribute to these changes. When cells with such modified or rearranged DNA subsequently divide, the abnormal genome and transformed phenotype may be reproduced, yielding groups or clusters of cells with a unique site(s) of HBV DNA integration (stage II). Continued division of such cells, under a variety of additional host factors or selection pressures, may ultimately lead to the development of an autonomously growing hepatic neoplasm (stage III).

This conceptual model, which is entirely speculative, requires integration of the HBV genome as an initial event in the transformation process but requires neither the expression of specific viral genes nor even the presence of HBV DNA in the eventual neoplasm (Fig. 8). If such a mechanism is shown to initiate the cellular transformation process, then the finding of integrated HBV DNA in a unique banding pattern in HBsAg$^+$/anti-HBe$^+$ carriers, especially in those persons who are no longer actively replicating virus, may have important implications in terms of risk for future development of HCC. This hypothesis is supported by recent unpublished reports from Japan of second and third recurrent hepatocellular carcinomas in HBV carriers who have undergone hepatic resection for removal of small primary liver neoplasms.

In summary, results of recent studies have shown that a significant proportion of long-term HBV carriers with continued viral replication may be serologically anti-HBe rather than HBeAg positive. Viral replication and secretion as detected by HBcAg in the liver and HBV DNA in serum appears to be suppressed or inactive in anti-HBe–positive carriers with normal liver histology but continues to be active in many anti-HBe–positive patients with chronic liver disease. Finally, uniquely integrated HBV DNA may be found in the liver genome even in the absence of active liver disease and after viral replication has ceased, and a speculative model is presented in which HBV-DNA integration serves as an initial event in the oncogenic transformation of hepatocytes.

ACKNOWLEDGMENTS

This research was supported in part by NIH grants AM-17609 and CA-32605, the Sarah Chait Memorial Foundation, the Gail I. Zuckerman Foundation, and the Marion Bessin Liver Research Center Fund.

REFERENCES

1. Brechot C, Pourcel C, Louise A, Rain B, Tiollais P: Nature 286:533–535, 1980.
2. Shafritz DA, Kew MC: Hepatology 1:1–8, 1981.
3. Brechot C, Hadchouel M, Scotto J, Fonck M, Potet F, Vyas G, Tiollais P: Proc Natl Acad Sci USA 78:3906–3910, 1981.

4. Shafritz DA, Shouval D, Sherman HI, Hadziyannis SJ, Kew MC: N Engl J Med 305:1067–1073, 1981.

5. Koshy R, Maupas P, Miller R, Hofschneider PH: J Gen Virol 57:95–102, 1981.

6. Gerin JL, Shih JRK, Hoyer BH: In Szmuness W, Alter HJ, Maynard JE (eds): "Viral Hepatitis— 1981 International Symposium." Philadelphia: Franklin Institute Press, 1982, pp 49–55.

7. Kam W, Rall L, Schmid R, Rutter WJ: In Szmuness W, Alter HJ, Maynard JE (eds): "Viral Hepatitis—1981 Symposium." Philadelphia: Franklin Institute Press, 1982, p 809.

8. Brechot C, Scotto J, Charnay P, Hadchouel M, Degos F, Trepo C, Tiollais P: Lancet 2:765–770, 1981.

9. Kam W, Rall LB, Smuckler EA, Schmid R, Rutter WJ: Proc Natl Acad Sci USA 79:7522–7526, 1982.

10. Bonino F, Hoyer B, Nelson J, Engle R, Verme G, Gerin J: Hepatology 1:386–391, 1981.

11. Beringer M, Hamer M, Hoyer B, Gerin JL: J Med Virol 9(1):57–68, 1982.

12. Weller IVD, Fowler MJF, Monjardino J, Thomas HC: J Med Virol 9(4):273–280, 1982.

13. Neurath AR, Shick N, Baker L, Krugman S: Proc Natl Acad Sci USA 79:4415–4419, 1982.

14. Lieberman HM, LaBrecque DR, Kew MC, Hadziyannis SJ, Shafritz DA: Hepatology 3:285–291, 1983.

15. Hadziyannis SJ, Lieberman HM, Karvountzis GG, Shafritz DA: Hepatology 3:656–662, 1983.

16. Hadziyannis SJ, Vissoulis C, Moussouros A, Afroudis A: Lancet 1:976–979, 1972.

17. Hadziyannis SJ, Giustozi A, Moussouros A, Merikas G: In Leevy CM (ed): "Diseases of the Liver and Biliary Tract." Fifth Quadr Meeting of IASL, 1974. Basel: S. Karger, 1976, pp 174–178.

18. Rogler CE, Summers J: J Virol 44:852–863, 1982.

19. Hadziyannis SJ, Gerber MA, Vissoulis C, Popper H: Arch Pathol 96:327–330, 1973.

20. Hadziyannis SJ: In Berk PD, Chalmers TC (eds): "Frontiers in Liver Disease." New York: Thieme-Stratton, 1981, pp 106–121.

21. Marion PL, Salazar FH, Alexander JJ, Robinson WS: J Virol 33:795–806, 1980.

22. Chakraborty PR, Ruiz-Opazo N, Shouval D, Shafritz DA: Nature 286:531–533, 1980.

23. Shafritz DA, Rogler CE: In Vyas GN, Dienstag JL, Hoofnagle JH (eds): "Viral Hepatitis and Liver Disease. Proceedings of the 1984 International Symposium on Viral Hepatitis." New York: Grune and Stratton, 1984, pp 225–243.

24. Shafritz DA, Arias IM: Hepatology 2:106–107, 1982.

25. Scullard GH, Pollard RB, Smith JT, Sacks SL, Gregory PB, Robinson WS, Merigan TC: J Infect Dis 143:772–783, 1981.

26. Szmuness W: Prog Med Virol 24:40–69, 1978.

27. Beasley RP, Lin C-C, Hwang L-Y, Chien C-S: Lancet 2:1129–1132, 1981.

28. Tooze J (ed): "DNA Tumor Viruses: Molecular Biology of Tumor Viruses," 2nd ed, Part 2. Cold Spring Harbor, NY: Cold Spring Harbor Laboratory, 1979.

29. Shin SI, Freedman VH, Risser R, Pollack R: Proc Natl Acad Sci USA 72:4435–4439, 1975.

Biochemical and Molecular Epidemiology of Cancer 271–282 (1986)

The Molecular Biology of Human Hepatitis B Virus Infection

George H. Yoakum, Brent E. Korba, Dimetris C. Boumpas, Dean L. Mann, and Curtis C. Harris

Laboratory of Human Carcinogenesis, Division of Cancer Etiology, NCI, Bethesda, Maryland 20892

Hepatitis B virus (HBV) infection is a serious world health problem that plays a primary role in viral hepatitis and is epidemiologically associated with liver cancer [1–3]. It is essential to develop direct and model experimental systems to study human HBV at the molecular level for both a fundamental understanding of the virus life cycle and the development of new intervention methods. The absence of an effective method for HBV propagation in tissue culture has led to the exploitation of several animal model systems; notably, the woodchuck (WHU) and chimpanzee models of HBV infection and pathology have been extensively studied [4–7]. Information about hepadenavirus pathology and the pattern of disease progression has been gained from these studies. However, the development of new methods of disease management for the HBV-infected human population will require interdisciplinary study of human HBV molecular biology to implement optimally the diagnostic and intervention capabilities that will be acquired with the insights and reagents generated from this approach.

Advancements in understanding the molecular biology of human HBV infection rely on technologic improvements in the following areas: 1) advances in genetic engineering methods, including the ability to transfect genes into various types of human cells in vitro [8,9; Yoakum et al, manuscript in preparation], 2) improved methods for growing normal human cells, including hepatocytes in vitro [10,11], and 3) the application of standard methods used in molecular biology (eg, Southern hybridization analysis) [12] to follow the life cycle of HBV infection in biological samples from chronically infected human populations [13–17; Yoakum et al, manuscript in preparation]. This approach to the study of HBV infection of human populations indicates that the nuclear capsid protein of HBV (HBcAg) can be cytolytic when overexpressed in epithelial cells [8]. The intricacies of gene expression that regulate HBcAg (*HBc* gene) are consistent with the biological role that the *HBc* gene

Received November 11, 1985.

© **1986 Alan R. Liss, Inc.**

product plays when observed in the cytoplasm rather than the nucleus of the human epithelial cell [8].

The detection of HBV infection in mixed populations of peripheral blood lymphocytes from patients with chronic active hepatitis [Yoakum et al, manuscript in preparation] suggests that immunologic function may be vulnerable during a critical time period when the chronic pattern of infection is beginning and/or a new sequela of infection is manifested. The virus may express the *HBc* gene, causing some subpopulations of infected lymphocytes to undergo lysis in response to the cytopathologic effects of the core antigen gene.

TRANSFECTION METHODS FOR CONSTRUCTION OF RECOMBINANT HUMAN CELLS

To understand the pathogenesis of disease caused by HBV, it is advantageous to study the effects of HBV genes in model human cell systems. Because of the current lack of an effective method to infect human cells in vitro with HBV, genetic studies of HBV gene expression require that HBV DNA be efficiently transfected into human cells. The important features of an in vitro genetic transfection system include 1) an efficient nontoxic means to introduce genetic information to recipient cells, 2) a suitable cell type for gene transfection and, 3) vectors with a dominant genetic marker whose expression permits selection of covalently linked genes under study independent of the expression of gene(s) being analyzed.

The $CaPO_4$:DNA transfection method is extremely toxic for normal human bronchial epithelial cells (NHBE) and also for a number of human carcinoma cell lines. Therefore, a protoplast fusion method was developed to transfect DNA carried on plasmids in *Escherichia coli* into various types of human cells at frequencies greater than 10^{-3} [8,9; Yoakum et al, manuscript in preparation]. Using this method, a stable HBV-carrying human recombinant cell line with an HBV gene structure was constructed, and this recombinant cell line (GTC2) was used for studies of HBV gene expression. This permitted the first study of HBV core antigen (*HBc*) gene expression in a human cell without the other HBV genes being present. The *HBc* gene was transiently expressed in 70 to 90% of transfected recipient cells for 6 to 12 days, and gpt^+ (guanine phosphoribosyl transferase/HBc$^+$) cells were selected at frequencies greater than 10^{-3} (Table I). The immediate response of the recipient cells to high frequency transfection provides a genetic test for cytopathologic effects that can be followed by analysis of the factors that regulate *HBc* gene expression in the stable gpt^+/HBc^+ population.

STUDIES OF HBV GENES IN MODEL SYSTEMS

The two most studied gene products of HBV, the surface antigen (HBsAg) and the core antigen (HBcAg), play different roles during HBV infection. The relationship of the serologic data to viral hepatitis suggests that the constitutively regulated HBsAg gene (*HBs*) [18] is required for expansion of the focus of viral infection because anti-HBs antibodies are required for disease protection by immunization and resolution during recovery [19]. In contrast, antibodies against the HBV core gene (*HBc*) product do not consistently appear during disease recovery and are frequently associated with virus replication and infectivity of patients' sera [20]. The importance of HBV core

TABLE I. Transfection of Human Epithelial Cells by Protoplast Fusion

Recipient cell designation	Plasmid	Genotype	Selection		Frequency of transfection	
			gpt^+	neo^+	Protoplast fusion	$CaPO_4$:DNA (3–125 mM Ca^{2+})
GTC1	pSV2gpt	gpt^+	+	−	3.2×10^{-3}	$<10^{-5}$
GTC2	pKYC200	gpt^+, HBc^+	+	−	3.1×10^{-3}	
GTC10	pSV2neo	neo^+	−	+	3.4×10^{-3}	$<10^{-5}$

The frequency of transfection of human cells (NCI H292) with pSV2-derived plasmids. Transfection was achieved by protoplast fusion with *Escherichia coli* strain HB101 carrying pSV2-derived plasmids and was determined after selection for gpt^+ or neo^+ expression. The growth rates of human cells in culture and frequency of gpt^+ transfectants were measured by using the clonal growth assay. Those colonies capable of eight divisions in gpt^+ selection or four divisions during neo^+ selection are stably transfected for these marker genes. The fraction of colonies continuing to grow as described above indicates the frequency of transfection for each experiment. Clonal isolation and continued passage indicates that greater than 90% of these colonies are genetically stable. The frequencies listed are averages of three experiments; the lower limit for detection is 10^{-5}.

gene (*HBc*) expression to the pathologic process during HBV infection is indicated by the cytopathologic effects that occur as a consequence of induced *HBc* gene expression in human epithelial cells [8]. Recent isolation of the X-region coding sequence of HBV has permitted the expression of this sequence in *Escherichia coli*, isolation of the X-gene product, and identification of antibodies to the X-gene product in the sera of patients with hepatocellular carcinoma (HPC) [21].

The application of molecular biology to clinical problems related to HBV infection has followed the isolation of HBV DNA on plasmids for sequence analysis [22–26], genetic transfection, and expression in procaryotic, mammalian, and human cells. The expression of the HBs gene in procaryotes has permitted the development of yeast cells carrying *HBs*/yeast chimeric plasmids that produce immunologically active HBsAg particles for the production of HBV vaccine. These recombinant yeasts produce unglycosylated HBsAg that aggregates to form 20 to 22 nm particles capable of eliciting a theoretically protective titer of anti-HBsAg antibodies in humans [27].

ANALYSIS OF HBV CORE GENE EXPRESSION IN HUMAN CELLS

NCI H292 cells stably carrying the pKYC200 plasmid (GTC2) were isolated by selection for the expression of the gpt^+ gene (Table I). The transfected genes have remained stably integrated after more than 30 passages of GTC2 cells in RPMI 1640 medium containing 10% fetal bovine serum (FBS) (HUT medium). The gpt^+ GTC2 cell line was used to test for the physical presence of the *HBc* gene and to ascertain the factors regulating the expression of the *HBc* gene. To detect the physical presence of pKYC200 sequences in GTC2 cells, high molecular weight DNA was isolated from cell nuclei for Southern blot analysis. GTC2 DNA was probed with pAM6 DNA after Bam HI/Hpa II or Gam HI/Msp I restriction enzyme digests to detect the presence of pKCY200 sequences in nuclear DNA. The pAM6 probe detected sequences between 0.9 and 10 kbp, and no hybridization to NCI H292 DNA was observed (Fig. 1). Hybridization analysis indicates that nuclear DNA from GTC2 cells contains sequences for pKYC200 after transfection and selection for the gpt^+ marker and that such cell lines may be mapped for gene-specific response to 5'-azacytidine treatment.

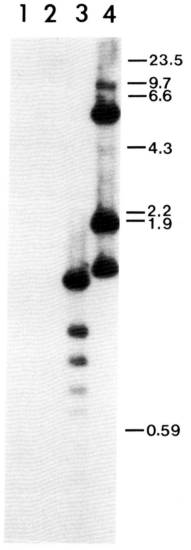

Fig. 1. Southern blot analysis of nuclear DNA from gpt$^+$ GTC2 cultures. Nuclei were isolated from gpt$^+$/HBc$^+$ GTC2 and NCI H292 cells, and high molecular weight DNA was purified for restriction digestion, electrophoresis, and hybridization with ^{32}P-labeled pAM6 DNA. The HBV probe revealed the presence of HBV sequences by hybridization to several bands ranging in size from 0.9 to 10.0 kbp. Lane 1 is Msp I/Bam HI and lane 2 Hpa II/Bam HI digests of parental DNA (NCI H292). Lane 3 is Msp I/Bam HI and lane 4 Hpa II/Bam HI digests of GTC2 DNA.

Treatment of GTC2 cells with 5'-azacytidine enhances production of HBcAg [4]. The cytotoxic effect of *HBc* induction in GTC2 cells causes an initial increase in HBcAg production at four to six divisions after cells are treated with 5'-azacytidine (primary culture, P_0). This increase reaches a maximum at approximately eight to ten divisions after treatment P_1 [8]. This long delay between 5'-azacytidine treatment and induced *HBc* gene expression [8, 28] suggested a mechanism involving a competitive interaction between remethylation and RNA synthesis by "activated" transcription complexes for access to the demethylated promoter region. Therefore, we initiated studies to determine the relative importance of demethylation at two specific sites relevant to the *HBc* gene [28]. The methylation status of an *Hpa*II site located in the promoter region of the *HBc* gene (HpaII^{-280}) can be resolved by determining the stoichiometric ratio of specific fragments after digestion, gel electrophoresis, and Southern hybridization [28]. Treatment with 5'-azacytidine decreases the degree of cytosine methylation at the HpaII^{-280} site as indicated by the loss of the 1,854 bp Bam HI-Hpa II and 975 bp Ava I-Hpa II fragments (Fig. 1; Table II). The twofold increase in the number of 1,683 bp BAM HI-Hpa II fragments that resulted from demethylation of the internal cytosine at HpaII^{-280} occurred when *HBc* gene expression was maximum (Table II; Fig. 2). The twofold increase in the number of Ava I-Hpa II fragments (866 to 868 bp) was also due to demethylation at HpaII^{-280}. The greater importance of HpaII^{-280} with respect to HpaII^{+479} is shown further by the small increase in the 759 bp fragment predicted by demethylation of both sites (Fig. 1). Hypomethylation at the HpaII^{+479} site was occasionally detected by these assays. However, methylation at HpaII^{+479} was variable in individual digests and random with respect to *HBc* gene expression, which indicates that methylation at HpaII^{+479} was not related to *HBc* gene expression.

Demethylation at the HpaII^{-280} site in the *HBc* gene promoter region was required for maximum production of HBcAg when GTC2 cells were cultured in L4-5S growth medium. The site-specific methylation pattern of GTC2 DNA was the same for cells subcultured in RPMI 1640 medium with 10% FBS (HUT medium) or LHC-

TABLE II. Measurement by Densitometry of Relative Amounts of GTC2 DNA Restriction Fragments*

Culture medium	Passage number[a]	P/N ratio	Relative amounts of Bam HI-Hpa II fragments (base pairs)				Sizes of Ava I-Hpa II fragments (base paris)			Total genomic 5'-methyl cytosine
			1,854	1,683	924 to 930	759	975	866 to 868	759	
HUT	NT	1.8 ± 0.2	43 ± 2	31 ± 1	22 ± 3	4 ± 1	61 ± 3	30 ± 2	9 ± 3	2.66 ± 0.17
L4-5S	NT	2.4 ± 0.2	41 ± 4	28 ± 3	22 ± 3	9 ± 1	57 ± 6	26 ± 5	17 ± 4	2.62 ± 0.13
L4-5S	P$_0$	2.7 ± 0.2	11 ± 3	53 ± 1	26 ± 3	10 ± 3	28 ± 4	49 ± 4	23 ± 1	0.45 ± 0.18
L4-5S	P$_1$	3.8 ± 0.5	4 ± 1	61 ± 6	19 ± 3	12 ± 4	8 ± 1	68 ± 2	24 ± 2	2.81 ± 0.20
L4-5S	P$_2$	2.0 ± 0.2	38	31	22	9	41	33	26	

*Southern hybridization autoradiographs were analyzed on a scanning-integrating densitometer (Beckman model Du-8). Relative areas (percent) are indicated for the different fragments generated by Bam HI-Hpa II or Ava I-Hpa II digestion of the 1,854 bp HBV fragment in GTC2 DNA. Values are the average (± SEM) of at least two measurements from two separate experiments. Statistical analysis was not possible for passage 2 after cells were treated with 5'-azacytidine because only two samples were used. The ratios of positive to negative (P/N) values for HBcAg was determined in sonicated cell extracts by radioimmunoassay [8]. A P/N ratio of 2.1 or greater is considered a positive response in the radioimmunoassay. Each passage represents approximately four to five cell divisions. P$_0$, primary (treated) culture; P$_1$, passage 1 (maximum HBcAg production); P$_2$, passage 2 (postcytotoxic response); NT, control cultures not treated with 5'-azacytidine. The total amount of 5'-methylcytosine in the genome after treatment of line GTC2 cells with 5'-azacytidine was determined as previously described [10].
[a]After treatment with 5 μM 5'-azacytidine.

4 medium [29] with 5% FBS (L4-5S medium) (Table II). Although hypomethylation of HpaII^{-280} increased *HBc* gene expression when cell cultures were grown in L4-5S medium, HUT medium did not support induced or basal levels of expression of the *HBc* gene after GTC2 cells were treated with 5'-azacytidine (Fig. 2) [8,28]. Steroid

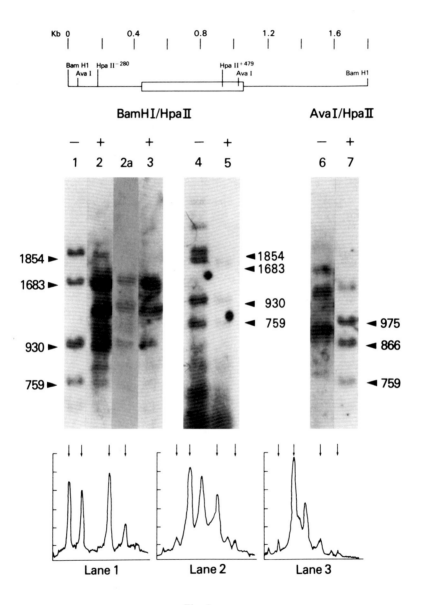

Fig. 2

hormones, growth factors, trace metals, and bovine pituitary extract were added to L4-5S medium but not to HUT medium [29].

To determine the temporal relationship of HpaII^{-280} demethylation to increased *HBc* gene transcription, whole cell RNA was extracted from GTC2 cells at various times after treatment with 5'-azacytidine and analyzed by hybridization to the 1,854 bp Bam HI HBV fragment (Fig. 2). The amount of 5'-methylcytosine in the genome of GTC2 DNA was measured [30] before cells were treated with 5'-azacytidine, at P_0, and at P_1 to determine overall changes in methylation during this experiment (Table II). The amount of 5'-methylcytosine was minimum at P_0 and returned to normal by P_1 (Table II), when site-specific demethylation at HpaII^{-280} and *HBc* gene expression were maximum (Table II; Fig. 2). The *HBc*-specific transcripts in extracts from GTC2 cells grown in HUT medium were nearly undetectable, which is consistent with the low amounts of HBcAg produced under this growth condition. GTC2 cells grown in L4-5S medium produced 30 times more *HBc*-specific transcripts. Treatment with 5'-azacytidine further increased the number of transcripts by a factor of about 5. Virtually no *HBc*-specific RNA was detected in postcytotoxic response cultures (P_2) or in cultures treated with 5'-azacytidine that were maintained in HUT medium (Fig. 2). Although the number of transcripts specifically derived from the *gpt* gene was about twice as high for cells grown in L4-5S medium as for those grown in HUT medium, 5'-azacytidine treatment did not appreciably increase (less than a factor of 2) the level of *gpt* gene transcription. This is consistent with other experiments, indicating that the SV40 early promoter is not induced by hypomethylation [31]. That cells must grow in L4-5S medium for gene expression to be induced by 5'-azacytidine indicates a nutritional or hormonal regulation *HBc* gene expression.

A mechanism for 5'-azacytidine induction by HpaII^{-280} hypomethylation of the *HBc* gene must take into account the following: 1) induction of *HBc* gene expression by 5'-azacytidine requires approximately six to ten cell divisions before reaching a maximum; 2) the cell death caused by treatment with 5'-azacytidine ends after the first passage of treated cultures; 3) the degree of cytosine methylation in the genome is lowest at P_0, and induced *HBc* gene expression is highest at P_1 when the overall degree of genomic methylation has returned to normal; and 4) more than 90% of

---

Fig. 2. Assay for site-specific demethylation of HBV DNA. GTC2 cultures were grown in HUT medium and plated ($\sim 10^4$ cells per cm^2) in HUT medium 24 hr before 5 μM 5'-azacytidine was added. After 24 hr, the treatment medium was replaced with L4-5S or HUT. Cells were subcultured at 6 to 7 day intervals (four to five cell divisions). DNA ($\sim$ 10 to 20 μg per lane) was digested with five- to tenfold excess of Hpa II and either Bam HI or Ava I (Boehringer Mannheim). The location of relevant sites for Hpa II maping of the 1,854 bp Bam HI fragment that contains the *HBc* gene from plasmid pKYC200 [8] is shown above the gel. The *HBc* gene-coding sequences are expanded to indicate the size relation of the gene to various products of digested GTC2 DNA. Southern hybridization analysis of GTC2 DNA was conducted with ^{32}P-labeled pAM6 probe DNA. The probe hybridized to GTC2 DNA digested with Bam HI-Hpa II (lanes 1 to 5) or with Ava I-Hpa II (lanes 6 and 7). Lanes 1, 4, and 6 contain DNA from GTC2 cells grown in L4-5S medium, and lanes 2, 3, 5, and 7 contain DNA from cells in parallel cultures treated with 5 μM 5'-azacytidine and grown for eight to ten divisions in L4-5S medium. The arrows indicate bands described above. Lanes 2 and 2a show the range of film exposures used to compare various bands by densitometric measurements; the 1,854 bp fragment can be measured at the exposure density for lane 2, but other bands are overexposed (lane 2a). Integrated areas under densitometric tracings (shown below the gel) similar to those in lanes 1 to 3 were used to determine the relative amount of DNA for the fragments listed in Table II. Molecular sizes for the bands are in kilobases.

GTC2 cells induced by 5′-azacytidine express HBcAg when induction of the *HBc* gene reaches a maximum, as shown by immunofluorescence [8]. The induction of a specific gene in 90% of the cells must involve an indirect mechanism, because a lethal dose of 5′-azacytidine would be required to demethylate simultaneously a single site in so large a portion of the cell population. If treatment with 5′-azacytidine is followed by a reduced capacity of the cell to methylate the $HpaII^{-280}$ site during the recovery of normal degrees of generalized methylation, the pattern of treatment, hypomethylation, and induction of the *HBc* gene expression would follow the sequence observed. This would occur if the initiation of activated transcription reduced the ability of the DNA cytosine methylase to maintain the methylation state at $HpaII^{-280}$ by exclusion.

HBV MOLECULAR BIOLOGY AND PATIENT STUDIES

The most readily available method for direct application of molecular biology methods to patient studies has been nucleic acid hybridization methods to detect viral sequences and transcripts in patients' tissues. The detection of HBV sequences in a variety of nonhepatic tissues from infected patients, including bone marrow [13], bile duct, endothelial, smooth muscle cells [32], placenta, kidney, and lymphocytes [13–17,33; Yoakum et al, manuscript in preparation], indicates that HBV infection involves cells with different embryonic origin and tissues of varied anatomical structure and function. These findings are striking since HBV was previously considered to be strictly an hepatotrophic virus with detectable virions in patients' sera [34–37] during viremia, and these results suggest widespread dissemination of the virus to include infection of nonhepatic tissues. The pathological consequences for chronically infected patients and the role played by infection of lymphocytes and placental tissues in disease transmission are important areas for investigation.

The presence of infective HBV in lymphocytes has been tested for in 109 people with chronic active hepatitis (CAH), four with AIDS, two with AIDS-related syndrome, and 36 control group persons, 16 of whom had serologically and clinically cleared the HBV infection, and 16 volunteers with no previous history of HBV infection (Yoakum et al, manuscript in preparation). The nucleic acids were isolated from the lymphocytes of these patients and analyzed by Southern hybridization of DNA and slot-blot analysis of lymphocyte RNA. Approximately one third of the CAH patients tested were positive for HBV DNA and RNA (Yoakum et al, unpublished results), and Southern hybridization analysis of CAH and AIDS patients indicates that HBV DNA is present in its intact replicative form detectable as discrete bands of DNA (Fig. 3).

DISCUSSION

HBc Gene Expression

The presence of replicative HBV in CAH and AIDS lymphocytes implicates the lymphocytes as a potential target cell that may quiescently harbor the virus and act as a reservoir for future cycles of active hepatitis infection and transmission of the disease. Regulation of the *HBc* gene may be critical to host cell viability because of the cytotoxicity of *HBc* gene expression. Although several HPC cell lines have been

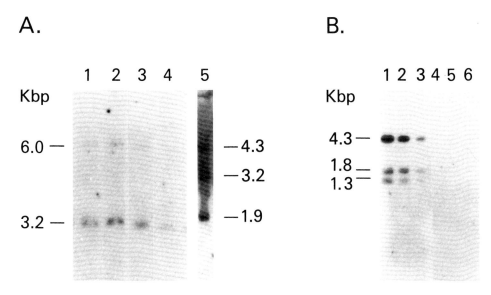

Fig. 3. A) Southern hybridization analysis of undigested lymphocyte DNA from AIDS patients (lanes 1 through 4) and from CAH patients (lane 5). B) Positive and negative control samples: Lanes 1 through 3 contain Bam HI-digested pAM6 DNA (this plasmid contains one complete copy of HBV DNA) loaded at 100 pg (lane 1), 30 pg (lane 2), and 3 pg (lane 3). Lane 4 contains 10 μg of undigested DNA from the lymphocytes of a volunteer with no history of HBV infection. Lane 5 contains 10 μg of undigested DNA from human lung lymph node tissue taken at autopsy. The tissue samples assayed in lanes 4–6 were from persons with no prior history of HBV infection.

isolated that carry multiple HBV genomic inserts, only PLC/PRF/5 and GTC2 cells treated with 5′-azacytidine grown in LHC-4 medium are known to express the *HBc* gene in vitro [28]. Hepatocellular carcinoma cells containing HBV express the *HBs* gene constitutively, producing the HBV surface antigen, HBsAg, without cytopathologic effects [18]. The sequences coding for HBcAg in PLC/PRF/5 cells are highly methylated, whereas HBV virion DNA and HBV DNA extracted from liver samples of infected patients are unmethylated [38]. The contrasting methylation pattern of the *HBc* gene in cells carrying HBV integrated as a provirus in the human genome and in HBV DNA extracted from virions and tissues of acutely infected patients suggests that methylation of HpaII^{-280} in the 5′-flanking region of the *HBc* gene may be important to the viability of host cells. Thus, host factors regulating *HBc* gene expression may have a pivotal role in establishing the intricacies of HBV host range and the variations in susceptibility that are related to nutrition, sex, age, and immunologic abnormalities.

Hypothesis of Hepatocellular Carcinogenesis

We have proposed that the preneoplastic and neoplastic hepatocytes attain resistance to mediators of cell distribution (thus having a survival advantage) and undergo proliferation during the repetitive cycles of the regenerative phase of CAH (Figs. 3, 4). This hypothesis of selective clonal cell expansion is consistent with

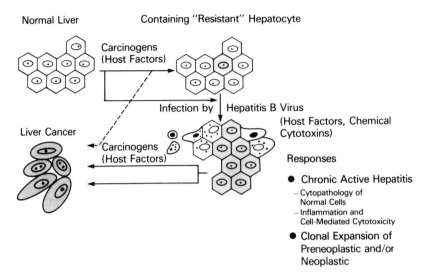

Fig. 4.   A hypothesis concerning the cocarcinogenicity of heptitis B virus in human liver carcinogenesis is schematically shown.

concepts derived from studies using animal models of liver carcinogenesis [39–42]. Following an initiating dose of a genotoxic agent, a "programmed" response is triggered, producing a cellular phenotype that has a survival-growth advantage, including resistance to the cytotoxicity of environmental chemicals and/or their metabolites and to the cytopathology related to HBV infection. This clone(s) of resistant cells expands in response to an endogenous proliferative factor(s) following partial hepatectomy and/or cell destruction of the nonresistant, normal cells by chemical and microbial toxins and by a host-mediated cytopathic response. In this context, CAH can be considered a "viral partial hepatectomy." The contributions of cytotoxicity used by mycotoxins (eg, aflatoxins from Aspergillus and trichothecene toxins from Fusarium) and/or alcoholic beverages and of subsequent liver regeneration may also be important, especially in patients with certain nutritional deficiencies.

What is the mechanism(s) for producing a resistant phenotype in CAH? Several possibilities seem plausible (Table III). The first general type of mechanism would be genetic control of the HBV genome integrated into PHC cells and their precursor cells. Methylation of the integrated HBV genome by the resistant hepatocytes could inhibit transcription of HBV mRNA and expression of HBV gene products, including those on the cell surface and those (eg, HBcAg) that may be cytotoxic [43]. This mechanism is compatible with data showing an inverse relationship between methylation level and expression of certain viral and nonviral genes. Recent studies using Alexander hepatocellular carconima cells and HBcAg gene transfected human cells have also shown that HBcAg expression is partly controlled by methylation [38,43]. Rearrangements of and mutations in the integrated HBV genome caused by exposure to chemical carcinogens are other genetic mechanisms that warrant investigation. PHC cells arising by these mechanisms would contain HBV genomic sequences in their DNA, but expression of the integrated HBV genome, especially the HBcAg gene, would be restricted, a predication that is consistent with the immunocytochem-

TABLE III. Putative Selective Clonal Expansion Factors in Human Liver Carcinogenesis*

Cell destruction mechanisms in nonneoplastic cells	Cell resistance mechanisms in preneoplastic and neoplastic cells
Lymphocyte-mediated cytotoxicity	Methylation of hepatitis B virus genome (eg, HBcAg gene)
Intracellular cytotoxicity by B core antigen	Rearrangement of hepatitis B genome
Environmental chemical "cytotoxins"	Mutations caused by chemical carcinogens in the integrated hepatitis B virus genome
Mycotoxins (eg, aflatoxins, trichotecenes)	Noninfectivity of the hepatocytes by hepatitis B virus (eg, receptor modification)
Alcoholic beverages	Restricted replication of proviral hepatitis B virus
Others	Increased detoxification of environmental chemical "cytotoxins"

*Nutritional, hormonal, and inherited host factors may play important roles.

ical observations demonstrating a reduction in HBsAg and HBcAg in dysplastic and neoplastic hepatocytes.

Because not all PHC contain integrated HBV sequences, we also propose a second general mechanism in which resistance to the cytopathological effects of HBV infection would be due to "noninfectivity" of and/or restriction of proviral replication in the carcinogen-altered hepatocytes. For example, the presumed membrane receptor for HBV could be blocked by HBsAG or modified by other mechanisms. In addition, restriction by a putative repressor protein of HBV replication and/or integration into the host cell DNA could be envisioned as mechanisms. One would also predict that attempts to infect these hepatocellular carcinoma cells with HBV in vitro would be unsuccessful.

This multifactoral hypothesis can be directly tested both in the duck [39] and woodchuck models of liver carcinogenesis [40] and in models using cultured and xenotransplated human hepatocytes [39,46,48]. Restriction enzyme analysis of the hepatitis B virus genome integrated into the DNA of three human hepatocellular carcinoma cell lines has revealed that the hepatitis B virus core antigen gene is partially or completely deleted. This finding is consistent with the proposed model described above.

REFERENCES

1. Gust I: In Szmuness W, Alter HJ, Maynarn JE (eds): "Viral Hepatitis." Philadelphia: Franklin Institute Press, 1982, pp 129–143.
2. Blumberg BS, London WT: N Engl J Med 304:782–784, 1981.
3. Harris CC, Sun T-T: Carcinogenesis 5:697–701, 1984.
4. Gerin JL: In Chisari FV (ed): "Advances in Hepatitis Research." New York: Masson Publishing USA, Inc., 1984, pp 40–48.
5. Popper H, Shih JWK, Gerin JL, Wong DC, Hoyer BH, London WT, Sly DL, Purcell RH: Hepatology 1:91–98, 1981.
6. Ponzetto A, Cote PJ, Ford EC, Engle R, Cicmanec J, Shapiro M, Purcell RH, Gerin JL: Virus Res 2:301–315, 1985.
7. Robinson WS, Marion P, Feitelson M, Siddiqui A: In Szmuness W, Alter HJ, Maynard JE (eds): "Viral Hepatitis." Philadelphia: Franklin Institute Press, 1982, pp 57–68.
8. Yoakum GH, Korba BE, Lechner JF, Tokiwa T, Gazdar AF, Seeley T, Siegel M, Leeman L, Autrup H, Harris CC: Science 222:385–389, 1983.

9. Yoakum GH: Biotechniques 2:24–30, 1984.

10. Lechner JF, Hangen A, McClendon IA, Pettis EW: In Vitro 18:633–642, 1982.

11. Leffert HL, Koch KS, Skelly H: In Barnes DW, Sirbasku DA, Sato GH (eds): "Methods for Serum-Free Culture of Epithelial and Fibroblastic Cells." New York: Alan R. Liss, Inc., 1984, pp 43–55.

12. Southern EM: J Mol Biol 98:503–510, 1975.

13. Romet-Lemonne JL, Elfassi E, Haseltine W, Essex M: Lancet 2:732, 1983.

14. Romet-Lemonne JL, McLane MF, Elfassi E, Haseltine W, Azocar J, Essex M: Science 221:667–669, 1983.

15. Lie-Injo LE, Balasegaram M, Lopez CG, Herrera AR: DNA 2:301–308, 1983.

16. Pontisso P, Poon MC, Tiollais P, Brechot C: Br Med J 288:1563–1566, 1984.

17. Chong-Jim O, Jenk-Ling D: Lancet 3:395–396, 1984.

18. Cattaneo R, Will N, Hernandez N, Schaller H: Nature 305:336–338, 1983.

19. McAleer WJ, Buynak EB, Maigetter RZ, et al: Nature 307:178–180, 1984.

20. Burrell CJ, Gowans EJ, Rowland R, et al: Hepatology 4:20–243, 1984.

21. Moriarity AK, Hoyer BH, Wai-Keu Shih J, et al: Proc Natl Acad Sci USA 78(4):2606–2610, 1981.

22. Burrell CJ, MacKay P, Greenway PH, et al: Nature 279:43–47, 1979.

23. Snisky JJ, Siddiqui A, Robinson WS, Cohen SN: Nature 279:346–348, 1979.

24. Valenzuela P, Gray P, Quiroga M, et al: Nature 280:815–819, 1979.

25. Charnay P, Pourcel C, Louise A, et al: Proc Natl Acad Sci USA 76(5):2222–2226, 1979.

26. Fujiyama A, Miyanohara A, Nozaki C, et al: Nucleic Acids Res 11:4601–4610, 1983.

27. Scolnick EM, McLean AA, West DJ, et al: JAMA 251:2812–2815, 1984.

28. Korba BE, Wilson VL, Yoakum GH: Science 228:1103–1105, 1985.

29. Lechner JF, McClendon IA, LaVeck MA, et al: Cancer Res 43:5915–5922, 1983.

30. Wilson VL, Jones PA: Cell 32:239–246, 1983.

31. Graessmann M, et al: Proc Natl Acad Sci USA 80:6470–6474, 1983.

32. Blum HE, Stowring L, Figus A, Montgomery CK, Haase AT, Vyas GN: Proc Natl Acad Sci USA 80:6682–6685, 1983.

33. Laure F, Zagury D, Saimot AG, et al: Science 229:561–563, 1985.

34. Bonino F, Hoyer B, Nelson J, et al: Hepatology 1:386–391, 1981.

35. Weller IVD, Fowler MJF, Monjardino J, Thomas HC: J Med Virol 9(4):273–280, 1982.

36. Beringer M, Hamer M, Hoyer B, Gerin JL: J Med Virol 9(1):57–68, 1982.

37. Kam W, Rall LB, Smuckler EA, Schmid R, Rutter WJ: Proc Natl Acad Sci USA 79:7522–7526, 1982.

38. Miller RA, Robinson WS: Proc Natl Acad Sci USA 80:2534–2538, 1983.

39. Sun T, Wang N: In Harris CC, Autrup H (eds): "Human Carcinogenesis." New York: Academic Press, 1983, pp 757–780.

40. Snyder RL, Tyler G, Summers J: Am J Pathol 107:422–425, 1980.

41. Popper H, Gerber MA, Thung SN: Hepatology 2:1S–9S, 1982.

42. Finkelstein SD, Lee G, Medline A, Tatematsu M, Makowka L, Farber E: Am J Pathol 110:119–126, 1983.

43. Yoakum GH, Korba BE, Lechner JF, Tokiwa T, Gazdar AF, Seeley T, Siegel M, Leeman L, Autrup H, Harris CC: Science 222:385–388, 1984.

44. Ehrlich M, Wang RYH: Science 212:1350–1357, 1981.

45. Miller RH, Robinson WS: Proc Natl Acad Sci USA 80:2534–2538, 1983.

46. Strom SC, Jirtle RL, Jones RS, Novicki DL, Rosenberg MR, Novotny A, Irons G, McLain JR, Michalopoulos G: JNCI 68:771, 1982.

47. Michalopoulos G, Strom SC, Novotony AR, Novicki DL, Jirtle RL: In Webber MM, Sekeley L (eds): "In Vitro Models for Cancer Research." New York: CRC Press, Vol 2 (in press).

48. Koike K, Kobayashi M, Mizusawa H, Yoshida E, Yaginuma K, Taira M: Nucleic Acids Res 11:5391–5402, 1983.

Biochemical and Molecular Epidemiology of Cancer 283–292 (1986)

Strategies and Current Trends of Etiologic Prevention of Liver Cancer

Sun Tsung-tang, Chu Yuan-rong, Hsia Chu-chieh, Wei Yao-peng, and Wu Shao-ming

Cancer Institute, Chinese Academy of Medical Sciences, Beijing, (S.T.-t., H.C.-c., W.S.-m.) and Qidong Liver Cancer Institute, Jiangsu Province, (C.Y.-r., W.Y.-p.), China

Primary hepatocellular carcinoma (PHC), the major primary malignancy of the liver, is among the top 10 most common cancers in the world [1]. It constitutes a global health issue when the closely associated HBV-linked chronic hepatitis is also taken into consideration [2,3]. Although surgical intervention at the asymptomatic stage through early detection among peoples at high risk may significantly increase the survival rate [4], etiologic prevention, aiming at the control of causative factors, should constitute the key approach to the ultimate control of liver cancer and the underlying chronic hepatitis [2,3]. Current efforts have successfully identified HBV and aflatoxins to be the most probable etiologic agents of liver cancer; accordingly, preventive strategy based on vaccination and also on control of mycotoxin exposure have been formulated, especially for people at increased risk [2,3]. In the present article, strategic considerations and rationale of conducting early, universal immunization of newborns in areas of liver cancer prevalence will be presented with some preliminary results of a pilot study in this direction. In addition, the recent development of techniques that permit the determination of individual aflatoxin exposure for field monitoring will also be updated in the direction of fascilitating longitudinal studies, which may give conclusive evidence on the carcinogenic role of aflatoxins among people at high risk to subsequent development of liver cancer.

PREVENTIVE APPROACH TO PHC THROUGH UNIVERSAL IMMUNIZATION OF NEWBORNS

Prospective epidemiologic studies have consistently demonstrated that there is a very high risk for hepatocellular carcinoma to occur with the HBsAg carrier state [5–7]. Such studies strongly indicate the causal relationship of HBV and liver cancer. HBV is thus considered to be second (to tobacco [cigarette smoking]) among the

Received June 7, 1985.

© **1986 Alan R. Liss, Inc.**

known human carcinogens [2]. At present, the only practical way of achieving widespread effective control of HBV infection is active immunization. No effective means to terminate chronic carrier state are available or are expected in the near future. It is logical to consider the possibility of using immunization against HBV infection to achieve the goal of PHC as well as HBV-linked chronic liver disease prevention. Since newborn infants are known to respond quite well to polypeptide immunogens such as HBV vaccines [2,8, Chu et al, manuscript in preparation], immunization at an earlier age is desirable to achieve a higher protection rate.

Since the target population to receive immunization against HBV infection will be newborns in areas of endemicity, the impact on liver cancer incidence will become evident 30 to 35 years after the start of a vaccination study on a reasonable scale. This expectation is based on the assumption that close association of HBV with PHC, which has been prospectively observed mainly [7] or exclusively [5,6] among middle-aged persons, can be extended to the younger age groups. Such extrapolation may not be correct. In accordance with the multifactorial origin of liver cancer, hepatocarcinogenesis at earlier ages may be the result of overexposure to chemical carcinogens, such as mycotoxins. A clear answer to the question raised above is important both for the rational design of prevention studies and also for a better understanding of the carcinogenic process of human liver cancer.

For these purposes, a consecutive series of 55 pathologically diagnosed PHC patients below the age of 30 from areas of prevalence was carefully studied through an immunohistological approach for HBsAg as a marker of HBV infection. The pathological features of these hepatomas were found to be quite similar to those seen in older patients. PAP immunochemical staining using two independent diagnostic kits for HBsAg demonstrated clear-cut and consistent findings that 96% (53/55) of these young patients were HBV infected; HBsAg was demonstrated in the cytoplasm of noncancerous hepatocytes. Its distribution in cytoplasm may be diffuse, peripheral, or in the form of inclusion bodies. In 10 cases of young PHC patients of similar ages from the Beijing area, eight were found to be positive for HBsAg following parallel staining. These data (Table I, Fig. 1) proved that there was very close association of PHC with HBV infection among young patients from areas of high and lower incidence [9]. Even though aflatoxin exposure was known to be significantly increased among local inhabitants in an area of liver cancer prevalence [3,10], liver cancer was rarely seen among noncarriers below 30 years of age, who constitute about 85% of the young population. The incidence of liver cancer among them is below 1 per 10^5 per annum. If immunization can greatly reduce HBV infection in the population vaccinated, its impact on liver cancer incidence will most likely include the young

TABLE I. HBV Status and Liver Disease Background of PHC Patients Under 30 Years of Age in a High Incidence Area*

	Percentage
Chronic hepatitis	100 (55/55)
Cirrhosis	53 (29/55)
HBsAg in hepatocytes	96 (53/55)

*This is a consecutive series of pathologically diagnosed young PHC patients in Qidong County, China. The presence of HBsAg in hepatocyte cytoplasm was identified by PAP immunostaining technique. Adapted from Xia et al [9].

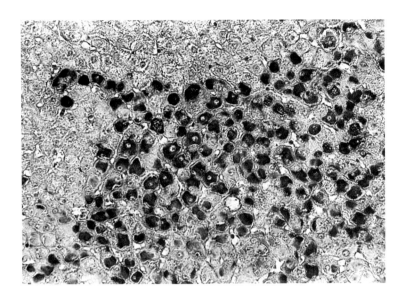

Fig. 1. HBsAg in hepatocytes of noncancerous liver tissue from a young PHC patient. Cytoplasmic HBsAg, inclusion type, demonstrated by PAP immunohistochemical technique. Section counterstained by hematoxylin and eosin. ×200.

generation and be observed within 30 to 35 years, provided the study groups are of sufficient scale.

The same study on young PHC patients also demonstrated that all had chronic liver disease. As shown in Table I, 100% (55/55) got chronic hepatitis, and about two thirds of them (40/55) had chronic active manifestations, diagnosed on pathological criteria (Fig. 2). The pictures of varying degrees of liver cell necrosis, inflammatory cell infiltration, and hyperplasia were quite similar to those observed previously among early PHC patients, mostly over 35 years of age [11]. However, cirrhosis occurred less often in the young patients. This fact indicates that cirrhosis per se is not directly related to the carcinogenic process and is the tissue reaction gradually accumulated in response to the damage of hepatocytes. It is the persistent though usually fluctuating process of liver cell damage and regeneration that plays an important role in hepatocarcinogenesis. The long process of hepatic pathology development was found to be closely associated with serological expression of transaminase abnormalities and α-fetoprotein elevations, reflecting liver cell damage and regeneration [1,2]. The invariable occurrence of chronic hepatitis as a premalignant stage constitutes the medical basis for selecting the reduction of HBV-related chronic liver disease with serological manifestations characterized above as the medium term endpoint of the effectiveness of the vaccination program. This will shorten the observation period of such a long program from 30 years or more to about 10 years. This endpoint, if achieved, will have two important implications: First, it reflects the control of a serious disease, which is at least 10 times more frequent than liver cancer per se. Second, it is a reliable indicator of a subsequent fall in the rate of liver cancer in the vaccinated generation, because our observations on hundreds of PHC patients

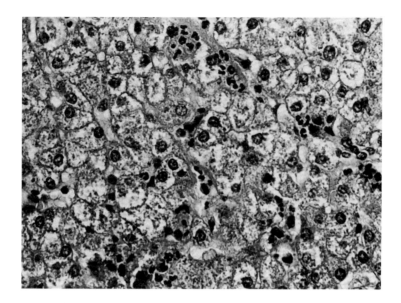

Fig. 2. Chronic active hepatitis in a 15-year-old PHC patient. Focal necrosis, inflammatory cell infiltration, and balooning degeneration of hepatocytes were seen in the hematoxylin and eosin-stained section. ×200.

demonstrated the fact that if there is no underlying chronic hepatitis then there is virtually no hepatoma [13].

Universal immunization will certainly provide the most effective and widespread protection against HBV among the population. However, HBV vaccines at present are still very expensive and not easily available. Before the advent of a DNA recombinant vaccine, public concern about the possibility of introducing extraneous infectious agents and proteins from plasma-derived sources should be considered. We need scientific rationale on the basis of which decisions can be made to adopt either universal immunization or selective vaccination of e antigen-positive mothers' children, who are known to be at highly risk to become carriers [14,15].

To resolve this issue, 121 pairs of randomly selected mothers and their children of 3 to 4 years of age were tested for their HBV infection status. They are natural inhabitants of Qidong County, China, known to have a high incidence rate of liver cancer. All assays were performed by using solid phase radioimmunoassays with reference standards of either HBsAg or anti-HBs quantitated at the same time in each experiment. The main results are shown in Tables II and III (Chu and Sun, unpublished data). Qidong County is an endemic area of HBV infection. Eighty-five percent of these young mothers, mostly around 25 years of age, had clearly measurable levels of either HBsAg or anti-HBs, indicating a high infection rate among the young female adults. Using similar indicators, 41% of their young children had already been infected. If additional markers were used, the percentage may further increase. It should be noted that the children (ages of 3 to 4 years) had 15.7% positively rate of serum HBsAg, already attaining the level of their mothers. These data clearly demonstrate that HBV infection occurs at early ages among the local people of a high incidence area. Analysis of the infection status of the 19 HBsAg-positive children's

TABLE II. HBV Infection Status of Mothers and Their Children in a PHC High Incidence Area*

	Percentage	
	Mothers	Children
Positivity rate of serum HBsAg	16.5 (20/121)	15.7 (19/121)
Serum anti-HBs over 10 mIU/ml	68.3 (41/60)	25.0 (15/60)

*One hundred twenty-one mothers were randomly selected from Qidong County, China. Children were 3 to 4 years old. RIA were done using Abbotts kits at detectability levels of 0.5 BU/ml for HBsAg and 5 mIU/ml for anti-HBs in serum (Chu and Sun, unpublished data).

TABLE III. Infection Status of Mothers Whose Young Children Were HBsAg Positive*

Status		
Children	Mothers	Percentage
HBsAg positive	Carriers	26.3 (5/19)
HBsAg positive	Noncarriers	73.7 (14/19)

*Experimental conditions were similar to those in Table II. Approximately 73.7% HBsAg-positive children were born by noncarrier mothers (Chu and Sun, unpublished data).

mothers showed that more than two thirds of the surface antigen-positive children came from noncarrier mothers. These data demonstrate that early horizontal transmission is the major mode of transmission of HBV infection in the population. This is also consistent with the data on the antigen positivity rate of young pregnant women. This was found to be around 4% of a relatively large series of mothers as measured by sensitive radioimmunoassays [Sun et al, manuscript in preparation]. There is no doubt that children from e antigen-positive mothers are at high risk of HBV infection, and selective immunization of such an infant group is logical either in a population with a very low carrier rate or in a population with a higher incidence but limited availability of vaccines. To achieve maximum protection of the population from HBV infection and to permit evaluation of impact on incidence rates of liver cancer and chronic hepatitis in areas of prevalence, the strategy of universal immunization by HBV vaccines of all newborns soon after delivery should be adopted to control the major early horizontal mode of transmitting HBV infection.

Implementation of such a strategic approach requires a large amount of investment to obtain sufficient quantities of qualified vaccines, which are still expensive and limited in availability. This poses an economic problem in the developing countries, many of which are prevalent in HBV infection and liver cancer. To alleviate the economic pressure of implementing a vaccination program on the basis of universal immunization, the possibility of using HBV vaccines at reduced doses should be explored. Although the usual dosage of vaccine in recommended regimens have been proven to be very effective in adults [16], in children [17], and also in newborns [18], they were based on empirical observations rather than on more rigid dose-response relationships in different age groups. Therefore, the possibility exists that vaccine dosages at significantly lower levels might still be located in the plateau region of the response curve, whereas the small amount of impurities in the vaccine preparation might be brought to the zone of very low response. The latter point deserves consideration too because a vaccination program against HBV infection might cover a very large number of people, and new generations may constitute the target population.

To address the issue mentioned above, a medium scale trial of universal immunizations of newborns with low dosages of HBV vaccine was done in Qidong County, China in September 1983. The vaccine used was HBVax, donated by Merck, Sharp & Dohme. Four groups of approximately 400 infants in each had received either 5 or 2.5 μg vaccine per shot in the usual three dose regimen given at 0, 1, and 6 months after delivery, with or without additional HBIG given soon after delivery to those born by carrier mothers. The detailed results of Sun et al will be published elsewhere. Some of the relevant data will be cited here.

This pilot study covers a defined natural population of 214,343 rural people of the endemic Qidong County. All newborns in several small townships were vaccinated within 30 min after birth. Over 95% of all newborns in the study period in the defined population were vaccinated and followed. Allocations to different protocols of immunization including a control group of similar size, were decided by drawing lots to insure randomization on a community level and to select a control group fairly when there was a limited supply of vaccine.

By using RIA kits made by Abbotts, the HBV infection status of mothers of different groups, including the control, were found to be quite close. Their carrier rate centered around 14%, and their e antigen positivity rate was about 4% of the population tested. Serum assays performed at 6.5 months after birth, 2 weeks after the third dose of vaccine, showed that there was a significant fall of the HBsAg positivity rate among all the vaccinee groups, being around 1.5% in contrast to the 7.7% level of the control. A protection rate of 80% at the 6 month period was achieved among infants receiving either 5 or 2.5 μg of HBVax in the three dose regimen. The antibody levels against surface antigen were also found to be significantly raised in the vaccinee groups. Eighty percent or more of the vaccinees at the 6 month period had serum anti-HBs exceeding the value of 20 m IU/ml. The 6 month data of this pilot study appear to be encouraging; however, only results after longer periods of observation will determine whether a low dose approach will provide levels of protection comparable to the conventional regimens.

The pilot study will provide rationale for designing and implementing a subsequent large-scale vaccination study program to address the critical question: Can vaccination against HBV prevent liver cancer? If the answer is yes, then two major conclusions can be drawn. One is theoretical, which says that HBV is definitely the major causative agent of liver cancer. The second is a pragmatic one, which says that vaccination offers the best way to control liver cancer. However, if the answer is no, we cannot exclude the etiologic role of HBV in hepatocarcinogenesis. This is because a small percentage of newborn vaccinees may be refractory to immunizations as a result of either very early infection or some inherent susceptibility to HBV infection, such as low immunologic responsiveness to this virus. Such infants have already been observed in the pilot study mentioned. This percentage is small compared to the general population but large enough to exceed the number of candidates to develop liver cancer. If because of some unknown mechanisms these carriers are especially at risk to develop PHC, the carrier rate but not the incidence rate of liver cancer will significantly be reduced following the immunization program. Therefore, it is necessary to conduct a well-designed vaccination study to give the final answer. It is worthwhile to stress again that PHC occurred invariably in the background of chronic hepatitis (mostly HBV linked) patients of all age groups. A significant reduction of the morbidity rate of chronic hepatitis among the vaccinees will reliably predict the significant fall in the incidence rate of liver cancer in the future.

PROSPECTIVE STUDY ON THE HEPATOCARCINOGENIC ROLE OF AFLATOXIN THROUGH INDIVIDUAL MONITORING

Aflatoxin has long been implicated as an important human hepatocarcinogen mainly on the basis of epidemiologic studies of correlations between the amount of aflatoxin in the ingested food and the liver cancer rate in the areas studied [19]. Further progress requires the conduction of longitudinal studies, which can provide conclusive evidence to establish aflatoxin as a human carcinogen. This process had been impeded because of the lack of tests suitable for measuring individual exposure to aflatoxin [20]. The recent use of antibodies for concentration and immunoassay, which made possible the measurement of short-term individual exposure to aflatoxin, has promoted the conduction of such prospective studies. Studies along this direction on aflatoxins will be briefly summarized and updated.

Development of immunoassay techniques for aflatoxin B_1 and M_1 provided simple and sensitive methods for their measurement [21,22]. However, these tests are also sensitive to nonspecific interference when biological samples are analyzed. Such background noise practically limits the potential increase of sensitivity. Immunoconcentration through the use of small affinity columns coupled with polyclonal or monoclonal antibodies against B_1 or M_1 can specifically concentrate aflatoxins and greatly increase the signal to noise ratio of the detected samples [23]. Thus, aflatoxin M_1 at a level of 1 pg/ml in a 24 hr urine specimen can be detected [10].

Using affinity columns possessing broad spectrum reactivity against various aflatoxins, including their metabolites, it was found that M_1 (AFM_1) in free form is the major metabolite stably excreted in human urine following increased exposure (Fig. 3). In case of drinking contaminated alcoholic beverages, 1.5 to 4% of ingested AFB_1 was converted into AFM_1 in the first 24 hr urine. AFM_1 in urine quickly fell

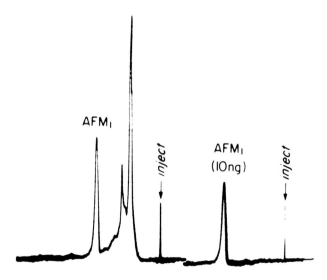

Fig. 3. HPLC profile of AFM_1 in a 24-hr urine sample from a healthy Qidong inhabitant. Urine was first concentrated 1,000-fold by affinity column. HPLC column: c18 u-Bondapak; mobile phase: 50% methanol in water; flow rate: 0.8 ml/min; fluorescence detector: Spectro-Glo of Gilsons. In wet seasons, the output may be 10-fold or more.

below the limit of detection (below 1 pg/ml) within 3 days after the removal of either contaminated rice or beverage. Therefore, urinary AFM_1 can be regarded as a chemical dosimetric indicator quantitatively reflecting short-term individual exposure to ingested aflatoxins [24].

Using urinary AFM_1 as an indicator of individual exposure, it was found recently that in high incidence areas of liver cancer, exposure to aflatoxin was significantly higher than in areas of lower risk [10]. The major source of contamination was corn or rice, especially corn. Local alcoholic beverages also contribute some, but to a much lesser extent. If 2% was chosen to be the conversion ratio of AFM_1 from AFB_1, probably 10% of the local inhabitants had a cumulative dose of aflatoxin exposure exceeding 1 mg/year per individual [10]. These observations were confirmed by subsequent extended studies, the results of which are shown in Table IV. Although the cumulative exposure calculated was not so high as to reach the level of inducing liver cancer in monkeys by aflatoxin alone [25], such exposure may cause profound changes in hepatocytes, whose turnover was greatly increased in the long pathologic process of chronic active hepatitis [3].

Qualitative and quantitative needs from field studies for antibodies against major members of aflatoxins promoted the establishment of monoclonals that have high affinity toward aflatoxins of special interest. AW_1 was the first monoclonal antibody developed that avidly bound AFB_1 [23]. Affinity columns coupled with AW_1 effectively concentrated AFB_1 directly from contaminated alcoholic beverages as well as from simple extracts of rice and corns [23,24]. Recently, a monoclonal of relatively high affinity toward AFM_1, AW11, was cloned. It was successfully used in radioimmunoassay of AFM_1 using tritiated AFB_1 as the labeled antigen and also in immunoconcentration of AFM_1 in human urine [Sun et al, manuscript in preparation]. In addition, several other monoclonals were developed with different spectrums of reactivity. The battery of monoclonals so far developed against aflatoxins seems to meet the demand for field monitoring of short-term individual exposure to the relevant carcinogen. In the meantime, the immunoassay technique was also refined to make it simple, sensitive, and suitable for field use [26].

The presently available technical system described above for measuring individual exposure to aflatoxins has fascilitated the implementation of prospective studies on high risk people, aiming at relating cumulative individual exposure to subsequent risk of PHC. The carcinogenic role of aflatoxin can thus be clearly defined. Such studies have been started or actively planned in China [3] and in other Asian and African countries [20]. In addition to these studies, the currently planned PHC prevention trial in which large scale vaccination against HBV infection will be carried

TABLE IV. Urinary Excretion of AFM_1 From People at Different Risk to PHC*

	Percentage	
	Over 5 ng per 24 hr	Over 10 ng per 24 hr
Beijing, normal	0 (0/24)	0 (0/24)
Qidong, normal	23 (9/40)	18 (7/40)
Qidong, CAH[a]	42 (28/66)	27 (18/66)

*Twenty-four hour urine was first concentrated by affinity column and then analyzed by HPLC and RIA parallelly [Wu and Sun, unpublished data].
[a]CAH chronic active hepatitis patients.

out, as presented in the first section of this paper, would be strengthened if aflatoxin monitoring studies are included concurrently to determine the possible contribution of aflatoxin exposure to the overall incidence of PHC in the target population of these expensive trials [20].

A trial of prevention through vaccination, aimed at identifying HBV as the main causative agent and immunization as the main control measure, a longitudinal study through aflatoxin monitoring, aimed at identifying AFB_1 as an important carcinogen, and the search for ways to reduce AFB_1 exposure constitute the major trends of current research on the etiology of human PHC. Probably 10 years will be needed for such studies to reach some important conclusions. The sharper the focus on causative factors of a human cancer, the better orientated will be the research on the mechanisms of its carcinogenesis. Human hepatocellular carcinoma is obviously such an example.

ACKNOWLEDGMENTS

This work was supported by the Ministry of Health of the Peoples Republic of China, the Cancer Research Institute of New York City, and the Cancer Unit of WHO Geneva.

REFERENCES

1. Muir C, Stazewski J: In Curtis C. Harris (ed): "Biochemical and Molecular Epidemiology of Cancer." New York: Alan R. Liss, Inc., (this volume).
2. "Prevention of Liver Cancer." World Health Organization Technical Report Series 691. Geneva: World Health Organization, 1983.
3. Sun T, Chu Y: J Cell Physiol Suppl 3:39, 1984.
4. Sun T, Huang X: In Mirand EA, Hutchinson WB, Mihich E (eds): "13th International Cancer Congress, Part D: Research and Treatment." New York: Alan R. Liss, Inc., 1983, pp 57–66.
5. Beasley RP, Hwang LY, Lin CC, Chien CS: Lancet 2:1129, 1981.
6. Sakuma K, Takahara T, Okuda K, Tsuda F, Mayumi M: Gastroenterology 83:114, 1982.
7. Lu J, Li W, Qin C, Nee C, Huang F: Chin J Oncol 5:406, 1983.
8. Huang LY, Beasley RP, Lee GC, Lan CC, Roan CH, Huang FY, Cheng CL: "1984 International Symposium on Viral Hepatitis." San Francisco, Abstract 9A/6, New York: Grunne and Stratton, 1984.
9. Xia Q, Wang N, Li T, Shao L, Li Y, Zhang S, Sun Z(T): Chin J Oncol 6:413, 1984.
10. Wu S, Sun Z(T), Wei Y, Ku G, Lu Z, Liu G: Chin J Oncol 6:163, 1984.
11. Sun Z(T), Chu Y, Wang L, Xia Q, Zhang Y: In Essex M, Todaro G, zur Hausen H (eds): "Viruses in Naturally Occurring Cancer." Cold Spring Harbor, NY: Cold Spring Harbor Laboratory, 1980, pp 471–480.
12. Harris CC, Sun T: Carcinogenesis 5:697, 1984.
13. Sun T, Wang N: In Harris CC, Autrup H: "Human Carcinogenesis." New York: Academic Press, 1983, pp 753–776.
14. Stevens CE, Beasley RP, Tsui J, Lee WC: N Engl J Med 292:771, 1975.
15. Okada K, Yamada T, Miyakawa Y, Mayumi M: J Pediatr 87:360, 1975.
16. Szmuness W, Stevens CE, Harley EJ, Zang EA, Oleszko WR, William DC, Sadovsky R, Morrison JM, Keller A: N Engl J Med 303:833, 1980.
17. Maupas P, Chiron JP, Barin F, Coursaget P, Gordeau A, Perrin J, Denis F, Diop Mar I: Lancet 1:288, 1981.
18. Deinhardt F, Gust ID: Bull WHO 60:661, 1982.
19. Linsell CA, Peers FG: In Hiatt HH, Watson JD, Winsten JA (eds): "Origin of Human Cancer, Book A." Cold Spring Harbor, NY: Cold Spring Harbor Laboratory, 1976, pp. 549–556.
20. Garner C, Ryder R, Montesano R: Cancer Res 45:922, 1985.

21. Langone JJ, Vunakis HV: JNCI 56:591, 1976.
22. Chu FS, Ueno I: Appl Environ Microsc 33:1125, 1977.
23. Sun Z(T), Wu Y, Wu S: Chin J Oncol 5:401, 1983.
24. Sun Z(T), Wu S, Wu Y: Acta Acad Med Sinicae 5:344, 1983.
25. Sieber SM, Adamson RH: In Chandra P (ed): "Antiviral Mechanism in the Control of Neoplasm." New York: Plenum, 1978, pp 455–480.
26. Martin CN, Garner RC, Tursi F, Garner JV, Whittle HC, Ryder R, Sizaret P: In Berlin A, Draper M, Hemminki K (eds): "Monitoring Human Exposure to Carcinogenic and Mutagenic Agents." Lyon: IARC Scientific Publications No.59, (in press).

Biochemical and Molecular Epidemiology of Cancer 293–301 (1986)

HTLV: The Family of Human T Lymphotropic Retroviruses and Their Role in Leukemia and AIDS

Marjorie Robert-Guroff and Robert C. Gallo

Laboratory of Tumor Cell Biology, National Cancer Institute, Bethesda, Maryland 20205

In 1980, the isolation of the first human retrovirus from cells of a patient with an aggressive malignancy of mature T cells was reported [1]. This virus was first termed the *human T-cell leukemia/lymphoma virus* (HTLV) and was to become the prototype virus (HTLV-I) of a larger family of human T-lymphotropic retroviruses. Since the publication of that finding, numerous isolations of HTLV-I have been made and the closely related viruses HTLV-II and HTLV-III have been discovered [2–4]. The purpose of this chapter is to describe this HTLV family and the larger "super-family" of similar viruses within the animal kingdom and to outline the current status of our knowledge concerning the disease associations of the viruses and the biologic and biochemical mechanisms involved in their interaction with host cells and in their induction of disease.

THE FAMILY OF HTLV AND THE SUPER-FAMILY OF RELATED VIRUSES

At the present time, the HTLV family consists of the three subtypes mentioned above. Within these subgroups, variants exist but in general do not exhibit sufficient differences to be distinguished immunologically from each other. The characteristics that these viruses share and their significant differences are summarized in Table I. It is clear that HTLV-I and HTLV-II are more like each other than they are to HTLV-III; however, the latter family member shares numerous structural, biochemical, genetic, and biological properties in common with HTLV-I and HTLV-II and, most importantly, the human host. It has become apparent that HTLV family members can also be grouped together with certain animal retroviruses by these same criteria. Figure 1 illustrates the grouping of this "super-family" of related retroviruses. Several important points can be made. The most unusual feature these viruses have in common is the property of *trans*-acting transcriptional (TAT) activation [5,6], a function of extra coding sequences within each virus not including the *gag*, *pol*, and

Received September 25, 1985.

© **1986 Alan R. Liss, Inc.**

TABLE I. Similarities Between HTLV-I, HTLV-II, and HTLV-III

Evolutionary features
  1. Relationship to simian retroviruses (STLV-I, STLV-III) in Old World Monkeys
  2. Presumed origin in Africa
Biological features
  1. Are human exogenous retroviruses
  2. Are lymphotropic, with particular affinity for $T4^+$ cells
  3. Induce syncitia in vitro
  4. Inhibit T-cell function in vitro
  5. Exert immunosuppressive effects in vivo
  6. Are transmitted via blood, sexual contact, and congenitally
Biochemical features
  1. Size of major core protein (24,000 molecular weight)
  2. Common p24 epitopes
  3. Properties of reverse transcriptase (100,000 molecular weight, preference for Mg^{2+} cation)
  4. No phosphoprotein adjacent to amino-terminal *gag* protein
Genomic features
  1. Trans-acting transcriptional activation of viral LTR
  2. Extra genes in addition to *gag*, *pol*, and *env*
  3. Double splicing mechanism generating 3′ mRNA of about 2 Kb
  4. Stretch of nucleotide sequence homology in *gag-pol* region and in LTRs

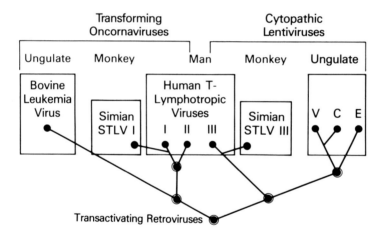

Fig. 1. HTLVs and their "super-family" of related retroviruses. STLV-I and STLV-III, Simian T-lymphotropic virus type I and type III; V, visna virus; E, equine infectious anemia virus; C, caprine arthritis and encephalitis virus.

env gene sequences which comprise the usual retroviral genetic component [7–9] (see below). (This function has not yet been identified for STLV-III, but is predicted to occur based on numerous other similarities.) The branch points and relationships depicted in Figure 1 are based on various criteria. The viruses to the left in Figure 1 are more immunologically related to one another, with HTLV-I and HTLV-II sharing the most homology, then STLV-I, and finally bovine leukemia virus (BLV). These viruses all infect T cells, have similar genetic and protein structure, and have similar morphology by electron microscopy. HTLV-III is boxed with HTLV-I and HTLV-II based on its common host species, T-cell tropism, similar structure of some proteins, and, of course, the TAT function. HTLV-III diverges from HTLV-I and HTLV-II in

its predominant cytopathic effect, altered gross morphology, and minimal immunologic cross-reactivity. In these latter properties it resembles the lenti viruses, and in
fact sequence homology with the visna virus has been reported [10]. Furthermore,
the recently isolated STLV-III has been shown to be immunologically closely related
to HTLV-III [11,12]. It is of some interest that this super-family of viruses contains
on both sides of the tree viruses from ungulates, monkeys, and humans. In addition,
it is becoming apparent that these viruses cause similar disease manifestations, with
those on the left side of the tree having predominantly proliferative effects and those
on the right having predominantly cytopathic ones (see Fig. 1). Other properties in
common must await further elucidation of biochemical, biologic, and immunologic
parameters.

DISTRIBUTION OF HTLV FAMILY MEMBERS

Not discussed above is another feature the HTLV family members share: a
probable African origin. Extensive seroepidemiologic studies have been carried out
to localize areas endemic for viral infection, to delineate populations at greatest risk
for infection, to trace the evolution and natural history of the viral infections, and to
identify populations suitable for preventive measures when they become available.
The distribution of HTLV-I is very broad [for review, see 13]. The most highly
endemic areas include southwestern Japan, the Caribbean basin and countries surrounding it, and many parts of Africa, although pockets of infection extend even to
the Arctic regions [14]. We find of great significance the fact that the distribution of
HTLV-III, while more restricted than that of HTLV-I, overlaps that of HTLV-I in
Africa, but has not yet entered the general population on other continents except for
groups at risk for development of the acquired immune deficiency syndrome (AIDS).
Taken together with the knowledge that retroviruses related to both HTLV-I and
HTLV-III have been isolated from old world primates [11,15,16], the case for an
African origin of all the HTLV family members becomes more compelling. It must
be pointed out, however, that the distribution of HTLV-II has not yet been elucidated.
Serologic evidence of infection by this virus has not been obtained for any healthy
normal population to date. The only group in which HTLV-II antibody prevalence
has been demonstrated has been in intravenous drug abusers, both in England [17]
and in New York (Robert-Guroff et al, submitted for publication). HTLV-II isolates
have been obtained from a patient with hairy cell leukemia [2] and from a New York
drug addict [18]. No association of this virus with additional patients who have hairy
cell leukemia has been detected.

The question of the origin of the HTLV family has more than academic interest.
The elucidation of the evolution of viral mutants can help in understanding biologic
effects of the virus by comparison with related animal viruses whose properties have
been studied for some time. In addition, if HTLV-III, for example, originated in
Africa, it may be that some African populations have adapted to the viral infection,
or the original virus strain may have been less virulent. This speculation is based on
the high prevalence of low titer antibodies to HTLV-III detected in children in Uganda
in the early 1970s [19]. Studies of other even earlier collections of African sera would
be very informative in this regard. If an early virus strain were less virulent, study of
such an isolate might provide clues for the treatment and prevention of present-day
intractable infections.

BIOLOGIC EFFECTS OF HTLV FAMILY MEMBERS

The study of HTLV provides a stimulating intellectual and scientific challenge because of the disparate biologic effects caused by the related agents on a cellular system normally devoted to combatting exogenous infectious agents. It is also precisely for this reason that the challenge to the medical community to provide treatment and preventative measures for HTLV infection is great. Superficially, HTLV-I and HTLV-II are understood to cause proliferation of T cells and hence to lead to unrestrained T-cell growth and malignancy in the form of leukemias and lymphomas. On the other hand, HTLV-III exerts a profound cytopathic effect on the T cells it infects, leading to cell death and consequent immune dysfunction in hosts depleted of effector cells. More in-depth studies have shown that HTLV-I and HTLV-II also have mild cytopathic effects and evidence is accumulating that they also exert immune suppressive effects. These effects have been demonstrated in vitro where T cells have shown loss of cytotoxic function as well as unrestrained proliferation without proper HLA restriction following infection [20]. More recent studies have shown that HTLV-infected cells, all of which express class II MHC antigens (HLA-D/DR or Ia), react nondiscriminantly to all known allelic variants of human HLA-D/DR antigens [21]. It has been proposed that autostimulation by a self-Ia determinant may both induce proliferation of HTLV-infected cells and lead to possible autoimmune effects [21]. In addition, serologic studies have suggested that some immunosuppressive effects occur in vivo in response to viral infection. This latter evidence includes serologic studies of healthy individuals and patients with various diseases from Miyazaki, Japan, where patients on infectious disease wards exhibited a higher prevalence of antibodies to HTLV-I than the general healthy population or than patients in other wards [22]. More recent evidence includes studies of New York drug addicts, where those with antibodies to HTLV-I or HTLV-II, regardless of their HTLV-III antibody status, were more likely to also have soft tissue infections than drug addicts lacking these antibodies (Robert-Guroff et al, unpublished information). Whether HTLV-III can also immortalize cells if the cytopathic effect were obliterated is not known. In any case, the mechanisms by which these disparate effects are caused, by viruses with similar genomes and protein products, must be elucidated.

MECHANISMS OF HTLV-INDUCED BIOLOGIC EFFECTS

It has been suggested, based on analogy to other retroviral systems, that the transmembrane protein, p21 for HTLV-I and HTLV-II and gp41 for HTLV-III, may be able directly to exert immune suppressive effects. This phenomenon has been described for the feline leukemia virus (FeLV) system [23,24], in which the transmembrane protein is designated *p15E*, although the biochemical mechanism by which this could occur is not known. A direct test of this hypothesis awaits either the purification of the HTLV transmembrane proteins or, alternatively, their synthesis or production by genetic engineering methodology. If this viral gene product exerts such an effect, the means by which the effect is augmented will still need to be elucidated.

A second proposed mechanism concerns the Il-2 (TCGF) receptor, whose expression on the surface of T cells is induced and/or enhanced following infection by HTLV [25,26]. While originally it was thought that a mechanism of T-cell proliferation might involve an autocrine model, with HTLV-I–infected cells bearing

Il-2 receptors responding to their own secretion of TCGF, it was subsequently learned that unlike the earliest cases examined, the majority of HTLV-I-infected cells do not produce TCGF [27]. It remains a possibility, however, that the TCGF receptor expressed on the surface of infected cells is altered in some way so as to have greater affinity for the growth factor, to respond to another or additional growth factor(s), or to require no triggering at all by a factor but rather to respond to some other exogenous stimulus. These questions will continue to be investigated.

Recently, an attractive mechanism proposed to explain in part some of the biologic effects of HTLV family members invokes the protein product of the extra genetic information present in the viruses [5–7], originally termed the *pX region* [28] but more recently the *TAT gene* [8,9]. It is this genetic sequence that is believed to encode the trans-acting transcriptional activation function common to the HTLV family members and to the larger super-family of HTLV-related viruses. This function provides a model (Fig. 2) for the activation of either viral or cellular genes responsible for T-cell proliferation or cytopathic effect leading to cell death. Because it is a trans-acting function, a single integration site for biologic effect is not necessary. Elucidation of the viral or cellular gene products activated by such a TAT function in HTLV-infected cells has become a crucial step in understanding the biologic effects of the HTLV family members. A recent development that will aid immensely in determining the molecular and biochemical mechanisms underlying the biologic effects of HTLV-III was the transfection of a cloned, full-length HTLV-III proviral DNA into human cord blood cells with resultant infection and cytopathic effect [29]. The clone and mutants derived from it will be invaluable in determining subgenomic regions responsible for certain viral functions.

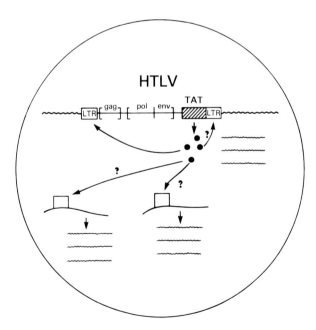

Fig. 2.   A model for transformation by HTLV invoking trans-acting transcriptional activation of viral and cellular genes by the protein product of the TAT gene.

THERAPEUTIC APPROACHES IN HTLV INFECTIONS

Because of the major differences in the biologic effects of the proliferative versus the cytopathic HTLV family members, approaches to treatment of the diseases induced by the viruses of necessity must be quite different. HTLV-I causes an aggressive malignancy of mature T cells of which the OKT4-positive cell is the primary target. Therapeutic approaches must take into account the fact that the infected individual possesses integrated provirus in the cellular genomic component that may become activated at any time. Effective agents for therapy might include any that are directed against a viral or a viral induced antigen on the infected cells. Recently, the development of a human monoclonal antibody against the major envelope glycoprotein of HTLV-I (Matsushita et al, submitted for publication) suggests a possible means of treating patients both directly with cytotoxic antibody and with antibody coupled to toxic substances to direct the drug to the appropriate cell. This approach requires that the infected cells express viral envelope at the time of treatment. It may be possible to activate the leukemic cells in vivo with some supplemental treatment to induce synthesis of the viral antigen, thereby rendering the cells susceptible to such an antienvelope reagent. Other monoclonal antibodies to "tumor-specific" antigens expressed on the surface of HTLV-I–infected cells might also be similarly used therapeutically. While a number of antigens normally present on the surface of T cells are expressed at higher levels on HTLV-I–infected cells, antibodies to these surface markers presumably would not be appropriate for treatment unless the antigens would have greater affinity for immunologic reagents or would be altered slightly, rendering them immunologically distinguishable from normal cellular antigens.

In HTLV-III infection, cell to cell spread of the virus is more important than with HTLV-I or HTLV-II because the cells continually die out, effectively eliminating the majority of potentially latent, provirus-containing cells. The virus, therefore, must continually reinfect new cells for the disease manifestations to be maintained. Therapeutic agents directed at inhibiting cell to cell spread of the virus have thus become prime candidates for effective intervention. It is likely that whatever drug is used for this type of treatment, the ability of the provirus to integrate into the host genome will require that treatment be continued with some regularity for the lifetime of an individual. The possibility that certain drugs may become ineffective with time is real, and combinations of agents may be necessary. In addition, prolonged therapy requires that the drugs used exhibit minimal toxic effect. One of the initial targets for inhibiting viral infectivity has been the reverse transcriptase. Current reverse transcriptase inhibitors under most intense investigation as potential anti-HTLV-III agents include suramin [30] and HPA23 [31]. Other agents with potential antiviral activity are also being investigated, such as recombinant human interferon alfa-A [32]. It also seems apparent that subsequent to antiviral therapy, additional regimens must include reconstitution of the immune system, perhaps by bone marrow transplant, to restore normal functioning.

Recently the discovery that HTLV-III induces neutralizing antibodies in infected individuals [33,34] raises the possibility of using passive antibody therapy in combatting AIDS. Initial studies have suggested that neutralizing antibody titers fluctuate inversely with severity of disease manifestation in infected individuals [34] (Table II). However, it must be firmly established that such antibodies, which apparently act by

TABLE II. HTLV-III Neutralizing Antibody in AIDS and ARC Patients and Others at Risk

Serum source	Antibodies to HTLV-III antigens		HTLV-III neutralizing antibody			
	No. positive/ No. tested	% Positive	No. positive/ No. tested	% Positive	Range of titer	Geometric mean titer ± SEM
Adult AIDS patients	288/297	97	21/35	60	10–520	44 ± 10
Pediatric AIDS patients	IP[a]		3/9	33	80–180	117 ± 28
Adult ARC patients	327/360	91	28/35	80	17–560	88 ± 16
Healthy homosexuals	96/235	41	2/12[b]	17	130–340	210 ± 101
Healthy heterosexuals	0/238	0	0/20	0		

[a]IP, in progress.
[b]Two of the 12 sera were also positive for HTLV-III antibodies by ELISA and Western blot assays. A third serum showed weak reactivity with HTLV-III p24.

blocking attachment of the virus to a cell surface receptor via the envelope glycoprotein, actually exert an in vivo protective effect. Monoclonal antibodies against the neutralizing epitope of the virus might then be used in therapeutic approaches.

PREVENTATIVE MEASURES FOR COMBATTING HTLV INFECTIONS

The first step in designing effective measures to control the spread of the various HTLV family members is to understand thoroughly the modes of transmission of the viruses, to delineate populations at risk, and to elucidate the natural history of the viruses and the course of progression of the diseases they induce. Studies of this nature have been underway for some time, and much information has been gained. To summarize briefly, all the HTLV family members appear to be transmitted only by close contact, resulting in cell to cell contact of infected and recipient cells. Thus, intimate sexual contact and intimate contact with blood or blood products would encompass the primary routes of transmission. Practices including sexual promiscuity and intravenous drug abuse, as we have seen in the AIDS epidemic, will therefore result in greater risk of infection because of greater likelihood of contact with infected cells. The possible role of insects as vectors spreading any of the HTLV family members has not been explored, although several seroepidemiologic studies on HTLV-I prevalence have shown an increased prevalence in populations where mosquitos or various parasites are abundant [14,35–37]. The areas endemic for HTLV-I infection have been largely elucidated, as have the risk groups for HTLV-III infection. One important question for all three viruses is the degree of maternal–infant transmission of virus. Any vaccine approach must clearly occur prior to any natural infection. Because of the virulence and rapidity of HTLV-III–induced disease, the majority of vaccine efforts are currently focused on this disease. However, in concept, similar vaccines would also be effective for HTLV-I or HTLV-II. One main obstacle in designing effective HTLV-III vaccines is the necessity for first determining whether the observed variability in the HTLV-III genome [38] results in variability in immunologic response or whether common epitopes exist among various HTLV-III isolates that elicit appropriate neutralizing antibodies with "group specificity." If, for example, natural HTLV-III neutralizing antibodies select for viral mutants in vivo, similarly to the situation with visna virus [39], then production of a broadly specific vaccine will be much more difficult.

Current attempts to design appropriate vaccines are focusing on several approaches, including the use of ISCOM preparations of viral envelope proteins [40], vaccinia virus–HTLV-III recombinants [41,42], and antiidiotypes to relevant viral antigenic determinants [43]. Genetically engineered peptides of appropriate viral genetic regions are being actively pursued, both as probes for pinpointing genetic regions encoding relevant biologic functions and subsequently as possibly effective vaccine preparations. Surely one of these efforts, or a conceptually new approach, must succeed. We can then be afforded protection against a so far intractable disease and can as well apply the lessons learned with HTLV-III to prevention of other human retrovirus infections.

REFERENCES

1. Poiesz BJ, Ruscetti FW, Gazdar AF, Bunn PA, Minna JD, Gallo RC: Proc Natl Acad Sci USA 77:7415, 1980.
2. Kalyanaraman VS, Sarngadharan MG, Robert-Guroff M, Miyoshi I, Blayney D, Golde D, Gallo RC: Science 218:571, 1982.
3. Popovic M, Sarngadharan MG, Read E, Gallo RC: Science 224:497, 1984.
4. Gallo RC, Salahuddin SZ, Popovic M, Shearer GM, Kaplan M, Haynes BF, Palker TJ, Redfield R, Oleske J, Safai B, White G, Foster P, Markham PD: Science 224:500, 1984.
5. Sodroski JG, Rosen CA, Haseltine WA: Science 225:381, 1984.
6. Sodroski J, Rosen C, Wong-Staal F, Salahuddin SZ, Popovic M, Arya S, Gallo RC, Haseltine WA: Science 227:171, 1985.
7. Haseltine WA, Sodroski J, Patarca R, Briggs D, Perkins D, Wong-Staal F: Science 225:419, 1984.
8. Arya SK, Guo C, Josephs SF, Wong-Staal F: Science 229:69, 1985.
9. Sodroski J, Patarca R, Rosen C, Wong-Staal F, Haseltine W: Science 229:74, 1985.
10. Gonda MA, Wong-Staal F, Gallo RC, Clements JE, Narayan O, Gilden RV: Science 227:173, 1985.
11. Daniel MD, Letvin NL, King NW, Kannagi M, Sehgal PK, Hunt RD, Kanki PJ, Essex M, Desrosiers RC: Science 228:1201, 1985.
12. Kanki PJ, McLane MF, King NW Jr., Letvin NL, Hunt RD, Sehgal P, Daniel MD, Desrosiers RC, Essex M: Science 228:1199, 1985.
13. Robert-Guroff M, Markham PD, Popovic M, Gallo RC: In Vogt P (ed): "Current Topics in Microbiology and Immunology." Berlin: Springer-Verlag, 1985, Vol 115, p 7.
14. Robert-Guroff M, Clark J, Lanier AP, Beckman G, Melbye M, Ebbesen P, Blattner WA, Gallo RC: Int J Cancer 36:651, 1985.
15. Miyoshi I, Yoshimoto S, Fujishita M, Ohtsuki Y, Taguchi H, Shiraishi Y, Akagi T, Minezawa M: Gann 74:323, 1983.
16. Guo H-G, Wong-Staal F, Gallo RC: Science 223:1195, 1984.
17. Tedder RS, Shanson DC, Jeffries DJ, Cheingsong-Popov R, Clapham P, Dalgleish A, Nagy K, Weiss RA: Lancet 2:125, 1984.
18. Hahn BH, Popovic M, Kalyanaraman VS, Shaw GM, LoMonico A, Weiss SH, Wong-Staal F, Gallo RC: In Gottlieb MS, Groopman JE (eds): "Acquired Immune Deficiency Syndrome" (UCLA Symposia on Molecular and Cellular Biology, New Series, Vol. 16). New York: Alan R. Liss, Inc., 1984, p 73.
19. Saxinger WC, Levine PH, Dean AG, De Thé G, Moghissi J, Laurent F, Hoh M, Sarngadharan MG, Gallo RC: Science 227:1036, 1985.
20. Popovic M, Flomenberg N, Volkman DJ, Mann D, Fauci AS, Dupont B, Gallo RC: Science 226:459, 1984.
21. Suciu-Foca N, Rubinstein P, Popovic M, Gallo RC, King DW: Nature 312:275, 1984.
22. Essex M, McLane MF, Tachibana N, Francis DP, Lee TH: In Gallo RC, Essex ME, Gross L (eds): "Human T-Cell Leukemia/Lymphoma Virus." Cold Spring Harbor, NY: Cold Spring Harbor Laboratory, 1984, p 355.

23. Mathes LE, Olsen RG, Hebebrand LC, Hoover EA, Schaller JP, Adams PW, Nichols WS: Cancer Res 29:950, 1979.
24. Copelan EA, Rinehart JJ, Lewis M, Mathes L, Olsen R, Sagone A: J Immunol 131:2017, 1983.
25. Mann DL, Popovic M, Murray C, Neuland C, Strong DM, Sarin P, Gallo RC, Blattner WA: J Immunol 131:2021, 1983.
26. Mann DL, Popovic M, Sarin P, Murray C, Reitz MS, Strong DM, Haynes BF, Gallo RC, Blattner WA: Nature 305:58, 1983.
27. Arya SK, Wong-Staal F, Gallo RC: Science 223:1086, 1984.
28. Seiki M, Hattori S, Hirayama Y, Yoshida M: Proc Natl Acad Sci USA 80:3618, 1983.
29. Fisher AG, Collalti E, Ratner L, Gallo RC, Wong-Staal F: Nature 316:262, 1985.
30. Mitsuya H, Popovic M, Yarchoan R, Matsushita S, Gallo RC, Broder S: Science 226:172, 1984.
31. Rozenbaum W, Dormont D, Spire B, Vilmer E, Gentilini M, Griscelli C, Montagnier L, Barre-Sinoussi F, Chermann JC: Lancet 1:450, 1985.
32. Ho DD, Hartshorn KL, Rota TR, Andrews CA, Kaplan JC, Schooley RI, Hirsch MS: Lancet 1:602, 1985.
33. Weiss RA, Clapham PR, Cheingsong-Popov R, Dalgleish AG, Carne CA, Weller IVD, Tedder RS: Nature 316:69, 1985.
34. Robert-Guroff M, Brown M, Gallo RC: Nature 316:72, 1985.
35. Tajima K, Fujita K, Tsukidate S, Oda T, Tominage S, Suchi T, Hinuma Y: Gann 74:188, 1983.
36. Biggar RJ, Saxinger C, Gardiner C, Collins WE, Levine PH, Clark JW, Nkrumah FK, Blattner WA: Int J Cancer 34:215, 1984.
37. Merino F, Robert-Guroff M, Clark J, Biondo-Bracho M, Blattner WA, Gallo RC: Int J Cancer 34:501, 1984.
38. Shaw GM, Hahn BH, Arya SK, Groopman JE, Gallo RC, Wong-Staal F: Science 226:1165, 1984.
39. Narayan O, Clements JE, Griffin DE, Wolinsky JS: Infect Immun 32:1045, 1981.
40. Morein B, Sundquist B, Hoglund S, Dalsgaard K, Osterhaus A: Nature 308:457, 1984.
41. Smith GL, Mackett M, Moss B: Nature 302:490, 1983.
42. Smith GL, Murphy BR, Moss B: Proc Natl Acad Sci USA 80:7155, 1983.
43. Jerne NK: In Schnurr I (ed): "Idiotypes—What They Said at the Time." Discussion at Les Baux-de-Provence, April 2–3, 1976. Basel, Switzerland: Basel Institute of Immunology, 1980, p 1.

Biochemical and Molecular Epidemiology of Cancer 303–311 (1986)

DNA Adduct Formation and Removal in Human Cancer Patients

Miriam C. Poirier, Eddie Reed, Robert F. Ozols, and Stuart H. Yuspa

National Cancer Institute, National Institutes of Health, Bethesda, Maryland 20205

cis-Diamminedichloroplatinum (II) (*cis*-DDP) is a remarkably potent chemotherapeutic agent, the cytocidal effects of which are caused by drug-DNA interactions. One such interaction results in the formation of an intrastrand N^7-deoxy(GpG)-diammineplatinum adduct, which, in cultured cells, comprises a major fraction of the total DNA-bound platinum and is slowly removed. We have elicited a polyclonal antibody specific for this adduct and developed an enzyme-linked immunosorbent assay (ELISA) capable of detecting 25 attomol of adduct/μg DNA or one adduct in 10^8 nucleotides. Because the antibody is specific for DNAs modified with certain chemotherapeutically effective *cis*-reacting analogs of *cis*-DDP, structurally similar bidentate intrastrand adducts are believed to play a role in the tumoricidal efficacy of these compounds. Using the anti-*cis*-DDP–DNA–ELISA we have analyzed 223 samples of DNA extracted from nucleated peripheral blood cells (buffy coat) of controls and of testicular and ovarian cancer patients at multiple times during *cis*-DDP treatment. Of these, all 23 samples from untreated controls were never positive, and 46% of the 200 samples from *cis*-DDP–treated patients were positive. Patients on their first course of chemotherapy receiving *cis*-DDP on 21 or 28 day cycles (5 days of drug infusion followed by 2 or 3 drug-free wk) accumulated DNA adducts as a function of dose and increasing cycle number. Thus, the removal time for measurable adducts formed during one cycle may be more than 28 days. An analysis of disease response data for 47 patients showed that individuals forming high levels of *cis*-DDP adducts (>200 attomol/μg DNA) were more likely to undergo complete remissions than those forming fewer adducts or no adducts at all. It is anticipated that the ability to monitor a quantitative biologic effect of *cis*-DDP exposure in uman cancer patients may allow the clinician to titrate *cis*-DDP dose for chemotherapeutic efficacy while attempting to minimize immediate toxicity and the threat of a second malignancy.

Key words: *cis*-diamminedichloroplatinum (II), DNA adducts, ELISA, human biomonitoring, cancer patients

Among the most effective chemotherapeutic agents currently available are a series of platinum coordination complexes, the prototype of which is *cis*-diamminedichloroplatinum (II) (*cis*-DDP) [1]. Treatment with this compound has resulted in 80–90% cure rates for testicular cancer and approximately a 20% cure rate for

Received April 25, 1985.

© **1986 Alan R. Liss, Inc.**

advanced ovarian cancer [2,3]. The biological activity appears to be mediated through chemical alterations of DNA that, in cultured cells, correlate directly with cytotoxicity [4]. To exhibit antitumor activity a compound must have *cis* leaving groups, either chlorides or hydrolyzable ester linkages, since the corresponding *trans* compounds are not effective [1]. Several types of adducts have been characterized in *cis*-DDP–exposed DNA [5], and some of the same adducts have been shown to form in exposed cultured cells. Interstrand DNA–DNA and DNA–protein crosslinks were among the earliest lesions identified and have been studied extensively by methods such as alkaline elution [4,6]. They comprise about 1% of total platinum bound to DNA and are almost completely removed by 72 hr after exposure. A major adduct is the intrastrand N^7-d(GpG)-diammineplatinum, which comprises 40–60% of the total Pt bound to DNA initially after exposure [7,8] and is removed only slowly over a period of days [7]. Other types of DNA damage are a short-lived monoadduct, which may be a precursor of the bidentate adduct, an N^7-d(GpXpG)-diammineplatinum adduct, which is a very small proportion of the total, and an N^7-d(GpA)-diammineplatinum adduct, which has not been extensively studied in vivo [7–9].

The development of antisera specific for carcinogen-DNA adducts has made possible determination of attomol (10^{-18} M) quantities of carcinogen bound to DNA in biological samples [10]. A unique feature of this technology is the ability to use quantitative immunoassays such as radioimmunoassay (RIA) and enzyme-linked immunosorbent assay (ELISA) to measure the extent of DNA modification by nonradio-labeled compounds. The high degree of sensitivity and specificity of these assays suggested that they might by useful in monitoring human populations for evidence of chemical exposure. An early attempt to measure benzo(a)pyrene-DNA adducts in pulmonary tissue from lung cancer patients [11] demonstrated that such studies would be feasible but difficult. In particular, smoking history questionnaires failed to yield reliable data on individual doses of hydrocarbon exposure. In addition, it was difficult to identify unexposed individuals (controls), possibly because of the ubiquitous nature of hydrocarbon exposure. In searching for a more uniform group in which to continue the validation of this approach, we chose cancer patients receiving *cis*-DDP chemotherapy. We anticipated that measuring DNA adduct levels might give the clinician an indicator of biologically effective dose, thus allowing more effective treatment on an individual basis. In addition, since the dosages and treatment regimens for exposed individuals would be known and since unintentional exposure would not be expected, validation of the assay would be much more straightforward. Finally, we anticipated a relationship between adduct formation and tumor response and hoped to investigate the long-term effects of DNA adduct formation by monitoring patients for the duration of their lifetime. Since *cis*-DDP is carcinogenic in rodents [12], the possibility exists that it may be identified as a human carcinogen.

MATERIALS AND METHODS

cis-DDP Administration and Blood Sample Preparation

We studied human cancer patients who were being treated for either ovarian or testicular cancer by the Medicine Branch of the National Cancer Institute. *cis*-DDP and carboplatinum (CBDCA) therapy were given as part of approved experimental protocols, and the doses varied between 20 mg/M^2/day $\times$ 5 and 40 mg/M^2/day $\times$ 5 for the former and was 400 mg/M^2/day $\times$ 2 for the latter. Control groups were untreated normal volunteers and patients on nonplatinum combination chemotherapy for non-Hodgkin lymphoma. In addition, some of the patients were studied for adducts prior to receiving *cis*-DDP and therefore served as their own controls. Platinum drug chemotherapy was given in courses of three to five cycles. In each cycle *cis*-DDP was administered as a 30 min daily intravenous infusion on each of 5 consecutive days, and CBDCA was a continuous 48 hr infusion. The drug-free interval was 2–3 weeks for *cis*-DDP and 5 weeks for CBDCA. On the morning following the last day of drug infusion (day 6 or 3), 30–50 ml of blood was obtained by routine venipuncture, centrifuged (20 min, 5,000 g, 4°C), and the nucleated cells (the buffy coat cells) were aspirated and frozen at −20°C until DNA isolation.

Epidermal Cell Culture and *cis*-DDP Exposure

Primary BALB/c mouse epidermal cells were prepared from newborn mouse skin as described [13]. Seeded in 150 mm dishes at a density of 2.5×10^7 per dish, cells were maintained as a basal cell population in Eagle's minimal essential medium with 8% fetal calf serum and 0.05 mM Ca^{2+} for 3 days. Exposure to 100 μM *cis*-DDP was for 4 hr in the culture medium, after which time plates were frozen until DNA extraction.

DNA Preparation and ELISA

DNA was extracted from frozen pellets of nucleated blood cells and cultured keratinocytes and isolated by CsCl centrifugation [14] within 1 month of the time the cells were frozen. DNAs were dialyzed against water and quantitated by absorbance at 260 nm. Samples were assayed for *cis*-DDP–DNA adducts by ELISA as previously reported [15,16]. The ELISA standard curve 50% inhibition was established at 10 $\pm$ 4 fmole (mean $\pm$ range) of platinum (atomic absorption spectroscopy performed by S.J. Lippard) in standard immunogen *cis*-DDP–DNA [15]. Biological samples were assayed as native DNA with 30–35 μg DNA per microtiter plate well and 35 μg of unmodified calf thymus DNA added to the standard curve wells. Each biological sample was assayed three times in triplicate wells by ELISA and not scored as positive unless the percentage of inhibition was 20% or more.

Data Analysis

Adduct analyses were performed on 223 samples from a total of 88 individuals. Patients receiving platinum drugs were studied one or more times during their course of chemotherapy. Individuals in the control groups were generally studied only once. Statistical significance was calculated by the two-sided chi square test as described by Armitage [17].

RESULTS
Antiserum Specificity

The antiserum used in these studies was elicited against calf thymus DNA modified to 5% with *cis*-DDP [16]. Specificity is directed toward the combination of platinum drug and DNA, and, as is usually the case with this type of antiserum, there is no specificity for unmodified DNA or the *cis*-DDP alone. Since the individual nucleoside adducts are not recognized by the antibody (M. Poirier, unpublished observations), adduct competition could not be used to assess directly the antibody specificity. However, a number of indirect experiments have yielded information concerning the antigenic determinants. Studies with *cis*-DDP–modified homopolymers [poly(dG)·(dC)] and heteropolymers [poly(dGdC)] demonstrated that the homopolymer was recognized by the antibody almost as well as the immunogen DNA, and the heteropolymer was not recognized at all [18]. This suggested that the antibody is primarily specific for the bidentate intrastrand N^7-d(GpG)-diammineplatinum adduct formed on adjacent deoxyguanosines. In addition, a series of *cis*-DDP analogs were used to modify calf thymus DNA, and the resulting modified DNAs were assayed competitively in the ELISA. The results [18] demonstrated that DNAs modified with compounds having *cis*-reacting leaving groups (chlorides or ester linkages) were recognized by the antiserum even though the *cis*-ammine groups had undergone a variety of substitutions. In general, DNAs modified with clinically active *cis*-DDP analogs were readily recognized by the anti-*cis*-DDP–DNA (Table I). Thus, the antiserum is specific for DNA modified on adjacent deoxyguanosines through displacement of *cis*-chloride leaving groups and recognizes adducts from clinically effective *cis*-DDP analogs having various ammine substitutions.

The antiserum recognizes modified DNAs from several biological sources, including cultured cells, rats, and mice exposed to *cis*-DDP. Early experiments were performed with the L1210 tumor line, which had been shown to be sensitive to the tumoricidal effects of *cis*-DDP. Adducts were quantitated in cells grown in suspension culture and as mouse ascites in vivo after exposure of either the cultures or the mouse to *cis*-DDP [16]. Conversely, DNA adducts formed by *trans*-DDP in L1210 cultures were not recognized by the antiserum [16]. Subsequently, adducts have been measured in *cis*-DDP–exposed cultured mouse keratinocytes (Fig. 1) and human ovarian cell lines (E. Reed and R.F. Ozols, unpublished data). In addition, measurable adduct levels have been observed in kidneys and gonads of Sprague-Dawley rats [15] and in kidneys, ascites, and solid tumor of nude mice bearing a human ovarian carcinoma (E. Reed and R.F. Ozols, unpublished data). Since recognized adducts appeared to form in a wide variety of biological systems and since in no case did untreated controls give false positives, we expected that human cancer patients might also form antibody-recognized adducts and that the assay might be a useful tool to investigate biologically effective dose in humans. Figure 1 demonstrates that DNA extracted from the nucleated cells contained in 50 ml of peripheral blood from a patient

TABLE I. Chemotherapeutic Efficacy of *cis*-DDP Analogs That Form Adducts Measurable by Anti-*cis*-DDP–DNA Serum

cis-Ammine substitution	*cis*-Leaving groups	Clinical Activity	Clinical Name	ELISA 50% inhibition (fmole Pt)
(Ammine)$_2$	(Cl)$_2$	+ + + +	CISPLATIN	66
Methylenediammine	(Cl)$_2$	+		62
(Aminoisopropyl)$_2$	(Cl)$_2$	+	CHIP	210
1,2 diaminocyclohexyl	4-carboxylato	+ +	Pt(DACH)	45
(Ammine)$_2$	cyclobutane-carboxylato	+ + +	CBDCA[a]	NT[b]

[a]DNA modified in vitro was not available, but blood sample DNAs from patients receiving CBDCA are positive in the ELISA.
[b]NT, not tested.

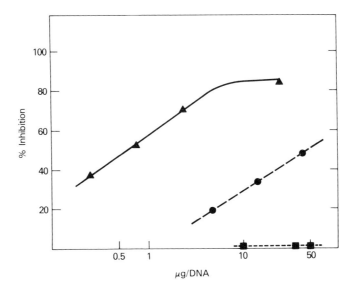

Fig. 1.   Competitive ELISA profiles in which increasing quantities of DNA from biological sources (abscissa) compete for anti-*cis*-DDP–DNA against standard immunogen *cis*-DDP–DNA coated on microtiter wells. [For description of ELISA procedure, see 15.] Sample DNAs that inhibit (ordinate) the antibody *cis*-DDP–DNA binding (antibody recognition) are from mouse keratinocytes exposed to 100 μM *cis*-DDP 4 hr in culture (▲) and from buffy coat cells of an ovarian cancer patient given 200 mg/M^2 of *cis*-DDP (●). DNA from a patient receiving nonplatinum chemotherapy (■) does not compete (no antibody recognition).

receiving *cis*-DDP was positive in the ELISA, and DNA prepared similarly from a patient receiving nonplatinum chemotherapy was negative. This finding indicated that a study in human cancer patients would be feasible.

Determination of *cis*-DDP–DNA Adducts in Cancer Patients

To date, 223 blood samples have been assayed from 88 individuals in the human patient study. Of these, all 23 samples from control groups were negative in the ELISA. Of the remaining 200 samples from 78 patients undergoing platinum drug therapy, 46% were positive in the ELISA. Since analysis of the data from 100 blood samples drawn at various times during the drug infusion indicated that adducts accumulated during drug administration (E. Reed et al, submitted for publication), all subsequent samples were taken after drug infusion. Therefore, of the 200 samples, 127 samples were obtained the morning after the last day of drug infusion; this was day 6 for the *cis*-DDP–treated patients and day 3 for those receiving CBDCA. Of the 127 postinfusion samples, 76 (or 60%) were positive. The data presented in Figure 2 and Table II are an analysis of only these samples.

ELISA data from the postinfusion blood DNAs are shown in Figure 2. Samples were from testicular and ovarian cancer patients receiving therapy on five different treatment protocols (for description of protocols, see Fig. 2). When clinical efficacy of the protocol was compared with ELISA results, the data indicated that groups having the highest fraction of samples positive in the ELISA (shown in Fig. 2) were most likely to achieve remission of the disease. For example, the PVB and PVBV groups are both testicular cancer patients receiving chemotherapy for the first time

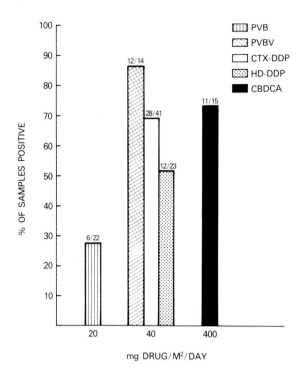

Fig. 2. ELISA results from 127 postinfusion blood samples grouped by treatment. Percentage of samples positive (ordinate) is plotted as a function of dose (abscissa) for each group. The groups are as follows: PVB, testicular cancer patients receiving velban, bleomycin, and 20 mg/M^2/day $\times$ 5 of *cis*-DDP on 21 day cycles; PVBV, testicular cancer patients receiving vinblastine, bleomycin, epipodophyllotoxin, and 40 mg/M^2/day $\times$ 5 of *cis*-DDP on 28 day cycles; CTX-DDP, ovarian cancer patients receiving cytoxan and 40 mg/M^2/day $\times$ 5 of *cis*-DDP on 28 day cycles; HD-DDP, ovarian cancer patients receiving 40 mg/M^2/day $\times$ 5 of *cis*-DDP as single agent therapy on 28 day cycles; and CBDCA, ovarian cancer patients receiving 400 mg/M^2/day $\times$ 2 of CBDCA single agent therapy on 28 day cycles. The first three groups of patients are receiving chemotherapy for the first time. The HD-DDP and CBDCA groups have previously failed platinum and/or other chemotherapy.

but are being given two different *cis*-DDP doses, 20 and 40 mg/M^2/day $\times$ 5. These patients all began treatment with advanced disease, and, clinically, the more aggressive regimen (PVBV) produced more complete remissions than PVB [19]. In addition, a higher percentage of blood samples from the PVBV patients were positive in the ELISA, as compared to samples from patients on the less-aggressive PVB regimen, (Fig. 2). Also shown in Figure 2 are ELISA data from the CTX-DDP and HD-DDP groups, which are ovarian cancer patients. The former group is receiving chemotherapy for the first time, and the latter comprises individuals who have failed previous chemotherapy. As a group, the CTX-DDP patients are more likely to achieve remission than the resistant HD-DDP patients. Disease response data for the individuals from whom we have obtained blood samples show 10 complete remissions and four failures in the CTX-DDP group and eight failures with only one complete remission in the HD-DDP group. The CTX-DDP patients also had a higher percentage of samples positive in the ELISA (Fig. 2). The last patient group shown in Figure 2 had previously failed chemotherapy containing platinum and other drugs (like those given

HD-DDP) and are receiving CBDCA, a less toxic second-generation *cis*-DDP analog. The dose of 800 mg/M^2 of CBDCA given over 2 days is equivalent to 648 mg/M^2 of *cis*-DDP. Preliminary clinical results suggest that these individuals are responding better than the HD-DDP group. In the ELISA, all but one of the blood samples from CBDCA patients were positive (Fig. 2).

Another type of correlation that suggests that there is a positive relationship between adduct formation and disease response is shown in Table II. ELISA data from 37 ovarian cancer patients were tabulated by groups according to highest (peak) adduct level observed and were correlated with disease response data. Among those 13 individuals whose peak adduct level was $\geqslant 200$ attomol/μg DNA, there was a 61% incidence (8/13) of complete response. Conversely, 66% of those individuals who failed chemotherapy formed no measurable adducts (4/6). In addition, among the 24 individuals with adduct levels below 200 attomol/μg DNA there was a 50% incidence of chemotherapy failure. The data shown in Table II suggest that the ability to form intrastrand DNA adducts at levels greater than 200 amole/μg DNA does appear to correlate with likelihood of disease remission.

DISCUSSION

These investigations have demonstrated that the intrastrand deoxy-(GpG)-diammineplatinum, a major antigenic determinant of the anti-*cis*-DDP–DNA, is formed in a wide variety of biological systems. In addition, conformationally similar DNA adducts are formed in vivo and in vitro upon interaction of a number of chemotherapeutically effective *cis*-DDP analogs with DNA. The formation of this adduct has been shown previously to correlate with cytotoxicity in cell culture [4; E. Reed, unpublished data] and now appears to be associated with remission of neoplastic disease in human cancer patients. Dose-response analysis also indicates that increasing doses of *cis*-platinum drugs result in an increase in adduct formation among patients who form adducts. Thus, the immunologic approach described here may serve as a prototype for measurements of exposure to other environmentally and occupationally hazardous compounds that damage DNA.

As a clinical study, the cancer patient results have yielded some insights regarding *cis*-DDP–DNA interactions that may be related to mechanisms of platinum drug chemotherapeutic efficacy. Accumulation of recognizable adducts occurs in human blood cell DNA both during the 5 days of drug infusion and during successive 1 month treatment cycles [15; E. Reed et al, submitted for publication], suggesting that

TABLE II. Correlation Between Peak Adduct Level and Disease Response in Buffy Coat Cell DNA Samples From 37 Ovarian Cancer Patients

	Attomols of adduct/μg DNA			Trend analysis (p value, two-sided chi square test)
	>200	1–200	0	
Total number of patients	13	18	6	
Disease response				
Complete response	8 (61%)	4 (22%)	1 (17%)	0.026
Partial response	4 (31%)	6 (33%)	1 (17%)	—
No response	1 (8%)	8 (44%)	4 (66%)	0.007

the half-life for removal of adduct is at least 28 days. In addition, adducts have been detected in human kidney DNA obtained at autopsy from a cancer patient last exposed several months previously (T. Fasy and M. Poirier, unpublished data). Relatively slow removal of *cis*-DDP adducts has been observed in cultured mammalian cells [7] and rat kidney DNA [15], suggesting that persistence of the intrastrand d(GpG) adduct may be a consistent phenomenon in mammalian systems.

Another prominent feature of these studies is the observation that not all of the patients receiving platinum drugs form adducts. A small fraction of individuals do not show evidence of adduct formation even though the cumulative total *cis*-DDP dosage approaches 900 mg/M^2. This may be the result of a gradually developing resistance or a specific genetically controlled biochemical environment. A similar phenomenon has been observed in rodents. About 20% of Sprague-Dawley rats do not readily form DNA adducts in kidneys and gonads, do not accumulate tissue-bound platinum, and do not appear to undergo kidney toxicity. Since the variability among these animals can be reduced, but not eliminated, by overnight fasting, it is possible that metabolism may be partially responsible for these differences. Thus, by analogy, unknown factors within the patient population may modulate adduct formation and contribute to the variability in disease response.

Current experimentation in both the human and animal models has provided new data regarding *cis*-DDP–DNA interactions. Continued study in animal models and patient populations may result in improved drug treatment protocols and methods to augment adduct formation in the target tissue without increasing toxicity. In addition, if *cis*-DDP is shown to be a human carcinogen we will have accumulated valuable information concerning the processing of DNA damage in humans during the early stages of neoplastic initiation.

ACKNOWLEDGMENTS

The *cis*-DDP–DNA immunogen and standard compounds for this study were obtained from Prof. Stephen J. Lippard. Assay of human blood samples was begun in collaboration with Leonard A. Zwelling. Statistical tests were performed by Robert Tarone. The technical assistance of Elroy Patterson and Dung Nguyen is gratefully appreciated.

REFERENCES

1. Litterst CL, Reed E: In Kaiser HE (ed): "Comparative Aspects of Cancer Treatment." Oxford: Pergamon, Vol 196, 1986 (in press).
2. Paulson DF, Einhorn L, Peckham M, Williams SD: In DeVita VT, Hellman S, Rosenberg SA (eds): "Cancer." Philadelphia: Lippincott, 1982, pp 786–822.
3. Young RC, Von Hoff DD, Gormley P, Makuch R, Cassidy J, Howser D, Bull JM: Cancer Treat Rep 63:1539, 1979.
4. Plooy ACM, van Dijk M, Lohman PHM: Cancer Res 44:2043, 1984.
5. Dijt FJ, Canters GW, den Hartog JHJ, Marcelis ATM, Reedijk J: J Am Chem Soc 106:3644, 1984.
6. Zwelling LA: In Lippard SJ (ed): "Platinum, Gold and Other Metal Chemotherapeutic Agents." Washington: American Chemical Society, 1983, pp 27–50.
7. Plooy ACM, Fichtinger-Shepman AMJ, Schutte HH, van Dijk M, Lohman PHM: Carcinogenesis 6:561, 1985.
8. Eastman A: Proc Am Assoc Cancer Res 25:367, 1984.
9. Fichtinger-Shepman AMJ, Lohman PHM, Reedijk J: Nucleic Acids Res 10:5345, 1982.

10. Poirier MC: Environ Mutagen 6:879, 1984.

11. Perera FP, Poirier MC, Yuspa SH, Nakayama J, Jaretzki A, Curnen MM, Knowles DM, Weinstein IB: Carcinogenesis 3:1405, 1982.

12. Leopold WR, Miller EC, Miller JA: Cancer Res 39:913, 1979.

13. Yuspa SH, Harris CC: Exp Cell Res 86:95, 1974.

14. Lieberman MW, Poirier MC: Cancer Res 33:2097, 1973.

15. Poirier MC, Reed E, Zwelling LA, Ozols RF, Litterst CL, Yuspa SH: Env Health Persp 62:89, 1985.

16. Poirier MC, Lippard SJ, Zwelling LA, Ushay HM, Kerrigan D, Thill CC, Santella RM, Grunberger D, Yuspa SH: Proc Natl Acad Sci USA 79:6443, 1982.

17. Armitage P: "Statistical Methods in Medical Research." Oxford: Blackwell, 1971.

18. Lippard SJ, Ushay HM, Merkel CM, Poirier MC: Biochemistry 22:5165, 1983.

19. Ozols RF, Deisseroth AB, Javadpour N, Barlock A, Messerschmidt GL, Young RC: Cancer 51:1803, 1983.

Biochemical and Molecular Epidemiology of Cancer 313–322 (1986)

Hormonal, Infectious, and Nutritional Aspects of Cancer of the Female Reproductive Tract

Robert N. Hoover

Environmental Epidemiology Branch, Division of Cancer Etiology, National Cancer Institute, Bethesda, Maryland 20205

Two malignancies of the female reproductive tract, endometrial cancer and cancer of the uterine cervix, seem to be ideal candidates for intensive interdisciplinary collaboration between epidemiologists and laboratory scientists. Epidemiologic, clinical, and laboratory research on endometrial cancer have led to a relatively unified theory of how a variety of risk factors might operate to influence the risk of this disease. While this "estrogenic-etiology" theory has been extensively developed, a number of questions about key biological mechanisms remain unanswered. The level of development of epidemiologic methods and laboratory adjuncts relevant to these questions suggests that interdisciplinary studies targeted on some of these issues might advance substantially our understanding of hormonal and nutritional aspects of carcinogenesis. Recent epidemiologic research on cervical cancer has produced a number of often interrelated leads (sexual, hormonal, chemical, and nutritional) to etiologic factors. At the same time, technological advances have permitted laboratory investigators to suggest specific testable hypotheses for the biochemical and/or molecular basis of these factors. The epidemiologic and pathological complexities of cervical cancer and the sophistication of the laboratory assays would seem to require close collaboration between epidemiologists and laboratory scientists for these hypotheses to be explored adequately.

Key words: endometrial cancer, cervical cancer, epidemiology, hormones, nutrition, viruses

The term *biochemical epidemiology* is rapidly becoming one of the more frequently used and abused phrases in the area of etiologic research on cancer. As a concept, it engenders almost universal enthusiasm among those considering it. Curiously enough, however, given the stature of those who discuss it, this enthusiasm is infrequently focused and rarely critical. Part of this stems from a lack of any consistent definition of what biochemical epidemiology is and is not. It often means different things to laboratory scientists, clinicians, and epidemiologists and is often defined differently by the same individual depending the topic under discussion and with whom it is being discussed.

Received June 10, 1985.

© **1986 Alan R. Liss, Inc.**

In general, I believe it is incumbent upon epidemiologists to perceive of biochemical epidemiology in one of its more restrictive definitions. Under these definitions, biochemical epidemiology would not include simply a series of laboratory measurements (no matter how elegant) on groups of humans, some of whom may have or may be at high risk of malignancy and others who may not. Rather, under the more restrictive definition, biochemical epidemiology is the incorporation of laboratory measurements into traditional, rigorous epidemiologic designs to enhance the value of both the epidemiologic investigation and the interpretation of the laboratory results. By this definition then, besides the usual criteria for good laboratory and epidemiologic research, there would be at least four additional requirements (two laboratory and two epidemiologic) to conduct a high-quality interdisciplinary investigation. First of all, the laboratory test would have to be adequately developed and standardized. Much of the current enthusiasm for interdisciplinary studies relates to avant-garde laboratory assays that are on the cutting edge of laboratory research and are neither well developed nor standardized when they are suggested for incorporation into human studies. Second, the laboratory assays suggested need to be applicable to the practical demands of epidemiologic investigations. With the rapid advances in technology, this is becoming less of problem than it has been in the past. However, it is still the case that for a laboratory adjunct to be useful in epidemiologic investigations the material required needs to be obtainable relatively simply in field situations, and the assays themselves need to be relatively simple and inexpensive so that they can be performed on large numbers of subjects. A requirement on the epidemiologic side is the ability to identify, target, and focus on a population that will be relevant for a study of the risk factor or biologic process on which the laboratory assays are focused. In addition, the investigation needs to ensure that there is adequate control for all sources of bias and confounding of the laboratory assays as well as those for the more traditional epidemiologic risk factors.

For all of these reasons, under this working definition of "biochemical epidemiology," to conduct a high-quality investigation is a challenging enterprise that can be very difficult both scientifically and in a practical sense, and it is often expensive. Because of this, there is a need to be selective and to focus resources (both scientific and monetary) on those issues and hypotheses that are developed enough to test robustly and for which the likelihood of a high scientific yield exists no matter what the results of the investigation.

Fortunately, for many reasons there are a substantial number of such opportunities in the area of malignancies of the reproductive tract. For the purpose of this discussion I will focus on two sites that offer a variety of such possibilities, endometrial cancer and cancer of the uterine cervix. I have chosen endometrial cancer because it is a site for which we have detailed insights into possible mechanisms of carcinogenesis based on a substantial amount of epidemiologic and clinical/laboratory research. While these disciplines have focused on some of the same issues, they have usually done so separately and, thus, there is also an apparent opportunity for major advances in our understanding of several key issues in carcinogenesis (including hormones and diet) by judiciously combining disciplines and working together on these issues. Cancer of the uterine cervix is particularly important in this area because of the number of epidemiologic leads to etiologic factors for which there has recently been both more specific hypotheses formulated and for which the technology exists to address these questions in an interdisciplinary manner.

ENDOMETRIAL CANCER

A number of independent risk factors have been well established epidemiologically for endometrial cancer. Several medical conditions are related to increased risk of endometrial cancer. Included are functional (estrogen secreting) ovarian tumors [1], the Stein-Leventhal syndrome [2], diabetes, and hypertension [3]. In addition, several reproductive risk factors are related to increased risk, most notably nulliparity and a late age at natural menopause [4]. Dietary-related factors seem also to be important. Obesity is a well-recognized risk factor for the development of endometrial cancer [5]. In addition, vegetarians experience a decreased risk of endometrial cancer, which may or may not be independent of weight [6,7]. Exogenous hormones have also been related to the risk of endometrial cancer. The use of menopausal estrogens [8] and sequential oral contraceptives [9,10] increases the risk of endometrial cancer, while the use of combination oral contraceptives results in a diminished risk [10–14]. Finally, age-related influences on endometrial cancer risk are somewhat different than for a number of other tumors, even a number of other hormonally related tumors. Specifically, endometrial cancer is extremely rare under age 45, but the risk rises precipitously among women in their late 40s and 50s in a much more dramatic fashion than for other tumors (Fig. 1) [15].

While epidemiologists were defining and quantifying these risk factors for the disease, clinical and laboratory investigations were being focused on these same conditions, resulting in a fairly unified theory of how these risk factors were influencing the risk of endometrial cancer (Fig. 2) [16,17]. Over half of these risk factors are associated either directly or through some as yet undetermined mechanism with increased levels of circulating estrogens, particularly so-called free or not protein-bound estrogens. Both the age effect and the use of combination oral contraceptives are felt to modify in some manner the increased risk associated with increased estrogen level through the modulating effects of progestogens. Finally, while nulliparity, diabetes, hypertension, and race have not been directly related to increased levels of circulating estrogens when controlled for the other factors, or for differences in

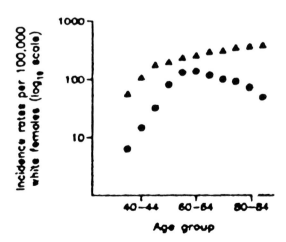

Fig. 1.   Average annual breast cancer (▲) and endometrial cancer (●) incidence rates for white females (SEER data, 1973–1977).

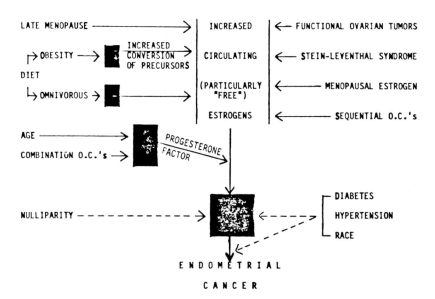

Fig. 2.   Risk factors for endometrial cancer and their possible modes of action.

progesterone levels, it is quite possible that these risk factors operate through a basic hormonal mechanism that has yet to be defined.

Given our knowledge of most human malignancy, the amount of information we have on this tumor concerning risk factors and the intermediate steps between these factors and endometrial cancer is substantial. However, this also serves to point up more specifically what we do not know and to whet one's appetite for the ability to unlock these unknown areas. Some issues that need to be resolved are strictly epidemiologic or strictly laboratory. Examples on the epidemiologic side are: How truly independent are some of these risk factors, particularly diabetes, hypertension, and obesity? How much of the racial effect is artifact caused by differential hysterectomy rates or ascertainment bias, and how much is "real"? How is the risk of endometrial cancer associated with menopausal estrogen use altered by the addition of a progestational drug to the regimen? How much of the disease in a defined population is accounted for by the aggregate of all of these risk factors?

However, most of the issues with respect to endometrial carcinogenesis can seemingly only be addressed adequately by truly interdisciplinary studies incorporating features of epidemiologic design along with appropriate laboratory adjuncts. These efforts could be directed specifically toward the black boxes on Figure 2 relating to the mechanisms by which certain risk factors operate.

Obesity is a well-established risk factor for endometrial cancer. It is also well established that obesity is related to increased peripheral conversion of precursors to circulating estrogens [18]. However, the manner in which this occurs is still unclear. There are very few data to address the issue of when in a woman's life the development of obesity is most important. In one preliminary effort with small numbers of observations, weight reduction from teenage obesity levels did not seem to have a large impact on adult endometrial cancer risk [19]. Laboratory observations in this general area have also shown that while weight reduction is associated with some decrease in total circulating estrogens, the increased conversion of precursors is apparently not much altered by such weight reduction [20]. This is bolstered by in vitro assays demonstrating increased conversion of precursors by fat samples from endometrial cancer cases compared to the fat samples from controls [21]. All of this raises the question of exactly how peripheral conversion of precursors to free estrogens is influenced by the numbers of adipocytes, their content in terms of type of fat, or some other factor. The observation that vegetarians experience a lower risk of endometrial cancer and have lower levels of free estrogens, even after control for indices of body fat, raises similar questions about possible mechanisms [22].

It has been speculated that the relative protection associated with being premenopausal and with the use of a combination of oral contraceptives operates through some type of progesterone mechanism that interferes with the estrogen etiology of endometrial cancer. The mechanism involved, however, remains unclear, although several have been proposed [16]. A key to an understanding of the mechanism will certainly involve a clarification of the currently conflicting epidemiologic evidence on the effect of cessation of use of combination oral contraceptives [12,13]. Two studies [12,13] noted that the "protection" was more substantial among current users and subsided somewhat with cessation. However, one study implied that the protection in fact was transitory [12], while the other still noted substantial protection a number of years after stopping [13].

Perhaps the most important of the black boxes in Figure 2 is the precise mechanism by which increased circulating estrogens produce endometrial cancer. To date, several possible mechanisms have been proposed. These include the possibility that estrogens are complete carcinogens themselves, that estrogens act as promotors in the classical laboratory sense of promotion, or that the increased risk of malignancy is simply due to the growth stimulation produced by estrogens that offers a greater opportunity for abnormal cells to arise or for carcinogens to act on vulnerable genetic material. The current epidemiologic evidence by itself does not allow the distinction of promotion from growth stimulation. However, the evidence can at least partially address the issue of distinguishing an early stage from a relatively late stage effect. Most notably, the increased risk associated with menopausal estrogen use shows up approximately 2 years after the onset of such use [23,24], and the risk declines progressively with each passing year after cessation of use [23,25]. As noted previously, the protective effect associated with combination oral contraceptives shows a similar pattern. The abrupt onset of risk with menopausal age can also be construed as a very rapid effect. Together these observations would argue fairly persuasively that estrogens act at a relatively late stage in the process of carcinogenesis.

If one chooses to embrace the tumor promotion model for estrogens and endometrial cancer, one has to deal with the dilemma of speculating about what the initiator could be. Thus far, no risk factors that would fall into this category are readily apparent, although admittedly they have not been well pursued by epidemiologic investigations.

Pursuit of these general issues translates to pursuit of a number of more specific questions, such as: How much of the effect of the epidemiologic risk factors is accounted for by the estrogen effect? Is there a dose effect for circulating estrogens that is similar regardless of source? How much of the increased circulating estrogen effect is due to free versus bound estrogen, and is there any difference in effect between major estrogens? How lasting is the exogenous estrogen effect on both disease and hormonal metabolism? What is the mechanism of action on hormonal status and endometrial cancer risk of the oral contraceptives? Are the few risk factors not yet related to a hormonal etiology actually related to hormonal metabolism in some way? How much of the obesity effect is simply calories and how much is source of calories, and, further, how much of the effect is related to the number of fat cells versus their content or type of fat? What is the mechanism of action of the increased circulating estrogen levels? If the mechanism is that of promotion, what are the initiating agents?

As I noted, addressing these issues in a high-quality manner would seem to require a combination of formal epidemiologic approaches with the incorporation of a number of laboratory adjuncts. Specifically, what would seem to be desirable would be a study of a large series of incident cases from a defined population, along with a large sample of controls who were representative of this same population. The study would involve extensive assessments of dietary patterns including major lifetime changes, anthropometric data throughout life, reproductive and medicinal risk factors, and probing for other relevant exposures. The laboratory adjuncts to such a study would include serum and urinary hormones, fat biopsies, and a variety of assays on fresh tumor material. It would seem that both the epidemiologic capabilities and the appropriate laboratory assays are developed enough to support such an investigation.

CANCERS OF THE UTERINE CERVIX

Our level of insight into mechanisms of carcinogenesis for the uterine cervix is certainly a long way from that of endometrial cancer. However, for some time a diverse number of risk factors have been repeatedly demonstrated for cancers of the uterine cervix. More recently, many more specific hypotheses have been proffered to explain the basis for these risk factors. In addition, recent advances in technology enable a number of these more specific hypotheses to be addressed directly in the context of epidemiologic investigations. Two noteworthy features of this disease make the interdisciplinary approach particularly attractive. First of all, most cervical cancer risk factors, and the hypotheses proffered concerning their mechanisms, are highly interrelated. Second, the disease presents some very complex problems in the areas of pathology and epidemiology. These two features of cervical cancer seem to insure that further advances toward more specific etiologic factors and mechanisms can probably only be made through interdisciplinary studies. On the other hand, these same features make such investigations very difficult to do well and to interpret appropriately.

Historically, several risk factors for this disease have been well known for some time. From the first observations relating to the frequency of this disease among married women and its absence among nuns [26] it has been suspected that this could be a sexually transmitted disease. Two of the more powerful risk factors that are routinely identified for this disease are an increased risk with increased numbers of sexual partners and an increased risk with earlier ages at first coitus [27,28]. Recently, these findings have been augmented by demonstration of the so-called male factor for this disease. Specifically, among women who have had only one sex partner, the risk of cervical cancer is directly related to various indicators of sexual promiscuity for this male partner [29]. Another long-recognized risk factor for this disease is socioeconomic status. Those in the lowest social classes experience approximately twice the risk of disease as those in the highest. A substantial portion of this relationship appears to be independent of the sexual factors previously mentioned.

More recently, three new risk factors for this disease have been proposed along with supporting data. High-quality epidemiologic investigations of oral contraception have produced a remarkably consistent impression that risk of cervical cancer increased with increased use of oral contraceptives [28,30–34]. This has been true whether the endpoint was dysplasia, carcinoma in situ, or invasive carcinoma. It was also true that a twofold excess risk has been noted for long-term use in both case-control studies and cohort investigations. Also recently, suggestions were made from descriptive, correlational studies that cigarette smoking might be a risk factor for cancers of the uterine cervix [35]. While there was some initial concern that this was only an apparent relationship because of the confounding influences of socioeconomic status and sexual factors, several analytic studies focused on this issue have indicated an excess risk of cervical cancer associated with cigarette smoking that is apparently independent of these other risk factors [28,36–38]. There is, however, a fair amount of inconsistency, including some lack of persuasive dose-response relationships, making a causal interpretation somewhat speculative at this time. Last among the more recent candidates for cervical cancer risk factors has been various micronutrient deficiencies. Since the malignancies of the uterine cervix are primarily squamous cell carcinomas of epithelial tissue, the theoretical speculation about a protective role for vitamin A and/or carotene seems to be applicable to these malignancies. Indeed, several studies have found that indices of vitamin A and carotene intake in the diet or serum were inversely related to the risk of cervical cancer [39–41]. Another study has suggested that vitamin C might also be relatively more common among the controls rather than the cases and, therefore, might be a biologically important protective factor against this malignancy [42].

As our knowledge of cervical cancer risk factors has evolved, more specific hypotheses have been suggested to explain the mechanisms through which some of these factors might operate. With the advent of these more specific hypotheses has also come the realization of how interrelated a number of these issues really are. In the area of infectious agents, infections with a variety of sexually transmitted agents have been related to elevated risks of cervical neoplasia. This is not surprising, since this is what one would expect simply on the basis of a relationship between promiscuity and risk of this tumor. The salient question is whether any one or several of these infectious agents are responsible for the associations of risk with the sexual factors, or are they merely a reflection of these risk factors. Much epidemiologic and laboratory effort has been directed toward evaluating this question. Historically, most of the interest has been in herpesvirus type II [43]. A number of early results suggested a relationship, while several failed to find such. Much of the early work was severely hampered by difficulties in the assays used to detect antibodies and a resulting wide variation in prevalence rates from study to study. A major concern was also whether these infections actually preceded the neoplastic process or whether neoplastic tissue was simply a more receptive host for this virus. To address these questions, a large prospective study was initiated in Czechoslovakia over 9 years ago [44]. Sera were obtained from women, who were followed for various conditions over this 9-year period. A case-control study within this cohort was reported last year [45]. Controls were matched to the cases of cervical neoplasia on the basis of age, age at first intercourse, number of sexual partners, smoking habits, and therapeutic procedures. No difference was found between the cases and controls in the level of antibody to herpes simplex virus type II by either of two laboratory assays. Another prospective study that started about the same time to follow women who were exposed in utero to DES also provided the opportunity to collect serum in a prospective manner [46]. Recent results from this study also indicate no difference in the levels of antibody to herpes simplex virus type II in either the sera collected at entry or that obtained at time of diagnosis [47]. Curiously enough, there was a difference in antibodies to herpes simplex virus type I between cases and controls in the sera collected at both times.

The candidate virus that has generated the most recent enthusiasm for an etiologic role in cervical neoplasia is the papilloma virus [48]. Adequate assessments have been made more difficult by the lack of antibody assays for the appropriate strains. However, a substantial amount of biochemical and molecular evidence has pointed toward a role for this virus. Since this is a topic of another paper in this session I will not go extensively into the evidence. It may be of some interest, however, to note that one of the hypothesized roles for this virus is that of a tumor promotor, perhaps promoting the effects of other infectious agents [49]. The recent results from the follow-up of the DES-exposed cohort indicate a 17-fold increased risk of cervical neoplasia for women with histological evidence of papilloma infection at the time of diagnosis [47]. None of these histological changes were present in the biopsy material obtained from a subset of these cases prior to diagnosis. This may indicate that if this virus has a role, it is likely to be involved at the latter stages of the carcinogenesis process. It also emphasizes the need to document whether the infection preceded the tumor, or whether neoplastic tissue is somehow more receptive to viral infection.

Possible mechanisms for the association with cigarette smoking have also recently been suggested. In a study from the American Health Foundation, it was noted that cervical mucus among smokers reflected the levels of cotinine seen in the serum and that the levels of nicotine were in fact more concentrated than those seen in the serum [50]. A logical next step would be to look for tobacco carcinogen-DNA adducts in cervical cancer specimens.

A number of the micronutrient hypotheses have also become more specific and more focused, some taking into account the apparent interrelationships between a number of these risk factors. One of the more provocative findings has been the observation that oral contraceptive users have lower serum and red blood cell folate levels than nonusers and that contraceptive users who also have cervical dysplasia have even lower levels [51]. These low levels are also accompanied by megaloblastic changes in the cervical epithelium. In a placebo-controlled trial of folic acid supplements in women with varying degrees of cervical dysplasia the dysplasia progressively improved among the group receiving folic acid and remained approximately the same among the placebo group [51]. A number of interesting questions are raised by these observations. Is risk of neoplasia associated with oral contraceptives caused by an accompanying folic acid deficiency, or are these independent or perhaps interactive risk factors? Is folic acid a factor in neoplasia among women who are not oral contraceptive users? The recent findings or diminshed induced chromosomal breaks at fragile sites near oncogenes following supplementation with folic acid makes these observations even more provocative for their etiologic and mechanistic possibilities [52].

In summary, we certainly do not have the depth of knowledge of possible mechanisms of carcinogenesis for cancers of the uterine cervix that we have for endometrial cancer. However, a substantial number of risk factors are known for cervical cancer. Recently, a number of more specific, mechanistically oriented hypotheses have been suggested to explain these risk factors. In addition, recent advances in technology have enabled a number of these more specific hypotheses to be addressed in epidemiologic studies.

It is appropriate for an epidemiologist to conclude a discussion of cervical cancer with a comment on the complexities of studying this disease. The neoplastic state itself is a complex one, which offers many intermediate endpoints between mild dysplasia and invasive malignancy. Many studies focus on early neoplastic states without recognizing that the progressive transition from one stage to another is not universal, and the diagnosis of many of these entities themselves is dependent on participation in screening programs. In addition, the majority of the risk factors and the hypotheses proposed to explain them are highly interrelated, offering numerous possibilities for spurious associations if other variables are not adequately controlled. An illustration of this latter point comes from preliminary analyses of a five-center study of invasive cancers of the uterine cervix (Table I) (L. Brinton, personal communication). In the crude data there appeared to be little or no association of risk with use of oral contraceptives. However, after introducing appropriate control for seven separate risk factors for cervical cancer, a significant trend of increasing risk with increasing duration of oral contraceptive use emerged. Indeed a substantial amount of this dramatic change was brought about by control for a distinctly nonbiological risk factor, that is, interval from diagnosis to last pap smear. Patients who have developed invasive cervical cancer tend not to have been participants in active screening. Therefore, the disease is related to relatively long intervals to last pap smear. Conversely, oral contraceptive users tend to be screened by pap smear relatively frequently because of their frequent contacts with the medical care system. Thus, there is a distinct possibility for negative confounding, and the failure to find a true association because of the confounding by this medical-care variable. This is apparently what happened in this instance.

Thus, because of the complexity of the disease and virtually all aspects of studies designed to address its risks factors, it appears that further advances toward specific etiologic factors and mechanisms will only be possible through interdisciplinary studies. It is just as clear that for the same reasons such investigations will be very difficult to do well and to interpret appropriately.

TABLE I. Relative Risks for Invasive Cervical Cancer by Years of Oral Contraceptive Use: Preliminary Results From a Case-Control Study in Five Geographic US Areas

Years of pill use	Age-adjusted RR	Adjusted[a] RR[1]
None	1.00	1.00
<5	0.78	1.29
5–9	1.16	2.00
10+	1.26	1.84

[a]Adjusted for age, race, number of sexual partners, age at first intercourse, interval since last pap smear, years smoked, history of a nonspecific genital infection or sore, and education.

REFERENCES

1. Waard F de: Acta Endocrinol 29:279, 1958.
2. Jackson RL, Dockerty MB: Am J Obstet Gynecol 73:161, 1957.
3. Wynder EL, Escher GC, Mantel N: Cancer 19:489, 1966.
4. Elwood JM, Cole P, Rothman KJ, Kaplan SD: JNCI 59:1055, 1977.
5. MacMahon B: Gynecol Oncol 2:122, 1974.
6. Phillips RL: Cancer Res 35:3513, 1975.
7. Armstrong BK: "Origins of Human Cancer." Cold Spring Harbor, NY: Cold Spring Harbor, 1977, pp 557–565.
8. International Agency for Research on Cancer: "Evaluation of the Carcinogenic Risk of Chemicals to Humans." Lyon, Switzerland: IARC, 1979, Vol 21, pp 95–102.
9. Silverberg SG, Makowski EL: Obstet Gynecol 46:503, 1975.
10. Weiss NS, Savyetz TA: N Engl J Med 302:551, 1980.
11. Kaufman DW, Shapiro S, Slone D, et al: N Engl J Med 303:1045, 1980.
12. Hulka BS, Chambless LE, Kaufman DG, et al: JAMA 247:475, 1982.
13. Centers for Disease Control: JAMA 249:1600, 1983.
14. Henderson BE, Casagrande JT, Pike MC: Br J Cancer 47:749, 1983.
15. Surveillance Epidemiology End Results: "Incidence and Mortality Data: 1973–77." U.S. Department of Health and Human Services, Monograph 57. Washington, D.C.: U.S. Government Printing Office, 1981.
16. Henderson BE, Ross RK, et al: Cancer Res 42:3232, 1982.
17. Kirschner MA, Schneider G, et al: Cancer Res 42:3281, 1982.
18. Siiteri PK, McDonald PC: "Handbook of Physiology." Washington, D.C.: American Physiological Society, 1973, pp 615–629.
19. Blitzer PH, Blitzer EC, Rimm AA: Prev Med 5:20, 1976.
20. Takalsi HK, Siiteri PK, Williams J, et al: Int J Obes 2:386, 1978.
21. Schindler AE, Exbert A, Friedrich E: J Clin Endocrinol Metab 35:627, 1972.
22. Armstrong BK, Brown JB, Clarke HT, et al: JNCI 67:761, 1981.
23. Weiss NS, Szekely DR, English DR, et al: JAMA 242:261, 1979.
24. Gray LA, Christopherson WM, Hoover RN: Obstet Gynecol 49:385, 1977.
25. Shapiro S, Kaufman DW, Slone D, et al: N Engl J Med 303:485, 1980.
26. Rigoni-Stern DG: Serv Progr Pathol Ther Ser 2:507, 1842.
27. Rotkin ID: Cancer Res 33:1353, 1973.
28. Harris RWC, Brinton LA, Cowdell RH, et al: Br J Cancer 42:359, 1980.
29. Buckley JD, Harris RWC, Doll R, et al: Lancet 2:1010, 1981.
30. Ory HW, Conger SB, Naib Z, Taylor CW, et al: "Pharmacology of Steroid Contraceptive Drugs." New York: Dover Press, 1977.
31. Peritz E, Ramcharan S, Frank S, et al: Am J Epidemiol 106:462, 1977.
32. Stern E, Forsythe AB, Youkeles L, Coffelt CF: Science 196:1460, 1977.
33. Vessey MP, Lawless M, McPherson K, Yeates D: Lancet 2:930, 1983.
34. WHO Collaborative Study of Neoplasia and Steroid Contraceptives: Br Med J 290:961, 1985.
35. Winklestein W Jr.: Am J Epidemiol 106:257, 1977.
36. Clarke ER, Morgan RW, Newman AM: Am J Epidemiol 115:59, 1982.
37. Lyon JL, Gardner JW, West DW, et al: Am J Public Health 73:588, 1983.
38. Greenberg ER, Vessey M, McPherson K, Yeates D: Br J Cancer 51:139, 1985.
39. Marshall JR, Graham S, Byers T, et al: JNCI 70:847, 1983.
40. LaVecchia C, Franceschi S, Decarli A, et al: Int J Cancer 34:319, 1984.
41. Bernstein A, Harris B: Am J Obstet Gynecol 148:309, 1984.
42. Wassertheil-Smoller S, Romney SL, et al: Am J Epidemiol 114:714, 1981.
43. Melnick JL, Adam E: Prog Exp Tumor Res 21:49, 1978.
44. Vonka V, Kanka J, Jelinek J, et al: Int J Cancer 33:49, 1984.
45. Vonka V, Kanka J, Hirsch I, et al: Int J Cancer 33:61, 1984.
46. Robboy SJ, Noller KL, O'Brien P, et al: JAMA 252:2979, 1984.
47. Adam E, Kaufman RH, Adler-Storthz K, et al: Int J Cancer 35:19, 1985.
48. Zur Hausen H, Gissman L, Schlehofer JR: Prog Med Virol 30:170, 1984.
49. Zur Hausen H: Lancet 2:1370, 1982.
50. Sasson IM, Haley NJ, Hoffman D, et al: N Engl J Med 312:315, 1985.
51. Butterworth CE Jr., Hatch KD, Gore H, et al: Am J Clin Nutr 35:73, 1982.
52. Yunis JJ, Soreng AL: Science 226:1199, 1984.

Biochemical and Molecular Epidemiology of Cancer 323–344 (1986)

Molecular Epidemiology and Oncogenicity of Human Cytomegalovirus

Eng-Shang Huang, Michelle G. Davis, John F. Baskar, and Shu-Mei Huong

Lineberger Cancer Research Center, Department of Medicine (E-S.H) and Department of Microbiology and Immunology (E-S.H., J.F.B., M.G.D., S.-M.H.), University of North Carolina at Chapel Hill, Chapel Hill, North Carolina 27514

Human cytomegalovirus (HCMV) is a ubiquitous human pathogen with a great degree of biological and structural similarities to other herpesviruses, and it has been classified as one of the five human herpesviruses. Clinically, it can cause a variety of manifestations ranging from asymptomatic subclinical infection to severe intrauterine infection leading to fetal death, developmental abnormality, and mental retardation, postprofusion syndrome, and interstitial pneumonitis in immunosuppressed organ transplant and immunocompromised patients [Weller, 1971]. Like other herpesviruses, it causes persistent as well as latent infections. Its ubiquitous presentation and often asymptomatic interaction with the human host frequently lead scientists to overlook its unique pathogenicity and possible oncogenicity. Therefore, it is somewhat difficult to convince scientists to believe that this virus has oncogenic potential comparable to that of other herpesviruses.

In this communication we will discuss the molecular epidemiology of CMV infection and the molecular biology of the virus-host interaction, emphasizing the fact that CMV should be considered to be an oncogenic DNA virus.

GENOMIC POLYMORPHISM OF HUMAN CMV

Human CMV is a double-stranded DNA virus with a genome of 150 million daltons, about 240 kb, and approximately 50% larger than the genome of herpes simplex virus. Intact viral DNA is composed of two covalently bonded components, L and S components, with four symmetrical arrangements, as described for herpes simplex virus (HSV) DNA [Kilpatrick and Huang, 1977]. Similar to HSV, the transcription of CMV genome is also cascadely regulated in three distinct phases [Stinski, 1978]. But, in contrast to HSV, CMV has a prolonged interval of early phase gene expression. The replication cycle of CMV is about 10 times longer than that of herpes simplex virus.

Received September 12, 1985.

© **1986 Alan R. Liss, Inc.**

DNA-DNA reassociation kinetics studies revealed that human CMV strains share at least 80% of sequence homology with prototype strain AD-169 [Huang et al, 1976]. The degree of homology existing among CMV strains is greater than that between HSV I and HSV II, which is about 50% [Kieff et al, 1972]. Although each isolate shares a relatively high degree of DNA sequence homology, they could not obviously have been classified into subgroups or subtypes [Huang et al, 1980b]. HCMV has extreme genomic and antigenic polymorphisms. The genomic polymorphism of CMV can be demonstrated by the restriction enzyme fragmentation of purified viral DNA and the analysis of the fragmentation product by agarose gel electrophoresis [Kilpatrick et al, 1976; Huang et al, 1976]. Viral DNA was labeled in culture with ^{32}P and was subjected to restriction enzyme fragmentation and agarose gel electrophoresis. As shown in Figure 1, each CMV isolate has its own distinct identity in DNA restriction pattern. No epidemiologically unrelated strains share an identical DNA restriction pattern. Identical patterns could be demonstrated in the case of recurrent infection and in viruses isolated from a pregnant woman and her offspring [Huang et al, 1980a,b]. The antigenic polymorphism of CMV strains can be demonstrated by complement fixation [Huang et al, 1976], neutralization test [Weller et al, 1960], and electroimmunodiffusion [Sweet et al, 1979]. But CMV strains cannot be distinguished by SDS-polyacrylamide gel polypeptide composition analysis [Gupta et al, 1977]. The restriction enzyme analysis of viral DNA has therefore become the most powerful tool with which to study the epidemiology and transmission of human cytomegalovirus infection.

PREVALENCE OF CMV INFECTION IN THE GENERAL POPULATION

The prevalence of CMV complement-fixing antibody in the adult population in different regions of the world ranges from 40% in Europe to close to 100% in Africa and the Far East [Krech, 1973; Ho, 1982]. In general, the rate of CMV infection is somewhat related to the social economic status of the population and, to a certain extent, to the geographic location. The prevalence is lower in Europe, Australia, and certain parts of America and significantly higher in underdeveloped countries. In certain regions of the Far East and Africa almost every adult has acquired CMV infection before age 35; in fact, approximately 15–20% of pregnant women and 15–20% of children under 1 year of age in the Far East are constantly shedding virus in the cervix and urine, respectively [Numazaki et al, 1970; Alexander, 1967]; in the United States virus is shed by about 5–7%. The prevalence of complement-fixing antibodies according to age group in the Washington, DC area was shown by Rowe et al [1956] and summarized by Ho [1982]. Approximately 71% of cord blood showed positive CMV CF antigen; this reflects the existence of maternal antibodies in the newborn. By the age of 6 to 23 months, 14% of the infants and babies had been exposed to CMV infection through perinatal infection. An additional 17% was added during 2 to 4 years of age at the nursery stage. At the high school level, 45% of the teenagers had CMV infection. In general, approximately 81% of adults by the age of 35 years or more in the Washington, DC area had been exposed to CMV infection. The prevalences of positive CF antibody samples from London and Sweden are significantly lower than that in the Washington, DC area [Ho, 1982].

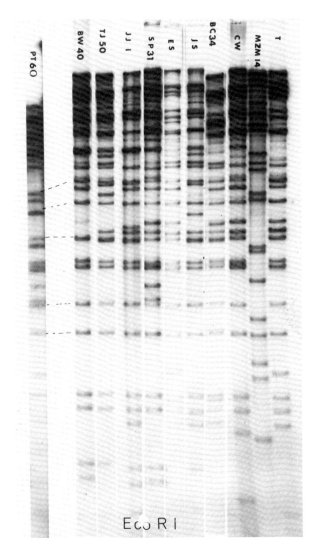

Fig. 1. Restriction enzyme analysis of virus DNA from various CMV isolates. Purified ^{32}P-labeled CMV DNAs were digested with restriction enzyme EcRI and then subjected to 1% agarose gel electrophoresis. Strain MZM 14 is a chimpanzee CMV shown for comparison. Others are human clinical isolates. Viral DNA polymorphism is evident.

MODES OF TRANSMISSION OF HUMAN CYTOMEGALOVIRUS

There are many ways that CMV can be transmitted from one individual to another in the entire human life cycle. Transplacental infection and infection via the endometrium resulting in congenital CMV infection is the common mode of transmission in the early stages of human life. Congenital infection occurs in about 1–2.5% of infants [Starr et al, 1970; Stagno et al, 1980] in the United States. This was determined by the isolation of CMV from urine of infants at birth. Around 20–30% of children became perinatally infected, as indicated by excreting CMV in urine at the age of 3 months. This perinatal infection resulted mainly from infection inside the genital tract of the mother during delivery. In addition, breast milk may be an important vehicle for virus transmission, because CMV has been frequently isolated from human milk [Stagno et al, 1980]. Up to the age of 6 months about 35–56% of children in the Far East and Finland and 8–13% in England and the United States excreted virus in urine.

We have studied the virus strains isolated from recurrent infected pregnant women during the consecutive gestation periods and virus from their offspring [Huang et al, 1980a,b]. It is extremely interesting that CMV recurrent infection frequently occurs in women during their pregnancies. The excretion of virus from the cervix usually becomes undetectable after delivery of the baby but is recurrent in the following gestation. Among 10 cases we studied, eight of the recurrent infections showed identical DNA restriction patterns in repeat CMV isolates [Huang et al, 1980a,b]. In another two cases, one infection with minor modification in the EcoRI pattern but with identical BamHI restriction patterns was found; the difference in the EcoRI pattern was possibly due to incomplete EcoRI enzyme digestion. Another one had more obvious distinction in EcoRI patterns between 1972 and 1973 isolates; it is possible that a new virus strain or a new recombinant strain was introduced in 1973 in this woman. These data indicate that the majority of maternal recurrent infection is due to the reactivation of the preexisting latent virus, and a small portion of recurrent infection might be due to the reintroduction of a new virus strain. In a study of the DNA restriction patterns of viruses isolated from consecutive congenitally infected infants, we found that in most cases viruses recovered from the mothers were identical to those recovered from their congenitally or neonatally infected babies, and viruses from congenitally infected infants born 2 to 4 years apart to the same mothers have identical restriction enzyme patterns [Huang et al, 1980a,b]. These data clearly explain the reactivation and the mother-to-offspring modes of CMV transmission in congenital and perinatal infection.

Reynolds et al [1973] studied the correlation of maternal cervical CMV secretion and CMV infection in babies. They found that only 4% of babies born of nonsecretors became infected, while 37% of babies born of CMV secretors (at trimester) became infected. In infants whose mothers shed virus postpartum and at trimester, the CMV infection rate was 57%. None of the babies of women who shed CMV in the urine was infected. Therefore, it is suggested that the uterine cervix is an important site of virus source in perinatal CMV infection of infants [Reynolds et al, 1973; Ho, 1982].

There are two very interesting studies on CMV transmission in newborn nurseries. First, Spector and Spector [1980], using restriction endonuclease analysis, found a pair of monozygotic twins who were infected with different strains of CMV at 6 and 9 weeks of age; neither of these viruses were from their mother because she was seronegative until 6 months after delivery. The babies were hospitalized for 4 months because of premature rupture of amnionic membrane and cesarean birth. A second interesting case was a CMV outbreak in a nursery reported by Gurevich and Cunha [1981]. In this case, a female infant with congenital CMV disease was admitted to a neonatal intensive care unit for only 8 hr. After this short period of admission, four infants in this intensive care unit became infected. Of them, two died because of the disseminated CMV infection. Two were twins with a seronegative mother. These two episodes clearly indicate that CMV infection and transmission occur commonly in the infant nursery.

Sexual transmission plays an important role in the transmission of CMV infection in teenagers and the adult population. This is based on the fact that CMV has been demonstrated in the uterine cervix, in saliva, and even in human semen [Lang and Kummer, 1972, 1975]. Jordan et al [1973] reported that 16 out of 120 (13.3%) women suspected of having venereal disease had cervical CMV infection. In a VD clinic in England, Willmott [1975] studied 531 females and found that 6.6% were positive for CMV. Recently, Handsfield et al [1985] in Seattle reported that viruses with identical restriction enzyme patterns have been isolated from two couples of male and female sexual partners. This indicates that heterosexual contact can be considered a common mode of transmission among young adults.

CMV infection is extremely frequent among homosexual men. In one study, Drew et al [1981; Drew, 1983] found that 30% of homosexual males in the San Francisco area actively shed CMV in urine or in semen. In our study of CMV infection among asymptomatic homosexual males in the Research Triangle Park in North Carolina, we found that CMV could be repeatedly isolated from semen of 30% (13 out of 40) of homosexual males examined. Virus particles could be demonstrated inside the sperm head as well as in the extracellular fluid (Fig. 2). Thirteen CMV isolates from this group were subjected to DNA restriction enzyme analysis. Results revealed that among these isolates, four (345-6, 7, SE, OTT) from four different individuals share one kind of DNA restriction pattern, while an additional pair (345-10 and 345-16) shares another identical pattern but is different from the former group. In the first group, two isolates came from a pair of sexual partners and another two came from two subjects who did not know each other. The sharing of identical DNA restriction patterns indicates the epidemiological relatedness of virus strains and implies sexual transmission of cytomegalovirus infection among this group of subjects (Fig. 3) [Huang, 1984; Huang, manuscript in preparation].

Finally, CMV can be transmitted by means of blood transfusions and organ transplantations. Quite a few studies on CMV infection have been reported, and a number of these reports provided conclusive data to support the possibility that blood transfusions are a source of CMV infection [Ho, 1982]. Paloheimo et al [1968] studied 63 open heart surgery patients who received an average of 7.6 units of blood that was positive for CMV infection by serology CF test. Thirty percent of the patients showed CMV infection after transfusion as detected by seroconversion or rising antibody titer. Among them the primary infection occurred in 10 out of 17 seronegative patients (59%) and secondary infection in nine out of 36 seropositive individuals (25%). Henle et al [1970] performed a similar study in Philadelphia and Helsinki. Fifty-three out of the 152 open heart surgery patients studied showed evidence of CMV infection. Primary infection occurred in 36 out of 61 seronegative patients (59%) and secondary infection occurred in 17 out of 91 seropositive patients. In this study Henle et al [1970] also found that the number of units of blood transfused was related to the rate of CMV infection. Ho [1982] has summarized data from 12 studies on a total of 1,550 recipients with moderate to large numbers of transfusion and from these 14% became infected; primary infection occurred in 139 out of 740 seronegative patients, and secondary infection occurred in 76 out of 800 seropositive patients. Because CMV has been demonstrated in blood from normal individuals as well as from organ recipients, it is believed that CMV is commonly transmitted via blood transfusion.

Cytomegalovirus infection is also a common complication in organ transplantation [Rubin et al, 1977]. Virus is often found in patients with interstitial pneumonia

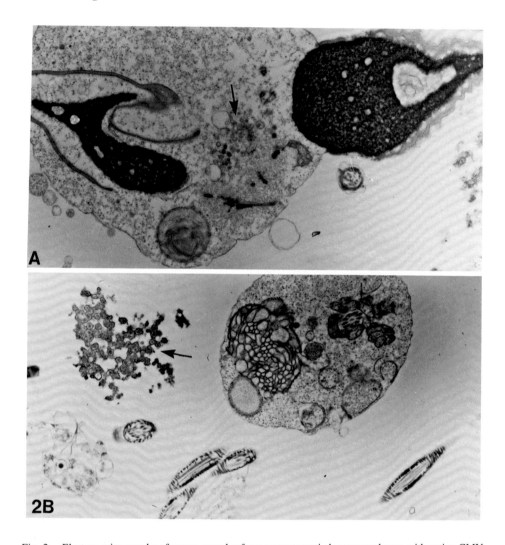

Fig. 2.   Electron micrographs of semen samples from asymptomatic homosexual men with active CMV infection. A) Intracellular location of viral particles (arrow); B) extracellular viral particles (arrow).

after transplantation. To understand the potential source of cytomegalovirus infection we have analyzed, in collaboration with Dr. Drew Winston, virus strains isolated from 18 patients having bone marrow transplantation. Among them four patients who had asymptomatic excretion of CMV in urine before transplantation subsequently developed CMV infection with syndromes of pneumonia (two patients), fever (one), and viruria (one). In each patient, the CMV infection that developed after transplantation was caused by a virus strain genetically identical to the isolate detected in urine before transplantation. CMV isolates from different sites in the same patient (urine, buffy coat, and lung) were identical, but CMV isolates from different patients were not [Winston et al, 1985]. In another separate study, we analyzed one pair of viruses isolated from a blood donor and a recipient who became infected with CMV subsequent to transfusion. The restriction enzyme analysis indicated that the virus isolated

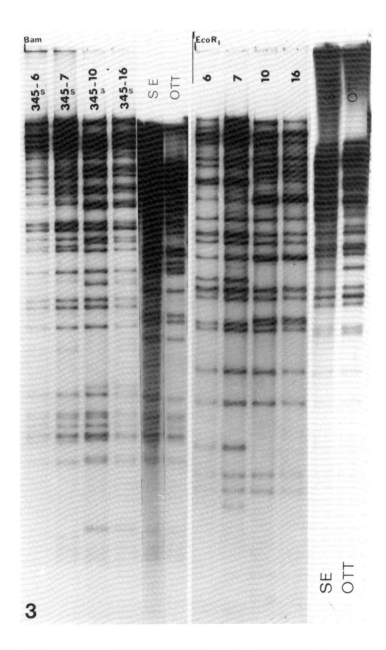

Fig. 3.   Restriction enzyme analysis of viral DNA from various CMV isolates from semen of asymptomatic homosexual men. Viral DNAs were subjected to BamHI (left) and EcoRI restriction enzyme digestion (right). Viral strains 345-6, 345-7, SE, and OTT share identical restriction patterns, while strains 345-10 and 345-16 are identical.

from the recipient was not genetically related to the strain isolated from the donor [Huang et al, 1980b]. These results imply that active infections in organ transplants are more likely caused by the reactivation of the recipient's latent virus via a graft versus host reaction. Nevertheless, transmission of virus from organ donor or from blood donors to recipient by donor's organ has been implied at least in renal allograft. It is therefore reasonable to assume that the reactivation of latent virus and the transmission of CMV to recipient via donor blood or donor organ both play important roles in active CMV infection in organ transplants.

CYTOMEGALOVIRUS INFECTION AND IMPAIRMENT OF CELLULAR IMMUNITY

Cytomegalovirus infection may produce immunosuppression in human beings. It induces transient abnormality in cellular immune function in healthy persons [Rinaldo et al, 1977, 1980]. Lymphocytes from patients with acute CMV mononucleosis showed a remarkable decrease in responsiveness to certain mitogens, such as pokeweed mitogen and concanavalin A. Analysis of lymphocyte T-cell subpopulations revealed a reversal in the ratio of T-helper to T-suppressor cells during human CMV infection [Carney et al, 1981]. The alternations in T-lymphocyte subsets are suggested to be responsible for the lymphocyte hyporesponses to selective mitogens. In certain patients with CMV mononucleosis, the T-lymphocyte subset ratios were found to be abnormal for more than 10 months [Carney et al, 1981; Reinherz et al, 1980]. During convalescence, the T-helper lymphocyte function increased, suppressor T cell decreased, and Con A responses returned to normal. The impairment of T-lymphocyte function by human CMV infection is obvious. It is possible that prolonged CMV infection may lead to immunodeficiency with abnormal helper and suppressor T-cell ratios. Hypothetically, certain tumors or virus-induced transformed cells might, therefore, fully express under such conditions. In addition, CMV infection has been found to be associated with leukopenia, which in turn leads to the predisposition of the patient to other opportunistic infection [Carney et al, 1981].

ONCOGENICITY OF HUMAN CYTOMEGALOVIRUS

One of our major concerns in addition to the aspects of infectious diseases and immune impairment during CMV infection is the potential oncogenicity of human CMV. Several lines of observation imply that human CMV might have oncogenic potential comparable to that of other herpesviruses. These observations encompass the essential information ranging from the basic biochemical and biological interaction between CMV and its infected hosts to the molecular epidemiological analysis of viral markers in human tumors and suggest a possible role of CMV in human malignancies.

Ability of Human CMV To Stimulate Cellular Macromolecular Synthesis in Virus-Infected Cells

In general, in oncogenic papovavirus and adenovirus systems, the ability of virus to induce cellular macromolecular synthesis, such as DNA, RNA, and enzymes related to nucleic acid metabolism, has been found to correlate with viral transformation and oncogenic potential. In herpesviruses, the oncogenic herpes simplex type

2 was found capable of stimulating cellular DNA synthesis under nonpermissive conditions [Melvin and Kucera, 1975; Yamanishi et al, 1975]. The DNA synthesis of well-differentiated peripheral lymphocytes was stimulated by Epstein-Barr virus (EBV) infection, and the ability of EBV to immortalize the lymphocyte was found to correlate with the ability of EBV to stimulate cellular DNA synthesis in EBV-infected cord blood cells [Gerber and Hoyer, 1971; Miller et al, 1974]. Similarly, CMV is able to stimulate cellular DNA synthesis in virus-infected permissive (human fibroblast) and nonpermissive (hamster and NIH3T3) cells [DeMarchi and Kaplan, 1977; St. Jeor et al, 1974]. Boldogh et al [1978a,b] found that the ability of HCMV to stimulate cellular DNA synthesis was dependent on the expression of very early CMV gene function and was relatively resistant to UV irradiation. Besides the stimulation of cellular DNA synthesis, Tanaka et al [1975] and Furukawa et al [1975, 1976] reported that cellular mRNA, tRNA, ribosomal RNA, and mitochondria DNA synthesis were also greatly stimulated in CMV-infected permissive and nonpermissive cells.

Kamata et al [1978] discovered that one of the chromatin-associated factors induced in human embryonic lung cells at very early stages of CMV infection stimulated template activity of cell chromatin. This factor coincided with a major component of immediate-early antigen synthesized within 1 hr after infection. As a consequence of derepression of host cell transcription, numerous cellular enzymes have been found to be markedly enhanced in CMV-infected permissive and nonpermissive cells. These include thymidine kinase (TK) [Estes and Huang, 1977; Zavada et al, 1976], DNA polymerase [Huang, 1975; Hirai et al, 1976], DNA-dependent RNA polymerase [Tanaka et al, 1978], ornithine decarboxylase [Isom, 1979], plasminogen activator [Yamanishi and Rapp, 1979], and exonuclease and topoisomerase (our unpublished data).

In HCMV-infected cells the stimulation of cell DNA synthesis is preceded by dramatic increases in TK and DNA polymerase activities. The stimulation of TK activity appeared as early as 12 hr after infection and peaked between 24 and 48 hr after infection. Both cytosol and mitochondrial TK were greatly stimulated, but the stimulation of the mitochondrial enzyme was to a lesser extent. Characterization of these enzymes with respect to phosphate donor specificity, pH optimum, thermostability, salt inhibition, and electromobility did not reveal any significant distinction from that of the noninfected cell, indicating that these enzymes are probably of cellular origin [Estes and Huang, 1977].

Infection of WI-38 human fibroblasts with HCMV leads not only to the stimulation of host cell DNA α- and β-polymerase syntheses but also to the induction of a novel virus-specific DNA polymerase. This novel virus-specific DNA polymerase did exhibit unique column chromatographic behavior, template specificity, and salt and drug sensitivities distinct from that of host cell α and β enzymes [Huang, 1975]. The virus-stimulated α and β DNA polymerases did not show characteristics distinct from those of mock-infected cells. The roles of the newly synthesized (or stimulated) host cell DNA polymerases with respect to the stimulation of cellular DNA and the involvement in viral DNA synthesis are still unclear.

Ornithine decarboxylase is an enzyme involved in the first rate-limiting reaction in the biosynthesis of protamine. This enzyme level is usually low in normal stationary phase cells, but increases remarkably upon infection of cells with oncogenic viruses. Its activity is high in tumor tissues and in virus-transformed cells. The activity of this enzyme and the rate of its biosynthesis are closely linked to DNA synthesis. In

HCMV-infected human embryonic cells, Isom [1979] has found that the ornithine decarboxylase activity was dramatically stimulated 12 hr after infection. This stimulation was not inhibited by the addition of polyamine, but was reversibly inhibited by the viral DNA synthesis inhibitor phosphonoacetate.

One additional biochemical indicator closely related to malignant transformation is the plasminogen activator. The plasminogen activator is an enzyme that is able to convert plasminogen into plasmin, which in turn degrades and hydrolyzes the fibrin. Transformation of cells by oncogenic DNA and RNA viruses frequently leads to the expression of high levels of plasminogen activator [Ossowski et al, 1974; Unkelass et al, 1973; Yamanishi and Rapp, 1979]. Infection of human and hamster cells with UV-inactivated HCMV also led to the stimulation of plasminogen activator synthesis [Yamanishi and Rapp, 1979]. This stimulation of plasminogen activator in HCMV-infected cells does not require viral DNA synthesis. Therefore, it is hypothesized that the stimulation of the plasminogen activator synthesis is an early gene function of human CMV.

In brief, instead of shutting down the host cell macromolecule synthesis, HCMV is able to stimulate the synthesis of numerous enzymes related to cell proliferation. Enzymes studied include TK, DNA polymerase, DNase, topoisomerase, ornithine decarboxylase, plasminogen activator, and so forth, as described above. The ability to stimulate the synthesis of these enzymes meets the biochemical criteria for the oncogenic potential of this virus.

Morphological Transformation of Mammalian Cells In Vitro by CMV

The concept of oncogenicity of HCMV can be further supported by the ability of HCMV to transform various mammalian cell cultures morphologically in vitro. Albrecht and Rapp [1973] first demonstrated, as Boldogh et al [1978a] did later, that UV-irradiated HCMV was able morphologically to transform hamster embryonic fibroblasts. The transformed cell lines were found to be oncogenic in golden Syrian hamsters. Tumors produced in hamsters were poorly differentiated malignant fibrosarcomas and could be continuously subcultured both in vivo and in vitro indefinitely. Boldogh et al [1978a,b] were able to demonstrate that CMV-transformed hamster cell lines and the cell lines developed from induced tumors did bear CMV-specific cytoplasmic and surface antigen(s) but not infectious virus. The status of CMV genome in these transformed cells is still unclear. After long periods of in vitro subcultivation the viral genome was undetectable by DNA-DNA reassociation kinetics analysis with a sensitivity of 0.1 viral genome equivalent per cell [Huang et al, 1983].

Nelson et al [1982] have recently infected NIH3T3 cells with cloned AD-169 strain CMV DNA fragments to identify the transforming region of HCMV. From mapping and transfection experiments they found that the transforming region was in the 2.9 kb subfragment of the HindIII-E fragment with map units between 0.123 and 0.14 on the DNA molecule of the AD-169 strain CMV. Transformed murine cells selected by 1.2% methylcellulose had high replicating efficiency and were tumorigenic in Balb/c nude mice. However, in their preliminary experiments, they were not able to detect viral DNA sequences homologous to the transforming HindIII-E fragment with analysis sensitivity of 0.5 copy of HindIII-E fragment per cell. Through the study of a series of deletion mutants of plasmid pCM4000 recombinants constructed by exonuclease III and S1 nuclease sequential digestion of the 2.9 kb HindIII-XbaI transforming fragment, Nelson et al [1984] were able to designate and to define the transforming region to the size of 172 bp between 489 and 317 bases from the HindIII site of plasmid pCM4000 DNA. This implies that morphological transformation of NIH3T3 cells can be achieved by small pieces of DNA without any obvious open reading frame. The DNA sequence of this small transforming sequence reveals that a stem-like hairpin structure resembling that of bacteria insertion elements exists within this short transforming DNA. A similar type of DNA sequence arrangement also exists in HSV I and II transforming DNA segments. Therefore, a hit-and-run mechanism for HCMV and HSV transformation has been suggested by Galloway and McDougall [1983].

In Syrian hamster embryo (SHE) cell systems, Clanton et al [1983] were also able to transform SHE cells morphologically with the Towne strain CMV XbaI-E fragment. This Towne XbaI-E DNA fragment was found to be homologous to BglII-transforming fragments N and C of HSV II but lacked homology to the 2.9 kb subfragment of HindIII-E, as demonstrated by Nelson et al [1982]. This Towne strain XbaI-E fragment was also found to be able to transform NIH3T3 cells. The resulting transformed cells were also oncogenic in athymic NIH nude mice.

In human cell systems, spontaneous release of HCMV from cell lines derived from human tissues has been reported [Rapp et al, 1975]. A virus strain, called *Major* (or Mj) was spontaneously released from a prostate cell line derived from a child. This prostate cell line grew in vitro to a passage level well above the expected life span. Geder et al [1976] speculated that CMV gene function might play a certain role in extending the life span of this human prostate cell line beyond the normal level. They further studied the transforming ability of the Mj strain CMV by low multiplicity (0.001 PFU per cell) infections of human embryonic lung (HEL) cells with this virus. After a crisis period, foci of morphologically transformed cells appeared. Two transformed cell lines were established. Both cell lines were tumorigenic in athymic nude mice. CMV-specific membrane antigens could be detected in these transformed cells by immunofluorescence tests with human convalescent serum or by cytotoxicity tests using spleen cells from hamsters bearing isographs of CMV transformed cells. Perinuclear and paranuclear fluorescence were also observed in most of the transformed cells when anticomplement immunofluorescence techniques were applied. Viral DNA had been found in transformed cells at 0.3 genome equivalents per cell at early passage (p48) but became undetectable after prolonged cultivation in vitro [Huang et al, 1983].

In human HEL fibroblasts we were able to obtain transformation foci when total XbaI or HindIII (but not EcoRI) digested HCMV DNA were used for transformation. The subconfluent (70–80%) HEL cells were transfected with XbaI CMV DNA by calcium phosphate precipitation and dimethyl sulfoxide (DMSO) treatment. On the fifth day after transfection the transfected cells were reseeded at low density in minimum essential medium with 3% fetal calf serum. The medium was changed three times a week. Cultures were monitored for morphologically transformed loci at 6–7 weeks. A tumor promoter agent, 12-O-tetradecanoyl-phorbol-13-acetate (TPA), was also used in our CMV transformation study to test whether CMV-initiated transformation requires a cocarcinogen or a promoting factor to facilitate the transformation event. Some transfected cultures and various controls were then treated with TPA at 25 ng/ml for 24 hr at 18 or 35 days after transfection.

In the absence of TPA treatment, the XbaI fragment-transfected culture yielded morphologically transformed foci at a frequency of approximately 1 per 10^6 cells when HEL cells were transfected with 2.5×10^{-6} μg per cell of XbaI DNA fragments. The TPA-treated culture yielded five to six transforming foci per 10^6 cells. No transforming foci have been found in cells transfected with sonicated CMV DNA either in the presence or in the absence of TPA. TPA or DMSO treatment alone did not induce any morphologically transformed foci in HEL cultures [Huang et al, 1983].

CMV-specific antigens and viral-specific mRNA could be detected in transformed foci by an anticomplement immunofluorescent test (ACIF) and by in situ DNA-RNA cytohybridization. Three continuous transformed cell lines, designated as *BH19, BH21*, and *BH47*, were established from cultures transfected with XbaI fragments and subsequently treated with TPA. These transformed cell lines were able to grow in soft agar, and they were also able to grow to high densities with short doubling times in medium containing a low serum concentration (2% fetal calf serum). These transformed cell lines are morphologically epithelial combined with short fibroblast in nature and are able to induce fibrosarcomas in athymic nude mice.

The tumorigenicity of these transformed cells was increased significantly by subsequent passages in nude mice. Metastases consisting of poorly differentiated fibrosarcomas could be found in the lung, liver, and spleen of these animals. The cell lines derived from these tumors still bear some virus-specific polypeptides that appear in the original transformed cells. The karyotype of these tumor cells still retains characteristics similar to that of the original transformed cells.

The TPA treatment appears crucial for CMV DNA fragments to immortalize the morphologically transformed human cells. Without TPA treatment cells from the CMV-transformed foci frequently cease multiplication after one or two subcultivations. The mechanism of the establishment of CMV-induced transformation, therefore, appears similar to that of other carcinogen-involved multiphase processes [Bereblum, 1978]. Hypothetically, we speculate that in the human cell HCMV is capable of initiating malignant transformation, but the maintenance of this malignant state might require the presence of a cocarcinogen, such as a tumor promoting agent. Treatment of HCMV DNA fragment-transfected NIH3T3 cells with TPA was not necessary in the experiment of Nelson et al [1982]. It was suggested that the promotion events fulfilled by TPA in HEL cells must reside endogenously in NIH3T3 cells. This might also explain the high frequency of transformation of NIH3T3 cells by numerous tumor viruses.

In contrast to CMV DNA fragment transformation of human fibroblasts, we were also able to establish CMV-transformed cell lines by low multiplicity infection and extensive subcultivation of HEL cells with strains BT1757 and Towne CMV without TPA treatment. Cell lines derived from BT1757 (2E, 4D, 5B, 6H, and 7E) and from Towne (LH1, LH2, and LH5) share similar biological characteristics as those derived from DNA fragment-transformed cells and are all tumorigenic in athymic nude mice. This suggests that the continuous induction of cellular mitotic activity or cellular macromolecule synthesis by frequent subcultivation might function as tumor promoter activity in assisting CMV in the immortalization of HEL cells.

THE ASSOCIATION OF CYTOMEGALOVIRUS INFECTION WITH HUMAN MALIGNANCIES

The major setback in the epidemiological analysis of the association of CMV with human cancers is the ubiquitous distribution of CMV and the high prevalence of

CMV antibodies in the asymptomatic control population. It is extremely difficult to conclude with biostatistical approaches whether CMV has a causal association with a particular cancer. Therefore, the data presented here from our studies and that of others, merely reflect an epidemiological association other than etiological association. To date, human CMV has been associated with Kaposi sarcoma [Giraldo et al, 1972a,b, 1975, 1978, 1980; Boldogh et al, 1981], prostatic adenocarcinoma [Sanford et al, 1977; Boldogh et al, 1983], adenocarcinoma of the colon [Roche and Huang, 1977; Huang and Roche, 1978; Roche et al, 1981], and cervical cancer [Melnick et al, 1978; Huang et al, 1983].

Kaposi Sarcoma

Kaposi sarcoma (KS) is a multifocal idiopathic pigmented hemorrhagic sarcoma with an extremely obscure nature. This previously rare tumor, first described in 1872 by the Hungarian dermatologist Dr. M. Kaposi [1872], is occurring with increasing frequency in patients with acquired immunodeficiency syndrome (AIDS). KS is characterized by the appearance of multicentric, hyperpigmented, vascular cutaneous nodules usually localized to the lower extremities but may involve lymph nodes and internal organs [Kaposi, 1872; Taylor et al, 1971; Safai and Good, 1981; Kungu and Gates, 1981]. Kaposi sarcoma is classified into three groups: classic, endemic, and epidemic. Before 1950, KS was a rare tumor occurring mainly in elderly white men with Mediterranean or Jewish ethnic origin; it occurred in 0.02 to 0.06 per 100,000 persons per year in the United States. Rare cases have been found in people of other races and ethnic backgrounds; KS in this group is referred to as classic KS. Classic KS is often relatively benign and has a protracted course.

With the advent of organ transplantation, an increased incidence of Kaposi sarcoma was observed in transplant recipients who received immunosuppressive therapy and in patients with malignancies and autoimmune diseases who received antimetabolites and corticosteroids [Klepp et al, 1978; Stribling et al, 1978; Penn, 1979]. These patients' ages ranged from 23 to 59 years (mean age 42 years), and the male to female ratio was 2.3:1. In one study, Harwood et al [1979] reported that all 12 of the renal transplant recipients who developed KS were either of Jewish or Mediterranean background. This indicates a role for genetic factors in susceptibility to this tumor. Widespread dissemination with visceral involvement is often seen in this group. It is noteworthy that organ transplant recipients also have a high incidence of cytomegalovirus infection.

Endemic KS occurs among the black population in equatorial Africa, such as in Zaire and Uganda, with the geographical clustering similar to Burkitt lymphoma. Approximately 9% of all tumors reported in Uganda are Kaposi sarcomas. African KS is not restricted to older men. It occurs in young adults between the ages of 25 and 45 years, with a male to female ratio of 17:1 [Taylor et al, 1971; Kungu and Gates, 1981; Friedman-Kien and Ostreicher, 1984]. Although the benign form of the disease is the most common, the more aggressive disseminated Kaposi sarcoma is also observed. The generalized lymphadenopathic form of KS, which has a high mortality, is also frequently seen in this endemic area in black children between the ages of 2 and 15 years [Taylor et al, 1971].

Since 1979 more than 3,500 cases of disseminated Kaposi sarcoma have been diagnosed in patients with AIDS in the United States. This type of Kaposi sarcoma is referred to as *epidemic Kaposi sarcoma* to distinguish it from the classic KS seen in elderly Europeans and North Americans and the endemic KS seen in Africa. Epidemic Kaposi sarcoma occurs primarily among homosexual and bisexual men, hemophiliacs and drug addicts who are much younger (mean age 38 years) than patients with classic KS. Epidemic Kaposi sarcoma is frequently associated with opportunistic infections such as CMV and pneumocystis carinii pneumonia. This new epidemic KS is a more widely disseminated tumor with mucocutaneous, lymph node, and visceral involvement [Safai and Good, 1981; Friedman-Kien and Ostreicher, 1984; Drew et al, 1982]. The early involvement of lymph nodes and visceral organs is similar to that seen in the lymphadenopathic and rapidly fatal form of KS that occurs endemically in African children.

The etiology of Kaposi sarcoma is still unclear and is expected to be multifactorial. Host characteristics, such as a genetic predisposition, an immunocompromised state, and also infectious agents and environmental factors (such as life-style) perhaps all play important roles in the development of this disease.

Among the infectious agents, cytomegalovirus was found to be the most common in patients with Kaposi sarcoma [Drew et al, 1982; Giraldo et al, 1978]. Dr. G. Giraldo and Dr. E. Beth spent a great deal of effort in searching for a viral agent associated with this tumor. In cell lines derived from KS biopsy specimens from a Zairian patient, they isolated a CMV strain, termed *K9V*. The CMV strain K9V was further analyzed by DNA restriction fragmentation and was found to share significant homology with the transforming CMV strain Major (Mj), which was spontaneously released from a prostate cell line established in Dr. F. Rapp's laboratory [Huang, 1984].

Giraldo and his colleagues also performed an extensive seroepidemiologic analysis of European and American KS patients that revealed a specific association with CMV, but not EBV, HSV I, or HSV II. African patients with a similar clinical course also had high titers of antibody to CMV. However, since CMV infections occur commonly in healthy Africans, a biostatistical significance could not be established in these patients [Giraldo et al, 1978].

In collaboration with Dr. Giraldo and his colleagues, we have examined classic and endemic KS tumor biopsy specimens for the existence of CMV-specific nucleic acid sequences and viral-specific macromolecules by DNA reassociation kinetics analysis, in situ hybridization, and immunofluorescence testing. In one set of studies, viral DNA and RNA could be detected in five out of 10 tumor biopsy specimens, and virus-specific antigens could be demonstrated in 80% of the specimens. In contrast, no HSV II or EBV DNA sequences or their viral-specific macromolecules could be detected. CMV DNA levels ranged from 0.25 to 1 genome equivalent per cell [Giraldo et al, 1980; Boldogh et al, 1981].

In a study of homosexual men with KS, Drew et al [1982] found that CMV could be isolated from body secretions, semen, or blood in seven of nine patients. CMV-specific antigens could be detected by immunofluorescence in KS tissues from six of nine patients, and CMV RNA was detected in two of three patients tested by in situ nucleic acid hybridization. In collaboration with Dr. McDougall, Fenoglio et al [1982] also demonstrated the existence of CMV RNA in KS cells derived from biopsy tissue. On the other hand, negative data have been reported by Rüger et al [1984], who used less sensitive Southern blot hybridization with a subgenomic DNA probe.

The association of CMV with KS has been suggested by seroepidemiological and molecular biological studies. Additional supporting evidence for the etiological role of CMV in KS is based on the oncogenicity of CMV as demonstrated by in vitro experiments. At the present time, more conclusive evidence is needed to prove the etiological role of CMV in KS.

Prostatic Adenocarcinoma and Benign Hypertrophy of the Prostate

Adenocarcinoma and benign hypertrophy of the prostate are two of the most common illnesses of the American male. The etiologies of these diseases are still unknown. Some studies suggest that these diseases may be related to an endocrine imbalance, but, to date, no conclusions have been made [Rubin, 1969]. Some preliminary observations imply that HSV and human CMV might play some role in the induction of prostatic adenocarcinoma. Lymphocytes from patients with prostatic adenocarcinoma were cytotoxic to CMV-infected and CMV-transformed cells that bore CMV-specific membrane antigens [Sanford et al, 1977]. The peripheral lymphocytes from 84% of patients with prostatic carcinoma were able to kill CMV-transformed cells. In addition, sera from prostatic carcinoma patients were able to block the specific cytotoxicity generated by their lymphocytes [Sanford et al, 1977]. These cellular immunologic data strongly suggest the association of CMV infection with the development of adenocarcinoma of the prostate, and the long-term persistence of an oncogenic CMV strain (Major) in a cell line derived from prostatic tissue [Rapp et al, 1975] makes this speculation more attractive.

To obtain more conclusive information, we have performed a molecular epidemiologic study to investigate the existence of viral DNA and viral-specific macromolecules in normal, benign hypertrophy and adenocarcinoma of the prostate. Surgically removed specimens from 13 normal, nine benign hypertrophy of the prostate (BHP), and 10 prostatic adenocarcinoma (ACP) patients were analyzed for the presence of CMV and HSV type II DNA, viral-specific RNA, and antigens by DNA-DNA reassociation kinetics analysis, in situ nucleic acid hybridization, and ACIF, respectively [Boldogh et al, 1983]. Experimental results showed three of nine (33%) BHP, four of 10 (40%) ACP, and only two of 13 (15.4%) normal prostates carried CMV DNA and/or CMV-specific macromolecules. HSV II-specific products were also found in two of 10 (20%) prostatic tumors and in one of 13 normal prostates (8%). It is worth noting that 60% of the prostatic tumors showed the existence of herpes group viral macromolecules (CMV or HSV II). Although the number of specimens studied here is not sufficient to make any biostatistical conclusion, it does encourage us to have a closer look at the possible etiological role of herpes group virus infections in prostatic adenocarcinoma and in benign hypertrophy of the prostate.

Cervical Cancer

There are considerable seroepidemiologic and biologic data that suggest a strong causal association between HSV II and cervical cancer [Rawls et al, 1973; Nahmias et al, 1974]. HSV II DNA, mRNA, and viral-specific protein markers have been found in human cervical cancer, in exfoliated tumor cells, and in cells undergoing neoplastic change [Frenkel et al, 1972; McDougall et al, 1980; Dressman et al, 1980], and, more recently, human papillomavirus (HPV) DNA sequences (such as HPV types 6, 11, 16, and 18) have been found at some frequency in cancer and precancerous lesions of human uterine cervix [Green et al, 1982; Gissman et al, 1982, 1983; Durst et al, 1983]. At the present time, there are no seroepidemiological data to prove the association of papilloma with cervical cancer. The seroepidemiological data from some geographic areas did not always support the close association of HSV II with cervical cancer. Meanwhile, not all women with cervical cancer had serological evidence of HSV II infection [Melnick et al, 1978; Alexander, 1973]. HCMV frequently has been found in cervices and vaginal discharge, especially in Asia where the association of HSV II and cervical cancer is not very common. Virus was isolated from cervical tumor biopsy tissue (our unpublished data) and from cell cultures derived from tumor biopsy tissue [Melnick et al, 1978]. In view of the oncogenic potential of CMV as demonstrated in vitro, we believe that CMV could play a role in the process of cervical malignancy.

In view of the seroepidemiologic link between HSV II and cervical cancer and the frequent existence of papilloma viral DNA in cervical carcinoma, zur Hausen [1982] proposed that genital cancers, including cervical cancer and penile carcinoma, result from a "promoting" papilloma infection and initiating events, frequently caused by herpes simplex infection. To strengthen this hypothesis, we add cytomegalovirus to the list of initiators or cofactors in this event.

We have performed a molecular epidemiologic survey of CMV DNA in cervical cancer and in normal cervices from various geographic regions by nucleic acid hybridization to investigate the possible association of CMV with cervical malignancy. In collaboration with Dr. E. Russell Alexander, we examined eight cervical cancers and six normal cervix specimens from Taiwan. CMV DNA was found in seven of eight (88%) cancer specimens at a level between 0.4 and 6.6 genome equivalents per cell, while three of six (50%) normal cervices showed positive at 0.2 to 1 genome per cell. Infectious CMV was isolated from one tumor specimen that carried CMV DNA at 6.6 genomes per cell. No HSV II sequence could be detected in these cervical cancers and normal cervices from Taiwan [Huang et al, 1983].

As for specimens from Africa (in collaboration with Dr. G. De-Thé), we found CMV DNA sequence in nine of 19 cervical cancers and in five of 10 normal cervices at 0.1 to 1 and 0.5 to 1 genome equivalent per cell, respectively. HSV II DNA was found in one of 12 cervical cancers and in one of four normal cervices. In specimens from Finland and the United States, HCMV DNA was detected in one of 11 and in two of 13 cervical cancers, respectively. No HSV II DNA was detected in either normal or cervical cancerous specimens from Finland and the United States. The CMV DNA positive rate is significantly lower in specimens from Finland and the United States compared with that from Taiwan and Africa. This might reflect the socioeconomic status of each population. Nevertheless, the frequency of the positive CMV rate in cervical cancer was higher than that of HSV II, and the rate of CMV-positive specimens in cervical cancers from Taiwan was also higher than that of normal cervices. However, the number of specimens studied was limited. It is essential to examine more specimens to compile conclusive data. Again, with the ubiquitous nature of CMV, it is extremely difficult to presume any causal association, especially with cervical cancer; nevertheless, we cannot overlook the possibility. Based on the extremely high frequency of positive CMV DNA in both cervices and cervical cancers, we can at least conclude that the human cervix might be a site for latent CMV infection.

Carcinoma of the Colon

Through extensive epidemiologic analysis, it was suggested that environmental, as well as genetic, factors might play important roles in the initiation of colon cancer.

However, the precise nature of the factors or genes involved is still undetermined. By cytologic observation and virus isolation, CMV has been detected in the intestinal wall of patients with ulcerative colitis [Powell et al, 1961; Levine et al, 1964], a disease suspected of being associated with colon cancer [Farmer et al, 1973]. By nucleic acid hybridization techniques, in collaboration with Dr. J.K. Roche of Duke University, we have shown the presence of viral DNA sequence in the diseased bowel of patients with ulcerative colitis, familial polyposis, and carcinoma of the colon. In contrast, results were negative for the CMV genome in the bowel of Crohn disease patients [Roche and Huang, 1977; Roche et al, 1981; Huang and Roche, 1978]; such patients have little or no increase in cancer risk. Although CMV was detected in a majority of patients with colon cancers, we have found that it frequently exists in some histologically normal and nonneoplastic diseased tissues of colon cancer patients. These observations make the interpretation of the association of CMV with colon cancer extremely difficult. It is more likely that the detected CMV was probably latent or harbored in the intestinal tissues of the majority of the patients. The fact that this virus is widely distributed also does not rule out a possible oncogenic role, since the close association of virus with host cells may give the virus an excellent opportunity to induce neoplastic transformation of its host during its long-term persistence.

CONCLUSIONS

The oncogenic potential of HCMV is strongly suggested by its ability to stimulate the synthesis of cellular macromolecules, such as DNA, RNA, and the enzymes associated with cell proliferation, and by its ability to transform human and other mammalian cells in vitro. CMV-transformed human and other mammalian cells were found tumorigenic in athymic nude mice. Although CMV DNA, RNA, and virus-specific antigens were found frequently in KS, prostatic adenocarcinoma, cervical, and colon cancers, its causal and etiologic roles with these cancers are still unclear. The possibilities of the preferential replication of CMV in these neoplastic tissues and the reactivation of latent virus in patients with malignancy still exist. Because of widespread CMV infections, it is very difficult to conclude that there is a causal association between CMV and human malignancies using sero- or molecular epidemiologic approaches. Nevertheless, the connection between CMV and some human malignancies is impossible to dismiss.

ACKNOWLEDGMENTS

We thank Drs. E. Russell Alexander, G. de-Thé, J. Roche, G. Giraldo, and T.I. Malinin for their collaboration and for providing tumor specimens, and we thank Barbara Leonard for manuscript preparation.

This project was supported by grants from NCI (CA21773) and NIAID (AI12712 and AI-15036).

REFERENCES

1. Albrecht T, Rapp F: Malignant transformation of hamster embryo fibroblasts following exposure to ultraviolet-irradiated human cytomegalovirus. Virology 55:53–61, 1973.
2. Alexander ER: Maternal and neonatal infection with cytomegalovirus in Taiwan. Pediatr Res 1:210, 1967.

3. Alexander ER: Possible etiologies of cancer of the cervix other than herpesviruses. Cancer Res 33:1486–1496, 1973.
4. Bereblum I: Established principles and unresolved problems in carcinogenesis. 60:723–726, 1978.
5. Boldogh I, Baskar JF, Mar EC, Huang ES: Human cytomegalovirus and herpes simplex type 2 virus in normal and adenocarcinomatous prostate glands. JNCI 70:819–825, 1983.
6. Boldogh I, Beth E, Huang ES, Kyalwazi KS, Giraldo G: Kaposi's sarcoma. IV. Detection of CMV DNA, CMV RNA and CMNA in tumor biopsies. Int J Cancer 28:469–474, 1981.
7. Boldogh I, Gonczol E, Gartner L, Vaczi L: Stimulation of host DNA synthesis and induction of early antigens by ultraviolet light irradiated human cytomegalovirus. Arch Virol 58:289–299, 1978a.
8. Boldogh I, Gonczol E, Vaczi L: Transformation of hamster embryonic fibroblast cell by UV-irradiated human cytomegalovirus. Acta Microbiol Hung 25:269–275, 1978b.
9. Carney WP, Rubin RH, Hoffmann RA, Hansen WP, Healey K, Hirsch MS: Analysis of T cell subsets in cytomegalovirus mononucleosis. J Immunol 126:2114–2116, 1981.
10. Clanton DJ, Jariwalla RJ, Kress C, Rosenthal LJ: Neoplastic transformation by a cloned human cytomegalovirus DNA fragment uniquely homologous to one of the transforming regions of herpes simplex virus type 2. Proc Natl Acad Sci USA 80:3826–3830, 1983.
11. DeMarchi JM, Kaplan AS: The role of defective cytomegalovirus particles in the induction of host cell DNA synthesis. Virology 82:93–99, 1977.
12. Dressman GR, Burek J, Adam E, Kaufman RH, Melnick JL, Powell KL, Purifoy DJM: Expression of herpesvirus-induced antigens in human cervical cancer. Nature 283:591–593, 1980.
13. Drew WL: Sexual transmission of CMV and its relationship to Kaposi's sarcoma in homosexual men. BD:OAS 20(1):121–129.
14. Drew WL, Conant MA, Miner RC, Huang ES, Ziegler JL, Groundwater JR, Gullett JH, et al: Cytomegalovirus and Kaposi's sarcoma in young homosexual men. Lancet 2:125–127, 1982.
15. Drew WL, Mintz L, Miner RC, Sands M, Ketterer B: Prevalence of cytomegalovirus infection in homosexual men. J Infect Dis 143:188–192, 1981.
16. Durst M, Gissmann L, Ikenberg H, zur Hausen H: A papilloma DNA from a cervical carcinoma and its prevalence in cancer biopsy samples from different geographic regions. Proc Natl Acad Sci USA 80:3812–3815, 1983.
17. Estes HE, Huang ES: Stimulation of cellular thymidine kinases by human cytomegalovirus. J Virol 24:13–21, 1977.
18. Farmer GW, Vincent MM, Fuccillo DA: Viral investigations in ulcerative colitis and regional enteritis. Gastroenterology 65:8–18, 1973.
19. Fenoglio CM, Oster MW, Gerfo PL, Reynolds T, Edelson R, Patterson JAK, et al: Kaposis sarcoma following chemotherapy for testicular cancer in a homosexual man: Demonstration of cytomegalovirus RNA in sarcoma cells. Hum Pathol 15:955–959, 1982.
20. Frenkel N, Roizman B, Cassai E, Nahmias A: A DNA fragment of herpes simplex 2 and its transcription in human cervical cancer tissue. Proc Natl Acad Sci USA 69:3784–3789, 1972.
21. Friedman-Kien AE, Ostreicher R: Overview of classical and epidemic Kaposi's sarcoma. In Friedman-Kien AE, Laurenstein LJ (eds): "AIDS, the Epidemic of Kaposi's Sarcoma and Opportunistic Infections." New York: Masson Publishing Co., 1984, pp 23–26.
22. Furukawa T, Sakuma S, Plotkin SA: Human Cytomegalovirus infection of WI-38 cells stimulates mitochondrial DNA synthesis. Nature 262:414–416, 1976.
23. Furukawa T, Tanaka S, Plotkin SA: Stimulation of macromolecular synthesis in guinea pig cell by human CMV. Proc Soc Exp Biol Med 148:211–214, 1975.
24. Galloway D, McDougall JK: The oncogenic potential of herpes simplex viruses: Evidence for a "hit-and-run" mechanism. Nature 302:21–24, 1983.
25. Geder L, Lausch R, O'Neill F, Rapp F: Oncogenic transformation of human embryo lung cells by human cytomegalovirus. Science 192:1134–1137, 1976.
26. Gerber P, Hoyer BH: Induction of cellular DNA synthesis in human leukocytes by Epstein-Barr virus. Nature 231:46–47, 1971.
27. Giraldo G, Beth E, Coeur P, Vogel CL, Dhru DS: Kaposi's sarcoma: A new model in the search for viruses associated with human malignancies. JNCI 49:1495–1507, 1972a.
28. Giraldo G, Beth E, Haguenau F: Herpes-type virus particles in tissue culture of Kaposi's sarcoma from different geographic regions. JNCI 49:1509–1513, 1972b.
29. Giraldo G, Beth E, Henle W, Henle G, Mike V, Safai B, Huraux JM, McHardy J, de-Thé G: Antibody patterns to herpesviruses in Kaposi's sarcoma II. Serological association of American Kaposi's sarcoma with cytomegalovirus. Int J Cancer 22:126–131, 1978.

30. Giraldo G, Beth E, Huang ES: Kaposi's sarcoma and its relationship to cytomegalovirus (CMV). III. CMV DNA and CMV early antigens in Kaposi's sarcoma. Int J Cancer 26:23–29, 1980.

31. Giraldo G, Beth E, Kourilsky FM, Henle W, Henle G, Mike V, et al: Antibody patterns to herpesvirus in Kaposi's sarcoma: Serological association of European Kaposi's sarcoma with cytomegalovirus. Int J Cancer 15:839–848, 1975.

32. Gissmann L, de Villiers EM, zur Hausen H: Analysis of human genital warts (condyloma acuminatum) and other genital tumors for human papilloma virus type 6 DNA. Int J Cancer 29:143–146, 1982.

33. Gissmann L, Wolnick L, Ikenberg H, Koldenovsky U, Schnurch HG, zur Hausen H: Human papilloma type 6 and 11. DNA sequence in genital and laryngeal papilloma and in some cervical cancers. Proc Natl Acad Sci USA 80:560–563, 1983.

34. Green M, Brackmann KH, Sanders PR, Loewenstein PM, Freel JH, Eisenber M, Switlyk SA: Isolation of a papilloma virus from a patient with epidermodysplasia verruciformis: Presence of related viral DNA genomes in human urogenital tumor. Proc Natl Acad Sci USA 79:4437–4441, 1982.

35. Gupta P, St Jeor S, Rapp F: Comparison of the polypeptides of several strains of human cytomegalovirus. J Gen Virol 34:447–454, 1977.

36. Gurevich I, Cunha BA: Non-parental transmission of cytomegalovirus in a neonatal intensive care unit. Lancet 2:222–224, 1981.

37. Handsfield HH, Chandler SH, Caine VA, Meyers JD, Carey L, Medeiros E, McDougall JK: Cytomegalovirus infection in sex partners: Evidence for sexual transmission. J Infect Dis 151:344–348, 1985.

38. Harwood AR, Osoba D, Hofstader SL, et al: Kaposi's sarcoma in recipients of renal transplants. Am J Med 67:759–765, 1979.

39. Henle W, Henle G, Scriba M, Joyner CR, Harrison FS, Von Essen J, Paloheimo J, Klemola E: Antibody responses to the Epstein-Barr virus and cytomegalovirus after open heart and other surgery. N Engl J Med 282:1068–1074, 1970.

40. Hirai K, Furukawa T, Plotkin SA: Induction of DNA polymerase in WI-38 and guinea pig cells infected with human cytomegalovirus (HCMV). Virology 70:251–255, 1976.

41. Ho M: "Cytomegalovirus, Biology and Infection." New York: Plenum Publishing Co., 1982, pp 79–104.

42. Huang ES: Human cytomegalovirus. III. Virus-induced DNA polymerase. J Virol 16:298–310, 1975.

43. Huang ES: The role of cytomegalovirus infection in Kaposi's sarcoma. In Friedman-Kien AE, Laurenstein LJ (eds): "AIDS, the Epidemic of Kaposi's Sarcoma and Opportunistic Infections." New York: Masson Publishing Co., 1984, pp 111–126.

44. Huang ES, Alford CA Jr., Reynolds DW, Stagno S, Pass RF: Molecular epidemiology of CMV infection in women and their infants. N Engl J Med 303:958–962, 1980a.

45. Huang ES, Boldogh I, Mar EC: Human cytomegaloviruses: Evidence for possible association with human cancer. In Philips LA (ed): "Viruses Associated With Human Cancer." New York: Marcel Dekker, 1983, pp 161–193.

46. Huang ES, Huong SM, Tegmeier GE, Alford CA Jr.: Cytomegalovirus: Genetic variation of viral genomes. Ann NY Acad Sci 354:332–342, 1980b.

47. Huang ES, Kilpatrick BA, Huang YT, Pagano JS: Detection of human cytomegalovirus and analysis of strain variation. Yale J Biol Med 49:29–43, 1976.

48. Huang ES, Roche JK: Cytomegalovirus DNA and adenocarcinoma of the colon: Evidence for latent viral infection. Lancet 1:957–960, 1978.

49. Isom HJ: Stimulation of ornithine decarboxylase by human cytomegalovirus. J Gen Virol 42:265–278, 1979.

50. Jordan MC, Rousseau WE, Noble GR, Stewart JA, Chin TDY: Association of cervical cytomegaloviruses with venereal disease. N Engl J Med 288:932–934, 1973.

51. Kamata T, Tanaka S, Watanabe Y: Human cytomegalovirus-induced chromatin factors responsible for changes in template activity and structure of infected cell chromatin. Virology 90:197–208, 1978.

52. Kaposi M: Idiopathisches multiples Pigmentsarcom der Haut. Arch Dermatol Syph Berl 4:265–273, 1872.

53. Kieff ED, Hoyes B, Bachenheimer SL, Roizman B: Genetic relatedness of type 1 and 2 herpes simplex viruses. J Virol 9:738–745, 1972.

54. Kilpatrick BA, Huang ES: Human cytomegalovirus genome: Partial denaturation map and organization of genome sequences. J Virol 24:261–276, 1977.

55. Kilpatrick BA, Huang ES, Pagano JS: Analysis of cytomegalovirus genomes with restriction endonuclease HindIII and EcoRI. J Virol 18:1095–1105, 1976.

56. Klepp O, Dahl O, Stenwig JT: Association of Kaposi's sarcoma and prior immunosuppressive therapy: A 5 year material of Kaposi's sarcoma in Norway. Cancer 42:2626–2630, 1978.

57. Krech U: Complement-fixing antibodies against cytomegaloviruses in different parts of the world. Bull WHO 49:103–106, 1973.

58. Kungu A, Gates DG: Kaposi's sarcoma in Kenya: A retrospective clinicopathological study. Antibiotics Chemother 29:38–55, 1981.

59. Lang DJ, Kummer JF: Demonstration of cytomegalovirus in semen. N Engl J Med 287:756–758, 1972.

60. Lang DJ, Kummer JF: Cytomegalovirus in semen: Observations in selected population. J Infect Dis 132:472–473, 1975.

61. Levine RS, Wanner NF, Johnson CF: Cytomegalic inclusion disease in the gastrointestinal tract of adults. Ann Surg 159:35–48, 1964.

62. McDougall JK, Galloway DA, Fenoglio CM: Cervical carcinoma: Detection of herpes simplex virus RNA in cells undergoing neoplastic change. Int J Cancer 25:1–8, 1980.

63. Melnick JL, Lewis R, Wimberly I, Kaufman RH, Adams E: Association of cytomegalovirus (CMV) infection with cervical cancer: Isolation of CMV from cell cultures derived from cervical biopsy. Int Virol 10:115–119, 1978.

64. Melvin P, Kucera LS: Induction of human cell DNA synthesis by herpes simplex virus type 2. J Virol 15:534–539, 1975.

65. Miller G, Robinson J, Heston L, Lipman M: Differences between laboratory strains of Epstein-Barr virus based on immortalization, abortive infection and interference. Proc Natl Acad Sci USA 71:4006–4010, 1974.

66. Nahmias AJ, Naib ZM, Josey WE: Epidemiological studies relating genital herpetic infection to cervical cancer. Cancer Res 34:1111–1117, 1974.

67. Nelson JA, Fleckenstein B, Galloway DA, McDougall JK: Transformation of NIH3T3 cells with cloned fragments of human cytomegalovirus strain AD169. J Virol 43:83–91, 1982.

68. Nelson JA, Fleckenstein B, Jahn G, Galloway DA, McDougall J: Structure of the transforming region of human cytomegalovirus AD169. J Virol 49:109–115, 1984.

69. Numazaki Y, Yano Y, Morizuka T, Takai S, Ishida N: Primary infection with human cytomegalovirus: Virus isolation from healthy and pregnant women. Am J Epidemiol 91:410–417, 1970.

70. Ossowski L, Quigley JP, Reich E: Fibrinolysis associated with oncogenic transformation: Morphological correlates. J Biol Chem 249:4312–4320, 1974.

71. Paloheimo JA, Von Essen R, Klemola E, Kaariainen L, Siltanen P: Subclinical cytomegalovirus infections and cytomegalovirus mononucleosis after open-heart surgery. Am J Cardiol 22:624–630, 1968.

72. Penn I: Kaposi's sarcoma in organ transplant recipients. Report of 20 cases. Transplantation 27:8–11, 1979.

73. Powell RD, Warner NE, Levine RS, Kirsner JB: Cytomegalic inclusion disease and ulcerative colitis. Am J Med 30:334–340, 1961.

74. Rapp F, Geder L, Murasko D, Lausch R, Ladda R, Huang ES, Webber MM: Long-term persistence of cytomegalovirus genome in cultured human cells of prostatic origin. J Virol 16:982–990, 1975.

75. Rawls WE, Adam E, Melnick JL: An analysis of seroepidemiological studies of herpesvirus type 2 and carcinoma of cervix. Cancer Res 33:1477–1482, 1973.

76. Reinherz EL, O'Brien C, Rosenthal P, Schlossman SF: The cellular basis for viral induced immunodeficiency: Analysis by monoclonal antibodies. J Immunol 125:1269–1274, 1980.

77. Reynolds DW, Stagno S, Hosty TS, Tiller M, Alford CA Jr.: Maternal cytomegalovirus excretion and perinatal infection. N Engl J Med 289:1–5, 1973.

78. Rinaldo CR Jr., Black PH, Hirsch MS: Interactions of cytomegalovirus with leukocytes from patients with mononucleosis due to cytomegalovirus. J Infect Dis 136:667–678, 1977.

79. Rinaldo CR Jr., Carney WP, Richter BS, Black PH, Hirsch MS: Mechanism of immunosuppression in cytomegaloviral mononucleosis. J Infect Dis 141:488–495, 1980.

80. Roche JK, Cheng KS, Huang ES, Lang DL: Cytomegalovirus: Detection in human colonic and circulating mononuclear cells in association with gastrointestinal disease. Int J Cancer 27:659–667, 1981.

81. Roche JK, Huang ES: Viral DNA in inflammatory bowel disease: CMV-bearing cells as a target in immune-mediated enterocytolysis. Gastroenterology 72:228–233, 1977.
82. Rowe WP, Hartley JW, Waterman S, Turner HL, Huebner RJ: Cytopathogenic agent resembling human salivary gland virus recovered from tissue cultures of human adenoids. Proc Soc Exp Biol Med 92:418–424, 1956.
83. Rubin P: Cancer of urogenital tract: Prostatic cancer: Current concepts in cancer. JAMA 210:322–323;1072–1073, 1969.
84. Rubin RH, Cosimi AB, Tolkoff-Rubin NE, Russell PS, Hirsch MS: Infectious disease syndromes attributable to cytomegalovirus and their significance among renal transplant recipients. Transplantation 24:458–464, 1977.
85. Rüger R, Colimon R, Fleckenstein B: Search for DNA sequences of human cytomegalovirus in Kaposi's sarcoma tissues with cloned probes: Preliminary report. Antibiotics Chemther 32:43–47, 1984.
86. Safai B, Good R: Kaposi's sarcoma: A review and recent development. CA 31:2–12, 1981.
87. Sanford EJ, Dagen JE, Geder L, Rohner JT, Rapp E: Lymphocyte reactivity against virally transformed cells in patients with urologic cancer. J Urol 118:809–810, 1977.
88. Spector SA, Spector DH: Use of restriction endonuclease mapping to document nosocomial acquisition of cytomegalovirus by monozygotic twins: In Nahmias AJ, Dowle WR, Schinazi RF (eds): "International Conference on Human Herpesviruses: Atlanta 1980. The Human Herpesvirus: An Interdisciplinary Prospective." New York: Elsevier, 1980, p 609.
89. St. Jeor S, Albrecht TB, Funk FD, Rapp F: Stimulation of cellular DNA synthesis by human cytomegalovirus. J Virol 13:353–362, 1974.
90. Stagno S, Reynolds DW, Pass RF, Alford CA Jr.: Breast milk and the risk of cytomegalovirus infection. N Engl J Med 302:1073–1074, 1980.
91. Starr JG, Bart RD, Gold E: Inapparent congenital cytomegalovirus infection. N Engl J Med 282:1075–1078, 1970.
92. Stinski MF: Sequence of protein synthesis in cells infected by human cytomegalovirus: Early and late virus-induced polypeptides. J Virol 26:686–701, 1978.
93. Stribling J, Weitzner S, Smith GV: Kaposi's sarcoma in renal allograft recipients. Cancer 42:442–446, 1978.
94. Sweet GH, Tegtmeier GE, Bayer WL: Antigens of human cytomegalovirus: Electroimmuno-diffusion assay and comparison among strains. J Gen Virol 43:707–712, 1979.
95. Tanaka S, Furukawa T, Plotkin SA: Human cytomegalovirus stimulates host cell RNA synthesis. J Virol 15:297–304, 1975.
96. Tanaka S, Ihara S, Watanabe Y: Human cytomegalovirus induces DNA-dependent RNA polymerase in human diploid cells. Virology 89:179–185, 1978.
97. Taylor JF, Templeton AC, Vogel CL, et al: Kaposi's sarcoma in Uganda: A clinical pathological study. Int J Cancer 8:122–135, 1971.
98. Unkeless JC, Tobia A, Ossowski L, Quigley JP, Rifkin PB, Reich E: An enzymatic function association with transformation of fibroblasts by oncogenic viruses. I. Chick embryo fibroblast cultures transformed by avian RNA tumor viruses. J Exp Med 137:85–111, 1973.
99. Weller TH: The cytomegaloviruses: Ubiquitous agents with protean clinical manifestations. N Engl J Med 285:203–214, 1971.
100. Weller TH, Hanshaw JB, Scott DE: Serologic differentiation of viruses responsible for cytomegalic inclusion disease. Virology 12:130–132, 1960.
101. Williams LL, Blakeslee JR, Huang ES: Isolation of a new strain of cytomegalovirus from explanted normal skin. J Gen Virol 47:519–523, 1980.
102. Willmott FE: Cytomegalovirus in female patients attending a VD clinic. Br J Vener Dis 51:278–280, 1975.
103. Winston DJ, Huang ES, Miller MJ, Lin CH, Ho WG, Gale RP, Champlin RE: Molecular epidemiology of cytomegalovirus infections associated with bone marrow transplantation. Ann Intern Med 102:16–20, 1985.
104. Yamanishi K, Ogino T, Takahashi M: Induction of cellular DNA synthesis by a temperature-sensitive mutant of herpes simplex virus type 2. Virology 67:450–462, 1975.
105. Yamanishi K, Rapp E: Production of plasminogen activator by human and hamster cells infected with human cytomegalovirus. J Virol 31:415–419, 1979.
106. Zavada V, Erban V, Rezacova D, Vonka V: Thymidine kinase in cytomegalovirus infected cells. Arch Virol 52:333–339, 1976.
107. zur Hausen H: Human genital cancer: Synergism between two virus infections or synergism between a virus infection and initiating events. Lancet ii:1370–1372, 1982.

Biochemical and Molecular Epidemiology of Cancer 345–353 (1986)

Molecular Epidemiology of Epstein-Barr Virus Infection: A Perspective

Joseph S. Pagano

Lineberger Cancer Research Center, School of Medicine, University of North Carolina, Chapel Hill, North Carolina 27514

Human herpesviruses, despite shifts in the evidence, continue to hold a leading position as candidates for oncogenic agents. Characteristically the viruses also cause latent infection. Proof of oncogenicity has been elusive because these viruses are universal infectious agents and because of the latent infection that they produce. There is as yet no clear path to distinguish molecular features of latency from the oncogenic relation.

Human herpesviruses are the first targets for effective antiviral drugs, which imparts an immediacy to understanding their role in cancer. The herpesvirus-encoded enzymes that activate or are inhibited by drugs such as Acyclovir raise the question whether it might be possible to abort virus-triggered cancers as well as acute infection. Also, the development of herpesvirus vaccines is accelerating so that prevention of these infections is becoming a realistic prospect.

Key words: human herpesviruses, herpesvirus-encoded enzymes, Burkitt's lymphoma, naso pharyngeal carcinoma

HUMAN HERPESVIRUSES AND CANCER

The five human herpesviruses exhibit a gradient of associations with malignancy. Varicella zoster virus is not associated with any cancer. An association between herpes simplex virus type 1 (HSV 1) and oral cancer is weak if it exists at all. A stronger association which has existed for years between herpes simplex virus type 2 (HSV 2) and carcinoma of the cervix seems to be fading. Although the virus inhabits the human cervix neither HSV genomes nor specific gene products have been found consistently in the carcinoma tissue or precancerous cells. The proposal that HSV 2 may work by a hit-and-run mechanism is difficult to establish because it is based on negative evidence. Moreover, analyses are clouded by the presence of latent as well as productive infection in the cervix. What we know about other oncogenic viruses tells us to expect that viral sequences and in some cases gene products persist

Received September 5, 1985.

© **1986 Alan R. Liss, Inc.**

not only in transformed cells and experimental tumors but also in vivo. Experimentally, although HSV 1 and HSV 2 can transform cells in vitro, the altered cells are rodent and not human [3]. Finally, from the epidemiologic vantage point, which is generally the starting point as well as the way toward proof of causation, the evidence linking HSV 2 infection with cervical cancer has failed to develop in the past decade. The association has been greatly weakened, even though belatedly, by the first prospective epidemiologic study of the issue; this study failed to disclose any link between HSV 2 infection and subsequent development of cervical cancer. There is tantalizing evidence linking human cytomegalovirus (CMV) infection with Kaposi's sarcoma (KS). In vivo KS has been linked with CMV infection in both Africa and in the United States. However, the finding of CMV DNA in sarcoma tissues has been inconsistent and not distinguished from latent or even productive infection [11]. Epidemiologically, the association is suggestive inasmuch as male homosexuals with AIDs have a high incidence of KS, whereas KS virtually never occurs in hemophiliac patients who contract AIDS; in the former group active CMV infection is common, but it is uncommon in hemophiliacs. In vitro transformation of human diploid fibroblasts by CMV DNA used together with a promotor substance has been achieved, and attempts are underway to transform human vascular endothelial cells with the virus and viral DNA [10]. One puzzle is that although CMV is a ubiquitous virus and exhibits broad tissue pleiotrophism the only strong association with a malignancy is restricted to one arising in vascular endothelial stem cells.

EPSTEIN-BARR VIRUS AND MALIGNANCY: BURKITT'S LYMPHOMA

Among the herpesviruses the Epstein-Barr virus (EBV) has continued to have the strongest associations with human malignancies. The evidence linking the virus with cancer of both lymphocytic and epithelial origin has strengthened but falls short of proof of causation. Why Burkitt's Lymphoma (BL) is endemic only in a belt across equatorial Africa has remained a great puzzle. In Kenya and in Uganda EBV genomes and gene products are found in over 99% of the tumors. In the rare nonendemic form of BL found in children in the United States the viral genome is found only occasionally—in 15% or less of the tumors. However, the potency of EBV as a transforming agent for human B lymphocytes in vitro together with the evidence that the virus can "immortalize" B lymphocytes in vivo causing polyclonal and leading even to monoclonal lymphocytic proliferation in immunosuppressed persons continues to fuel suspicions [1].

In equatorial Africa EBV infection occurs very early, with more than 90% of infants infected in the first year of life. The proclivity of infants with unusually high EBV antibody titers to develop BL seems to confer a special role on the virus in the genesis of BL. The peak age of onset of BL is 7 yr; until then virus infection remains inapparent. Since EBV infection occurs early in life in other underdeveloped areas some other factor must contribute to the pathogenesis of BL in Africa [1]. Malaria has been proposed to be a cofactor because malarial infection is both immunosuppressive for the T cell-mediated arm of the immune system at the same time it is a B-lymphocyte immunostimulant. Recently human T-cell leukemia virus type 3 (HTLV 3), which is prevalent as a subclinical infection in up to 70% of the population in equatorial Africa, where BL is common, has been suggested to be cofactor [12,14]. This is a provocative idea because BL has a relatively high frequency in patients with

AIDS in the United States. BL in AIDS seems to be associated more consistently with EBV than is the sporadic form of BL in the United States [5].

HTLV 3 infection cannot be the sole cofactor for BL endemicity since BL is an ancient disease in Africa, whereas sera collected from BL patients as recently as 1964 do not show HTLV 3 antibodies. Nevertheless, the notion that HTLV 3 infection may contribute to the pathogenesis of EBV-initiated BL is attractive. The incidence of BL with the authentic chromosomal translocations in patients with AIDS is impressive. Moreover, HTLV 3 and EBV may in some way interact to coinfect B cells. There is evidence that prior infection with EBV may enable HTLV 3 to gain access to B lymphocytes. Whether the dual infection in some way modulates the cytopathic effects of HTLV 3 so that there is a double stimulus for B lymphoproliferation is speculative at this point. So far HTLV 3 genomes have not been found in the B-cell lymphomas that arise in patients with AIDS [11,14].

All cases of BL, whether in endemic or nonendemic regions and whether in patients with AIDS or in others, exhibit the characteristic chromosomal anomalies that have been described in BL for some time: The t(8;14) translocation is the most common, and t(8,22) and t(2;8) translocations are also characteristic of BL. These translocations, which occur at fragile sites on the chromosomes, are adjacent to genes encoding various classes of immunoglobulins. The breakpoints in each case are also at the location of the *c-myc* oncogene. When the oncogene is translocated (t[8;14]) it comes under the influence of the molecular regulatory mechanism controlling immunogobulin gene expression, with the result that the oncogene becomes activated and constitutively expressed [7]. However, the *c-myc* oncogene does not need to be translocated to be activated, as in the case of the t(8;22) and t(2;8) translocations, in which instead the transcriptional regulatory sequences of the λ or κ loci translocate to sites near *c-myc* [13]. Oncogene transposition or activation seems to be crucial for the generation of BL, operating even in the non-EBV-associated American forms of BL. It is thought that EBV by virtue of its lymphoproliferative qualities increases the likelihood of such a translocation. However, these chromosomal translocations and their newly discovered molecular significance do not explain the endemic pattern of incidence of BL in Africa since they occur in BL everywhere.

The idea that certain strains of EBV might be oncogenic has been largely dismissed until recently. Different isolates of the various herpesviruses, especially HSV and CMV, each have unique restriction endonuclease cleavage patterns and can be distinguished. It was believed that EBV genomes do not display such heterogeneity and therefore that specific oncogenic strains of EBV did not exist. This idea may bear reexamination as it becomes evident that there is more heterogeneity than had been suspected in some segments of the EBV genome. However, preliminary analyses of EBV genomes in nasopharyngeal carcinoma (NPC) have failed to disclose a specific pattern in the HinF-I fragments of the U-2 section of the genome, now recognized to be variable as well as subject to deletion and substitution. This approach deserves further work. In any case it is now possible to trace strains of EBV by these unambiguous means to determine transmission patterns [15].

EBV AND NASOPHARYNGEAL CARCINOMA

The association of EBV with nasopharyngeal carcinoma (NPC) is if anything even more intriguing than the association with BL [2]. The malignancy arises in the posterior nasopharynx in the Waldeyer ring, an area rich in lymphocytes. The tumor is usually anaplastic, but about 10% exhibit a differentiated squamous morphology. The tumor spreads by local invasion and metastases to regional lymph nodes. Prognosis is strongly influenced by stage of disease so that early detection is very important. In stage I the response to chemotherapy and radiation permits a 70% 5-yr survival rate. Until recently only the undifferentiated (type 3) form of the tumor has been associated with EBV infection by reason of high titers of antibodies to EBV early antigen (EA-D) as well as to viral capsid antigen (VCA) and nuclear antigen (EBNA). The association derives strength from the consistent finding of EBV genomes in NPC from every part of the world regardless of whether the disease is endemic or sporadic in incidence. Recently EBV DNA and RNA have been demonstrated in type 1 differentiated NPC and in type 2 intermediate classification; in the type 1 histopathologic class EBV antibody titers are not distinctively elevated [6, 15].

The epidemiology of NPC presents some striking features. The peak ages for the disease are in midlife between 40 and 60 years, with a male preponderance. However, in North Africa the disease is reported to have a fairly high incidence in younger persons, in the second and third decades of life, as well as in the older age group. The disease exhibits a strong endemicity in South China, with an incidence approximately 1000-fold higher than the sporadic disease that occurs in the United States. Sporadic disease usually occurs in Western peoples in midlife. However, after the congenital malignancies NPC although rare is said to be the most common carcinoma in the first decade of life in the United States. NPC is also common in expatriate Chinese, but the incidence declines in second and subsequent generations of emigrants. The disease seems to be relatively common, occurring at an intermediate incidence level, in blacks in equatorial Africa, but it is also found in Algeria, Tunisia, and other North African countries in Caucasians. There is a high incidence of the disease in Alaskan eskimos.

The elevation of titers of EBV antibodies is not particularly useful from an epidemiologic point of view inasmuch as EBV antibodies are universal in normal populations, and the titers are not always high in patients with NPC. There is a positive correlation between EBV VCA and EA antibody titers and course of disease, with rising titers of EBV antibodies of IgG class suggesting relapsing disease. Much more valuable and intriguing are the EBV IgA responses that occur not only in patients with NPC but even before the disease occurs. In South China in the high risk groups the appearance of IgA antibodies to EBV VCA or EA augurs a sharply increased risk of NPC, with disease becoming apparent within 12 to 18 months. Most of these responses occur in apparently normal persons without evidence of disease even in biopsied tissue from Waldeyer ring, but some already have early cancer. This is the only known malignancy in which specific identified antibodies antedate and may herald the appearance of the disease.

Cofactors contributing to the high incidence of NPC in the endemic areas have been proposed, including regional flora such as the tung oil tree, which contains tumor-promoting substances, and genetic predisposition. Studies of HLA types found in patients with NPC suggest that a few selected types are associated with the occurrence of NPC. However, more decisive genetic analyses coming from studies of HLA patterns in members of the families of afflicted persons have not been carried out. In any case, if certain genotypes are more susceptible to NPC they must be found in three widely different population groups: South Chinese, Black Africans from the equatorial regions, and Caucasians on the north coast of Africa; all these groups have an elevated incidence of the tumor [6].

These remarkable phenomena open a broad field of opportunities for epidemiologic, molecular, clinical, and cancer control research. Exact incidence figures still need to be ascertained in both endemic and nonendemic regions. Other risk factors if there are any need to be identified to help predict whether NPC will actually occur in persons with the IgA responses. As the polypeptide constituents of the antigens evoking the responses are identified it may become possible to pinpoint responses to particular EBV polypeptides that have a stronger predictive value. On the molecular level much work needs to be done: Not even the origin of these antibody responses— whether caused by reactivation of virus replication in the oropharynx or by an antigenic stimulus arising in NPC progenitor cells—has been determined. For early detection biopsies of apparently normal tissue at Waldeyer ring may eventually yield evidence of viral genomes or their gene products in some meaningful pattern. Early detection methods might then be devised based not on conventional histopathology, since no cancer exists, but rather on molecular analyses carried out by Southern blot and Northern blot hybridizations to detect DNA or RNA and by Western blot analyses to detect specific viral proteins. Ultimately, if the IgA responses signal some kind of viral reactivation process it may be possible to intervene with antiviral agents such as Acyclovir and interferon.

EBV MOLECULAR ASPECTS

The EBV genome has a molecular weight of 100×10^6 daltons or 170 kilobase pairs [2]. Although the genome has four internal regions of direct repeated sequence and terminal iterations there is no homology between the terminal and internal repeats. Therefore, inversions or isomeric forms of the genome that are found with other herpesviruses do not exist. On the other hand, the EBV genome does exist both in cell lines and in human tissues infected with the virus in a circular episomal form. The episomes are circularized linear genomes that exist only intracellularly in both latently and productively infected cells. The episomes are present as nuclear constituents in a nucleosomal arrangement similar to cellular DNA. In contrast to the linear genomes, which become encapsidated and are replicated by virus specified DNA polymerase, the episomal form of the genome is maintained in cells in a regulated mode of replication tied to cell cycle and apparently mediated by cellular rather than viral DNA polymerases. The EBV episome is thought to be the molecular basis for latency, presenting as an ideal vehicle for the phenomenon of reactivation, which is so characteristic of herpetic infections. Latent EBV genomes can be activated at the level of transcription and translation going on in some cases to full-fledged replication. In addition, integrated forms of the EBV genome have been detected in a few cell lines. Whether such forms regularly occur in nature and whether they are specifically linked to malignant states is unknown. In any case, complete copies of the genome are inserted at nonunique sites in a setting of deletion and duplication of cellular DNA sequences at the insertion sites.

In the quest for the molecular features that distinguish latent from transforming functions there are two general approaches. The first involves the effort to identify transforming sequences within the EBV genome, which has thus far met with little success because of the difficulty of transfecting and transforming cells with segments of EBV DNA. More fruitful has been the analysis of transcriptional products in nonproductively transformed cells. This is an apposite approach inasmuch as the entire EBV genome is present as an episome in the infected cells. Since expression of the genome is strictly regulated there are likely to be specific messages keyed to the latent and oncogenic states as well as to virus production and reactivation. In non-productively infected Burkitt's lymphoma cell lines only a small portion of the genome is transcribed into messenger RNA, with at least four messages distinguished so far; some of the products of these messages have been identified, and the function of others is suspected. However, central questions persist, namely, which if any of these messages are peculiar to the latent state and which to the oncogenic state, since the lines analyzed are both transformed and latently infected [2].

A subsidiary approach has been the analysis of NPC tissues directly. These analyses reveal a general resemblance transcriptionally to latently infected BL cell lines; it is not yet possible to discern whether there are fine points of difference that may be peculiar to NPC, and it has not been possible to distinguish "latent" from "oncogenic" messages. One NPC analysis has revealed a different transcriptional pattern, which, compared with transcription found in completely latent infection, has been termed an *enhanced transcriptional state*. This transcriptional pattern resembles that found in latently infected cell lines, such as Raji, that have been exogenously induced into the synthesis of early antigen; such inductions stop short of viral replication. Enhanced transcription may be meaningful in that there are enhanced responses to EBV antigens in patients with NPC. Whether or not all NPCs at one time or another go through a phase of enhanced transcription and whether the genesis of the distinctive antibody responses in patients with NPC arises from the tumor itself are questions under investigation [6, 15].

PATHOGENESIS OF EPSTEIN-BARR VIRUS INFECTIONS

One of the long-standing puzzles posed by EBV has been the association of a lymphotrophic virus with a malignancy, NPC, which is epithelial in origin. In addition to NPC of the three histologic types, other malignancies of epithelial origin arising in the upper respiratory tract, including supraglottal and laryngeal tumors and thymic epithelial tumors, have been implicated. All four of these cancers may have a common embryonic origin. Also, evidence of virus has been found in the parotid gland, a probable replication site for EBV, and, in immunosuppressed persons with chronic EBV infection, in lung tissue. Recently, replication of virus has been detected in the tongue of persons afflicted with AIDS; the virus is in areas of hairy leukoplakia, a premalignant lesion. This may be an aberrant site of replication occurring only in the profoundly disordered setting of AIDS, or it may have significance for persons without AIDS, which is suggested by the recent finding of EBV DNA in some cancers of the tongue. Whether EBV has a role in the pathogenesis of lingual malignancies or whether tissue or organ restrictions are eased allowing replication of the virus in these conditions is unknown. In any case, EBV clearly interacts with epithelial cells as well as with lymphocytes [9].

A current view of the pathogenesis of EBV infection is that the virus initially infects epithelial cells in the oropharynx, where it replicates. Probably the virus gains access to the epithelial cells by using the same C2R receptors for the C2D component of complement that are receptors for EBV in B lymphocytes. Soon thereafter B lymphocytes also become infected with EBV, but these cells remain sites of latent infection in vivo. EBV-infected B cells not only circulate in the peripheral blood but they also probably find their way into a number of organs, including spleen, liver, bone marrow, and perhaps brain, where pathologic reactions take place in response to their presence. EBV-infected B lymphocytes bear a new virally encoded surface antigen, termed *lymphocyte-determined membrane antigen* (LYDMA), which is believed to be the target for cytotoxic T-lymphocyte responses manifested by the characteristic atypical lymphocyte response of infectious mononucleosis [8].

The evidence that EBV can infect human epithelial cells has accumulated slowly but now seems to be convincing. EBV DNA and RNA can be demonstrated directly by in situ cytohybridization with specific EBV DNA and cRNA probes in epithelial cells recovered from the oropharynx and parotid duct of patients with acute infectious mononucleosis. Moreover, EBV is capable of infecting, although with very low efficiency, primary human epithelial cells cultured in vitro; in these cells it appears that the viral replicative cycle takes place as indicated by EBV EA and VCA antigens as well as EBV DNA and EBNA, which are detectable after infection. Viral expression and replication may be linked to cell-cycle events or state of differentiation, which would help to explain the asynchronous character of infection of epithelial cells in the oropharynx and the persistent nature of the infection with long continued virus excretion. EBV neoplastic conditions may thus arise along three pathways: in the epithelial cells, which the virus primarily infects; through generation of polyclonal lymphoproliferation of latently infected B lymphocytes; or through the generation of diclonal or monoclonal cell lines with the characteristic chromosomal translocations discussed earlier that become altered and selected from polyclonal proliferating B lymphocytes [9].

ANTIVIRAL DRUGS

We can make predictions about the potential efficacy of antiviral drugs in the various stages of EBV infection states. Despite the lack of a distinctive EBV-encoded thymidine kinase (TK), Acyclovir is activated in EBV-infected cells by triphosphorylation of the drug to low levels. The drug triphosphate strongly inhibits the replication of EBV through a high affinity interaction with the EBV-encoded DNA polymerase. Acyclovir triphosphate acts as an inhibitor by competing with dGTP. However, the drug has no effect on the replication of EBV episomes in latently infected cell lines, presumably because these forms of the EBV genome are replicated by cellular rather than by viral DNA polymerase. The lack of effect of the drug on latent infection seems also to hold in vivo, not only for EBV but also the other human herpesviruses when they are in the latent state. In both EBV-infected cell lines and patients, administration of Acyclovir quickly suppresses but does not abolish infection, probably because of the incurable repository of cells containing EBV episomes. Some newer drugs have more persistent effects after administration in cellular models of EBV infection, but they too fail to cure the infection. Finally, immortalization or transformation of B lymphocytes by EBV is unimpeded by strongly inhibitory concentrations of Acyclovir [4].

Therefore, we would expect that Acyclovir would interfere with but not abolish oropharyngeal virus replication and excretion and that it would have no effect on NPC, BL, or polyclonal lymphoproliferation. A possible exception might be in the earliest phases of the development of NPC in which there is evidence of viral reactivation as signaled by the EBV IgA responses discussed earlier; if these responses are due to renewed replication of virus rather than simply an enhanced transcription with translation of additional gene products, but not viral replication and cell death, then administration of Acyclovir might interrupt virus-triggered effects. In the case of polyclonal lymphoproliferation, if this process requires continued recruitment of B lymphocytes by continuing infection of the cells, as the previously infected lymphocytes are eliminated by cytotoxic immune responses, then antiviral therapy may tip the balance in favor of the host [15]. Alternative therapeutic interventions might involve agents that do not have as their targets viral replication itself, but rather cell changes triggered by virus infection or synthesis of other virus-encoded polypeptides and enzymes such as ribonucleotide reductase. For the former type of intervention interferon may be of use, and for the latter approach the new antiviral drug, 2-acetylpyridine thiosemicarbazone (A723U), which is not a nucleoside analog and does not interfere directly with viral DNA replication, may provide the paradigm for treatment of this virus-triggered neoplasia.

CONCLUSIONS

Thirty years ago astute epidemiologic observations by Dennis Burkitt set in motion studies that led to the discovery of the Epstein-Barr virus. Subsequently, seroepidemiologic surveys established that EBV is the principal cause of infectious mononucleosis (IM). Molecular analyses of tissue specimens from patients with BL, NPC, and IM coupled with simple epidemiologic designs greatly strengthened the association of EBV with malignancy. In many ways the origins of our ideas about EBV-associated diseases were essentially epidemiologic. The primary need now is for more professional epidemiologic investigations—timely because of the availability of an expanded range of molecular markers.

In infectious mononucleosis transmission between partners can now be followed by comparison of restriction endonuclease patterns of EBV genomes found in cell lines established from peripheral blood and by exposure to virus excreted in the oropharynx. Such work should among other things better establish the ill-defined incubation period of IM. We also need to identify risk factors for IM (apart from age) and for the increasingly recognized complications. Finally, better definition of chronic mononucleosis and a prospective study of the likelihood of its development are needed. Similarly, we know nothing about the risk factors and immunologic markers for lymphoproliferative syndromes in allograft recipients, which might be coupled with investigation of the emergence of monoclonal disease in some of these patients.

In Burkitt's lymphoma some fresh and more plausible ideas about cofactors contributing to endemicity of BL are needed. Although HTLV 3 antibodies have apparently not been found in sera from patients with BL collected in 1964, the prevalence of HTLV 3 infection in the BL endemic region is tantalizing. We need firm incidence data on the occurrence of authenticated BL in AIDS in the United States and elsewhere in the world. We need to identify risk factors for BL in patients with AIDS and to address the question of whether pre-AIDS or asymptomatic HTLV 3 infection poses a risk of BL. In patients in whom lymphomas do develop an analysis of virus-specific markers, both EBV and HTLV 3, needs to be carried out.

For nasopharyngeal carcinoma, comparative genetic studies such as of HLA markers in the various racial stocks prone to NPC are still lacking. Genetic studies in those persons with IgA responses in whom NPC later does or does not develop might be revealing. More precise incidence figures and demographic profiles would help to identify other factors that may be contributing to the endemicity of NPC in South China and elsewhere. Improved data are needed to determine whether there actually are three levels of incidence of NPC, sporadic, endemic, and intermediate. Initiative for a new cancer control effort may arise from an analysis of possible molecular markers of incipient NPC in biopsied tissues from persons prone to development of the cancer. Finally, well-designed molecular epidemiologic surveys of other malignancies of epithelial origin in which EBV has become implicated should be considered. As the EBV transforming genes and their control elements become identified we can ask again whether there are specific disease-linked genomic variants or whether EBV-associated diseases are tied to differential gene expression—questions that bring to a focus the disciplines of epidemiology and molecular biology.

REFERENCES

1. de-Thé G, Geser A, Day N, Tukei P, Willams E, Beri D, Smith P, Dean A, Bornkamm G, Feorino P, Henle W: Nature 274:756–761, 1978.
2. Epstein MA, Achong BG (eds): "The Epstein-Barr Virus." New York: Springer Verlag, Inc., 1979.
3. Pagano JS, Lemon SM, The Herpesviruses. In Braude AI (ed): "Infectious Diseases and Medical Microbiology", Edition 2. Philadelphia: W.B. Saunders Co., 1986, pp 470–477.
4. Pagano JS, Datta AK: Am J Med [special issue] "Acyclovir Symposium". pp 18–26, 1982.
5. Ziegler J, Miner R, Rosenbaum E, Lennette E, Shillitoe E, Casavant C, Drew W, Mintz L, Gershow J, Greenspan J, Beckstead J, Yamamoto K: Lancet 2:631–633, 1982.
6. Prasad U, Ablashi D, Levine PH, Pearson G (eds): "Nasopharyngeal Carcinoma: Current Concepts." University Malaya Press: Kuala Lumpur, 1983.
7. Magrath I, Erikson J, Whang-Peng J, Sieverts H, Armstrong G, Benjamin D, Triche T, Alabaster O, Croce C: Science 222:1094–1098, 1983.
8. Notkins AL, Oldstone MBA (eds): "Concepts in Viral Pathogenesis." New York: Springer-Verlag, 1984, pp 307–314.
9. Sixbey J, Pagano JS: In Remington J, Swartz M (eds): "Current Clinical Topics in Infectious Diseases." New York: McGraw-Hill, 1984, Vol 4.
10. Plotkin SA, Michelson S, Pagano JS, Rapp F (eds): "CMV: Pathogenesis and Prevention of Human Infection." New York: Alan R. Liss, Inc., 1984.
11. Gottlieb MS, Groopman JE (eds): "Acquired Immune Deficiency Syndrome" UCLA Symposia, New Series, Vol 16. New York: Alan R. Liss, Inc., 1984.
12. Gallo R, Essex M, Gross L (eds): "Human T-Cell Leukemia/Lymphoma Virus: The Family of Human T-Lymphotropic Retroviruses: Their Role in Malignancies and Association with AIDS." Cold Spring Harbor, NY: Cold Spring Harbor Laboratory, 1984.
13. Croce C, Erikson J, Huebner K, Nishikura K: Science 227:1044–1047, 1985.
14. Wong-Staal F, Gallo RC: "Human T-Lymphotropic Retroviruses." Nature 317:395–403, 1985.
15. Levine PH, Ablashi DV, Pearson GR, Kottaridis SD (eds): "Progress in Medical Virology: EBV and Associated Diseases." Boston: Martinus Nijhoff Publ, 1985.

Biochemical and Molecular Epidemiology of Cancer 355–357 (1986)

Detection of Oncogenes and Viruses in Human Tissues and Cells

James K. McDougall

Fred Hutchinson Cancer Research Center, Seattle, Washington 98104

Molecular hybridization, which depends on the ability of single strands of nucleic acid to recognize and to base-pair with other strands of complementary sequence, has enabled significant advances to be made in the understanding of nuclear and chromosomal structure and gene expression. The techniques used employ purified nucleic acids from cells or viruses in the examination of sequence complexity by renaturation in solution or detection of complementary sequences immobilized on nitrocellulose membranes. From studies using these techniques we know that the eukaryotic genome contains not only unique sequences but also DNA sequences that are repeated many times. It was the recognition of such repeated gene sequences that led to the development of the in situ hybridization method. Although molecular hybridization in solution or on membranes can identify the different classes of DNA or RNA isolated from a particular cell population, we learn little about the relative distribution of the different sequences throughout the tissue or in individual cells. The development and interpretation of in situ hybridization methods depend on an understanding of the principles underlying the generally more controllable and quantitative procedures used in solution and filter hybridization methods.

The first part of this workshop dealt with applications of the in situ hybridization procedure to the detection of two viruses of major current interest, human T-cell lymphotropic virus type III (HTLV-III) and the human papilloma virus(es) (HPV), and the chromosomal localization of amplified oncogenes. A newly developed and simplified procedure for nonradioactive cytological hybridization was also discussed.

The use of ^{35}S-labeled RNA transcribed from cloned HTLV-III has enabled *Harper* (NIH) to detect virus-specific RNA in primary lymphocytes from patients with AIDS. The low frequency of cells positive for HTLV-III RNA (0.01% of cells) is consistent with results from Southern blot experiments. The use of a ^{35}S label allows a much shorter exposure time than can be achieved with the ^{3}H label used by *Emanuel* (Philadelphia) in studies of oncogene amplification. Advantages of a ^{3}H-labeled probe are the short path length of radioactive emission and the long half-life of the isotope. Therefore, it has been possible to localize amplified oncogene se-

Received May 13, 1985.

© **1986 Alan R. Liss, Inc.**

quences (c-*myc*, N-*myc*, and c-*abl* in these studies) to chromosomes and to propose that certain cytogenetically recognized chromosome abnormalities, eg, homogenously staining regions (HSRs), abnormally banded regions (ABRs), double minutes (DRs), and translocation sites, can be related to altered oncogene function or expression.

The development of nonradioactive probes for molecular hybridization provides a pathway for these procedures to become an accepted part of the armamentarium of diagnostic and pathology laboratories. The use of biotin-labeled DNA probes to detect HPV in human tissues was described by *Beckmann* (Seattle). A number of laboratories have recently shown that many anogenital tumors contain HPV DNA sequences and that particular HPV types are associated with different diseases. Using this method of in situ hybridization it is possible to study the distribution of HPV types in the cells of malignant and premalignant lesions. Retrospective studies on stored formalin-fixed, paraffin-embedded tissue sections is feasible with this procedure, as is hybridization to cells in diagnostic smears, enabling data to be collected on disease progression in relation to HPV type present. Further developments of the biotin-labeled probe hybridization procedure, described by *Brigati* (Hershey), allow hybridization results to be observed within 8 hr of section cutting. A reduced hybridization period, reduced probe concentration, and direct colorimetric detection of nucleic acid sequences provide further advantages to this procedure and will increase its usefulness in histochemical laboratories. The sensitivity of the method is sufficient for use in specific diagnoses of viral infection but will require further improvement to be of value in studies of viral latency and oncogenesis.

The second half of the workshop concerned the detection of oncogenes and their expression, amplification, and genetic polymorphism. DNA extracted from rat lung tumors induced by tetranitromethane (TNM) was shown to induce secondary transformants by transfection into NIH3T3 cells. An activated cellular homologue of the K-*ras* oncogene was detected in the secondary transfectants, as described by *Stowers* (NIEHS). Neither structural mutations nor amplification of the activated oncogene could be demonstrated in the different lung tumors. In a study of human lung cancer, *Cohen* (Louisiana State) examined genetic polymorphisms in the oncogenes H-*ras* and *fms* to determine if a specific oncogene polymorphism might be associated with familial clustering of malignancies. This type of approach will become of great value both in biochemical epidemiology and in determining progression of disease and the origin of cells involved in relapse of transplant recipients. Alitalo (Helsinki) described the amplification of c-*myc*, without rearrangement of the gene, in bone marrow cells of a patient with acute myeloid leukemia. Other oncogenes examined showed no evidence of rearrangement or amplification. The use of DNA-mediated gene transfer has enabled the identification of dominant cellular transforming genes as well as facilitating studies of viral sequences that can transform cells to malignancy. *Buonaguro* (Seattle) has produced transformants of NIH3T3 cells using a 558 base pair fragment of cytomegalovirus DNA. The cells derived from these transfections are tumorigenic in nude mice, and DNA extracted from the cell lines produces secondary transformants. The transforming fragment of CMV DNA does not encode a protein and therefore it is hypothesized that transformation may be achieved by activation or mutation of a cellular oncogene. In this case detection of the target sequence may be more important than detection of the transforming (initiating) viral sequence. The construction of recombinant libraries from transformed cell lines provides the best way to resolve such problems.

In summary, methods based on the original development of nitrocellulose blotting procedures by Southern [1] allow for detection of as small a fragment of viral nucleic acid as 200 base pairs per diploid cell in DNA extracted from human cells and can detect amplification of cellular genes, eg, oncogenes, during development and disease. The in situ hybridization method, originally developed by Pardue and Gall [2] and John et al [3] during studies of ribosomal gene localization to the "cap" region of oocytes of *Xenopus laevis*, has become a valuable tool in the detection of viral sequences and gene alterations in individual cells and the localization of genes on chromosomes. One caveat to be aware of, and of particular importance in studies of human tumors, is the need to purify probes free of vector (plasmid) and bacterial nucleic acid sequences to avoid nonspecific cross-hybridization with contaminating bacteria or plasmids.

REFERENCES

1. Southern EM: J Mol Biol 98:503, 1975.
2. Pardue ML, Gall JG: Proc Natl Acad Sci USA 64:600, 1969.
3. John HL, Birnsteil ML, Jones KW: Nature 223:582, 1969.

Biochemical and Molecular Epidemiology of Cancer 359–372 (1986)

Host Factors in Carcinogenesis: Carcinogen Metabolism and DNA Damage

Herman Autrup

Laboratory of Environmental Carcinogenesis, The Fibiger Institute, DK-2100 Copenhagen Ø, Denmark

Chemical carcinogens are biotransformed into their ultimate carcinogenic form by the cytochrome P-450 mixed function oxidase system. Variation in the composition and quantities of these cytochromes may be a determining factor in the host and organ susceptibility to the carcinogenic effects. Formation of carcinogen-DNA adducts is an important consequence of the reaction between the ultimate carcinogen and cellular DNA. The biological importance of these adducts is discussed.

Key words: carcinogen metabolism, cytochrome P-450, carcinogen-DNA adducts, polycyclic aromatic hydrocarbons, aromatic amines, aflatoxin, N-nitrosamines

Host factors play important roles in determining the risk of developing cancer. The very first step in the initiation of chemically induced cancer involves the biotransformation of chemical carcinogens into their ultimate forms. These metabolites are very reactive and react immediately with cellular macromolecules, especially DNA, under the formation of covalently bound adducts (Fig. 1). The formation of specific adducts has subsequently been associated with cytotoxicity, cell killing, mutagenesis, and transformation.

The importance of carcinogen metabolism in carcinogenesis has been suggested from animal studies based on the inducibility of arylhydrocarbon hydroxylase (AHH) [1]. Cytochrome P-450 (P-450)-dependent monooxygenases play a major role in the activation as well as the deactivation of chemical carcinogens. The P-450 enzyme system is composed of numerous isoenzymes, and the isoenzymes differ by substrate specificity and regio- and stereoselectivity. The enzyme system is mainly localized in the liver, but is also found in stratified epithelium and other surface epithelia that serve as barriers for the contact with environmental carcinogens [2]. These observations suggest that the amount and the relative composition of the various isozymes of epithelial P-450 may be important determinants in both organ specificity and individual susceptibility exhibited by many carcinogens.

Received June 10, 1985.

© **1986 Alan R. Liss, Inc.**

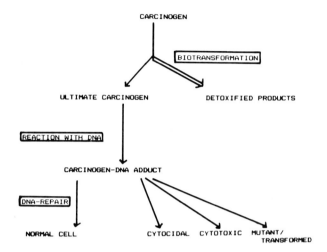

Fig. 1.   Host factors in chemical carcinogenesis.

The biological effective tissue dose of the carcinogens is the amount of the ultimate carcinogen reaching the target tissues or is formed in the tissues and can conveniently be measured as the amount of reaction product formed between the ultimate carcinogen and the cellular macromolecules, eg, DNA. Thus, the biological effective dose is dependent on the concentration of the carcinogens reaching the target tissues and on the composition of the P-450 isozymes. A wide interindividual variation and tissue variability in the ability to activate chemical carcinogens are seen both in different binding levels to tissue DNA [3,4] and in mutation frequency, when human cells or subcellular systems were used as the activation system in mutation assays [5,6]. Some primary DNA lesions have been associated with various cellular effects, and in general a good correlation has been established between the amount of adducts and the subsequent mutation or transformation frequencies. However, the adducts may be recognized by repair enzymes and eliminated before any cellular or genetic consequences can be realized. The persistency of the adducts is for some carcinogens more important than the initial level of adducts immediately following exposure. Cells lacking the ability to repair the DNA damage are more susceptible to the toxic and carcinogenic action of different carcinogens [7].

CYTOCHROME P-450 AND XENOBIOTIC METABOLISM AS INDICATORS FOR CANCER SUSCEPTIBILITY

Animal experiments have shown a positive correlation between the susceptibility to polycyclic aromatic hydrocarbons (PAH) carcinogenesis and the inducibility of P-450–associated AHH, rather than the basal AHH activity [1]. Inducibility has been shown to be under genetic control in mice, and it is suspected to be under genetic control in man [8]. Using this concept, several studies have reported a higher level of inducibility of AHH in mitogen-stimulated lymphocytes isolated from patients with lung cancer, laryngeal carcinoma, and cancer of the oral cavity than from noncancer patients [for review, see 9,10]. However, there are conflicting reports, and the high inducibility phenotype may be a consequence of the disease rather than one of the causative factors. Polymorphism in drug metabolism may be another in vivo assay for identifying individuals at high risk for chemically induced cancer. This phenomenon has long been recognized in pharmacology, where people have been reported to respond differently when treated with the same dose of a drug. These aberrant reactions are caused by deficiencies in the metabolism of the drug, possibly by a modification of the P-450 at the active sites. Genetic polymorphism has been reported for several drugs, including debrisoquine, sparteine, and phenformin, and all appear to involve the same allele [11]. Debrisoquine, an antihypertension drug, is metabolized by a specific but minor form of P-450, with 4-hydroxydebrisoquine as the predominant metabolite. Of the polymorphic drugs, debrisoquine has mostly been used for in vivo studies. Population studies indicate ethnic differences, and among Caucasians approximately one out of 10 has impaired metabolism. People with a metabolic ratio (debrisoquine/4-hydroxydebrisoquine) greater than 12.6 belong to the poor metabolizer group [11,12]. The frequency distribution shows a bimodal distribution. It has been assumed that poor metabolizers of debrisoquine may have a low rate of activation of the carcinogen and subsequent lower risk for developing cancer. However, in vitro studies indicate no association between the metabolism of 2-acetylaminofluorene (2-AAF) and other general substrates for mixed function oxidases and the amount of this type of P-450 isolated from both rat and human liver [13,14].

Case control studies of cancer patients with bronchial carcinoma, one cancer in which the involvement of chemical carcinogens has clearly been established, show that the cancer patient group had a much higher frequency of fast metabolizers than the control group, and by using the log values of the metabolic ratios the frequency distribution for the lung cancer patients showed that they were among the fastest metabolizers compared to the control group [15]. Similar results were reported for patients with liver cancer in Nigeria [2], where aflatoxin B_1 (AFB), a potent animal liver carcinogen, may play an important role in the induction of liver cancer in man [16]. In contrast, bladder cancer patients showed the normal distribution of debrisoquine phenotype [17]. However, another metabolic polymorphism has been observed in the case of bladder cancer [18]. Occupational exposure to aromatic amines has frequently been associated with increased risk for bladder cancer [19]. Aromatic amines are detoxified to less harmful compounds by acetylation of the amino group, and actually a higher proportion of bladder cancer patients belong to the slow acetylator type, which suggests that they are less efficient in the acetylation of aromatic amines to less toxic compounds.

Other attempts to phenotype people with respect to mixed function oxidase activities include measuring the clearance rate of antipyrine [20,21]. The biotransformation of antipyrine involves several of the P-450 isoenzymes [22]. Early studies showed that the clearance rate of antipyrine in man correlated with the inducibility of AHH in the lymphocytes [20], but the clearance rate did not correlate with the level of AHH activity in human liver biopsy specimens [23]. The latter results indicate that the antipyrene clearance rate may not be a reliable metabolic index of the ability of other organs, including the liver, to convert chemical carcinogens to their reactive intermediates. Animal studies support these results, as the serum antipyrine half-life in mice did not show any relationship to the S9-mediated mutagenicity of several different carcinogens [24].

An alternative and more specific approach to study individual ability to biotransform chemical carcinogens is to phenotype people with respect to the composition and quantity of the various P-450 isozymes. A total of 10 different P-450 isozymes have been isolated and purified from rat liver by affinity chromatography and have been characterized by immunological and biochemical methods [25,26]. Several human P-450 isozymes have been isolated from the liver and other organs [26–28], but their substrate specificity is not as well understood as that of rat liver P-450, although some of the human P-450's properties resemble that of the rats.

In the following discussion, the nomenclature of Ryan et al [29] will be used for rat P-450 and the Coon nomenclature [30] for rabbit P-450. Cytochromes P-450c and P-450d are the major 3-methylcholanthrene (MC)-inducible forms and P-450b, P-450e, and P-450h the phenobarbital (PB)-inducible isoenzymes in the rat. In untreated rat livers, P-450a (50%), P-450c (18%), and P-450e (16%) were the major isozymes [25]. Metabolic studies using either reconstituted systems with purified P-450 or monospecific antibodies against the P-450 isozymes as inhibitors in an enzyme reaction indicate that several P-450 isozymes are involved in the metabolism of the same substrate and at the same positions, although the kinetics may be different. The role of different P-450 isozymes in the metabolism of different carcinogens, especially benzo(a)-pyrene (BP), has been extensively studied (Table I). Using purified rabbit liver P-450 isozymes, Deutsch et al [31] showed that highly purified cytochrome P-450 exhibited different catalytic activity toward BP and BP 7,8-diol with respect to both the metabolic profile and the ability to produce the ultimate carcinogenic form of BP. The MC-inducible form (LM2) isozyme is more active than the BP-inducible form (LM4) in the conversion of BP to products that reacted with DNA, while P-450 LM4 is more active than LM2 with 7,8-diol as the substrate. The other rabbit liver P-450 isozymes gave intermediate results. Incubation of BP with LM4 in a reconstituted system did not produce any significant amounts of BP diols [32], suggesting that one single form of rabbit liver P-450 is not sufficient to convert BP to its ultimate

TABLE I. Substrate Specificity of Rat Cytochrome P-450

	P-450 isozymes			
	b	c	d	e
Benzo(a)pyrene (BP)				
DNA binding		+		
Mutation		+		
Deactivation	+			+
BP 7,8-diol				
Mutation	(+)	+		
Aromatic amines				
2-AAF and Trp-P-2				
Mutation		(+)	+	
Deactivation	+			+
Aflatoxin B_1				
DNA binding	+			
Mutation		+	+	
Deactivation		+	+	
Dimethylnitrosamine				
Mutation	−	−	−	−

+, isoenzyme involved; (+), partly involved; −, not involved.

carcinogen, BP 7,8-diol-9,10-epoxide, but that a combination of P-450 isozymes, in addition to expoxide hydrolase, is required. In contrast, when BP was incubated in a reconstituted system containing rat liver P-450c, the BP diols, including BP 7,8-diol, accounted for more than 65% of the total metabolites [33]. This form of the P-450 is also the most important in the total metabolism of BP as shown by inhibition of the enzyme activity after addition of anti-MC-cytochrome P-450 immunogloblin to the reaction mixture [34]. It is interesting that 7,12-dimethylbenz(a)anthracene is metabolized to diols by P-450b and P-450c, although the proximate carcinogen, DMBA 3,4-diol, was not produced to any significant degree [33]. Noninduced microsomes produced the highest relative amount of the proximate carcinogen. The same results were observed with other PAHs, benzo(a)phenanthrene [35], and benz(a)anthracene (BA). The major BA diols formed by P-450c and P-450d are BA 5,6- and BA 8,9-diol [36]. Using a reconstituted P-450 system to activate BP and BP 7,8-diol in the Ames mutation assay, P-450c was the most efficient. BP and BP 7,8-diol were also good substrates for P-450d, whereas P-450b only produced one-third of the revertants produced by P-450c [37]. Of the rabbit liver P-450 isoenzymes, form LM6 was the most efficient in converting BP to mutagenic metabolites. The other rabbit P-450 forms only resulted in slight increase in mutation frequency [38].

Aromatic amines, another major group of chemical carcinogens, have been associated with the induction of bladder cancer in man. The ultimate carcinogenic forms of these compounds are N-hydroxylated products, whereas C-hydroxylation, in contrast, gives rise to less harmful compounds. Both metabolic pathways are mediated by the P-450–associated mixed function oxidases [39,40]. In a reconstituted system, rat liver P-450d is the major P-450 responsible for the N-oxidation of 2-acetylaminofluorene (2-AAF) [41,42], but the N-oxidation product only accounts for a small percentage of the total metabolites produced by P-450d. Other rat P-450 isozymes are also involved in the N-oxidation. In contrast, only rabbit liver P-450 LM4 is involved in the N-oxidation, but, as in the case of rat liver P-450d, LM4 is also catalyzing oxidations at other sites of the AAF molecule [40]. When mutagenesis in the Ames test was used as an endpoint for the activation of aromatic amines, the MC-inducible forms of P-450 (P-450c and P-450d) are the most active for 2-AAF [43], 2-aminofluorene [37], 4-aminobiphenyl [44], and Trp-P-2 [37,43,45]. This is consistent with the hypothesis that N-hydroxy metabolites are the most mutagenic metabolites of aromatic amines. Rabbit liver LM4 was also the most active form in the metabolism of 2-aminoanthracene to mutagenic products [38]. Aflatoxin B_1, a suspected liver carcinogen in man, is activated through an epoxide at the 8,9 position in the furan ring [46]. Detoxification of AFB involves the formation of hydroxylated products or demethylation at the anisol group [47]. In a reconstituted system, highly purified rat liver P-450b has been demonstrated to be the major P-450 involved in formation of the epoxide and the subsequent binding of AFB to DNA [48]. This isozyme was severalfold more active than any other P-450. Ueno et al [49] have reported that AFB was specifically activated into a DNA binding form by P-450 I-a. This form was induced by PCB and had an absorption peak of 450.0 nm in the CO difference spectrum. The MC-inducible forms P-450c and P-450d were mostly involved in the biotransformation of AFB_1 to AFM_1 [48]. In contrast, Yoshizawa et al [50] did not demonstrate any significant selectivity of any P-450 in the binding of AFB_1 to DNA. This observation was supported by Robertson et al [37], who reported that P-450c and P-450d metabolized AFB_1 into mutagenic metabolites in the Ames test to a higher extent than did P-450b.

Very few studies have been reported on the involvement of P-450 in the activation of N-nitrosamines. The ultimate carcinogenic metabolites are carbonium ions formed by initial hydroxylation at the C-carbon atom next to the nitrosogroup. Robertson et al [37] and Masson et al [51] have reported that rat P-450 isozymes are apparently not involved in the conversion of dimethylnitrosamine to its mutagenic form. N-nitroso-2,6-dimethylmorpholine, a potent pancreatic carcinogen in hamster, is metabolized to its proximate carcinogenic form, N-nitroso (2-hydroxypropyl) (2-oxopropyl) amine by rabbit liver P-450 LM2 and LM3a [52]. LM3a also had high N-demethylase activity [53].

The complexity of the P-450 forms involved in the activation and deactivation of different types of chemical carcinogens suggests that no common determinant of P-450 could be used to identify individuals who may have a higher risk for developing cancer caused by chemical exposure. A fingerprinting, both qualitative and quantitative, of the various P-450 forms in a specific tissue may serve as an indicator. However, knowledge of the tissue distribution and the kinetic parameters will be required to complete this kind of analysis. An isozyme analysis of the P-450 forms in one organ may not be representative for the other organs that are targets for the carcinogenic effect. A complicating factor in this type of analysis is that environmetal exposure, including the carcinogens themselves, affects the absolute and relative amounts of P-450 [54–56]. This inducibility of P-450 may by itself be the most important factor in determining higher risk to individuals, because it may represent a means to protect the organism against toxic exogenous compounds.

Different approaches have been taken to identify and quantitate the various forms of P-450. Monoclonal antibodies directed against P-450 isolated from induced rat and rabbit livers have been developed. As the functional and structural properties of P-450 are highly conserved through the species, at least some of the antibodies produced against animal P-450 forms recognize the human P-450 forms [27,28,57,58].

Antibodies can be used either as enzyme inhibitors for quantitative measurements of the contribution of a specific P-450 to the total activity of the tissue or as antibodies in a radioimmunoassay or the ELIZA assay. Fujino et al [59] have used a monoclonal antibody (Mab) 1-7-1, produced against rat liver P-450c/d, to study the effect on AHH activity and on ethoxycoumarin deethylase (ECD) activity in human placenta. Mab 1-7-1 inhibited totally the AHH activity and part of the ECD activity in placentas from smoking mothers, but the Mab had little or no effect on the activities in placenta from nonsmokers. Animal experiments have shown that 87% of the liver AHH and 39% of the ECD activity were mediated by the P-450 against which the antibody was raised. The results suggest that more than one form of P-450 can deethylate ethoxycoumarin and that both are present in human tissues. In normal and hydrocarbon-induced monocytes and in the liver, Mab 1-7-1 did not have any effect on either AHH or ECD activities, whereas the activity was inhibited about 50% in control and hydrocarbon-stimulated lymphocytes. An antibody against rat liver P-450 (UT-H) did inhibit the metabolism of debrisoquine by human liver microsomes [60].

Other methods to determine the amount of the P-450 independent of the functional activities are antibody-directed radioimmunoassay, enzyme-lined immunosorbent assay [61–63], and immunoblotting [27,28,62]. The latter method has been used to quantitate human liver and lung P-450 using antisera raised to purified human liver P-450 [27] and to human colon P-450 [28].

Recent developments in molecular biology have made it possible to understand the molecular mechanism underlying the multiplicity and the selective induction of the P-450 isozymes. This technology may provide another approach to fingerprinting the types and amounts of P-450 expressed in a given tissue by using DNA probes of the different P-450 genes. The genes for rat liver P-450c [64], P-450d [65,66], and P-450b [67,68] and forms of MC-inducible mouse liver P-450 [69] and rabbit P-450 [70] have been cloned. The cloned genes have been used to study the regulation of the expression of P-450 after induction with traditional P-450 inducers [71,72] and to study the developmental expression of mRNA [73]. By using specific parts of the cloned DNA sequences for Southern blot analysis Kawajiri et al [66] were able to distinguish between the two very closely related forms P-450c and P-450d. These preliminary results indicate that specific probes are more accurate than monoclonal antibodies to fingerprint an individual's P-450. Significant sequence homology exists among the mouse, rat, and rabbit P-450 structural genes, making them applicable in human systems as well. A 85% homology has been reported between rat and human P-450c [73]. Although in the near future we may be able to phenotype individuals for their P-450 pattern, its value in risk evaluation remains doubtful. It is clear that no specific P-450 is responsible for the activation of all carcinogens. An isozyme form that is mainly responsible for the activation of one carcinogen may be a form that deactivates other types of chemical carcinogens. In some cases more than one form of P-450 and additional enzyme activities are required for the formation of the ultimate carcinogens. Fingerprinting could therefore only be used to assess the potential risk of an individual to a particular compound, unless sophisticated computer programs are developed that take into consideration the organ distribution, types, quantities, and kinetic parameters for the single enzymes. The kinetic parameters may also be dependent on the substrate concentration, making this type of analysis even more complex.

As the tertiary structure of the P-450 is very important for substrate binding, a mutation in the coding region of the binding site may significantly affect enzymatic activity [75]. A study of gene polymorphism in either the structural and/or the regulatory genes may therefore be an interesting approach to identify people at high risk. Although gene polymorphism has been observed in both genes in rat liver P-450c no polymorphism was observed in human placental DNA [74–76].

CARCINOGEN-DNA ADDUCTS AS MEASURES FOR CARCINOGEN ACTIVATION

The reaction between the ultimate carcinogen and DNA gives rise to the formation of a covalent-bound complex—an adduct—which has long been considered an important and essential step in the chemical induction of cancer. Brooks and Lawley [77] reported in 1964 a good correlation between the carcinogenic potency of different aromatic polycyclic hydrocarbons in mouse skin and the extent to which they bound covalently to cellular DNA in the target tissues. However, this observation is apparently not valid for all classes of carcinogens. Neumann [78] has reported that for 4-amino-stilbene no correlation existed between initial DNA binding, initial adduct pattern, persistency of DNA adducts, accumulation and persistency of adducts after repeated doses, and the tissue susceptibility. A large literature has accumulated concerning the structure of the products formed between the carcinogen and DNA, as well as the biochemical and biological consequences of this interaction.

The major carcinogen-DNA adducts have been identified from the most common carcinogens, including PAH, nitrosamines, and aromatic amines [78]. Reaction between the ultimate carcinogens and DNA occur at nearly all possible sites in the DNA, including the triphosphate ester, although some specific positions are preferentially attacked by the strongly reactive metabolites. Most of the detectable reaction with DNA takes place between the guanine base and the carcinogens, and an interesting specificity appears between the various classes of carcinogen. PAH "bay-region" diolepoxides generally react with the 2-amino group, aromatic amine N-oxides with the C8 position, and alkylating compounds and aflatoxin B_1 with the N7 position. These are the major adducts formed both in vivo in experimental animals treated with the carcinogen and in human cells in vitro treated with radiolabeled carcinogens [2]. The major adduct formed after incubating the cells or subcellular fractions with DNA and chemical carcinogens is illustrated in Table II. With all carcinogens a great number of carcinogen-DNA interactions occur, and a study of their biological effects may be difficult. In addition, biologically important DNA modifications may have escaped detections because of insufficient sensitivity of the analytical procedures. The classic example is the alkylation of the 06 position of guanine or 04 position in thymidine [80]. Another potential source of misunderstanding is that for some carcinogens biological effects may be a result of the generation of apurinic or apyrimidinic sites rather than the adducts themselves. The apurinic/apyrimidinic sites can be generated either spontaneously or enzymatically [81,82].

Benzo(a)pyrene and other PAHs are activated by a multistep enzymatic process to diolepoxides that reacts with the 2-amino group of guanine, eg, the major BP-DNA adduct has been identified as trans-(7R)-N^2-(10[7β, 8α, 9α-trihydroxy-7,8,9,10-tetrahydrobenzo(a)pyrene]yl)deoxyguanosine. The stereochemistry of the PAH diolepoxide is very important for the biological activity of the diolepoxides [83]. The amounts of BP-DNA adducts have been associated with skin carcinogenesis in mice [84,85] and mutation frequency in hamster V-79 cells [86]. The amounts of total adducts are correlated to the transformation frequency in C3H 10T½ C18 cells and mutation frequency in Salmonella T100 [87]. A wide-range linear response curve for DNA binding was observed for BP, administered both orally [88] and by skin

TABLE II. Carcinogen-DNA Adducts Detected in Intact Cellular Systems

Carcinogen	Ultimate form	Major site	Minor site
Aflatoxin B	Epoxide	7-Gua	
Aromatic amines	N-Oxide		
2-Acetylaminofluorene		8-Gua	N2-Gua
2-Naphthylamine		8-Gua, N6-Ade	N2-Gua
N,N-Dimethylaminoazobenzene		8-Gua	N2-Gua
Nitrosamines	Carbonium		
Dimethylnitrosamine		7-Gua	06-Gua
Diethylnitrosamine		06- & N7-Gua	04-Thy
Polycyclic aromatic hydrocarbons			
Benzo(a)pyrene	Epoxide	N2-Gua	
7,12-Dimethylbenz(a)anthracene		N2-Gua	N6-Ade
Nitrocompounds			
4-Nitroquinoline-1-oxide	N-Oxide	8-Gua	N2-Gua
1-Nitropyrene	N-Oxide	8-Gua	

painting [89]. In a bacterial system, the major mutational lesion after exposure to BP diolepoxide is a base pair substitution changing a GC pair to a TA pair and to a lesser extent an AT to TA transversion [90]. This is the type of mutation seen in the 12th codon of the activated c-Ha-ras oncogene isolated from human tumor cells. When the ultimate carcinogen of BP was reacted in vitro with the nontransforming cellular oncogene it became transforming in the NIH 3T3 transformation assay. Assuming uniform distribution of the adducts, 100% transforming activity was obtained at 2.3 adducts per DNA strand [91].

The ultimate carcinogenic form of the aromatic amines and their acetylated derivatives, an N-oxide, reacts generally with the 8 position of guanine and is linked through the amino group of the carcinogens. Some rearrangement of the ultimate carcinogen occurs, and adducts formed between the exocyclic 2-amino group in guanine and the ortho position to the amino group is generally detected with all aromatic amines. The C8 adducts of AAF comprise 90% of the DNA adducts bound to DNA both in cultured cells and in animals. These adducts can be either acetylated or deacetylated products, with the deacetylated form being the most persistent [92]. In the Ames system a good correlation exists between the number of C8 modifications and the number of revertants/survivors. It has been calculated, assuming random distribution of the carcinogen-DNA modifications, that one modification per genome will result in one mutant per 2.25×10^6 bacteria [93–95]. Similar correlations exist between other C8 adducts and mutation frequency in TA1538.

2,3-Dihydro-2-(N7-guanyl)3-hydroxyaflatoxin B_1 was the major DNA adduct formed both in vivo and in vitro [96,97] after AFB treatment. No correlation was observed between the amount or persistence of this particular DNA adduct, but repeated administration of AFB to rats, at a regimen shown to produce a high incidence of liver cancer, caused accumulation of aflatoxin B_1-formamidopyrimidine [98]. These products are formed by the ring scission of the imidazole ring of guanine. It has also been suggested that apurinic sites formed by the release of the adducts are associated with some of the biological phenomena [99]. This suggestion has been supported by a base substitution analysis in Escherichia coli, where it was observed that activated AFB specifically induced GC to TA transversion. This type of mutation can best be explained by an apurinic site [100]. The released product, AFB-Gua, has been detected in rat urine after exposure to AFB and in human urine in people living in areas of high risk for liver cancer [101,102]. Modification in vitro of nontransforming DNA—in the NIH 3T3 system—with AFB did result in transforming activity [103].

The ultimate carcinogenic forms of N-nitrosamines and many direct acting carcinogens are carbonium ions that preferentially react with the 7 position of guanine. Depending on the stability and chemical reactivity of the carbonium ions, they will react with oxygen atoms, eg, 06 in guanine and 04 in thymidine [80]. The important role of 06 alkylation rather than the major product was first described by Goth and Rajewski [104], who observed that 06 ethylguanine was the persistent lesion in rat brain DNA that correlated with tumor incidence. In the case of alkylating compounds the persistency of the 06 adducts becomes more important in determining the organ and species specificity. The 06 alkyl modification is removed by the enzyme 06 methylguanine DNA methyltransferase. The presence of this enzyme is very important for both the cytotoxic and the transforming activities of alkylating agents in human cells [105]. The enzyme in mammalian cells is very specific for the 06 lesion

TABLE III. Methods to Detect Carcinogen-DNA Modifications

Assay	Estimate of sensitivity (adducts/bases)
Immunological	
RIA	1/10E4
ELIZA-Competitive	1/10E (6–7)
Immunoblot	1/10E6
Biochemical	
^{32}P Postlabeling	1/10E(6–9)
Physical	
Synchronous fluorescence	1/10E6

and does not repair other 0 alkyl products, so it is no surprise that it is 04 ethylthymidine and not 06 ethylguanine that accumulates in rat hepatocyte DNA after continuous exposure to diethylnitrosamine [106]. A positive association between the amount of 04 ethylthymidine and the preneoplastic lesion, GGT-positive foci, was reported [106]. The mutagenicity of 06 methylguanine has been studied in *E coli*, showing that this lesion induced exclusively GC to AT transitions. This mutation was only observed if the methyltransferase system was depleted or missing [106]. Construction of plasmids containing specific carcinogen-modified bases at specific sites may be a very interesting and important tool for a better understanding of the role specific adducts play in the carcinogenic process [108,109].

Generally, for all the carcinogens mentioned, specific carcinogen-DNA adducts have been shown to persist for long periods of time and could accumulate during long-term exposure. The persistence of the DNA adducts is not only of academic interest but could also have a practical implication, because they may be used as a quantitative measure of exposure.

Several new technologies have been developed to identify and quantitate carcinogen-DNA adducts (Table III) [110]. The most promising approach is the immunological methods, as they are very specific for a particular modification. In recent years a large number of polyclonal and monoclonal antibodies have been produced against both individual adducts and modified DNA covering the whole spectrum of modifications by the most frequently applied experimental carcinogens [111]. These antibodies can be used in RIA, ELIZA, USERIA, and immunoblot methods. These procedures have been used in studies of, for example, the persistence of a specific adduct. Polyclonal antisera against BPDE-modified DNA have also been used in preliminary population studies. Antigenicity in DNA has been demonstrated both in lung tissue and lymphocytes from lung cancer patients [112] and in occupationally exposed groups of roofers and foundry workers [113], but it is very difficult to make any conclusion on cancer risk based on these observations. Furthermore, the adduct level is measured mainly in the lymphocytes, a cell type not susceptible to the carcinogenic action of BP, and at present there have been no studies comparing the binding level in the target organs with the lymphocytes.

CONCLUSIONS

Two different approaches to identify individuals with a higher cancer risk after exposure to chemical carcinogens are emerging. One method is metabolic phenotyping with respect to a particular drug. This method is not invasive and does not require any sophisticated analytical procedure. A better understanding between the polymorphism and its influence on the metabolism of specific carcinogens is essential to validate this procedure's applicability. It also appears to be limited to certain types of cancer, eg, lung cancer and hepatocellular carcinoma, although the etiological agents in these two types of cancer are quite different and require different forms of P-450 for activation to their ultimate forms. The second promising approach is the detection of carcinogen-DNA adducts. The adduct level is a function of exposure level, ability to activate/deactivate the carcinogen, and efficiency of the DNA repair system to repair that particular damage, and as such the best measure at the present time to identify exposed individuals. People with a high level of carcinogen-DNA adducts may be considered to be at a higher risk for developing cancer than individuals with no adducts. However, this measure only represents one step in the carcinogenic process. There are quite likely many other unknown factors that determine the development of tumors.

ACKNOWLEDGMENTS

The author thanks Dr. L. Dragsted for valuable comments during the preparation of this manuscript and Mrs. Birgit Elk for typing the manuscript.

REFERENCES

1. Kouri RE, Nebert DW: In Hiatt HH, Watson JD, Winsten JA (eds): "Origins of Human Cancer." Cold Spring Harbor, NY: Cold Spring Harbor Laboratory, 1977, p 811.
2. Autrup H: Drug Metab Rev 13:603, 1982.
3. Harris CC, Trump BF, Grafström RG, Autrup H: J Cell Biochem 18:285, 1982.
4. Autrup H, Harris CC: In Harris CC, Autrup H (eds): "Human Carcinogenesis." New York: Academic Press, 1983, p 169.
5. Harris CC, Hsu I-C, Trump BF, Selkirk JK: Nature 272:633, 1978.
6. Sabadie N, Richter-Reichhelm HB, Saracci R, Mohr U, Bartsch H: Int J Cancer 27:417, 1981.
7. McCormick JJ, Maher VM: In Harris CC, Autrup H (eds): "Human Carcinogenesis." New York: Academic Press, 1983, p 401.
8. Boobis AR, Nebert DW: Adv Enzyme Regul 15:339, 1977.
9. Gelboin HV: N Engl J Med 309:105, 1983.
10. Kouri RE, Levine AS, Edwards BK, McLemore TL, Vesell ES, Nebert DW: Banbury Rep 16:131, 1984.
11. Idle JR, Ritchie JC: In Harris CC, Autrup H (eds): "Human Carcinogenesis." New York: Academic Press, 1983, p 857.
12. Ritchie JC, Idle JR: In Bartsch H, Armstrong B (eds): "Host Factors in Carcinogenesis." Lyon: I.A.R.C., 1982, p 381.
13. McManus ME, Boobis AR, Minchin RF, Schwartz DM, Murray S, Davies DS, Thorgeirsson SS: Cancer Res 44:5692, 1984.
14. Boobis AR, Murray S, Hampden CE, Davies DS: Biochem Pharmacol 34:65, 1985.
15. Ayesh R, Idle JR, Ritchie JC, Crothers MJ, Hetzel MR: Nature 312:169, 1984.
16. Linsell CA, Peers FG: In Hiatt HH, Watson JD, Winsten JA (eds): "Origins of Human Cancer." Cold Spring Harbor, NY: Cold Spring Harbor Laboratory, 1977, p 549.
17. Cartwright RA, Philip PA, Rogers HJ, Glashan RW: Carcinogenesis 5:1191, 1984.
18. Cartwright RA: Banbury Rep 16:359, 1984.
19. Case RAM, Hosber ME, McDonald DB, Pearson JT: Br J Ind Med 11:75, 1954.
20. Kellermann G, Jett JR, Luyten-Kellermann M, Moses HL, Fontana RS: Cancer 45:1438, 1980.
21. Kalamegham R, Krishnaswamy K, Krishnamurthy S, Bhargava RNK: Clin Pharmacol Ther 25:67, 1979.

22. Penno IB, Dvorchik BH, Vesell ES: Proc Natl Acad Sci USA 78:5193, 1981.
23. Pelkonen O, Sotaniemi E, Tokola O, Ahokas JT: Drug Metab Dispos 8:218, 1980.
24. Roberfroid MB, Malaveille C, Hautefeuille A, Brun G, Vo TK, Bartsch H: Chem Biol Interact 47:175, 1983.
25. Guengerich FB, Dannan GA, Wright ST, Martin MV, Kaminsky LS: Biochemistry 21:6019, 1982.
26. Guengerich FP, Shimada T, Distlerath LM, Reilly PEB, Umbenhauer DR, Martin MV: In Harris CH (ed): "Biochemical and Molecular Epidemiology of Cancer." New York: Alan R. Liss, Inc., 1986.
27. Guengerich FP, Wang P, Davidson NK: Biochem 21:1698, 1982.
28. Strobel HW, Newaz SN, Fang W-F, Lau PP, Oshinsky RJ, Stralka DJ, Salley FF: In Rydström J, Montelius J, Bengtsson M (eds): "Extrahepatic Drug Metabolism and Chemical Carcinogenesis." Amsterdam: Elsevier, 1983, p 57.
29. Ryan DE, Iida S, Wood AW, Thomas PE, Lieber CS, Levin W: J Biol Chem 259:1239, 1984.
30. Koop DR, Morgan ET, Tarr GE, Coon MJ: J Biol Chem 256:10704, 1981.
31. Deutsch J, Leutz JC, Yang SK, Gelboin HV, Chiang YL, Vatsis KP, Coon MN: Proc Natl Acad Sci USA 75:3123, 1978.
32. Wiebel FJ, Selkirk JK, Gelboin HV, Haugen DA, Van der Hoeven TA, Coon MJ: Proc Natl Acad Sci USA 72:3917, 1975.
33. Wilson NM, Christou M, Turner CR, Wrighton SA, Jefcoate CR: Carcinogenesis 5:1475, 1984.
34. Hara E, Kawajiri K, Tagashira Y: Cancer Res 43:3604, 1983.
35. Ittah Y, Thakker DR, Levin W, Croisbt-Delcey M, Ryan DE, Thomas PE, Conney AH, Jerina DM: Chem Biol Interact 45:15, 1983.
36. van Bladeren PJ, Armstrong RN, Cobb D, Thakker DR, Ryan DE, Thomas PE, Sharma ND, Boyd DR, Levin W, Jerina DM: Biochem Biophys Res Commun 106:602, 1982.
37. Robertson IGC, Zeiger E, Goldstein JA: Carcinogenesis 4:93, 1983.
38. Norman RL, Muller-Eberhard U, Johnson EF: Biochem Biophys Res Commun 89:195, 1979.
39. McManus ME, Minchin RF, Sanderson N, Wirth PH, Thorgeirsson SS: Cancer Res 43:3720, 1983.
40. McManus ME, Minchin RF, Sanderson N, Schwartz D, Johnson EF, Thorgeirsson SS: Carcinogenesis 5:1717, 1984.
41. Lotlikar PD, Pandey RN, Clearfield MS, Paik SM: TOXLett 21:111, 1984.
42. Goldstein JA, Weaver R, Sundheimer DW: Cancer Res 44:3768, 1984.
43. Kawajiri K, Yonekawa H, Gotoh O, Watanabe J, Igarashi S, Tagashira Y: Cancer Res 43:819, 1983.
44. Masson HA, Ioannides C, Gorrod JW, Gibson GG: Carcinogenesis 4:1583, 1983.
45. Watanabe J, Kawajiri K, Yonekawa H, Nagao M, Tagashira Y: Biochem Biophys Res Commun 104:193, 1982.
46. Essigmann JM, Croy RG, Nadzan AM, Busby WF Jr., Reinhold VN, Buchi G, Wogan GN: Proc Natl Acad Sci USA 74:1870, 1977.
47. Wong ZA, Hsieh DPH: Toxicol Appl Pharmacol 55:115, 1980.
48. Bansal SK, Fung PH, Caballes L, Gurtoo HL: Proc Annu Meet Am Assoc Cancer Res 25:113, 1984.
49. Ueno Y, Ishii K, Omata Y, Kamataki T, Kato R: Carcinogenesis 4:1071, 1983.
50. Yoshizawa H, Uchimaru R, Kamataki T, Kato R, Yeno Y: Cancer Res 42:1120, 1982.
51. Masson HA, Ioannides C, Gibson GG: TOXLett 17:131, 1983.
52. Kokkinakis DM, Koop DR, Scarpelli DG, Coon MJ, Hollenberg PF: Cancer Res 45:619, 1985.
53. Yang CS, Tu YY, Koop DR, Coon MJ: Cancer Res 45:1140, 1985.
54. Vesell ES, Penno MB: Banbury Rep 16:117, 1984.
55. Conney AH, Buening MK, Fortner JG, Jerina DM, Birkett DJ: Excerpta Med Int Congr Ser 484:78, 1980.
56. Darby NJ, Burnet FR, Lodola A: Biochem Biophys Res Commun 119:382, 1984.
57. Wolf CR, Seilman S, Oesch F, Zmelizad Z, Adams DJ: "Sixth International Symposium on Microsomes and Drug Oxidation, Abstract." London: Taylor and Francis, 1984.
58. Song B-J, Fujino T, Park S-S, Friedman FK, Gelboin HV: J Biol Chem 259:1394, 1984.
59. Fujino T, Gottlieb K, Manchester DK, Park SS, West D, Gurtoo HL, Tarone RE, Gelboin HV: Cancer Res 44:3916, 1984.
60. Distlerath LM, Guengerich FP: Proc Natl Acad Sci USA 81:7348, 1984.

61. Seidel SL, Shawver LK, Shires TK: Arch Biochem Biophys 229:519, 1984.
62. Wolf CR, Moll E, Friedberg T, Oesch F, Buchmann A, Kuhlmann WD, Kunz HW: Carcinogenesis 5:993, 1984.
63. Payne M, Beaune P, Kremers P, Guengerich FP, Letawe-Goujon F, Gielen J: Biochem Biophys Res Commun 122:137, 1984.
64. Sogawa K, Gotoh O, Kawajiri K, Fujii-Kuriyama Y: Proc Natl Acad Sci USA 81:5066, 1984.
65. Kawajiri K, Gotoh O, Sogawa K, Tagashira Y, Muramatsu M, Fujii-Kuriyama Y: Proc Natl Acad Sci USA 81:1649, 1984.
66. Kawajiri K, Gotoh O, Tagashira Y, Sogawa K, Fujii-Kuriyama Y: J Biol Chem 259:10145, 1984.
67. Ravishankar H, Padmanaban G: J Biol Chem 260:1588, 1985.
68. Walz FG Jr., Vlasuk GP, Omiecinski CJ, Bresnick E, Thomas PE, Ryan DE, Levin W: J Biol Chem 257:4023, 1982.
69. Tukey RH, Nebert DW: Biochemistry 23:6003, 1984.
70. Leighton JK, Kemper B: J Biol Chem 259:11165, 1984.
71. Hines RN, Foldes RL, Levy JB, Omiecinski C, Ho K-L, Shen M-L, Bresnick E: Banbury Rep 16, 1984.
72. Tukey RH, Negishi M, Nebert DW: Mol Pharmacol 22:779, 1982.
73. Chen Y-T, Negishi M, Nebert DW: DNA 1:231, 1982.
74. Hines RN, Houser WH, Iversen PL, Foldes RL, Heiger W, Conrad RL, Bresnick E: Paper presented at UCLA Symposium on Biochemical and Molecular Epidemiology of Cancer, 1985.
75. Hankinson O, Andersen RD, Birren BW, Sander F, Negishi M, Nebert DW: J Biol Chem 260:1790, 1985.
76. Simmons DL, Kasper CB: J Biol Chem 258:9585, 1983.
77. Brookes P, Lawley PD: Nature 202:781, 1964.
78. Neumann H-G: Recent Results Cancer Res 84:77, 1983.
79. Singer B, Kusmierek JT: Annu Rev Biochem 52:655, 1982.
80. Pegg AE: Cancer Invest 2:223, 1984.
81. D'Andrea AD, Haseltine WA: Proc Natl Acad Sci USA 75:4120, 1978.
82. Sage E, Haseltine WA: J Biol Chem 259:11098, 1984.
83. Jerina DM, Michaud DP, Feldmann RJ, Armstrong RN, Vyas KP, Thakker DR, Yagi H, Thomas PE, Ryan DE, Levin W: In Sato R, Kato R (eds): "Microsomes, Drug Oxidations and Drug Toxicity." Tokyo: Japan Scientific Societies Press, 1982, p 195.
84. Alexandrov K, Ronas M, Bourgeois Y, Chouroulinkov I: Carcinogenesis 4:1655, 1983.
85. Nakayama J, Yuspa SH, Poirier MC: Cancer Res 44:4087, 1984.
86. Brookes P, Osborne MR: Carcinogenesis 3:1223, 1982.
87. Theall G, Weinstein IB, Grunberger D, Neshow S, Hatch G: Banbury Rep 13:231, 1982.
88. Dunn BP: Cancer Res 43:2654, 1983.
89. Shugart L, Holland JM, Rahn RO: Carcinogenesis 4:195, 1983.
90. Eisenstadt E, Warren AJ, Porter J, Atkins D, Miller JH: Proc Natl Acad Sci USA 79:1945, 1982.
91. Marshall CJ, Vousden KH, Phillips DH: Nature 310:586, 1984.
92. Poirier MC, Hunt JM, True B, Laishes BA, Young JF, Beland FA: Carcinogenesis 5:1591, 1984.
93. Beland FA, Djuric Z, Fifer EK, Heflich RH: J Cell Biochem 96:35, 1985.
94. Beland FA, Beranek DT, Dooley KL, Heflich RH, Kadlubar FF: Environ Health Perspect 49:125, 1983.
95. Beranek DT, White GL, Heflich RH, Beland FA: Proc Natl Acad Sci USA 79:5175, 1982.
96. Croy RG, Essigmann JM, Reinhold VN, Wogan GN: Proc Natl Acad Sci USA 75:1745, 1978.
97. Essigmann JM, Croy RG, Nadzan AM, Busby WF Jr., Reinhold VN, Büchi G, Wogan GN: Proc Natl Acad Sci 74:1870, 1977.
98. Croy RG, Wogan GR: JNCI 66:761, 1981.
99. Amstad PA, Wang TV, Cerutti PA: JNCI 70:135, 1983.
100. Foster PL, Eisenstadt E, Miller JH: Proc Natl Acad Sci USA 80:2695, 1983.
101. Donahue PR, Essigmann JM, Wogan GN: Banbury Rep 13:221, 1983.
102. Autrup H, Bradley KA, Shamsuddin AKM, Wakhisi J, Wasunna A: Carcinogenesis 4:1193, 1983.
103. Yang SS, Modali R, Taub JV, Yang GC: J Cell Biochem 96:32, 1985.
104. Goth R, Rajewsky MF: Proc Natl Acad Sci USA 71:639, 1974.
105. Domoradzki J, Pegg AE, Dolan ME, Maher VM, McCormick JJ: Carcinogenesis 5:1641, 1984.
106. Swenberg JA, Dyroff MC, Bedell MA, Popp JA, Huh N, Kirstein U, Rajewsky MF: Proc Natl Acad Sci USA 81:1692, 1984.

107. Loechler EL, Green CL, Essigmann JM: Proc Natl Acad Sci USA 81:6271, 1984.
108. Essigmann JM, Green CL, Loechler EL: J Cell Biochem 96:35, 1985.
109. Chambers RW, Fenwick RG, Cline SW, Tsang SS, Ireland L: J Cell Biochem 96:38, 1985.
110. Kriek E, Den Engelse L, Scherer E, Westra JG: Biochem Biophys Acta 738:181, 1984.
111. Poirier MC: Environ Mutagen 6:879, 1984.
112. Perera FP, Poirier MC, Yuspa SH, Nakyama J, Weinstein IB: Carcinogenesis 3:1405, 1982.
113. Shamsuddin AKM, Sinopoli NT, Hemminki K, Boesch RR, Harris CC: Cancer Res 45:66, 1985.

Biochemical and Molecular Epidemiology of Cancer 373–385 (1986)

Cancer-Prone Diseases and DNA Repair

Malcolm C. Paterson

Health Sciences Division, Chalk River Nuclear Laboratories, Chalk River, Ontario, Canada K0J 1J0

A promising approach to a better understanding of the human carcinogenic process is the investigation of molecular mechanisms governing mankind's genetic susceptibility to cancer. In view of the repertoire of hereditary disorders accompanied by increased risk of developing neoplasia [1], the human genome contains a number of loci, any one of which, in its mutated form, confers marked predisposition to malignancy. Indeed, the study of heritable variations in sensitivity to harmful environmental agents, termed *ecogenetics*, is rapidly emerging as a rewarding experimental tack for clarifying the cause and course of malignant transformation [eg, 2,3].

One of the most active branches of ecogenetic experimentation is the in vitro investigation of cultured cells derived from patients in whom excessive cancer occurrence is associated with an untoward response to a known environmental carcinogen [2–7]. These patients, for the most part, are afflicted with rare, clinically well-defined diseases characterized by a simple Mendelian monogenic mode of inheritance. Cells cultured from these subjects typically display enhanced sensitivity to the lethal action of the relevant environmental agent and, in some cases, anomalies in the ability to process—that is, to repair, bypass, or otherwise circumvent—damage inflicted on DNA by the same agent.

The archetypal disorder for these studies is xeroderma pigmentosum (XP). In this autosomal recessively transmitted affliction, marked propensity to sunlight-induced skin neoplasms and in vitro cellular hypersensitivity to the cytotoxic, mutagenic, and carcinogenic actions of ultraviolet (UV) rays are causally linked to deficiencies in enzymatic processes that repair or bypass UV-induced cyclobutyl pyrimidine dimers in DNA [3,5–7]. Somatic cell fusion analyses have thus far allocated fibroblast strains from some 120 unrelated patients to nine genetically

Malcolm C. Paterson's present address is Molecular Genetics and Carcinogenesis Laboratory, Department of Medicine, Cross Cancer Institute, 11560 University Avenue, Edmonton, Alberta, Canada T6G 1Z2.

Received September 3, 1985.

© **1986 Alan R. Liss, Inc.**

distinct groups on the basis of a biochemical complementation test, indicating extensive genetic heterogeneity in the disease. Over 80% of the strains have been assigned to eight mutually complementing groups, designated A to H. The prominent biochemical anomaly in each of these groups appears to be a malfunction in the ability to execute the nucleotide mode of excision repair active on pyrimidine dimers. The remaining XP strains have been lumped together to form a ninth complementation group, the so-called variant. Strains belonging to this latter group exhibit a marked deficiency in performing postreplication repair (also termed replicative or daughter-strand repair). This is a poorly defined process believed to be instrumental in enabling the de novo DNA synthesis machinery to retain base-sequence fidelity when replicating past dimers and other noncoding alterations in template DNA [for two schools of thought on this highly controversial system, see 7,8].

A second ecogenetic trait under active investigation is ataxia telangiectasia (AT), an ionizing radiation analog of XP in which proneness to lymphoreticular malignancies and hypersensitivity to X or γ rays are associated with suspected defects in the enzymatic processing (ie, repair or bypass) of lesions induced in DNA by free radical attack [3,4,9]. This autosomal recessive disorder appears to exhibit an even higher degree of genetic heterogeneity than XP, in that preliminary cell fusion analyses have identified at least five (and possibly nine) complementation groups in 17 unrelated AT families [3,10].

This workshop, "Cancer-Prone Diseases and DNA Repair," covered a potpourri of recent advances and current controversies in the study of DNA repair processes present in mammalian systems. Particular emphasis was placed on those repair systems occurring in humans as revealed by examining cultured cells from donors with XP, AT, or other cancer-prone diseases. Three major topics were addressed during the workshop by seven invited discussants:

Topic 1. Molecular Cloning of Human and Hamster DNA Repair Genes

A. "Molecular and cellular characterization of a human excision-repair gene." J.H.J. Hoeijmakers, Department of Cell Biology and Genetics, Erasmus University, Rotterdam, The Netherlands.
B. "Transfer of hamster repair gene(s) into excision-deficient XP cells." J.E. Cleaver, Laboratory of Radiobiology, University of California, San Francisco, California.

Topic 2. Some Recent Advances in DNA Repair Studies

A. "Novel model for pyrimidine dimer repair in human cells." M.C. Paterson, Health Sciences Division, Chalk River Nuclear Laboratories, Chalk River, Canada.
B. "Defective posttranslational protein modification in AT cells." U. Kuhnlein, Health Sciences Division, Chalk River Nuclear Laboratories, Chalk River, Canada.
C. "Correlation between O^6-alkylguanine-DNA alkyltransferase activity and resistance to the cytotoxic and mutagenic effects of alkylating agents in human cells." J.J. McCormick, Carcinogenesis Laboratory, Michigan State University, East Lansing, Michigan.
D. "Microheterogeneity in processing DNA damage in mammalian genomes." P.C. Hanawalt, Department of Biological Sciences, Stanford University, Stanford, California.

Topic 3. Some Current Controversies in DNA Repair Studies

A. "Role of poly(ADP-ribose) synthesis in repair: Fact and fiction." J.E. Cleaver, Laboratory of Radiobiology, University of California, San Francisco, California.

B. "Do pyrimidine dimers block replication forks?" H.J. Edenberg, Department of Biochemistry, Indiana University School of Medicine, Indianapolis, Indiana.

The presentations of the discussants, interspersed with comments from the convenor, are now summarized in turn.

MOLECULAR CLONING OF HUMAN AND HAMSTER DNA REPAIR GENES

The critical importance of fully functional DNA repair systems to the well-being of mankind has been evident since the seminal discovery by Cleaver [11] almost two decades ago that cultured fibroblasts from certain XP patients are defective in their ability to excise pyrimidine dimers. In the intervening period little advancement has been made in defining the precise enzymatic reactions mediating the multistep excision-repair process operative on these UV photoproducts. With the advent of molecular cloning technology, numerous laboratories have recently expended considerable effort in an attempt to clone genes responsible for this and other DNA repair systems. This experimental approach is expected to permit the isolation and characterization of the relevant genes and their products, thereby facilitating elucidation of the innermost workings of these repair processes.

Two of the leaders in this research area, namely, Jan Hoeijmakers, a member of the group led by Dirk Bootsma, and James Cleaver, reported their progress to date.

Molecular and Cellular Characterization of a Human Excision-Repair Gene

The studies of the Dutch group have been directed toward the identification of genes and proteins promoting dimer repair in human cells with the goal of providing an explanation for the primary defect in XP [12,13].

Hoeijmakers reported that, with the aid of a standard microneedle injection technique, he and his colleagues have detected factors in crude human cell extracts that temporarily compensate for the anomaly in fibroblast strains belonging to various excision-defective XP complementation groups (as judged by transient [<8 hr] restoration of UV-induced unscheduled DNA synthesis [UDS]). This correction of the repair defect was observed when extracts from complementary (but not homologous) XP cells were injected; hence, each complementation group is deficient in a specific factor.

In the two XP groups (A and G) examined further, the correction factors were inactivated by treatment with proteinase K, signifying that both activities are comprised, at least in part, of proteins. The XP group A correcting activity precipitated at between 30 and 60% ammonium sulfate saturation. The Dutch found that the same activity binds efficiently to DEAE cellulose and to UV-irradiated double-strand DNA attached to cellulose. The latter binding property greatly facilitated purification of the activity, as less than 1% of the total protein fraction in crude cellular extracts was retained by this affinity chromatographic method.

In an effort to clone genes complementary to those in different excision-defective XP strains, Hoeijmakers and coworkers have transfected simian virus 40

(SV40)-transformed XP A and F cell lines with genomic DNA that was 1) isolated from repair-proficient (HeLa) cells, 2) partially cleaved to an average size of 50 to 60 kilobase pairs (kbp), and 3) ligated to a molar excess of a dominant marker gene (*Escherichia coli gpt*) in a linearized plasmid. Although the dominant marker was transfected at high frequencies (one transformant per 10^3–10^4 cells), the Dutch were unable to obtain transformants that were repair proficient by coinsertion of a complementary gene. In contrast, substitution of the XP lines with a Chinese hamster ovary (CHO) repair-deficient line (43-3B; complementation group 2 of Thompson et al [14]) resulted in a high yield of repair-proficient transformants, thus permitting the cloning of the human gene complementary to those present in the repair-deficient CHO line. It is noteworthy that only a small amount of exogenous DNA was integrated in the genome of the XP cells compared to the CHO cells, thereby explaining, at least in part, the inability of the former cells to serve as recipients for repair genes in the transfection experiments.

As alluded to above, the Dutch group has recently cloned a human gene, designated *ERCC-1*, which overcomes the repair defect in 43-3B [13], a line displaying cross-hypersensitivity to the cytotoxic effects of UV radiation and mitomycin C (MMC) (measured by loss of colony-forming ability [CFA]) [15]. After transfection of *ERCC-1*, the repair capacity of 43-3B cells was restored to normal, as judged by three endpoints: dimer removal, UV-induced UDS, and post-UV or post-MMC CFA. Molecular characterization of the gene disclosed a DNA segment of ~15 kbp containing at least nine exons, which code for an mRNA transcript of 1.1 kb. *ERCC-1* has been found to be expressed constitutively in a variety of human cell types, suggesting that the gene performs a vital "housekeeping" function. Sequence analysis of an *ERCC-1* cDNA clone revealed an open frame for a protein of 273 amino acids. Southern blot analysis of a panel of human/rodent cell hybrids has permitted assignment of the gene to human chromosome 19. Other studies have demonstrated that *ERCC-1* is not deleted or grossly rearranged in strains belonging to XP groups A, C, F, and G, and that the gene is not able to enhance repair capability after transfection of virus-transformed XP A and F cell lines.

Bootsma's laboratory is presently investigating the function of the *ERCC-1* gene in repair and its effect when transfected in strains representing other XP complementation groups, as well as other human repair deficiency syndromes, especially Fanconi anemia.

Transfer of Hamster Repair Gene(s) Into Excision-Deficient XP Cells

Like Hoeijmakers, Cleaver reported that he has been unsuccessful in his attempts to clone repair genes in XP cells using a standard genomic DNA transfection technique. This failure led Cleaver and Karentz to adopt an alternative experimental approach that was designed to facilitate the integration of whole chromosomal fragments from repair-proficient CHO cells into the genome of XP cells. The objective of this approach was to clone into the defective XP cells rodent DNA sequences that promote the repair of UV-damaged DNA. To this end, cultures of XP group A cells and X ray-inactivated CHO cells were fused with polyethylene glycol, and the cultures were then exposed periodically to low-dose UV rays to select for UV-resistant hybrid colonies.

Several secondary and tertiary hybrids containing successively smaller quantities of rodent DNA have been selected for further investigation. DNA-DNA hybridization analyses, employing both whole genomic DNA and specific repetitive *"Alu"*-like sequences of hamster origin, indicated that the hybrids possess varying proportions of rodent DNA integrated into the hybrid genomes and are not the XP revertants. Moreover, no UV-resistant colonies were recovered from control cultures (eg, X-irradiated XP cells or unirradiated XP/irradiated XP fusions) subjected to the same UV selection procedure.

Efforts are currently underway in Cleaver's laboratory to clone, from the hybrid genomes of these XP/CHO lines, hamster DNA sequences responsible for the expression of excision-repair enzymes or other factors conferring resistance to the deleterious effects of UV radiation.

SOME RECENT ADVANCES IN DNA REPAIR STUDIES
A. Novel Model for Pyrimidine Dimer Repair in Human Cells

As noted in the Introduction, elucidation of the primary biochemical defect(s) in the different genetic forms of XP remains an elusive goal. As a case in point, notwithstanding the multiplicity of complementation groups, all excision repair-deficient XP strains seem to be blocked at the same stage (initial incision step) in the nucleotide repair mode acting on dimers. (Note that the current working models for this multistep excision-repair pathway have been derived primarily from the more extensive and sophisticated investigations possible in simple prokaryotic systems; for details, see Haseltine [16] and Sancar and Rupp [17]). In his presentation, Paterson described a series of experiments that promise not only to provide new insight into the basic enzymatic deficiency in some of these XP groups but also may lead to a better understanding of early reactions in dimer repair in normal cells.

The studies of Paterson and his colleagues were initiated in an effort to reconcile the longstanding inconsistency in the excision-repair properties of XP group D strains. The strains, although known to be severely, if not entirely, defective in recognizing dimer-containing sites (detected as UV-induced sites sensitive to the strand-incising activity of *Micrococcus luteus* UV endonuclease), nevertheless seemingly perform an appreciable amount of UV-stimulated UDS [3]. To account for these peculiar repair properties, it was reasoned that, following UV exposure, group D cells may act aberrantly on a fraction of the dimer-containing sites, inserting "repair" patches while failing to excise the photoproducts themselves. To test whether a portion of the dimer-containing sites are modified but not removed in XP D strains, the Chalk River group measured the photoreactivability (a well-established diagnostic probe of dimer authenticity) of such sites in DNA from normal and group D cells as a function of cell incubation time after UV exposure. Following post-UV (254 nm) incubation, the cultures were lysed; their isolated DNA was subjected to exhaustive enzymatic photoreactivation (PR; *Streptomyces griseus* photolyase plus visible light) to monomerize dimers, and was then analyzed for residual dimer-containing sites with an *M luteus* extract containing UV endonuclease activity. This protocol revealed the appearance of single-strand breaks in the DNA from UV-treated and incubated XP fibroblasts that were not seen in similarly treated normal fibroblasts [3,4]. The incidence of these peculiar sites, which were detected as strand nicks, peaked after 48 hr of post-UV incubation in the XP D strains; the maximal yield equalled 15% of the dimers initially introduced and corresponded to the residual capacity (15–20% of normal) of the same strains to perform UV-stimulated DNA repair replication. A similar accumulation of such novel sites was observed in XP group A cells, whereas groups C, E, or variant cells behaved like normal controls. The same incidence of sites was observed in XP A and D strains when the extracted DNA from post-UV-incubated cultures was subjected to photoenzymatic treatment alone, that is, without subsequent UV endonuclease treatment. This surprising observation led Paterson and coworkers to propose that during incubation of UV-treated strains from groups A and D the phosphodiester bond between the two dimer-forming pyrimidines may be ruptured and that at such altered sites individual DNA chains are then held together solely by the cyclobutane bridge joining the two pyrimidine bases. The excision-repair system presumably aborts at this stage in group A cells, since these cells carry out negligible repair synthesis; in contrast, the intradimer backbone cleavage in group D cells seems to be accompanied by the subsequent, presumably proximal, abortive insertion of a normal size patch.

These XP data raised the possibility that this heretofore undetected reaction may also take place in normal cells. To test this proposal, the Chalk River group photo-chemically reversed the dimer-containing excision fragments isolated from post-UV-incubated normal cells and thereby were able to observe the release of free thymidine and thymidine monophosphate, implying that the excised oligonucleotides do indeed contain a dimer, with an internal phosphodiester break, at one end.

Based on the above findings, Paterson put forward a new model for the repair of pyrimidine dimers in human cells. In this scheme, which is unlike that found in any other biological system studied to date, hydrolysis of the internal phosphodiester bond of dimerized pyrimidines constitutes the first step in the nucleotide excision-repair process that operates on these UV photoproducts. This reaction may then be followed by classical strand incision/lesion excision/repair synthesis/strand ligation reactions. Paterson speculated that the function of the putative pyrimidine dimer-DNA phosphodiesterase may be to produce a localized structural change at the dimer-containing site such that the site is then recognizable by a generalized "bulky lesion-repair complex" that possibly resembles the UVRABC excinuclease complex that acts in E coli on an array of chemically disparate defects in DNA [17]. It was further hypothesized that scission of the phosphodiester bond between dimerized pyrimidines may also serve to reduce regional conformational stress caused by the intradimer cyclobutane bridge, thus reinstating hydrogen bonding to adjoining base pairs and, in so doing, presumably promoting the fidelity of de novo DNA synthesis on a UV-damaged template. Research into these and other ramifications of the new model are in progress.

Defective Posttranslational Protein Modification in AT Cells

Kuhnlein described his provocative observations on DNA binding proteins associated with human DNA repair processes. His most recent work has focused on the major apurinic/apyrimidinic (AP) DNA binding protein present in cultured cells and placenta. Kuhnlein has purified the protein to near homogeneity from HeLa cells. This AP DNA binding activity and the major AP endonuclease activity presumably reside in the same protein since the two activities copurified through a series of chromatographic steps and the molecular weight of the binding protein (37.6 kilodal-tons [kd]) was similar to those reported previously for the AP endonuclease isolated from HeLa cells and placenta (MW = 41.0 and 37.0 kd, respectively). AP DNA binding, as measured in a glass filter binding assay, was inactivated by treatment of the protein with snake venom phosphodiesterase without loss of AP endonuclease activity, indicating that DNA binding is not necessarily a prerequisite for endonucleolytic cleavage. The phosphodiesterase treatment resulted in the formation of a new protein with a molecular weight reduced by 2.3 kd, which may represent the unmodified precursor protein. AP DNA binding also proved to be sensitive to dextranase; this activity might thus be mediated by a polysaccharide containing α-glucopyranose linkages in addition to phosphodiester bonds.

In follow-up experiments, Kuhnlein compared the properties of the AP endonuclease purified from the HeLa line with those of the same enzyme isolated from an SV40-transformed AT line designated AT5BIVA [for details, see 18]. Relative to its HeLa counterpart, the protein from the AT line had 1) a significantly higher molecular weight (AT, 38.9 kd; HeLa, 37.6 kd), 2) a three- to fourfold reduction in affinity for AP sites (dissociation equilibrium constant: HeLa, 7.8×10^{-11} M; AT, 28.3×10^{-11} M), and 3) a five- to tenfold enhancement in sensitivity to inactivation by phosphodiesterase. The latter two differences were also observed with the AP DNA binding protein from the nontransformed parental AT strain AT5BI, signifying that an altered AP endonuclease is characteristic of the AT genotype rather than SV40 transformation.

The AP endonuclease is not the only protein involved in DNA metabolism whose DNA binding activity is apparently dependent on a secondary phosphodiesterase-sensitive protein modification. In earlier studies [19,20], Kuhnlein and associates demonstrated that two others, namely, a protein that preferentially binds to DNA damaged by UV radiation, N-acetoxy-N-acetylaminofluorene (N-acetoxy-AAF) or cis-diamminedichloroplatinum(II), and a single-strand DNA binding protein whose activity is reduced or absent in XP group A strains, are also subject to inactivation by phosphodiesterase treatment.

These observations prompted Kuhnlein to hypothesize that the DNA interaction of a whole class of damage-recognizing proteins may be regulated by a similar type of posttranslational modification. As Kuhnlein further surmised, the findings raise the intriguing possibility that the primary defects in AT and XP (and perhaps other syndromes associated with faulty DNA metabolism) may reside in the process mediating this secondary modification rather than in the structural genes of particular DNA metabolizing enzymes. In short, protein modification processes are expected to reflect the interplay of many different enzymes and cellular metabolites, and defects in such processes may well explain the diversity of clinical abnormalities found in these Mendelian single-gene traits.

Correlation Between O^6-Alkylguanine-DNA Alkyltransferase Activity and Resistance to the Cytotoxic and Mutagenic Effects of Alkylating Agents in Human Cells

N-nitroso compounds, such as N-methyl-N'-nitro-N-nitrosoguanidine (MNNG) and ethylnitrosourea (ENU), form an array of reaction products in the DNA of living cells, including the addition of alkyl groups to the extranuclear O^6 atom of guanine. The repair of these O^6-alkylguanine (O^6-AlkGua) residues is accomplished in human cells, as in *E coli*, by the direct transfer of the offending alkyl group to a cysteine residue in the repair protein, termed *O^6-alkylguanine-DNA alkyltransferase* or *O^6-methylguanine-DNA methyltransferase* (MT) [21]. The reaction is unconventional among known DNA repair processes in that it is stoichiometric and suicidal rather than catalytic and regenerating. That is, the activity of each MT molecule is consumed upon S-alkylation of its acceptor cysteine residue. The study of the metabolic fate of O^6-AlkGua residues, as governed by MT activity, has received considerable attention in recent years because these lesions in particular have been strongly implicated in the mutagenic and carcinogenic potency of N-nitroso compounds [22].

McCormick described studies from his laboratory that further incriminate O^6-AlkGua residues as highly toxic defects in cellular DNA. Fibroblast strains from patients with familial polyposis coli (GM2355) and Gardner syndrome (2938, GM3314, and GM3948), two autosomal dominant disorders predisposing to colon cancer, were compared to those from clinically normal subjects for their response to the cytotoxic and mutagenic effects of MNNG and ENU. Using standard assays [23], cytotoxicity was assessed by loss of colony-forming ability while conversion to 6-thioguanine resistance served as a measure of mutagenicity. Three of the four strains from affected patients, namely 2398, GM2355, and GM3948, displayed a normal response to the cytotoxic and mutagenic actions of MNNG and ENU. In contrast, cells of the fourth strain (GM3314), as well as those from an evidently clinically normal fetus (GM0011), were inactivated and mutated at elevated rates by both agents.

To investigate a plausible biochemical basis of the increased sensitivity to MNNG and ENU observed in strains GM0011 and GM3314, McCormick and his collaborators measured constitutive levels of MT in sonicates of cultures of the various strains under study, adopting the assay procedure of and in collaboration with A. Pegg et al of Hershey Medical Center (Hershey, PA) [21]. The three strains exhibiting normal cytotoxic and mutagenic responses to both agents were shown to have normal MT activities, whereas the two hypersensitive strains contained nondetectable amounts of the O^6-alkyl-acceptor protein.

In an extension of this work, cultures of 1) an XP group A strain (XP12BE), 2) a second XP A strain transformed by SV40 virus (XP12ROSV), and 3) a normal strain transformed by the same virus (GM637) were compared with nontransformed normal controls for their lethal and mutagenic responses to the two N-nitroso agents and for their level of MT. The activity of the O^6-alkyl-acceptor protein proved to be normal in XP12BE cells, reduced in GM637 cells, and nondetectable in XP12RO. Similarly, when treated with MNNG for survival and mutation analyses, the XP12BE strain behaved like nontransformed normal controls, GM637 displayed an intermediate degree of sensitivity, and XP12ROSV was hypersensitive. (Note that the enhanced sensitivity to MNNG-induced cell inactivation and reduction in MT activity are two hallmarks of the Mer⁻ (*methyl repair* minus) phenotype, which is displayed by many human tumor and virus-transformed cell lines [24].) In contrast to the MNNG results, GM637 cells exhibited an intermediate response to ENU, whereas both XP12BE and XP12ROSV were sensitive.

On the basis of these combined data, McCormick postulated that O^6-alkylguanine and/or any other reaction product repaired by MT is a potentially lethal and mutagenic lesion and that nucleotide excision repair, which is malfunctional in XP cells, contributes to the repair of potentially lethal and mutagenic damage introduced by ENU.

In the ensuing discussion period, Michael Middlestadt (Chalk River) reported that he and M. Paterson had independently obtained data on a number of nontransformed human fibroblast strains that were in substantial agreement with those presented by McCormick. Simply put, their results suggested that faulty repair of O^6-

AlkGua lesions may be largely, if not completely, responsible for the hypersensitivity of these strains to either MNNG or N-methyl-N-nitrosourea (MNU). The strain GM0011, which they had previously reported to exhibit an in vitro age-dependent increase in MNU-induced killing [4], correspondingly demonstrated an in vitro age-dependent decrease in constitutive MT levels. Moreover, the relative MT deficiency also paralleled the relative degree of MNU-induced hypercytotoxicity in strains derived from the following subjects, all of whom are either afflicted with, or predisposed to, neoplasia: 1) members of a GS family in which MNNG hypercytotoxicity in vitro has been reported previously [25]; 2) a patient with Hodgkin's disease who developed multiple primary neoplasms subsequent to receiving conventional chemotherapy; 3) a patient suffering from acquired immune deficiency syndrome; and 4) a patient diagnosed with pelvic Ewing's sarcoma. Only those strains with severely depressed MT levels ($<10\%$ normal), that is, GS family proband, GM3314, and late passage GM0011, showed a moderate enhancement (approximately twofold) in sensitivity to the lethal effects of ENU and methyl methanesulfonate (MMS).

Microheterogeneity in Processing DNA Damage in Mammalian Genomes

Hanawalt reviewed three examples of intragenomic heterogeneity in the repair of mammalian DNA that have been discovered in his laboratory. He began with the reminder that biological endpoints, such as survival, do not necessarily correlate with measured levels of excision repair. For example, cultured·rodent cells typically exhibit relatively low levels of excision repair after UV irradiation but such cells survive as well as similarly irradiated repair-proficient human cells. However, XP group C cells do not survive UV irradiation as well as the rodent cells, even though they display overall levels of repair similar to that exhibited by rodent cells. Thus, two questions were posed by Hanawalt: 1) What is the abnormality in excision repair in XP C cells? 2) How do rodent cells manage to tolerate the persistence of 80% of the UV-induced pyrimidine dimers in their genomes?

The possibility that cells might be selective in the processing of particular functional and/or structural domains in their genetic material was raised, and it was pointed out that most of the methods currently used to study DNA repair are not intrinsically sensitive to intragenomic heterogeneity in distribution of repair sites or persisting damage. A method was developed by Mansbridge and Hanawalt [26] to test the proposal that the low level of repair occurring in XP C cells is confined to restricted domains of the genome. The hypothesis proved to be valid for the three different group C strains examined even when the possibility of cell population heterogeneity as an explanation was excluded by UDS analysis. These findings have now been confirmed and extended by Mullenders et al [27], who have provided evidence that the repair in XP C chromatin occurs in association with the nuclear matrix (actively transcribed genes?). The results have also been confirmed independently by Cleaver (reported during the workshop); in addition, Cleaver showed that repair heterogeneity is not characteristic of XP D cells. In summary, the primary defect in XP C cells would appear to reside in the ill-defined process that affords the excision-repair machinery accessibility to many domains in the genome rather than in the basic enzyme complex that incises accessible DNA at sites containing pyrimidine dimers and other bulky lesions.

The second example discussed by Hanawalt was that of the highly repetitive α DNA species found in all primates in heterochromatic (nontranscribed) chromatin near centromeres. In African green monkey kidney cells, the α DNA is in tandem arrays of about 450 units of 172 bp [H. Madhani and S.A. Leadon, unpublished observations], which can be readily isolated for repair studies [28]. It was demonstrated that in confluent cultures, α DNA is as proficiently repaired as bulk DNA for certain lesions (eg, pyrimidine dimers, thymine glycols, and damage induced by X rays, MMS, and dimethylsulfate) but not for others (eg, bulky chemical adducts induced by aflatoxin B_1 (AFB_1), angelicin, 8-methoxypsoralen, and N-acetoxy-AAF). Evidence was obtained for a different DNA structure and/or chromatin packing configuration in the α DNA compared to that in the bulk DNA [29,30]. Finally, it was shown that UV irradiation, before or after the introduction of AFB_1 adducts, causes repair in α DNA to be enhanced to the normal level [31]. Thus, the disruption produced by the presence of pyrimidine dimers in α chromatin evidently permits excision repair of these and other bulky lesions.

The third example given by Hanawalt was the recent discovery that repair of pyrimidine dimers in the active dihydrofolate reductase (DHFR) gene in CHO cells is much more efficient than in the overall genome [32]. In these studies the presence of pyrimidine dimers in defined restriction fragments within and upstream from the transcribed DHFR gene was detected by Southern analysis after treatment of the DNA with T4 endonuclease V, which incises DNA at dimer-containing sites. While two thirds of the dimers were removed from a fragment within the gene after 24 hr of post-UV (20 Jm^{-2}) incubation, less than 10% of the dimers were removed from a fragment 30 kbp upstream from the gene. Only 15% of the dimers were removed from the overall genome in these irradiated cells in the same 24 hr period. These results suggest that damage processing can vary according to the activity of the affected genomic sequences. The preferential repair of vital sequences (eg, "housekeeping" genes such as DHFR) may account for the UV resistance of CHO cells in spite of their low overall repair capacity. Hanawalt pointed out that these findings may have important implications for the use of rodent cells in risk assessment. It would be of interest to know how this phenomenon of differential repair in the CHO genome affects the probability of activation of a proto-oncogene at different sites that may be repaired more or less efficiently.

The overall conclusion from the interesting findings presented by Hanawalt is that the repair of damage in mammalian chromatin depends on the type and location of the lesions in the genome and on the functional state of the DNA at damaged sites. Clearly, it may be necessary to understand the "fine structure" of DNA repair in the mammalian genome to interpret the effects of DNA damage on particular biological endpoints, such as survival, mutagenesis, and carcinogenesis.

SOME CURRENT CONTROVERSIES IN DNA REPAIR STUDIES

Investigators of DNA repair, as in any other active field concerned with the innermost workings of a mammalian cell, are in the throes of attempting to resolve a number of controversial subjects. The latest views on two of the more contentious areas currently plaguing mammalian DNA repair studies, namely, the role of poly(ADP-ribosyl)ation in DNA repair and the mechanism of postreplication repair, were presented by a leading participant in each dispute.

Role of Poly(ADP-Ribose) Synthesis in Repair: Fact and Fiction

Recent years have seen the emergence of an attractive model in which poly(ADP-ribose) polymerization of chromatin is relegated a regulatory role in DNA repair (for details regarding the model and other information relevant to this section, see the discussion of Cleaver et al [33]). According to the model, poly(ADP-ribose) polymerase, a chromatin-bound enzyme that catalyzes the successive transfer of ADP-ribose units from NAD to nuclear proteins, is activated by strand breaks in DNA. Poly(ADP-ribosyl)ation serves to unwind the tightly packed nucleosomes and thus might render DNA damage-containing sites more accessible to repair or might regulate the activity of certain DNA repair enzymes. In particular, it is proposed that the activity of DNA ligase II is enhanced by poly(ADP-ribosyl)ation. Synthesis and degradation of poly(ADP-ribose) attached to ligase II might thereby modulate a dynamic balance between incision and ligation events.

After describing the model, Cleaver reviewed the large body of data often cited in support of it. He drew attention to the fact that the evidence derives almost exclusively from the use of benzamide analogs, particularly 3-aminobenzamide (3AB), as selective inhibitors of poly(ADP-ribose) polymerase. These chemicals potentiate the toxic effects of alkylating agents, increase DNA fragmentation in cells treated with alkylating agents or X rays, and enhance the level of repair synthesis without affecting the excision of alkylated bases. At first glance, then, the data are both consistent and complementary and the following scenario is attractive. Poly(ADP-ribose) synthesis specifically stimulates the activity of DNA ligase II. Consequently, inhibition of poly(ADP-ribose) polymerase and in turn the ligation step (by 3AB) causes strand breaks to persist that would permit nick translation at repair sites and thus increase repair synthesis.

However, Cleaver hastened to point out that upon closer examination, the evidence favoring the scenario given above is fraught with serious shortcomings and disturbing contradictions. First, the model proposes stimulation of ligase II by poly(ADP-ribosyl)ation, yet in other studies on purified proteins, such as topoisomerase I and retinal transductin, attachment of the polymer results in loss of activity. Second, the increased DNA fragmentation induced by 3AB is accompanied by increased repair synthesis in only a limited number of cell types, implying that these two effects are not necessarily related. Third, the responses of cells to 3AB appear much more pronounced when treated with alkylating agents than with other types of DNA-damaging agents. Fourth, Cleaver presented data from his own laboratory demonstrating that the enhanced repair synthesis commonly observed when human cells containing alkylation damage are incubated in the presence of 3AB is not associated with either the number or length of repair patches. And last but not least, he obtained paradoxical results when MMS-damaged human fibroblasts were incubated with a range of 3AB concentrations. At doses up to 1 μM, the chemical appeared to reduce the incidence of strand breaks, whereas at doses between 2–10 μM, strand breakage levels actually increased. At these excessive concentrations, 3AB is known to inhibit de novo synthesis of purines and in all probability induces other toxic side effects. It was further proposed that the well-documented increase in repair synthesis may simply reflect activation of nonspecific endonucleases.

In conclusion, Cleaver seriously questioned the validity of the current model involving poly(ADP-ribose) synthesis in DNA repair and, as has been most recently advocated by others, in gene expression during neoplastic transformation and differentiation.

Do Pyrimidine Dimers Block Replication Forks?

The mechanism(s) by which mammalian cells undergo de novo DNA synthesis on damaged template is steeped in controversy. Two models, delineating the most extreme views, are as follows: 1) upon encountering a lesion, such as a dimer, the replication apparatus skips past and reinitiates downstream, thus leaving a gap that is subsequently closed by de novo synthesis perhaps accompanied by reciprocal strand exchange of a short region opposite the noncoding lesion-containing site [8]; and 2) the replication machinery terminates prematurely upon reaching a lesion and then those abnormal termini (plus the normal ones) are in some manner joined in the formation of complete daughter strands [7].

Using SV40 DNA replicating episomally in cultured monkey cells as a model system, Edenberg described an intriguing line of experimentation designed to answer one of the key questions in resolving the validity of the two models: Does the presence of a pyrimidine dimer in the template strand block the movement of a replication fork or does the fork continue to advance (unwind), jumping past the dimer and thus leaving a gap in its wake? The experimental strategy adopted to address this question was to examine individual SV40 replicating intermediates by electron microscopy after cleavage of the origin of replication with a restriction enzyme. Since the SV40 genome replicates bidirectionally from a fixed origin, with the two forks advancing at approximately equal rates, the forks are normally equidistant from the origin, yielding symmetrical "H-shaped" molecules upon cleavage. Accordingly, if forks are not blocked by dimers, the molecules from post-UV-incubated cells should be symmetrical (although the molecules may contain single-strand regions behind each fork). On the other hand, if forks are blocked or delayed, asymmetrical H-shaped molecules should be observed, since in any one molecule the dimers are random and therefore likely to be found at different distances from the origin.

The results, although preliminary, indicate that while undamaged cells contain a preponderance of symmetrical H-shaped molecules (as predicted), asymmetrical forms are dominant in UV-damaged cells. These observations, in combination with earlier work on the same system [34], prompted Edenberg to advance a semidiscontinuous model for replication of DNA on damaged template. Namely, dimers in the template for the continuously synthesized strand block fork progression, whereas dimers in the template for the discontinuously synthesized strand merely block individual chains, ie, Okazaki fragments, and would therefore be expected to leave small gaps.

CONCLUSIONS

Although our insight into mammalian DNA damage and its metabolic processing lags well behind that in simpler prokaryotic organisms, the studies presented in this workshop raise expectations that significant advances along several experimental fronts may well be forthcoming in the near future. The progress in cloning putative human DNA repair genes reported here is particularly encouraging, as are the novel molecular and enzymological observations on the possible underlying defect(s) in the nucleotide mode of excision repair in XP cells.

ACKNOWLEDGMENTS

Research from the author's laboratory was financed in part by U.S. NCI contract NO1-CP-21029(Basic) with the Clinical and Environmental Epidemiology Branches, NCI, Bethesda, Maryland.

The author is grateful to the discussants for their helpful commentary on the manuscript and to V. Bjerkelund and K. Brown for excellent secretarial assistance.

REFERENCES

1. Mulvihill JJ: In Mulvihill JJ, Miller RW, Fraumeni JF Jr. (eds): "Genetics of Human Cancer." New York: Raven Press, 1977, pp 137–143.
2. Mulvihill JJ: Ann Intern Med 92:809, 1980.
3. Paterson MC, Gentner NE, Middlestadt MV, Weinfeld M: J Cell Physiol Suppl 3:45, 1984.
4. Paterson MC, Gentner NE, Middlestadt MV, Mirzayans R, Weinfeld M: In Castellani A (ed): "Epidemiology and Quantitation of Environmental Risk in Humans from Radiation and Other Agents." New York: Plenum Press, 1985, pp 235–267.
5. Kraemer KH: In Fitzpatrick TB, Eisen AZ, Wolff K, Freedberg IM, Austen KF (eds): "Update: Dermatology in General Medicine." New York: McGraw-Hill, 1983, pp 113–142.
6. Lehmann AR, Karran P: Int Rev Cytol 72:101, 1981.
7. Cleaver JE: J Environ Pathol Toxicol 3:53, 1980.
8. Lehmann AR: In Hanawalt PC, Friedberg EC, Fox CF (eds): "DNA Repair Mechanisms." New York: Academic Press, 1978, pp 517–518.
9. Hanawalt P, Painter R: In Gatti RA, Swift M (eds): "Ataxia-Telangiectasia: Genetics, Neuropathology, and Immunology of a Degenerative Disease of Childhood." New York: Alan R. Liss, Inc., 1985, pp 67–71.
10. Jaspers NGJ, Painter RB, Paterson MC, Kidson C, Inoue T: In Gatti RA, Swift M (eds): "Ataxia-Telangiectasia: Genetics, Neuropathology, and Immunology of a Degenerative Disease of Childhood." New York: Alan R. Liss, Inc., 1985, pp 147–162.
11. Cleaver JE: Nature 218:652, 1968.
12. de Jonge AJR, Vermeulen W, Klein B, Hoeijmakers JHJ: EMBO J 2:637, 1983.
13. Westerveld A, Hoeijmakers JHJ, van Duin M, de Wit J, Odijk H, Pastink A, Wood RD, Bootsma D: Nature 310:425, 1984.
14. Thompson LH, Busch DB, Brookman K, Mooney CL, Glaser DA: Proc Natl Acad Sci USA 78:3734, 1981.
15. Wood RD, Burki HJ: Mutat Res 95:505, 1982.
16. Haseltine WA: Cell 33:13, 1983.
17. Sancar A, Rupp WD: Cell 33:249, 1983.
18. Kuhnlein U: J Biol Chem (in press).
19. Tsang SS, Kuhnlein U: Biochim Biophys Acta 697:202, 1982.
20. Kuhnlein U, Tsang SS, Lokken O, Tong S, Twa D: Biosci Rep 3:667, 1983.
21. Pegg AE, Roberfroid M, von Bahr C, Foote RS, Mitra S, Bresil H, Likhachev A, Montesano R: Proc Natl Acad Sci USA 79:5162, 1982.
22. Lindahl T: Annu Rev Biochem 51:61, 1982.
23. Howell JN, Greene MH, Corner RC, Maher VM, McCormick JJ: Proc Natl Acad Sci USA 81:1179, 1984.
24. Yarosh DB, Foote RS, Mitra S, Day RS III: Carcinogenesis 4:199, 1983.
25. Paterson MC, Smith BP, Krush AJ, McKeen EA: Radiat Res 87:483, 1981.
26. Mansbridge JN, Hanawalt PC: In Friedberg EC, Bridges BR (eds): "Cellular Responses to DNA Damage." New York: Alan R. Liss, Inc., 1983, pp 197–207.
27. Mullenders LHF, van Kesteren AC, Bussmann CJM, van Zeeland AA, Natarajan AT: Mutat Res 141:75, 1984.
28. Zolan ME, Cortopassi GA, Smith CA, Hanawalt PC: Cell 28:613, 1982.
29. Zolan ME, Smith CA, Hanawalt PC: Biochemistry 23:63, 1984.
30. Leadon SA, Zolan ME, Hanawalt PC: Nucleic Acids Res 11:5675, 1983.
31. Leadon SA, Hanawalt PC: Carcinogenesis 5:1505, 1984.
32. Bohr VA, Smith CA, Mellon I, Okumoto D, Hanawalt PC: Cell 40:359, 1985.
33. Cleaver JE, Milam KM, Morgan WF: Radiat Res 101:16, 1985.
34. Edenberg HJ: Virology 128:298, 1984.

Biochemical and Molecular Epidemiology of Cancer 387–390 (1986)

Identification of Genes and Proteins Involved in Excision Repair of Human Cells

Jan H.J. Hoeijmakers, Andries Westerveld, Marcel van Duin,
Wim Vermeulen, Hannie Odijk, Jan de Wit, and Dirk Bootsma

Department of Cell Biology and Genetics, Erasmus Univerity, 3000 DR Rotterdam, The Netherlands

The autosomal, recessive disorder xeroderma pigmentosum (XP) is characterized by extreme sensitivity of the skin to sun exposure and predisposition to skin cancer [1,2]. The basic defect in most XP patients is thought to reside in an inefficient removal of UV-induced lesions in the DNA by excision repair [3]. The biochemical complexity of this process is amply illustrated by the fact that so far nine complementation groups within this syndrome have been identified [4,5]. Despite extensive research, none of the genes or proteins involved have been isolated.

Using a microinjection assay system we have identified components in crude cell extracts that transiently correct the defect in (injected) fibroblasts of all excision-deficient XP complementation groups, as indicated by temporary restoration of UV-induced unscheduled DNA synthesis (UDS; see Fig. 1) [6,7]. This correction is complementation group specific, since it is only found when extracts from complementing XP cells are injected [6,7].

After incubation of extracts with proteinase K the XP-A and XP-G correcting activities were lost, indicating that the complementation is due to proteins. The XP-A correcting protein was found to precipitate between 30 and 60% ammonium sulfate saturation (Table I). Furthermore this protein binds to DEAE-cellulose and to (UV-irradiated) double-strand (ds) DNA attached to cellulose. The latter affinity chromatography step allows a considerable purification, since less than 1% of the proteins applied to such columns is retained (Table II). It has to be established whether the XP-A correcting protein binds by itself or via other proteins to the UV-irradiated DNA and whether it also binds to nonirradiated (ds or ss) DNA. Similar experiments with the XP-G correcting protein are in progress.

As a direct approach toward molecular cloning of the XP correcting genes, we have performed transfection experiments of SV40 transformed XP-A (XP12ROSV40,

Received June 25, 1985.

© **1986 Alan R. Liss, Inc.**

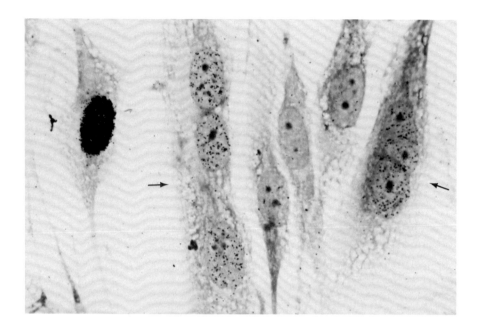

Fig. 1.   Micrograph of two XP25RO (XP-A) homopolykaryons (arrows) after microinjection of a Hela extract, followed by UV irradiation and assay for UDS. The monokaryons (one of which is in S phase) are not injected. The presence of silver grains above non-S phase nuclei indicates UV-induced UDS.

TABLE I. Purification of XP-A Correcting Protein by (NH₄)₂SO₄ Precipitation

	UDS (grains/nucleus)[a]
Hela extract	39 (±3)
Hela extract: Precipitate 30% saturation[b]	14 (±2)
Hela extract: Precipitate 30–60% saturation[b]	69 (±4)
Hela extract: Precipitate 60–90% saturation[b]	7 (±1)
Noninjected cells	4 (±1)

[a]SEM are given in parentheses.
[b]Precipitate dissolved in 40% of the original volume.

TABLE II. Purification of XP-A Correcting Protein by UV-DNA-Cellulose Affinity Chromatography

	Protein concentration (mg/ml)	% of input	UDS (grains/nucleus)[a]
Hela extract	50	100	76 (±7)
Nonbound fraction	42	84	4 (±1)
Bound fraction	0.7	0.7	24 (±2)

[a]UDS of noninjected cells: 3 (±1) grain/nucleus. SEM are given in parentheses.

XP20S[SV]) and XP-F (XP2YO[SV]) cell lines using genomic DNA fragments (about 50 kbp) from repair-proficient cells in vitro ligated to a molar excess of a dominant marker gene. Although high efficiencies were obtained for the transfer of the dominant marker (one stable transformant in 10^3–10^4 cells), we, and others, were unable to isolate transformants that were repair competent by coinsertion of the correcting gene. In contrast, the same approach applied to a repair-deficient CHO mutant yielded many repair-proficient transformants, which enabled the cloning of the human gene correcting the defects in this line [8]. A striking difference between the CHO and XP cells used is that only a small amount of exogenous DNA is integrated in the genome of XP cells compared to CHO cells. In Figure 2 the relative number of copies of dominant marker genes present in the genome of XP, CHO, and HeLa transformants is shown. Similar cell line-specific differences in stable uptake of exogenous sequences were observed with cotransfected carrier DNA. We presume that the small amounts of DNA integrated by the XP cells tested can explain at least in part the negative transfection results with these cells. An alternative approach for cloning XP correcting genes is offered by the finding of Legerski et al [9] that microinjection of polyA$^+$RNA of HeLa cells in XP-A and XP-G fibroblasts also transiently corrects the defect in these cells.

As mentioned above, we have recently cloned a human gene (designated *ERCC-1*) complementing the excision-repair defect of a UV- and mitomycin C (MM-

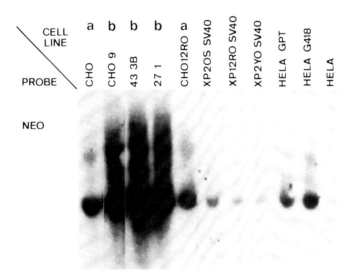

Fig. 2.   Southern blot analysis of the amount of exogenous DNA integrated after DNA transfection by various human and CHO cell lines. Ten petri dishes of each cell line were transfected with cos 43-34 DNA (containing pSV3gpt, pMCS [neomycin resistance], and the human repair gene *ERCC-1*) and mouse carrier DNA. After selection (CHO cells and Hela for gpt, XP cells and Hela for neomycin resistance), the pooled transformants of every cell line (in total 200–5,000 different clones) were grown in mass culture, and DNA was isolated, restricted with PstI, and, after gel electrophoresis (10 μg per lane) and transfer to nitrocellulose, hybridized with a ^{32}P-labeled probe for the neomycin resistance gene. The relative intensity of the bands reflects the relative average number of dominant marker gene copies integrated in the genome of every cell line. Similar results were obtained for insertion of pSV3gpt, *ERCC-1*, and mouse carrier DNA. CHO cells marked with a and b are derived from each other.

C)-sensitive CHO cell line (43-3B) [8]. After transfection, *ERCC-1* induces repair proficiency in 43-3B cells with respect to UV and MM-C survival, dimer removal, and UDS. Molecular characterization of this gene revealed that it consists of at least nine exons, spread over a region of about 15 kbp, and that it codes for an mRNA of 1.1 kb, which is constitutively expressed in a variety of human cells. In preliminary experiments we did not observe a drastic effect of UV irradiation of the cells on *ERCC-1* transcription. Sequence analysis of an *ERCC-1* cDNA clone revealed an open reading frame for a protein of 273 amino acids. Using Southern blot analysis of a panel of human/rodent cell hybrids, *ERCC-1* was assigned to human chromosome 19. ERCC-1 is not deleted or grossly rearranged in cell lines from XP complementation groups A, C, F, and G and does not induce repair proficiency after transfection to SV40 transformed XP-A and F fibroblasts. The relationship between *ERCC-1* and other XP complementation groups and other human syndromes associated with DNA repair defects, such as Fanconi anemia, is presently under investigation.

REFERENCES

1. Kraemer KH: In Fitzpatrick TB, Eisen AZ, Wolff K, Freedberg, IM, Austen KF (eds): "Update: Dermatology in General Medicine." New York: McGraw-Hill Book Company, 1983, p 113.
2. Friedberg EC: "DNA-Repair." New York: W.W. Freeman and Company, 1985.
3. Cleaver JE: Nature 218:652, 1968.
4. de Weerd-Kastelein EA, Keijzer W, Bootsma D: Nature [New Biol] 238:80, 1972.
5. Fischer E, Keijzer W, Thielmann HW, Popanda O, Bonert E, Edler L, Jung EG, Bootsma D: Mutat Res 145:217, 1985.
6. de Jonge AJR, Vermeulen W, Klein B, Hoeijmakers JHJ: EMBO J 2:637, 1983.
7. Hoeijmakers JHJ, Zwetsloot JCM, Vermeulen W, de Jonge AJR, Backendorf C, Klein B, Bootsma D: In Friedberg EC, Bridges BA (eds): "Cellular Responses to DNA Damage" UCLA Symposia on Molecular and Cellular Biology, New Series, Vol 11. New York: Alan R. Liss, Inc., 1983, p 173.
8. Westerveld A, Hoeijmakers JHJ, van Duin M, de Wit J, Odijk H, Pastink A, Wood RD, Bootsma D: Nature 310:425, 1984.
9. Legerski RJ, Brown DB, Peterson CA, Robberson DL: Proc Natl Acad Sci USA 81:5676, 1984.

Biochemical and Molecular Epidemiology of Cancer 391–395 (1986)

Isolation of the Molecular Clone of the *Neu* Oncogene From the B103 Rat Neuro/glioblastoma Cell Line

Mien-Chie Hung, Alan L. Schechter, Lalitha Vaidyanathan, David F. Stern, and Robert A. Weinberg

Whitehead Institute for Biomedical Research, Nine Cambridge Center and Department of Biology, Massachusetts Institute of Technology, Cambridge, Massachusetts 02142

The *neu* oncogene is a transforming gene carried in the genomes of a series of neuro/glioblastoma cell lines. Previously, we showed that the *neu* oncogene is homologous to *erb B* and also encodes a 185,000 dalton (p185) tumor antigen. We have constructed a cosmid library with DNA from a mouse transfectant that has acquired the *neu* oncogene via transfection. This library was screened, and several clones were obtained. Structural analysis by Southern blotting indicated one of the clones, cNeu 103, contained the restriction pattern specific to *neu*. Transfection of this clone onto monolayers of NIH 3T3 cells yielded numerous foci that, when examined, were shown to produce the novel tumor antigen p185. These data indicate we have isolated an intact and biologically active clone of the *neu* oncogene.

Key words: *neu*, oncogene, growth factor receptor

We have been investigating an oncogene (*neu*) that is carried in the genomes of several rat neuro/glioblastoma cell lines [1]. These cell lines were derived from tumors that were induced by transplacental injection of ethylnitrosourea (ENU) during the 15th day of gestation [2]. Employing this defined chemical regimen, the activation of *neu* in these induced tumors appears to be a frequent occurrence [3].

The *neu* oncogene is associated with the expression of tumor antigen, a 185,000 dalton protein (p185). NIH 3T3 cells that have acquired a *neu* oncogene via transfection synthesize the p185 protein, whereas NIH 3T3 cells that have been transformed by other oncogenes do not [4]. Characterization of the protein yielded some clues concerning the identity of the *neu* gene. The p185 protein was found to be a phosphorylated and glycosylated cell surface protein bearing many similarities to cell surface receptors.

The relationship between the EGF-r gene and *v-erb B* [5] sparked our attempts to find homology between *neu* and other known retroviral-associated oncogenes. The

Received April 17, 1985.

© **1986 Alan R. Liss, Inc.**

culmination of this work was the finding that the *neu* gene was homologous to *erb B* and that the tumor antigen, p185, was serologically related to the EGF-r [3].

The relationship between the *neu* and *c-erb B* genes was clarified when subsequent Southern analysis revealed that the normal and oncogenic forms of *neu* are distinct from the gene that encodes the EFG-r [6].

As an initial step toward defining the molecular alterations that have endowed the *neu* oncogene with its transforming potential, we have isolated, by molecular cloning, the *neu* oncogene from the B103 rat neuro/glioblastoma cell line. This clone of the *neu* oncogene is biologically intact as assayed by transfection onto NIH 3T3 cells and encodes the p185 tumor antigen.

MATERIALS AND METHODS
Construction and Screening of Cosmid Library

The cosmid library was constructed essentially according to the protocol of Ish-Horowitz and Burke [7]. The Eco R1-digested DNA from B103-1 was cloned into the Eco R1 site of the pSAE vector [8]. The library was screened according to published techniques [9], employing as probe a gel-purified SacI/PvuII fragment of avian erythroblastosis virus [10]. This fragment is *erb B* specific and reacts with DNA containing the *neu* oncogene [3].

Southern Analysis

Southern blot analysis was performed as previously described [3] with the exceptions of 50% formamide in the hybridization buffer and higher temperature (65°C) washes.

Immunoprecipitation

Immunoprecipitation of p185 was carried out with metabolically labeled ^{35}S-cysteine cell lysates as described in detail elsewhere [3].

Transfection of Cloned DNA

DNA transfection into mouse NIH 3T3 cells was carried out by the calcium phosphate precipitation technique of Graham and van der Eb [11] as modified by Anderson et al [12]. After 2 weeks, foci of morphologically transformed cells were scored and analyzed.

RESULTS AND DISCUSSION

We wished to obtain a clone of the *neu* oncogene that had maintained its transforming activity. Previous work showed that the entirety of the *neu* oncogene was contained within a large Eco R1 segment of approximately 33 kb in size [3]. Therefore, we wished to isolate by molecular cloning this Eco R1 segment, which should contain a biologically intact *neu* oncogene.

We constructed a cosmid library from Eco R1-digested genomic DNA. With the aid of a probe specific for *erb B* to screen the library, several positive colonies were picked. One was isolated to homogeneity. This clone, designated cNeu103, contains a 33 kb Eco R1 insert.

We wish to determine whether cNeu103 was capable of oncogenic transformation of NIH 3T3 cells. To that end, we transfected 1 μg of the cloned DNA by the calcium phosphate precipitation technique [12], and after 2 weeks we scored foci of transformed cells. Approximately 300 foci appeared on the monolayer of NIH 3T3 cells that had been transfected with the cNeu103 clone. These foci largely contained cells that were extremely refractile. Figure 1 shows a representative cell line derived from one such focus.

To prove that these foci of transformed cells contained the intact cNeu103 DNA and the encoded tumor antigen p185, we further analyzed these cells. Figure 2 shows a Southern analysis of the DNA and an immunoprecipitation analysis of the proteins from cell lines derived from four foci. These immunoprecipitations used the monoclonal antibody 16.4, which is specific for p185 [3]. The data indicated that all four foci contain both the transfected 33 kb Eco R1 segment of the *neu* clone, cNeu103, and the p185 protein, known to be encoded by this gene.

We have isolated the biologically active clone of the *neu* oncogene that was derived from the B103 neuro/glioblastoma cell line. This clone induces foci of NIH 3T3 cells containing the p185 with high efficiency. Moreover, it is indistinguishable from the *neu* gene that is present in the B103 cell line as judged by resistance to inactivation with endonuclease Eco R1 and sensitivity to BamH1 prior to transfection (data not shown). We are in the process of isolating the normal allele of the *neu* gene in similar fashion. In this way, we hope to generate the necessary reagents to determine the exact structural differences between the normal and oncogenic forms of *neu*.

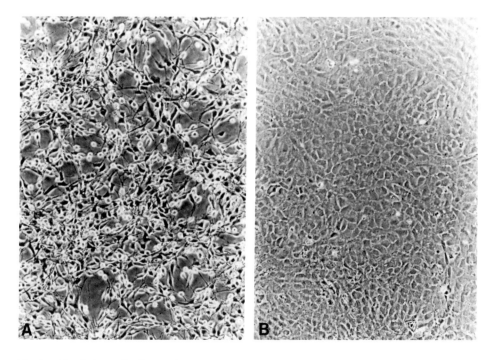

Fig. 1.   Morphology of cells transformed by cNeu103. A) cNeu103-12, a cell line derived by transfection of the *neu* oncogene clone. B) Untransfected recipient NIH 3T3 cells.

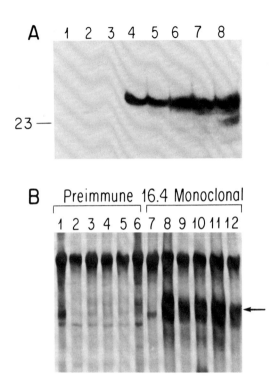

Fig. 2. A) Southern analysis of cNeu103-NIH transformants. DNA was isolated from the indicated sources and analyzed by Southern analysis as previously described [3], employing a 4.0 kb BamH1 segment of cNeu103 as probe. Lane 1, BDIX rat liver; lane 2, B103 neuro/glioblastoma; lane 3, NIH 3T3; lane 4, B103-1, primary transfectant of B103, transfectants of cNeu103; lane 5, cNeu103-3; lane 6, cNeu103-12; lane 7, cNeu103-13; lane 8, cNeu103-14. The position of 23 kb fragment from λ Hind III markers is shown on the left. B) Immunoprecipitation of p185. Lysates of ^{35}S-cysteine-labeled cells were incubated with either preimmune (lanes 1–7) or anti-p185 monoclonal antibody 16.4 (lanes 8–12) and subsequently precipitated and analyzed by SDS gel electrophoresis. Lanes 1, 7, NIH 3T3; lanes 2, 8, B103-1; lanes 3, 9, cNeu103-3; lanes 4, 10, cNeu103-12; lanes 5, 11, cNeu103-13; lanes 6, 12, cNeu103-14. The arrow shows the position of p185.

ACKNOWLEDGMENTS

M.-C.H. was supported by a postdoctoral fellowship from the Cancer Research Institute. A.L.S. and D.F.S. were supported by postdoctoral fellowships from the U.S. N.I.H. This work was supported by grants from the American Business Cancer Foundation and by N.I.H. grant CA 39964-01.

REFERENCES

1. Shih C, Padhy L, Murray M, Weinberg RA: Nature 290:261, 1981.
2. Schubert D: Nature 249:224, 1974.
3. Schechter AL, Stern DF, Vaidyanathan L, Decker S, Drebin J, Greene MI, Weinberg RA: Nature 312:513, 1984.
4. Padhy L, Shih C, Cowing D, Finkelstein R, Weinberg RA: Cell 28:865, 1982.
5. Downward J, Yarden Y, Mayes E, Scarce G, Totty N, Stockwell P, Ullrich A, Schlessinger J, Waterfield M: Nature 307:521, 1984.

6. Schechter AL, Hung M-C, Vaidyanathan L, Weinberg RA, Yang-Feng T, Franke U, Ullrich A, Coussens L: Science 229:976, 1985.
7. Ish-Horowitz D, Burke J: Nucleic Acids Res 9:2989, 1981.
8. Grosveld F, Lund F, Murray E, Mellor A, Flavell RA: Nucleic Acids Res 10:6715, 1982.
9. Maniatis T, Fritsch E, Sambrook J: "Molecular Cloning, A Laboratory Manual." Cold Spring Harbor, NY: Cold Spring Harbor Laboratory, 1982.
10. Vennstrom B, Fanshier L, Moscovici C, Bishop JM: J Virol 36:575, 1980.
11. Graham F, van der Eb J: Virology 52:456, 1973.
12. Anderson P, Goldfarb MP, Weinberg RA: Cell 16:63, 1979.

Biochemical and Molecular Epidemiology of Cancer 397–400 (1986)

Familial Clustering of Malignancies: Distribution of Ha-*ras* Restriction Fragment Length Polymorphism in Normal and High Risk Populations

J. Craig Cohen, Karen Buonagura, John Bickers, Gerald Berenson, and Henry Rothschild

Department of Medicine, Louisiana State University, School of Medicine, New Orleans, Louisiana 70112

In a study using deceased probands with lung cancer, a familial clustering of malignances was documented. In these families a significant positive correlation between relationship to the proband and the occurrence of lung cancer was demonstrated. This relationship was independent of smoking history. Of interest was the observation that several other types of cancer clustered in these families. These data suggest that a common genetic determinant is associated with an increased frequency of malignancy.

Key words: oncogene, lung cancer, cancer family syndrome

The occurrence of cancer sometimes among several members of the same family can be expected as a random event, inasmuch as about 22% of all persons die of cancer affecting different anatomic sites [1]. Sometimes, however, the presence of cancers among several generations and many members of the same family cannot always be explained simply by chance. The tendency to develop colon cancer in the presence of polyposis coli, for example, is inherited in simple Mendelian fashion [2,3]. Furthermore, some families exhibit extraordinary incidences of cancer at several different sites, such as the combination of breast cancer, brain cancer, sarcoma, leukemia, and Hodgkin's disease [2–4]. Pedigree analysis of several large families with high prevalences of cancers led Lynch and coworkers [5–7] to propose a genetic entity that was later called *cancer family syndrome*.

We recently showed an increased risk for lung cancer in first-degree relatives of lung cancer probands [8]. As presented in this article, further analyses of these data revealed the clustering of multiple cancers in these pedigrees. Examination of a restriction fragment length polymorphism in the Ha-*ras* oncogene in families with

Received August 7, 1985.

© **1986 Alan R. Liss, Inc.**

multiple cancers was then performed for possible association of cancer with a specific oncogene allele.

MATERIALS AND METHODS
Study Population

Probands for epidemiological studies were living, whites with primary lung cancers. All first-degree relatives were identified, and cancer history and pedigree data were obtained by telephone interviews and mail questionnaires [8]. When multiple lung cancers were found among first-degree relatives of the proband, the pedigree was extended to include second- and third-degree relatives.

Heparinized blood samples (279 total) were obtained from five pedigrees that had three or more cancers among first-degree relatives. These samples represented the high risk population. For comparison, 172 blood samples drawn from white school children (kindergarten and first grade) during a mass screening program were used.

Restriction Fragment Length Polymorphism (RFLP) Detection

DNA was extracted from lymphocytes isolated from heparinized blood samples. DNAs were digested with BamHI and fragments separated by electrophoresis on 0.8% agarose gels and trasferred to nitrocellulose sheets for hybridization with ^{32}P-labeled, cloned Ha-*ras* DNA for autoradiographic visualization as described previously [9].

RESULTS

The data presented in Table I establish the familial risk for lung cancer that appears in the over 40 age group. Of interest is the observation that overall there was an increased incidence of all cancers in the proband families. Further analysis of these data revealed that this difference was due to the occurrence of the less common malignancies (ie, excluding lung, breast, colon-rectum, prostate, and uterus that as a group occur at a frequency of greater than 10 per 100,000).

TABLE I. Distribution of Cancers Among First-Degree Relatives Stratified by Sex and Age

	Males				Females			
	Probands		Spouses		Probands		Spouses	
Population	No.	%	No.	%	No.	%	No.	%
Under 40	180	100	145	100	133	100	109	100
None	169	93.9	137	94.5	123	92.5	97	88.9
Lung	1	0.6	1	0.7	0	0.0	1	0.9
Other	10	5.6	7	4.8	10	7.5	11	10.1
Over 40	1,196	100	933	100	1,136	100	928	100
None	955	79.8	833	89.3	968	85.2	838	90.3
Lung	76	6.4[a]	30	3.2	26	2.3[b]	3	0.3
Other	165	13.8[c]	70	7.5	142	12.5[d]	87	9.4

[a]Relative risk estimate = 2.1 (P < 0.05).
[b]Relative risk estimate = 7.2 (P < 0.05).
[c]Relative risk estimate = 1.4 (P < 0.05).
[d]Relative risk estimate = 1.9 (P < 0.05).

Analysis of the Ha-*ras* RFLP in DNA samples obtained from pedigrees that had multiple lung and other cancers was compared to that of a matched normal population (Tables II, III).

The allelic frequency for both normal and high risk (cancer families) populations was determined for each of the four alleles distinguishable by BamHI digestion [10]. The alleles were designated A to D corresponding to 6.6, 6.8, 7.5, and 8.0 kb Ha-*ras*–specific fragments, respectively. No significant difference was noted between the normal and high risk populations (Table II).

Examination of the genotypic frequencies (Table III) for these populations yielded some interesting results. Significant differences ($P < 0.05$) in the frequencies of the AA and BC genotypes were observed.

DISCUSSION

In a retrospective epidemiological study using lung cancer probands a familial risk of lung and other cancers was demonstrated (Table I) [8]. These data suggest the presence of a susceptibility gene that generally influences the incidence of cancer. The gene could either 1) affect the ability of the immune system to respond to randomly arising transformed cells, 2) alter the tolerance to carcinogens such as cigarette smoke, or 3) represent a primary mutation in an oncogene.

As an initial step in evaluating the molecular basis for the observed familial clustering of cancers, the Ha-*ras* oncogene RFLP identified by BamHI digestion was studied in both families with a history of multiple malignancies, in first-degree relatives, and in a cross-sectional population. As shown in Table II, no differences were observed between normal and high risk populations for the four Ha-*ras* alleles. Differences in the genotypic frequency (Table III) were apparent, however. The higher frequency of the BC genotype was observed in the spouses who are not from high cancer families; therefore, it is likely that the more frequent occurrence of this allele was an aberration of the sample and not associated with malignancies. The occurrence of the AA genotype in spouses and normal populations was not signifi-

TABLE II. Allelic Frequency of c-Ha-*ras* Polymorphism in High Risk Population

Population	RFLP (%)				No. in sample
	A	B	C	D	
Whites	61.3	15.3	15.9	7.5	172
High risk	70.0	16.9	9.7	3.4	98
Cancers	80.0	15.0	5.0	—	10
Spouses	60.7	21.4	14.3	3.6	14

TABLE III. Genotype Frequency of c-Ha-*ras* Restriction Fragment Length Polymorphism in High Risk Population

Population	Genotype (%)										No. in sample
	AA	AB	AC	AD	BB	BC	BD	CC	CD	DD	
All whites	40.1	16.7	16.7	9.9	4.1	2.9	1.7	5.2	1.2	1.2	172
High risk	53.0	20.3	8.2	4.3	2.3	9.9	—	1.0	—	1.0	98
Cancers	70.0	20.0	—	—	—	10.0	—	—	—	—	10
Spouses	42.9	14.3	14.3	7.1	7.1	14.3	—	—	—	—	14

cantly different, and yet it occurred more frequently in the high risk than in the normal population. Further, it was the most often found genotype in the cancer patients.

Krontiris et al [10] reported that the polymorphism in the Ha-*ras* gene was due to multiple insertions of a repeated sequence, resulting in the higher molecular weight fragments (B, C, and D alleles). These investigators reported a more frequent occurrence of alleles with multiple insertions in nonfamilial cancer patients than in their normal population. Data from our study concerning familial cancers indicate that these insertions are negatively associated with cancer risk, because the AA genotype is found at an increased frequency in the high risk population and cancer patients derived from this population.

ACKNOWLEDGMENTS

This work was supported by NIH grants R01-CA-35686 and R01CA34823 and by funds from the National Heart, Lung and Blood Institute of the United States Public Health Service (HL02942 and HL21649) and the National Research and Demonstration Center—Arteriosclerosis (HL15103). Funding was also provided by the Optimist Leukemia Foundation of Louisiana, Inc.

REFERENCES

1. Cairns J: Sci Am 233:64–78, 1975.
2. Schimke RN: "Genetics and Cancer in Man." New York: Churchill and Livingstone, 1978.
3. Swift M: In Fraumeni JF (ed): "Cancer Epidemiology and Prevention." Philadelphia: WB Saunders, 1982.
4. Warthin AS: Arch Intern Med 12:546–555, 1913.
5. Lynch HT, Shaw MW, Magnuson CW, et al: Arch Intern Med 117:206–212, 1966.
6. Lynch HT: "Recent Advances in Cancer Research." New York: Springer Verlag, 1967, Vol 12.
7. Lynch HT, Krush AJ: Surg Gynecol Obstet 136:221–224, 1973.
8. Ooi WL, Elston RC, Chen VW, et al: JNCI (in press).
9. Cohen JC: Cell 19:653–662, 1980.
10. Krontiris TG, Dimartino NA, Colb M, Parkinson DR: Nature 313:369–374, 1985.

Biochemical and Molecular Epidemiology of Cancer 401–409 (1986)

Studies on the Mechanism of Transformation and Mutation by HSV-2

Curtis R. Brandt, Franco M. Buonaguro, James K. McDougall, and Denise A. Galloway

Tumor Biology Division, Fred Hutchinson Cancer Research Center, Seattle, Washington 98104

Transfection of NIH3T3 cells with a 232 nucleotide Sau3a fragment of the BglII N fragment of HSV-2 results in morphological transformation. This Sau3a fragment (m1.1) contains a potential stem-loop structure flanked by short, direct repeats reminiscent of insertion sequences. Several transformants were isolated and characterized with respect to morphology in culture, cloning efficiency in agarose, and tumorigenicity. DNA isolated from one transformant (m1.1F) is active in secondary transfections. HSV-2–specific DNA sequences are not detectable in any of the m1.1 transformants we have analyzed. Preliminary experiments on the ability of cloned HSV-2 DNA to induce 6 thioguanine mutants after transfection into NIH3T3 cells are also presented and suggest this system may be useful for mutation analysis.

Key words: transformation, herpes simplex type-2, mutation

Morphological transformation mediated by HSV appears to be fundamentally different than transformation induced by other double-strand DNA viruses that carry genes for transforming proteins expressed in cells [1]. Several HSV-specific antigens have been found in various transformed cells but no antigen is invariably expressed in all transformed cells [2–5]. Mapping of the transforming region of HSV-2 has identified two regions of the genome (BglII N and BglII C fragments) that could morphologically transform cells [6–8]. These two regions are different than the transforming region mapped in HSV-1 despite the fact that HSV-1 and HSV-2 have colinear genomes [6,9]. The picture is further complicated by reports that the sequences retained by transformants change with passage of cells. In addition, transformation persists in the absence of detectable viral sequences [10–15].

Transfection of the BglII N fragment of HSV-2 into rodent cells induces transformation when assayed by focus formation in low serum or colony formation in methyl cellulose [6,7]. These transformants show altered growth properties in culture, form tumors in nude mice, and BglII N sequences are retained in some of the cell

Received April 17, 1985.

© **1986 Alan R. Liss, Inc.**

lines. The corresponding region of HSV-1 does not transform rodent cells when assayed by the same methods.

Using deletion fragments of the HSV-2 BglII N fragment, we have recently localized the transforming region to a 737 nucleotide fragment (BC24), which maps at about 0.6 on the HSV-2 genome [16]. The nucleotide sequence of this fragment shows that a stem-loop structure can be formed within the BC24 sequence. This stem-loop structure is reminiscent of IS-like sequences in bacteria in that it has short, direct repeats at the base of the stem [17].

The most striking aspect of this potential stem-loop structure is that a similar structure exists in the transforming region of human cytomegalovirus (strain AD 169) [18] even though there is no sequence homology between HSV-2 and HCMV in these regions. A stem-loop structure cannot be formed from the HSV-1 sequence, which corresponds to the BC24 sequence of HSV-2. Experiments presented in this paper show that a 232 nucleotide fragment of HSV-2 DNA, which contains the stem-loop IS-like structure, transforms rodent cells in culture. We also characterize some of the transformation-related properties of cell lines established from transformed foci.

One mechanism consistent with the hit and run hypothesis is the induction of mutations in cellular genes by viral DNA. SV40 and adenovirus are mutagenic when introduced into cells [19–22]. Cells exposed to UV or neutral red-inactivated HSV-1 show higher rates of mutation to 6-thioguanine resistance. Partially inactivated HSV-1 was as potent a mutagen as the carcinogen 4-nitroquinoline-1-oxide [23]. We have been studying the rate of mutation to 6-thioguanine resistance after transfection of HSV-2 DNA into rodent cells. In this paper we present preliminary results that show NIH3T3 cells that can be transfected at high efficiency can be used to obtain 6-thioguanine–resistant mutants. Our preliminary results also suggest that transfected DNA is mutagenic in NIH3T3 cells.

MATERIALS AND METHODS
Cell Culture

NIH 3T3 cells were grown in Dulbecco's modification of Eagle's medium (DME: GIBCO, Grand Island, NY) containing 10% fetal calf serum (Hyclone, Logan, UT). Cells for transfection were taken from lots tested for background foci and stored in liquid nitrogen. They were passed no more than twice prior to transfection. Cloning efficiency in agar was tested as follows. Cells were trypsinized and counted. Aliquots containing 1×10^4 cells were pelleted and resuspended in 5 ml of $2 \times$ DME containing 20% FCS. The cells were mixed with 5 ml of 0.74% Noble agar at 42°C and plated in 100 mm plates on a layer of 0.9% Noble agar in $1 \times$ DME with 10% fetal calf serum. Fresh DME with 10% FCS was added every 4 days.

DNA Transfections, Focus Formation, and Tumorigenicity Assays

DNA transfections and focus formation assays were carried out as described previously [16]. To assay cells for tumorigenicity, cells were trypsinized, washed in phosphate-buffered saline (PBS), resuspended in 0.2 ml PBS, and injected subcutaneously into BALB/C nu/nu mice. Each mouse received 1×10^6 cells. Mice were checked weekly for tumors.

Construction of Recombinant Molecules

The construction of pmtrIIa and pBC24 has been described [16]. The clone m1.1 was constructed during sequencing of pBC24 and contains a 232 nucleotide

Sau3a fragment containing the IS-like element cloned into the BamHI sites of M13 mp7. Plasmid molecules and the M13 replicative form were isolated using alkaline lysis [24]. Figure 1 shows a map of the BglII N fragment of HSV-2 and the positions of the HSV sequences in pmtrIIa, pBC24, and m1.1

Isolation and Analysis of High Molecular Weight Cell DNA

High molecular weight cellular DNA was isolated from tissue culture plates as described previously [7]. DNAs were digested with restriction enzymes using conditions described by the manufacturer (BRL, Gaithersburg, MD or New England Biolabs, Beverly, MA) and electrophoresed in 0.7% agarose gels in TRIS-acetate buffer. Gene Screen Plus was used for Southern blots. Transfer and hybridization were carried out as described by the manufacturer (New England Nuclear, Boston, MA).

RESULTS

Transformation of NIH3T3 Cells by a Small Fragment of HSV-2 DNA That Contains an IS-Like Element

While sequencing the transforming BC24 fragment of HSV-2, we cloned in M13mp7 a 232 nucleotide Sau3a fragment that contains a sequence that has the potential to form a stem-loop flanked by short, direct repeats [16]. To determine if this short cloned sequence (m1.1) could transform NIH3T3 cells in a focus formation assay, we isolated double-strand m1.1RF and transfected it into NIH3T3 cells using calcium phosphate precipitation. We also transfected pmtrIIa and pBC24 as positive controls (see Fig. 1) and pBR322 and SstI-cut m1.1 RF as negative controls. Results are presented in Table I. As we reported previously [16], pmtrIIa and pBC24 form foci in NIH3T3 cells at about the same efficiency (9 and 12 foci, respectively). The m1.1RF also induced morphologically transformed foci at about the same efficiency as pmtrIIa and pBC24 (8 and 7 foci in two experiments). The plasmid pBR322 did

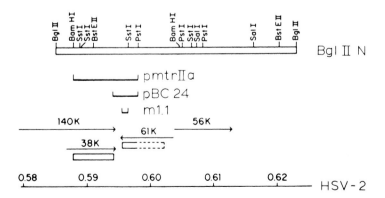

Fig. 1.   A map of the BglII N fragment showing the positions of the HSV-2 sequences used to transfect NIH3T3 cells. The restriction map is shown on the top. The locations of pmtrIIa, pBC24, and m1.1 sequences are shown below the restriction map. The bottom line shows the map coordinates on the HSV-2 genome.

TABLE I. Transformation of NIH3T3 Cells With Small Fragments of HSV-2 DNA

Experiment No.	pBR322	pmtrIIa	pBC24	m1.1	m1.1 SstI
1	1[a]	—	12	8	—
2	0	9	—	7	0

[a]Number of transformants per two 60 mm dishes of transfected cells.

not induce foci at an appreciable rate (1 and 0 foci in two separate experiments). These results show that the m1.1 RF can induce morphological transformation in cultured rodent cells.

Examination of the nucleotide sequence of m1.1 showed that an SstI restriction site exists in the loop of the potential stem-loop. When m1.1RF was digested with SstI and transfected into NIH3T3 cells, focus formation was reduced to background levels. This result suggests that the SstI site in the m1.1 sequence is important for morphological transformation. It also suggests that m13mp7 by itself does not induce focus formation.

Characterization of Cell Lines Established From Morphologically Transformed Foci

Three foci from the m1.1 transfection (m1.1B, m1.1C, and m1.1F) and one focus from a pBC24 transfection (NIH3B) were isolated for further study of their transformation-related properties. The morphologies of the cells in culture are shown in Figure 2. In culture, m1.1B and m1.1C cells are almost indistinguishable from NIH3T3 controls. There are few rounded refractile cells and the cells do not pile up extensively, although m1.1B and m1.1C grow to slightly higher saturation densities than NIH3T3 cells (data not shown). The cell lines NIH3B and m1.1F look typical of morphologically transformed cells. There are many round refractile cells and they grow in a disorganized pattern, crossing over each other.

Cloning efficiency in soft agar was determined by plating 1×10^4 cells in 100 mm dishes. After 2 to 3 weeks growth, colonies were counted. Results are presented in Table II. NIH3B and m1.1F were efficient at forming colonies (43 and 41%, respectively). Clones m1.1B and m1.1C were much less efficient at forming colonies (7.3 and 3.9%, respectively), while NIH3T3 controls were very inefficient (less than 0.43%). Several agarose clones were isolated, grown, and frozen for later analysis (see below).

Tumorigenicity was assayed by injecting 1×10^6 cells subcutaneously into nude mice. Results are presented in Table II. Two wks after injection, tumors were visible at the site of injection in all of the NIH3B- and m1.1B-injected mice (4+/4) and in two of four m1.1F-injected mice. At 5 wks, all of the m1.1F-injected mice had developed tumors at the site of injection. None of the tumors were metastatic. In contrast, none of the m1.1C- or NIH3T3-injected mice developed tumors. The tumors were excised and divided into portions. One small portion was processed for histological examination. Half of the remaining tumor was frozen at $-70°C$ and the other half was used to establish cell cultures. Histologically all of the tumors were fibrosarcomas.

m1.1F DNA Induces Secondary Transformants in NIH3T3 Cells

High molecular weight DNA was isolated from m1.1F cells, digested with several restriction enzymes, and used to induce secondary transformants. Results are

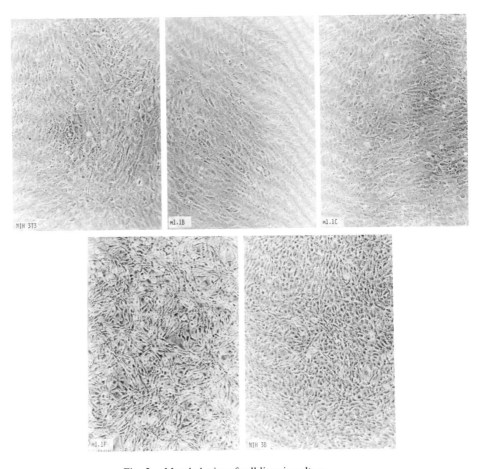

Fig. 2.   Morphologies of cell lines in culture.

TABLE II. Characteristics of Cell Lines Studied

Cell line	Transfected with	Cloning in soft agarose (%)	Tumori-genicity	Type of tumor	Metastasis	Cultures established
NIH3B	pBC24	43	4+/4	Fibrosarcoma	—	2+/4
m1.1B	m1.1	7.3	4+/4	Fibrosarcoma	—	4+/4
m1.1C[a]	m1.1	3.9	4−/4	—	—	ND
m1.1F	m1.1	41	4+/4	Fibrosarcoma	—	2+/4
NIH3T3[b]	—	0.43	4−/4+	—	—	—

[a]Two mice died of unknown causes. No visible tumors at time of death. Postmortems not done on these mice.
[b]One NIH3T3 mouse developed spontaneous fibromatosis over left eye.

TABLE III. Transfection of NIH3T3 Cells With 1.1F DNAs

Sample	Foci/microgram	Enhancement over background
Herring sperm	0.019	—
p1.1	0.143	7.50
1.1F BamHI	0.032	1.70
1.1F Pst	0.081	4.30
1.1F HindIII	0.084	4.40
1.1F-RI	0.039	2.05
1.1F-SstI	0.008	0.42
1.1F uncut[a]	0.013	0.68

[a]High molecular weight. DNA not sheared to reduce size.

presented in Table III. Herring sperm DNA gave a background of 0.019 foci per microgram of DNA. The positive control, p1.1 (the m1.1 Sau3a fragment cloned in pBR322) DNA, gave 0.143 foci per microgram of DNA, which was 7.5-fold above background. All of the restriction-digested samples were less efficient than p1.1 DNA. Of the enzymes used, PstI- and HindIII-digested m1.1F DNA gave the highest levels of secondary transfectants (4.3- and 4.4-fold over background, respectively). EcoRI and BamHI digested m1.1F DNA gave intermediate levels of secondary transfectants (2.05- and 1.7-fold over background, respectively). The m1.1 sequence has an SstI site in the loop of the potential stem-loop structure and cutting of m1.1 with SstI eliminates transformation (Table I). If the m1.1 sequence is necessary for transformation, then SstI-digested m1.1F DNA should not induce secondary transformants. This is the case, as SstI-cut m1.1F DNA had a transformation efficiency of 0.008 foci per microgram. This is less than half the background rate. This result may indicate that the 1.1 sequence is present and has introduced an SstI site relevant to morphological transformation. Alternatively, the cellular gene(s) altered by HSV transformation could contain an SstI site that would inactivate the function of the gene. Intact high molecular weight m1.1F DNA gave lower than background levels of secondary foci. High molecular weight DNA may not transfect efficiently.

Southern Blot Analysis of DNA From Primary Transfectants, Agarose Subclones, and Tumor Cell Lines

To determine if HSV-2–specific sequences are present in transformed cells, high molecular weight DNA was isolated from the primary transfectants, several agarose subclones, and several tumor cell lines described above. DNAs were digested, electrophoresed in 0.7% agarose, transferred to Gene Screen Plus, and hybridized to nick-translated concatemerized BC24 insert. Evidence for integration of HSV-2 DNA in primary transfectants has been difficult to obtain. Even under low stringency washing conditions and exposure to film for 9 days, we find no evidence for retention of HSV-2 sequences in the m1.1 transformants (data not shown).

Blots were washed to remove the BC24 probe and rehybridized with nick-translated M13mp7 DNA. Analysis of M13 sequences is complicated by the fact that we find endogenous mouse sequences that cross hybridize at low stringency with M13 probes. None of the transformants contained detectable vector sequences (data not shown).

Induction of 6-Thioguanine–Resistant Mutants

Our results from Southern blot analysis of the NIH3B and m1.1F primary transfectants, agarose subclones, and tumors are consistent with previous results that HSV-2 sequences are difficult to detect in transformed rodent cells and in cervical carcinomas [see 1]. Attempts to determine the mechanism of transformation are hampered by this fact and by the fact that we do not know the cellular target for transformation. We have begun a series of experiments designed to assess the effect of the HSV and CMV transforming regions and transfected DNA on a specific cellular gene. This will enable us to determine if alterations in the target gene are related to the transfected DNA.

Briefly, the system involves transfecting NIH3T3 cells with various DNAs and then selecting for 6-thioguanine–resistant mutants among the survivors of the treated populations. The details of these experiments will be published elsewhere.

Table IV shows the results from a preliminary experiment designed to determine if we could obtain mutants after transfecting DNAs into NIH3T3 cells. Our background mutation frequency in untreated NIH3T3 cells was 1.4×10^{-7}, which is in the range expected for a single gene in eukaryotic cells. The mutation frequency for pBR322 transfected cells was 6.7×10^{-7}, which is 4.8-fold above the background mutation frequency. We transfected three different doses of the HSV-2 mtrII containing plasmid pBC24. Two points can be made. First, there appears to be a small dose-response effect in the BC24/25 (25 μg/plate) and BC24/50 (50 μg/plate) samples. The BC24/25 sample had a mutation frequency of 1.0×10^{-6}, which is 7.1-fold higher than background. The mutation frequency in the BC24/50 sample is 1.6×10^{-6}, which is 1.6-fold higher than BC24/25 and 11.4-fold higher than background. The mutation frequency in the BC24/200 sample (9.5×10^{-7}) is lower than the BC24/25 sample. This may be due to the toxicity of large amounts of transfected DNA in NIH3T3 cells. We cannot say at present if pBC24 is more mutagenic than pBR322, since we only used 8 μg of pBR322 per plate in the transfection. The second point to be noted from the results is that the transfected DNAs clearly induce mutations at a higher frequency than background.

TABLE IV. Frequencies of 6-Thioguanine–Resistant Mutants in Transfected NIH3T3 Cells*

Sample	μgDNA transfected per plate	Foci	Surviving fraction	Mutation frequency	Enhancement over background	Enhancement over pBR322
Control[a]	—	1	6.7×10^6	1.4×10^{-7}	—	—
pBR322/8	8	3	4.45×10^6	6.7×10^{-7}	4.78	—
pBC24/25	25	3	3×10^6	1×10^{-6}	7.14	1.49
pBC25/50	50	5	2.95×10^6	1.6×10^{-6}	11.4	2.4
pBC24/200	200	3	3.15×10^6	9.5×10^{-7}	6.78	1.42

*NIH3T3 cells were passed in HAT medium for 2 weeks to reduce background. One hundred millimeter plates were seeded with 1.5×10^7 cells per plate and 24 hr later transfected as described previously [16]. After an additional 24 hr the plates were trypsinized and the cells seeded into roller bottles in DME with 10% fetal calf serum. The cells were passed twice during the next 8 days (1.5×10^7 cells reseeded at each pass). After an 8 day expression time, cells were trypsinized and 1.5×10^7 cells were seeded at a density of 5×10^5 cells/plate in DME with 10% fetal calf serum 0.1 mM 6-thioguanine. Resistant foci were counted 2 to 3 weeks later.
[a]NIH3T3 cells plated in 6-thioguanine without treatment.

Several mutants were isolated and expanded to analyze for alterations in the HGPRT gene using a cDNA clone for the mouse HGPRT gene (pHPT5) [25]. Three of six BC24 mutants show detectable alterations in the HGPRT gene upon Southern blot analysis (data not shown). None of the mutants have integrated pBC24 sequences (data not shown). These preliminary results are encouraging and we are continuing these studies to determine the mechanism by which HSV sequences can mutate cellular sequences.

DISCUSSION

The results presented here extend our previous observations that demonstrated that a 737 nucleotide fragment of HSV-2 DNA is able to transform NIH3T3 cells in culture [16]. We previously suggested that an IS-like element may be important in the mechanism of transformation. We have now shown that an even smaller 232 nucleotide fragment can transform cells. This 232 nucleotide fragment contains the IS-like sequence, strengthening our earlier conclusion that an IS-like element may be important for transformation.

This result provides at least some explanation for the routine failure to detect HSV-2 sequences in transformed cells and tumors. The m1.1 fragment constitutes 0.15% of the HSV-2 genome, which may be very difficult to detect by Southern blot. Future attempts to detect HSV-2 sequences in transformed cells and tumors must take this into account.

We have characterized several cell lines as to the transformation related properties. The BC24 transformant (NIH3B) has many round, refractile cells, which pile up and cross over one another in culture; NIH3B also clones in agar at high efficiency and is tumorigenic in nude mice. We had not previously tested pBC24 transformants for these properties. One of the m1.1 transformants (m1.1F) is similar to NIH3B in its properties. The other two m1.1F transformants m1.1B and m1.1C are different in some respects. In culture they are almost indistinguishable from NIH3T3 cells and they clone in soft agar at lower efficiencies than NIH3B and m1.1F. The transformant m1.1B forms tumors in nude mice while m1.1C does not. These results show that there is an extreme variability in transformation-related properties and that morphology in culture and cloning in soft agar do not necessarily correlate well with tumorigenicity.

How does the HSV-2 mtr region transform rodent cells? Many mechanisms can be postulated, several of which we are currently testing. One hypothesis, about which we present preliminary data, is that the HSV-2 transforming region could act as a mutagen. HSV-1 has been shown to induce mutations [23]. We are currently testing the mutagenic activity of DNA at the HGPRT locus and have presented some preliminary results suggesting that mutations do occur at a frequency higher than background. These results are too preliminary to conclude much about mutagenesis but the results suggest we now have a useful assay system. Mutants resistant to 6-thioguanine have altered hypoxanthine-guanine phosphoribosyl transferase, which is used in the salvage pathway for purine biosynthesis in eukaryotic cells [26]. The structural gene for murine HGPRT has been cloned and partially sequenced and cDNA probes are available [25,27]. These characteristics give us a powerful selection system and a way to identify the target gene and alterations that may have occurred in mutant cells.

ACKNOWLEDGMENTS

We thank Margaret Swain, Patsy Smith, and Angela Taeschner for technical assistance; Dr. C.T. Caskey for providing the pHPT5 cDNA clone; Dr. David Myerson for reading the pathology slides; and Toni Higgs for typing the manuscript. Support for this work came from a Public Health Research Service Award to C.B. (GM 09125), a World Health Organization Fellowship to F.B. (IARC/R. 1365), and grants from the National Cancer Institute to D.A.G. (CA26001) and J.K.M. (CA29350).

REFERENCES

1. Galloway DA, McDougall JK: Nature 301:21, 1983.
2. Reed CL, Cohen GH, Rapp F: J Virol 15:668, 1975.
3. Flannery VL, Courtney RJ, Schaffer PA: J Virol 21:284, 1977.
4. Suh M, Kessous A, Poirier N, Simard R: Virology 184:303, 1980.
5. Lewis JG, Kucera LS, Eberle R, Courtney RJ: J Virol 42:275, 1982.
6. Reyes GR, LaFemina R, Hayward SD, Hayward GS: Cold Spring Harbor Symp Quant Biol 44:629, 1979.
7. Galloway DA, McDougall JK: J Virol 38:749, 1981.
8. Jariwalla RJ, Aurelian L, Ts'O POP: Proc Natl Acad Sci USA 77:2279, 1980.
9. Camacho A, Spear PG: Cell 15:993, 1978.
10. Galloway DA, Copple CD, McDougall JK: Proc Natl Acad Sci USA 77:880, 1980.
11. Frenkel N, Locker H, Cox B, Roizman B, Rapp F: J Virol 18:885, 1976.
12. Copple CD, McDougall JK: Int J Cancer 17:501, 1976.
13. David DB, Kingsbury DB: J Virol 17:788, 1976.
14. Minson AC, Thouless ME, Elgin RP, Darby G: Int J Cancer 17:493, 1976.
15. Hampar B, Aaronson SA, Derge JG, Chakrabarty M, Showalter SD, Dunn CY: Proc Natl Acad Sci USA 73:646, 1976.
16. Galloway DA, Nelson JA, McDougall JK: Proc Natl Acad Sci USA 81:4736, 1984.
17. Kleckner N: Annu Rev Genet 15:341, 1981.
18. Nelson JA, Fleckenstein B, Jahn G, Galloway DA, McDougall JK: J Virol 49:109, 1984.
19. Bellet AJD, Younghusband HB: J Cell Physiol 101:33, 1979.
20. Lukash LL, Buzhievskaya TI, Varshaver NB, Shapiro MI: Somat Cell Genet 7:133, 1981.
21. Marengo C, Mbikay M, Weber J, Thirion JP: J Virol 38:184, 1981.
22. Paraskeva C, Roberts C, Biggs P, Gallimore PH: J Virol 46:131, 1983.
23. Schlehofer JR, zurHausen H: Virology 122:471, 1982.
24. Birnboim HC, Doly J: Nucleic Acids Res 7:1517, 1979.
25. Konecki DS, Brennand J, Fuscoe JC, Caskey CT, Chinault AC: Nucleic Acids Res 10:6763, 1982.
26. Caskey CT, Kruh GD: Cell 16:1, 1979.
27. Melton DW, Konecki DS, Brennand J, Caskey CT: Proc Natl Acad Sci USA 81:2147, 1984.

Biochemical and Molecular Epidemiology of Cancer 411–418 (1986)

Correlation Between O^6-Alkylguanine-DNA Alkyltransferase Activity and Resistance of Human Cells to the Cytotoxic and Mutagenic Effects of Methylating and Ethylating Agents

Veronica M. Maher, Jeanne Domoradzki, Rebecca C. Corner, and J. Justin McCormick

Carcinogenesis Laboratory, Department of Microbiology, and Department of Biochemistry, Michigan State University, East Lansing, Michigan 48824-1316

A series of cell lines derived from patients with a hereditary predisposition to colon cancer, ie, Gardner's syndrome (GS) and familial polyposis coli (FP), were compared with those of normal persons and of xeroderma pigmentosum (XP) patients for sensitivity to *N*-methyl-*N'*-nitro-*N*-nitrosoguanidine (MNNG) and *N*-ethyl-*N*-nitrosourea (ENU). They were also compared for their level of O^6-alkylguanine-DNA-alkyltransferase (MT) activity. Enzyme activity was determined from the ability of cell extracts to remove methyl groups from the O^6 position of guanine in a DNA substrate. The resistance of the various cell lines to the cytotoxic and mutagenic effects of MNNG was highly correlated with their MT activity. Cells with no detectable activity were extremely sensitive; those with intermediate levels showed intermediate sensitivity; those with high levels of MT were the most resistant, showing thresholds on their mutation curves and shoulders on their survival curves. The majority of the GS, FP, and XP cell lines showed normal sensitivity and normal levels of MT. Cells from one GS patient were very low in MT and sensitive to MNNG. However, cells from the GS patient's affected daughter were normal and had a normal amount of MT activity. When the normal level of MT in cells was decreased by exposure to exogenous O^6 methylguanine, the cells were abnormally sensitive to the induction of mutations by MNNG. Related studies comparing the cytotoxic and mutagenic effects of ENU in the various cell lines suggest that MT plays an important role in repair of potentially cytotoxic and mutagenic damage by ENU but that nucleotide excision repair also is involved.

Abbreviations used: ENU, N-ethyl-N-nitrosourea; FP, familial polyposis coli; GS, Gardner's syndrome; MNNG, N-methyl-N'-nitro-N-nitrosourea; MT, O^6-alkylguanine-DNA-alkytransferase; O^6MeG, O^6-methylguanine; XP, xeroderma pigmentosum.

Received August 20, 1985.

© **1986 Alan R. Liss, Inc.**

Key words: cell synchrony, DNA repair, O[6]-alkylguanine-DNA-alkyltransferase, mutagenesis, human cells, post replication repair, xeroderma pigmentosum

Familial polyposis coli (FP) is a rare genetic disease characterized by hundreds of adenomatous polyps in the colon and rectum that inevitably terminate in cancer unless surgically removed [1]. A related disease, Gardner's syndrome (GS), is also characterized by multiple polyps of the lower digestive tract that are predisposed to malignancy, but in addition, GS is associated with the appearance of multiple osteomas, fibromas, and sebaceous cysts [2]. A number of investigators have reported that fibroblasts derived from skin biopsies of such FP and GS patients are abnormal in their response to alkylating agents, including MNNG. Because methylating agents have been implicated in colon carcinogenesis [3], we wanted to see if fibroblasts from these patients were also abnormally sensitive to mutations induced by such carcinogens. A positive result would support the hypothesis that mutations occurring in the colon epithelial cells of these patients at an abnormally high frequency are a contributing factor in the disease.

We also wanted to compare the level of O[6]-alkylguanine-DNA-alkyltransferase (MT) activity in FP and GS cells with that of other human fibroblasts. MT, a protein acceptor molecule that removes alkyl groups from the O^6 position of guanine and transfers them to cysteine to form S-alkyl cysteine and to regenerate guanine [4–6], has been shown to be present constitutively in human fibroblasts [7]. Since O^6-methylguanine is considered to be the major lesion responsible for mutations induced by methylating agents in mammalian cells [8], including human cells [9], there was a possibility that GS and FP cells would be deficient in such a DNA repair system. Our results indicate that a low level of MT activity is highly correlated with sensitivity to both the cytotoxic and the mutagenic effects of MNNG but that abnormal levels of MT are not characteristic of all GS or FP cell lines.

MATERIALS AND METHODS
MT Assay

In collaboration with M. Eileen Dolan and Anthony E. Pegg of the Hershey Medical Center, Pennsylvania State University, we measured the level of MT activity in a series of human fibroblast cell lines [10]. In brief, the assay consists of preparing a DNA substrate containing radioactive methyl groups predominantly at the O^6 position of guanine [11,12] and exposing it to extracts of the cells to be tested. After the extract has removed the methyl groups from the DNA, the substrate is digested and analyzed by HPLC for the number of unrepaired O^6-methylguanine bases remaining. The MT activity is expressed as femtomole methyl removed per milligram of protein [10].

Cytoxicity and Mutagenicity Assays

For the investigation of the biologic effects of MNNG or ENU in these various cell lines, cytotoxicity was determined by measuring the survival of the colony-forming ability using our published methods [13]. Sensitivity to mutation induction was determined by measuring the increase in frequency of 6-thioguanine-resistant cells in the treated populations as previously described [13]. The frequencies are corrected for the background and for the cloning efficiency of the cells, which ranged from 40 to 80%.

RESULTS

Correlation Between MT Activity and Resistance to MNNG Cytotoxicity and Mutagenicity

The results of our investigation of MT activity showed that fibroblasts derived from foreskins of a series of normal newborn males contain a high level of MT activity, compared to bacterial cells or Chinese hamster cell lines of indefinite life span in culture. However, we identified three human cell lines that are virtually devoid of MT activity, one line with an intermediate level and two with somewhat more than the normal amount [10]. Examples are shown in Table I.

One of the cell lines virtually devoid of MT activity was an SV40 virus-transformed XP cell line (XP12ROSV), but another XP cell line from the same complementation group (group A) had a normal or somewhat higher than normal level. One of the GS cell lines (GM3314) showed very low activity, but the affected daughter of that patient (GM3948) showed a high level of MT. The cell line GM0011 was derived from an apparently normal fetus. The cell line with the intermediate level of MT (GM637) is an SV40 virus-transformed normal cell line.

These cell lines and additional cell lines were compared for their sensitivity to the cytotoxic and mutagenic effects of MNNG. As shown in Figure 1B, the mutation induction data fall into four groups. The three cell lines lacking MT activity are sensitive to very low doses of MNNG: The one with an intermediate amount of MT shows intermediate sensitivity; the lines with normal levels of MT are resistant to low doses and respond only after exposure to higher doses; and the two lines with the highest levels of MT appear to be slightly more resistant than normal to mutation induction by MNNG. The survival data (Fig. 1A) show a corresponding result, but the latter two cell lines are not more resistant than the cells with normal levels of MT. The data suggest that O[6]-methylguanine, or any other adduct specifically repaired by the MT protein, is a principal potentially cytotoxic and mutagenic lesion induced by MNNG. It should be noted that a human cell extract (from XP12BE cells) that was very proficient in removing methyl groups from the O[6] position of guanine did not remove methyl from the O[4] position of thymine in a poly dT·poly dA substrate [10].

TABLE I. Alkyltransferase Activity in Cell Extracts

Cell line	fmol methyl removed per mg protein[a]	Expressed as percent of normal cells
XP12BE	211	151
GM3948	208	
SL66	152	
GM2355	142	100
SL68	123	
GM637	96	69
GM0011	< 10	
GM3314	< 8	6
XP12ROSV	< 7	

[a]Each value is the mean of three or more determinations.

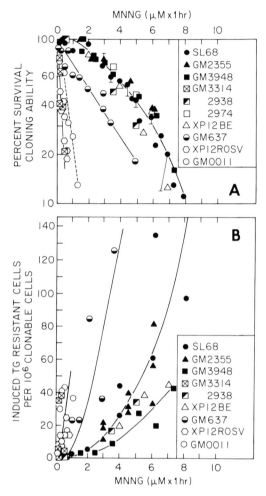

Fig. 1. Cytotoxicity (A) and mutagenicity (B) induced by MNNG in human fibroblast cell lines that differ in their level of MT activity. Reprinted from Domoradzki et al [10] with permission.

Effect of Depletion of MT Activity by Exogenous O^6-Methylguanine

Because there is always a possibility that other DNA repair systems were influencing these results, it was useful to be able to specifically manipulate the level of MT activity in the cells and then determine the effect on the frequency of mutations induced by MNNG and on cell survival. This was done by exposing fibroblasts with normal levels of MT activity (SL68) to exogenous O^6-methylguanine (O^6-MeG) in the medium for 15 or 24 hr. Table II shows the extent of the depletion that occurred [14]. The MT levels were reduced to between 21 and 42% of the control.

The four sets of MT-depleted cells receiving 0.4 mM O^6-MeG and their corresponding control populations were then challenged with MNNG. The results (Fig. 2) showed that if the level of MT was reduced, cells were more sensitive than the control cells to the induction of mutations by low doses of MNNG [14]. At doses high enough to cause a rapid increase in the frequency of mutants in the control

TABLE II. Effect of Exposure to Exogenous O^6-MeG for 15 or 24 hr on the Level of MT Activity in Human Cell Extracts

Experiment No.	Control population (MT activity; fmol removed per mg protein)[a]	O^6-MeG–exposed population		
		Dose O^6-MeG (mM)	MT activity (fmol removed per mg protein)[a]	Activity remaining (% of control)
I	272	0.4	108	40
II	210	0.4	80	38
III	480	0.4[b]	200	42
		0.8[b]	150	31
IV	317	0.4	66	21

[a]Each value is the mean of three determinations.
[b]15 hr exposure.

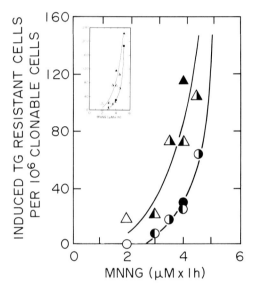

Fig. 2.   Mutagenicity of MNNG in cells with reduced levels of MT activity (triangles) or with normal levels (circles). Different shading of symbols designates different experiments. Reprinted from Domoradzki et al [14], with permission.

population, which had not been exposed to O^6-MeG, the difference between the two populations was less pronounced. If O^6-methylguanine is the principal potentially mutagenic lesion, this is the result one would expect, since at those doses, the supply of MT protein available for repair should be exhausted in both sets of cells.

In contrast to the mutation results, there was no significant difference between the two populations in their response to the killing effect of MNNG (data not shown). If O^6-methylguanine in DNA is a potentially cytotoxic lesion, an explanation for the lack of increased sensitivity in the MT-depleted cells is the following. Unlike the introduction of mutations, which is S phase dependent and essentially complete in a short period of time following exposure, cell death (loss of ability to form a colony) reflects a process that is not completed until much later. Regeneration of MT protein could have occurred rapidly enough to remove the methyl groups before their effect was made permanent.

To obtain information on the rate of regeneration, we measured the level of MT activity in extracts of cells exposed to exogenous O^6-MeG (0.4 mM) for 24 hr, but then allowed 7 to 24 additional hr incubation in normal culture medium lacking O^6-MeG. The results (Table III) indicated that by 7 hr the level of MT activity is 56% of normal [14]. This newly synthesized MT would be able to remove methyl groups from the DNA and prevent their exerting a cytotoxic effect.

Repair of ENU-Induced Lesions

Simon et al [15] in this laboratory showed earlier that XP12BE cells are significantly more sensitive than normal human fibroblasts to the cytotoxic and mutagenic effects of ENU. Yet this is one of the two cell lines with the highest levels of MT activity. If O^6-ethylguanine is the principal potentially cytotoxic or mutagenic lesion and is repaired solely by the action of the MT protein, one would not expect to find this difference in sensitivity between XP12BE cells and normal cells.

It is known that XP12BE cells are extremely deficient in rate of excision of lesions induced by ultraviolet light [16]. We and our collaborators showed they are incapable of excising DNA adducts produced by such bulky, multiringed structures as N-acetoxy-2-acetylaminofluorene [17] or the "anti" 7,8-diol-9,10-epoxide of benzo[a]pyrene [18]. Warren and Lawley [19] reported that bacteria deficient in excision of UV-induced lesions are slower than normal cells in repair of O^6-ethylguanine, but repair O^6-methylguanine at the normal rate. Therefore, it is possible that the ethyl group present in DNA at the O^6 position is large enough to distort the DNA molecule and to allow nucleotide excision repair processes to recognize the lesion.

If this hypothesis is valid and if human cells make use of both MT and nucleotide excision repair processes ("UV repair") to remove DNA damage induced by ethylating agents, this would explain our results with XP12BE cells. The hypothesis predicts that cell lines possessing MT but deficient in "UV repair," as well as cell lines deficient in MT but possessing normal "UV repair" should both be more sensitive to ENU than normal cells are. Furthermore, cells deficient in both kinds of repair processes should be even more sensitive than the above two kinds of cells.

We tested this hypothesis by comparing a series of such cell lines for their sensitivity to the killing and mutagenic action of ENU. The mutagenicity results (Fig. 3, bottom panel) support our prediction. SV40 virus-transformed normal cells (GM637), with normal UV repair but with only 69% as much MT, showed a response close to normal. The XP12BE cells, which totally lack UV repair but have abundant levels of MT, were abnormally sensitive. GM0011 cells with normal UV repair but lacking MT were abnormally sensitive, and XP12ROSV cells, which lack MT and carry out UV repair at a rate only ~5% that of normal, were the most sensitive of

TABLE III. Regeneration of MT Activity of Cell Extracts After Depletion by Exposure to Exogenous O^6-MeG

Experimental conditions	MT activity	
	fmol removed per mg protein	Percent of control
No exposure to O^6-MeG	283	100
24 hr of exogenous O^6-MeG (0.4 mM)	65	23
7 hr after removal of exogenous O^6-MeG	158	56
18 hr after removal of exogenous O^6-MeG	188	66

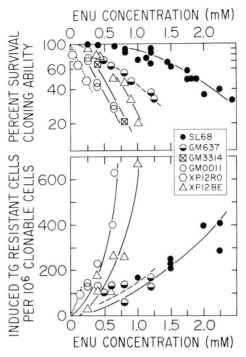

Fig. 3. Cytotoxicity and mutagenicity induced by ENU in human fibroblast cell lines that differ in their level of MT activity.

all to the mutagenic effect of ENU. In general, the survival data (Fig. 3, upper panel) also support the hypothesis, but the GM 637 cells showed somewhat greater sensitivity to killing by ENU than they showed toward its mutagenic effect.

DISCUSSION

The results of the MNNG studies in these human fibroblasts indicate that resistance to the biologic effects of MNNG is highly correlated with levels of MT activity. They also show that sensitivity to the cytotoxic or mutagenic effects of methylating agents is not a characteristic of the majority of GS or FP fibroblast cell lines tested.

The studies in which exogenous O^6-MeG was supplied to the cells to deplete the normal level of MT activity indicate that if the level decreases, cells are more at risk of mutations induced by methylating agents. Taken together with the data in Figure 1, these results support the hypothesis that in human fibroblasts, O^6-MeG is a principal cytotoxic and mutagenic DNA lesion.

The results of the ENU studies suggest that MT protein plays an important role in the repair of potentially cytotoxic and mutagenic damage, but nucleotide excision repair also is involved. These data showing correlations will need to be supported by studies of the rate of removal of particular DNA lesions by the various cell lines that lack one or the other of the two types of repair systems.

ACKNOWLEDGMENTS

We thank our collaborators, Dr. A.E. Pegg and M.E. Dolan, for the measurement on the MT activity of the various cells and Dr. Yenyun Wang for sharing results of biological studies with GM0011 cells. We thank Linda Stafford for technical assistance with mutagenicity studies and Laurie Wiest for assisting with the MT studies. This research was supported in part by DHHS grants CA21253 and CA18137 from the National Cancer Institute.

REFERENCES

1. McKusick VA: JAMA 182:271–277, 1962.
2. Gardner EJ, Richard RC: Am J Hum Genet 3:139–148, 1953.
3. "IARC, Monographs on the Evaluation of Carcinogenic Risk of Chemicals to Man." Lyon: International Agency for Research on Cancer, Vol 4, pp 145–151, 1974.
4. Olsson M, Lindahl T: J Biol Chem 225:10569–10571, 1980.
5. Foot RS, Mitra S, Pal BC: Biochem Biophys Res Commun 97:654–659, 1980.
6. Mehta JR, Ludlum DB, Renard A, Verly WG: Proc Natl Acad Sci USA 78:6766–6770, 1981.
7. Grafstrom RC, Pegg AE, Trump BF, Harris CC: Cancer Res 44:2855–2857, 1984.
8. Newbold RF, Warren W, Medcalf ASC, Amos J: Nature 283:596–599, 1980.
9. Medcalf ASC, Wade MH: Carcinogenesis 4:115–118, 1983.
10. Domoradzki J, Pegg AE, Dolan ME, Maher VM, McCormick JJ: Carcinogenesis 5:1641–1647, 1984.
11. Pegg AE, Wiest L, Foote RS, Mitra S, Perry W: J Biol Chem 258:2327–2333, 1983.
12. Pegg AE, Balog B: Cancer Res 39:5003–5010, 1979.
13. McCormick JJ, Maher VM: In Friedberg EC, Hanawalt PC (eds): "DNA Repair, A Laboratory Manual of Research Procedures." New York: Marcel Dekker, Vol 1B, pp 501–520, 1981.
14. Domoradzki J, Pegg AE, Dolan ME, Maher VM, McCormick JJ: Carcinogenesis 6:1823–1826, 1985.
15. Simon L, Hazard RM, Maher VM, McCormick JJ: Carcinogenesis 2:567–570, 1981.
16. Robbins JH, Kraemer KH, Lutzner MA, Festoff BM, Coon HG: Ann Intern Med 80:221–248, 1974.
17. Helflich RH, Hazard RM, Lommel L, Scribner JD, Maher VM, McCormick JJ: Chem Biol Interact 29:43–56, 1980.
18. Yang LL, Maher VM, McCormick JJ: Proc Natl Acad Sci USA 77:5933–5937, 1980.
19. Warren W, Lawley PD: Carcinogenesis 1:67–78, 1980.

Biochemical and Molecular Epidemiology of Cancer 419–426 (1986)

Cells From Xeroderma Pigmentosum Variants Are Abnormally Sensitive to Transformation by UV, but Their Excision Repair Is "Error Free"

J. Justin McCormick, Suzanne Kateley-Kohler, Masami Watanabe, and Veronica M. Maher

Carcinogenesis Laboratory, Department of Microbiology, and Department of Biochemistry, Michigan State University, East Lansing, Michigan 48824-1316

One class of xeroderma pigmentosum (XP) patients, known as XP variants, inherit the characteristic predisposition to sunlight-induced skin cancer, but unlike the majority of XP patients, their cells do not exhibit a deficiency in the rate of excision repair of ultraviolet (UV) radiation-induced DNA damage. XP variant cells are only slightly more sensitive to killing by 254 nm UV radiation or simulated sunlight. But they are much more sensitive than normal to the induction of mutations by these agents. Their sensitivity to UV-induced transformation to anchorage independence was investigated. Low doses of UV (2 to 4.5 J/m^2), doses that resulted in little or no measureable transformation in normal cells, caused a dose-dependent increase in the frequency of anchorage-independent XP variant cells. Doses of 6 to 8 J/m^2 were required to elicit a comparable response in the normal fibroblasts. Even when the two kinds of cells were compared at doses adjusted to give equal cytotoxicity, the frequency of transformation in the XP variant cells was higher than normal. Thus, their sensitivity to induction of anchorage independence paralleled their sensitivity to UV-induced mutations. To see if this was the result of an "error-prone" excision repair process, synchronized populations of cells were irradiated under conditions that allowed various lengths of time for excision repair before the onset of DNA synthesis (S phase) and assayed the frequency of 6-thioguanine–resistant cells induced. Both kinds of cells irradiated at the beginning of S phase showed high frequencies; those irradiated in

Abbreviations used: G_1, period in the cell cycle between mitosis and S phase or following G_0 but before S phase; G_0, resting, noncycling state (in this study, entrance into G_0 resulted from density inhibition of cell replication); NF, normal fibroblasts initiated from foreskin of normal neonates; S or S phase, semiconservative DNA synthesis period; TG, 6-thioguanine; XP, xeroderma pigmentosum.

Masami Watanabe's present address is Division of Radiation Biology, Faculty of Pharmaceutical Sciences, Kanazawa University, Kanazawa 920, Japan.

Received August 19, 1985.

© **1986 Alan R. Liss, Inc.**

early G_1, 12 hr prior to S, showed four times lower frequencies. However, for every time point, the frequency of mutants induced per dose of UV was significantly higher in the XP variant population than in the normal, suggesting that the XP variant cells have an abnormally error-prone process of replicating DNA on a template containing unexcised lesions or that normal cells by-pass many of such lesions using an error-free process.

Key words: XP variant, transformation, human cells, cell synchrony, error-free repair, anchorage independence, post replication repair

Xeroderma pigmentosum (XP) patients are characterized by a genetic predisposition to sunlight-induced skin cancer [1]. Skin fibroblasts from the majority of such patients are very deficient in nucleotide excision repair of DNA damage induced by 254 nm UV radiation [1–3] and are abnormally sensitive to the killing and mutagenic effects of UV [4–7] or simulated sunlight [7]. But cells from one set of XP patients, designated XP variants, carry out excision repair of UV-induced DNA damage at the normal rate [1,3,8], and yet, if exposed to sunlight, the patients develop the clinical characteristics of the disease. We and others showed previously that fibroblasts from XP variants are only slightly more sensitive than normal to the killing action of UV or simulated sunlight, but are much more sensitive to their mutagenic effect [7,9,10]. Because of the sensitivity of XP variant patients to sunlight-induced skin cancer, we compared fibroblasts from such patients with normal cells for sensitivity to the transforming effect of UV radiation. The results showed that these XP variant cells are, indeed, much more easily transformed to anchorage independence by low doses of UV than are normal cells. To see if this abnormal sensitivity resulted from mutations (errors) being introduced in the XP variant cells, we irradiated them under conditions that allowed various lengths of time for excision repair before DNA replication and measured the frequency of mutants induced. If excision repair in these cells were "error prone," allowing them time for excision before DNA replication should not reduce the frequency of mutants. If excision repair were "error free," the frequency of mutants should decrease with time allowed for excision before replication begins, just as it does in normal cells [4].

MATERIALS AND METHODS

Cells and Medium

XP variant cells, XP4BE, were obtained from the American Tissue Culture Collection; normal fibroblasts were initiated from foreskin material. Unless otherwise specified, the medium used was modified Ham's F10 medium lacking hypoxanthine, supplemented with 15% fetal bovine serum for XP4BE or 10% for normal cells.

Cell Synchronization

Cells were synchronized as previously described [4] by release from confluence and plating at a density of 10^4 cells per cm^2. The time of onset of S phase was determined using incorporation of tritiated thymidine as previously described [11].

UV Irradiation

Cells were irradiated attached to the surface of 100 mm diameter dishes. The medium was removed and the cells rinsed and irradiated with an incident dose of 0.1 or 0.2 J/m^2 per sec. After irradiation, they were refed with fresh medium and, unless treated at confluence (G_0 state), allowed to undergo cell replication in the original dishes.

Cytotoxicity Assay

The cytotoxic effect of irradiation was determined by comparing the cloning efficiency of the treated populations with that of the untreated controls [12]. Except for the confluent G_0 populations, cells were irradiated at cloning densities and allowed to form colonies in situ as described [12]. Those irradiated in G_0 were plated at cloning densities immediately or after the designated period of time postirradiation [11].

Transformation Protocol

Cells in exponential growth were plated into 100 mm diameter dishes at 1 to 5×10^5 cells per dish (10 dishes per dose) so that there was sufficient room for the surviving population to undergo cell replication for 5 days following UV irradiation without reaching confluence. A second series of dishes were plated at a twofold higher density. After irradiation cells were allowed to replicate exponentially. The denser populations were pooled on day 4 and 10^6 cells were plated at a lower density to continue multiplying for 4 or 5 additional days before being pooled and assayed for anchorage independence and/or TG resistance (day 8 or 9) as previously described [6,13]. On day 5 following irradiation, the set originally plated at the lower densities was pooled and assayed for anchorage independence.

Anchorage Independence Assay

The cells (5×10^4 or 10^5), suspended in 1.5 or 3 ml of Ham's F10 medium containing 0.33% Noble agar (top agar), were plated into 10 or more 60 mm diameter dishes containing 5 ml of freshly solidified bottom agar (made with the same medium, but containing 2% Noble agar). Additional medium was added weekly as needed to make up for evaporation. The dishes were incubated at 37°C in 3% CO_2 and 97% air in a humidity as close to 99% as possible. After 3 to 4 wks, the frequency of transformation was determined from the number of agar colonies with a diameter equal to or greater than 60 μm, as determined with an inverted microscope equipped with an ocular micrometer.

Mutagenesis Assay

The procedures for measuring the induction of mutations have been described [11,12]. Briefly, at the end of an 8–9 day expression period, cells were pooled and ~ 2×10^6 cells plated in TG medium at 400 cells/cm^2. The cloning efficiency of the cells at the time of selection was also determined. The mutant frequency was determined from the number of TG-resistant colonies corrected for the number of clonable cells plated. The cloning efficiency of the XP cells ranged from 16% to 45%; that of the normal cells ranged from 25% to 89%.

RESULTS
Sensitivity of XP Variants to UV Transformation

Figure 1 compares the sensitivity of the XP4BE variant cells with that of several normal cell lines to the cytotoxic, mutagenic, and transforming effects of UV. The

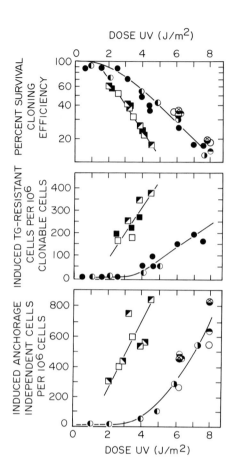

Fig. 1. Cytotoxicity, mutagenicity, and transforming activity of UV radiation in XP4BE variant cells (squares) and normal human fibroblasts (circles). Cells were irradiated in exponential growth. The frequency of TG-resistant cells was assayed after 8 or 9 days of expression and that of anchorage-independent cells after 5 to 9 days. The background frequencies of TG-resistant cells and AI cells have been subtracted. The frequencies of TG-resistant cells have been corrected for cloning efficiency. Reprinted from McCormick et al [13], with permission.

XP4BE cells were significantly more sensitive than normal to UV-induced transformation to anchorage independence. Low doses (2 to 4 J/m^2), which in the normal cells resulted in little or no increase in frequency of AI cells, gave a dose-dependent, linear increase in frequency of AI cells in the XP4BE population. These low doses also induced a linear, dose-dependent increase in the frequency of TG-resistant cells in the XP4BE population, but little or no increase in the normal cells. Even if the data for the XP4BE cells and the normal cells at doses that cause equal cytotoxicity, eg at a 37% survival dose, are compared, the frequency of transformation (AI cells) was significantly higher in the XP4BE cells than in the normal population. This relationship is also true for the mutation frequencies.

Evidence That Excision Repair in the Variant Cells is "Error Free"

Populations of normal and XP4BE cells in the G_0 state were released from confluence and assayed for the time of onset of S phase. The data in Figure 2 show

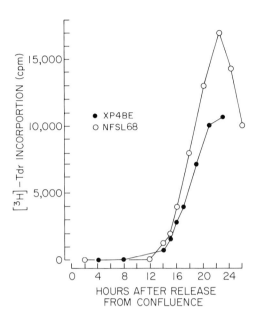

Fig. 2. Time of onset of DNA synthesis in cells synchronized by release from confluence. Reprinted from Watanabe et al [11], with permission.

that for normal cells and XP4BE cells plated at 10^4 cells/cm^2, DNA synthesis began after ~ 16 hr. Therefore, populations were released from confluence at different times so as simultaneously to irradiate one set of cells just at the onset of S phase (16 hr after release from G_0) and one set in early G_1, ~ 12 hr away from S phase (4 hr after release). Similarly, we arranged for cells to have 16 hr or more for excision repair before the onset of S phase by irradiating cells in the G_0 state (confluent) and plating them at lower density (10^4 cells/cm^2) immediately or after various periods of time in confluence.

The results (Fig. 3, lower panels) showed that allowing time for excision repair prior to S decreased the frequency of mutants in *both* kinds of cells. Cells treated just prior to the onset of S showed the highest frequencies. Cells treated in early G_1 at the same density 12 or 18 hr prior to the onset of DNA synthesis showed a much lower frequency of mutants. The frequencies were still lower when cells were irradiated in confluence (G_0) and allowed 24 or 48 hr for excision repair before onset of S phase. The data indicate that, just as in normal cells, excision repair of UV-induced lesions in XP4BE cells is essentially "error free," that is, excision decreases the frequency of mutants by eliminating potentially mutagenic lesions.

Nevertheless, comparison of the data in the left and right lower panels of Figure 3 indicates that UV-induced lesions remaining unexcised in the DNA of XP variant cells at the time they begin DNA synthesis always result in much higher frequency of induced mutants than in normal human cells.

The upper left panel of Figure 3 shows that synchronized populations of XP4BE cells irradiated in situ at cloning densities ~ 12 hr prior to S exhibited essentially the same survival as cells irradiated in situ just before S. In other words, unlike mutage-

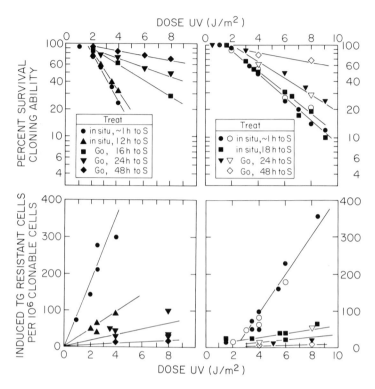

Fig. 3. Cytotoxicity and mutagenicity of UV in cells treated under conditions allowing various lengths of time postirradiation before the onset of S phase. Left panels, XP4BE cells; right panels, normal cells. The XP4BE cells were synchronized by release from confluence, plated at 10^4 cells/cm^2, and irradiated 16 hr later (1 hr to S) or 4 hr later (12 hr to S). Alternatively, they were irradiated at confluence and released immediately (16 hr to S) or after 8 hr (24 hr to S) or 32 hr (48 hr to S). The data for the normal cells shown were obtained using this same protocol (open symbols) or from populations plated at a density that allowed 24 hr before S began (closed symbols). Reprinted from Watanabe et al [11], with permission.

nicity, cytotoxicity is not S-phase dependent. This is also the result obtained with normal human cells (Fig. 3, upper right panel) [4]. Note, however, that the XP4BE cells irradiated at the G_1/S border or in early G_1 were slightly more sensitive than normal cells to killing by UV. This was reported earlier for asynchronously growing cells [7,9].

When irradiated in the G_0 state (at confluence) and immediately plated at cloning densities, both kinds of cells exhibited a higher survival than when plated at low densities and irradiated 4 to 6 hr later. In Figure 3, see curve labeled "16 h to S" for XP4BE cells (upper left panel) and "24 h to S" for normal cells (upper right panel). Part of this apparent "resistance" of cells irradiated in confluence can be attributed to a lower effective dose of UV caused by the crowding that occurs [cf, 4]. Holding XP4BE cells in the G_0 resting state for 8 hr (24 hr to S) or 32 hr (48 hr to S) before plating them at cloning density allowed time postirradiation for excision repair and resulted in still higher survival (Fig. 3, upper left panel), just as it does for the normal cells (Fig. 3, upper right panel). No such change in survival occurs in excision repair-deficient XP12BE cells [4,5]. Thus, excision repair that takes place before the XP4BE cells in G_0 are released to proceed through the cells cycle also decreases the lethal effects of UV.

DISCUSSION

XP4BE variant cells, like excision repair-deficient cells [6] can be transformed to anchorage independence by much lower doses of UV than are required for normal cells. Thus, their sensitivity to transformation parallels their sensitivity to UV-induced mutations. The inability of excision repair-deficient XP cells to remove UV-induced DNA damage at the normal rate could account for their abnormal sensitivity to mutations and transformation by UV. However, cells from XP variant patients, unlike cells from the majority of XP patients, have normal rates of excision repair [1–3]. The mechanism(s) responsible for the abnormal sensitivity of the XP variant cells to induction of mutations and anchorage independence by UV are not known. However, the data in Figure 3 suggest that excision repair in normal and XP variant cells is equally error free and that the abnormally high frequency of mutants induced by UV in the XP4BE cells is not the result of mutations being put in by the excision repair process.

Although the nature of the mechanism causing higher than normal frequencies of mutants (TG-resistant cells) in the XP variant cells is not known, the same mechanism could account for the higher frequency of transformed AI cells. We speculate that during DNA replication on a damaged template either the XP variant cells use an abnormally error-prone process to by-pass such lesions or normal cells possess a special error free mechanism for by-passing some of the UV induced lesions while using the same mechanism or process as the XP4BE cells for replicating past the remaining damage [11]. This would result in more mutations and, by analogy, more transformation events, being "fixed" (made permanent) in the XP variant cell per dose of UV than in normal cells.

Experimental evidence in support of either hypothesis is lacking. However, it is known that in XP variant cells, initiation and chain elongation are more readily blocked by pyrimidine dimers than in normal cells or in excision repair-deficient XP cells [14–16]. This is the case in spite of the XP variant cells' ability to carry out nucleotide excision repair at the normal rate [1–3].

In summary, the data indicate that XP variant cells, XP4BE, are abnormally sensitive to transformation to anchorage independence induced by UV when compared on the basis of an equal number of DNA lesions, but also when compared on the basis of equal cytotoxicity. This finding, taken together with data showing that this relationship is also true for mutation induction and that excision repair-deficient XP cells also are abnormally sensitive to transformation [6], supports the hypothesis that transformation to anchorage independence results from damage to DNA.

ACKNOWLEDGMENTS

We thank Carol Howland for typing this manuscript. The excellent technical assistance of Mechthild Howell, P. Ann Ryan, and Linda A. Stafford is gratefully acknowledged. This research was supported in part by DHHS NIH grants CA21289 and CA21253 from the National Cancer Institute and by a grant from the Women's Auxiliary of the Veterans of Foreign Wars.

REFERENCES

1. Robbins JH, Kraemer KH, Lutzner MA, Festoff BW, Coon HG: Ann Intern Med 80:221, 1974.
2. Cleaver JE, Bootsma B: Annu Rev Genet 9:19, 1975.
3. Zelle B, Lohman PH: Mutat Res 62:363, 1979.
4. Konze-Thomas B, Hazard RM, Maher VM, McCormick JJ: Mutat Res 94:421, 1982.
5. Maher VM, Dorney DJ, Mendrala AL, Konze-Thomas B, McCormick JJ: Mutat Res 62:311, 1979.
6. Maher VM, Rowan LA, Silinskas KC, Kateley SA, McCormick JJ: Proc Natl Acad Sci USA 79:2613, 1982.
7. Patton JD, Rowan LA, Mendrala AL, Howell JN, Maher VM, McCormick JJ: Photochem Photobiol 39:37, 1984.
8. Cleaver JE: J Invest Dermatol 58:124, 1972.
9. Maher VM, Ouellette LM, Curren RD, McCormick JJ: Nature 261:593, 1976.
10. Myhr BC, Turnbull D, DiPaolo JA: Mutat Res 62:341, 1979.
11. Watanabe M, Maher VM, McCormick JJ: Mutat Res 146:285, 1985.
12. McCormick JJ, Maher VM: In Friedberg EC, Hanawalt PC (eds): "DNA Repair, A Laboratory Manual of Research Procedures." New York: Marcel Dekker, 1981, pp 501–521.
13. McCormick JJ, Kateley-Kohler S, Watanabe M, Maher VM: Cancer Res 46:489, 1986.
14. Cleaver JE, Thomas GH, Park SD: Biochim Biophys Acta 564:122, 1979.
15. Kaufmann WK, Cleaver JE: J Mol Biol 149:171, 1981.
16. Park SK, Cleaver JE: Proc Natl Acad Sci USA 76:3927, 1979.

Biochemical and Molecular Epidemiology of Cancer 427–440 (1986)

Investigations on the DNA Lesions Responsible for Alkylating Agent-Induced Mutagenesis

Linda B. Couto, Edward L. Loechler, Calvert L. Green, and John M. Essigmann

Laboratory of Toxicology, Department of Applied Biological Sciences, Massachusetts Institute of Technology, Cambridge, Massachusetts 02139

The DNA lesions responsible for mutagenesis by methylating agents are examined from two perspectives. As one approach, a bacterial plasmid, pSTR2, containing the ribosomal S12 gene was used as the target for chemically induced mutagenesis by N-methyl-N-nitrosourea. After chemical treatment of plasmid and transformation of *Escherichia coli*, cells containing mutant progeny plasmids were selected by vitrue of their resistance to the antibiotic streptomycin. The frequency of streptomycin-resistant transformed cells was linearly dependent on the dose of alkylating agent to the plasmid. Treatment of alkylated plasmid with purified O^6-methylguanine DNA methyltransferase reduced the level of O^6-methylguanine by 99% without affecting the levels of other methylated purines. Transformation of *E coli* with alkylated plasmids treated with the methyltransferase reduced mutagenesis by 98% compared to controls not treated with the repair protein, indicating that lesions sensitive to *in vitro* repair by this protein (eg, O^6-methylguanine) were likely to have been responsible for mutagenesis. In the second part of this study, the role of O^6-methylguanine in mutagenesis was examined more specifically. An

Abbreviations used: O^6-MeGua, O^6-methylguanine; O^6-methylguanine-M13mp8, genome of M13mp8 in which the first guanine of the *Pst*I site was replaced with O^6-MeGua; MF, mutation frequency; AP, apurinic acid; ss, single stranded; ds, double stranded; LB, Luria broth; Gua, guanine; 3-MeAde, 3-methyladenine; 3-MeGua, 3-methylguanine; 7-MeGua, 7-methylguanine; O^4-MeThy, O^4-methylthymine; MNNG, N-methyl-N'-nitro-N-nitrosoguanidine; MNU, N-methyl-N-nitrosourea; MT, O^6-methylguanine DNA methyltransferase; Str, streptomycin; Str^R, streptomycin resistant; Str^S, streptomycin sensitive; Tc, tetracycline; Tc^R, tetracycline resistant; WT, wild type.

Linda B. Couto's present address is Department of Pathology, Stanford University School of Medicine, Stanford, CA 94305.

Edward L. Loechler's present address is Department of Biology, Boston University, Boston, MA 02215.

Calvert L. Green's present address is AMGen, Inc., Thousand Oaks, CA 91320-1789.

Received May 28, 1985.

© **1986 Alan R. Liss, Inc.**

oligonucleotide was synthesized containing O^6-methylguanine as the only modified base and, using recombinant DNA techniques, this oligonucleotide was built into the unique *PstI* site in the genome of the virus M13mp8. After introduction of this vector into *E coli*, progeny phage were produced, of which 0.4% were found to be mutated in their *PstI* site. To determine the impact of DNA repair on mutagenesis, levels of O^6-methylguanine DNA methyltransferase were depleted in host cells for viral replication by treatment with N-methyl-N′-nitro-N-nitrosoguanidine prior to uptake of the site-specifically modified genome. In these cells, the mutation frequency caused by O^6-methylguanine increased with increasing N-methyl-N′-nitro-N-nitrosoguanidine dose (the highest mutation frequency observed was approximately 20%). DNA sequence analysis of 60 mutant genomes revealed that O^6-methylguanine induced exclusively G to A transitions.

Key words: DNA repair, O^6-methylguanine, chemical mutagenesis

Chemical carcinogens are known to react at many nucleophilic sites on DNA, producing a broad spectrum of chemical-DNA lesions [1]. Some of these lesions are presumed to induce mutations, which in principle could initiate the carcinogenic process [2]. Determination of the lesion(s) responsible for the mutagenic and carcinogenic properties of a given chemical has been complicated by the fact that most carcinogens react with DNA to produce multiple DNA-bound forms. Probably the most extreme example of this is observed with methylating agents, which produce at least 15 different DNA adducts [1].

Methylating agents that react through a monomolecular nucleophilic substitution pathway (S_N1), eg, N-methyl-N-nitrosourea (MNU), can react at both nitrogen and oxygen atoms on the DNA molecule [3]. In contrast, methylating agents that interact through a bimolecular substitution pathway (S_N2), eg, methyl methanesulfonate, react very poorly at DNA oxygens, with the result that virtually all alkyl adducts form at nitrogen atoms. Chemicals reacting by the S_N1 pathway have been shown to be more mutagenic [1] and carcinogenic [3] than chemicals reacting by the S_N2 mechanism. In addition, mutagenesis by chemicals reacting by the S_N1 mechanism has been shown to be independent of induced error-prone repair processes [4,5]. Among other evidence, the higher mutagenic potency of S_N1-type methylating agents has been taken to indicate that the mutagenic activity of these agents is due principally to adducts involving DNA oxygens.

Of the numerous lesions produced by methylating agents, the adduct resulting from methylation at the O^6 position of guanine is thought to be principally responsible for mutagenesis. This lesion has been indirectly implicated with mutagenesis *in vivo* [6–8], and it has been shown to be directly responsible for mutagenesis when added as the deoxynucleoside triphosphate precursor for *in vitro* replication of bacteriophage [9] or plasmid [10] DNA. Because its formation fixes guanine in the enol tautomer, O^6-methylguanine (O^6-MeGua) has been predicted to cause mispairing with thymine [11], and this has been demonstrated *in vitro* [12–14]. Methylation at the O^4 position of thymine has also been shown to result in mispairing to guanine in *in vitro* systems [15,16], although the role of this adduct in *in vivo* mutagenesis has not yet been established. Nevertheless, O^4-ethylthymine has been shown to accumulate in hepatocyte DNA of rats experiencing chronic treatment with diethylnitrosamine, suggesting a possible role for this lesion in the initiation of the hepatocellular carcinomas produced by this treatment [17]. These data, together with other evidence, have pointed to methylation at the O^6 position of guanine and/or the O^4 position of thymine as likely significant chemical reactions in the mutagenicity induced by S_N1-type methylating agents.

We have developed two complementary experimental approaches for studying the roles that O^6-MeGua and O^4-methylthymine (O^4-MeThy) play in methylating agent mutagenesis. The first approach involves generalized mutagenesis of an extra-chromosomal vector by treatment of the naked DNA with a direct-acting methylating agent. This vector is a plasmid genome that contains a gene in which chemically induced forward mutations can be sensitively detected. The level of mutagenesis induced by chemical damage of the plasmid can be determined both before and after treatment of the plasmid with purified repair proteins known to remove selectively certain alkyl adducts. This analysis enables determination of the relative contribution to total mutagenesis of the lesions removed by *in vitro* repair. To define more precisely the relative involvement of individual lesions in mutagenesis, a second experimental approach is taken. Specifically, a short piece of DNA containing a known alkyl adduct is chemically synthesized. This modified oligonucleotide is inserted into a single-strand (ss) region created using recombinant DNA techniques at an exact site in the genome of a bacterial virus or plasmid. The monoadducted genome is then introduced into a bacterial host, where the single lesion is processed in a presumably normal manner by the cell's replication and repair systems. Finally, mutants generated by misreplication or misrepair of the adduct are selected and characterized. These studies establish the exact relationship between the structure of the adduct and the structure of the mutation it creates *in vivo*. In this article, we describe the use of these complementary approaches in an investigation of the lesions(s) responsible for mutagenesis induced by MNU.

MATERIALS AND METHODS
Cells, DNA Vectors, and Materials

Escherichia coli 6451 was obtained from D. Baltimore, Massachusetts Institute of Technology. Plasmid pKH47 was purchased from Bethesda Reasearch Laboratories; plasmid pNO1523 was obtained from D. Dean and M. Nomura, University of Wisconsin; plasmid pSTR2 was constructed in this laboratory. Plasmid pSTR2 contains the tetracycline resistance (Tc^R) gene of pKH47 and the *E coli rpsL* gene of pNO1523 (under the control of its natural promoter); the latter gene encodes a ribosomal protein (protein S12) that confers streptomycin sensitivity (Str^S) to the cell. The details of the construction of plasmid pSTR2 will be presented elsewere. ^{3}H-MNU was purchased from Amersham. Nonradioactively labeled MNU was the gift of G. Buchi, Massachusetts Institute of Technology, and the 19 Kdal fragment of *E coli* O^6-methylguanine DNA methyltransferase (MT) was the gift of B. Demple, Harvard University. The following base standards were purchased from commercial sources: guanine (Gua) and 7-methylguanine (7-MeGua) from Sigma Chemical Company (St. Louis, MO); 1-methyladenine (1-MeAde) and 6-methyladenine (6-MeAde) from Fluka, AG (Bucks, Switzerland); 3-methyladenine (3-MeAde) from Cyclo Chemicals (Los Angeles, CA); 3-methylguanine (3-MeGua) from Vega Biochemicals (Tucson, AZ); adenine (Ade) from P.L. Biochemicals (Milwaukee, WI); 7-methyladenine (7-MeAde) was provided by A. Chin, Battelle Memorial Institute (Columbus, OH). O^6-MeGua was the gift of P. Newberne, Massachusetts Institute of Technology. All other strains and materials were as previously described [18].

Methylation of Plasmid pSTR2 DNA

Plasmid DNA was methylated by MNU (0,15,25, and 50 mM) in 0.2 M Na cacodylate, pH 6.9, at 37°C for 1 hr at a DNA concentration of 0.3 μg/ml. In experiments using radiolabeled MNU, the specific activity was 0.16 Ci/mmol.

O^6-Methylguanine DNA Methyltransferase Treatment of Methylated pSTR2 DNA

Methylated plasmid (25 mM MNU) DNA (200 μg; 900 pmol O^6-MeGua) was incubated with 9,300 units of MT at 37°C for 30 min in 50 mM HEPES, pH 7.8, 15 mM DTT, 1 mM EDTA, and 50 μM spermidine, in a total volume of 13.7 ml. In a parallel control reaction, methylated plasmid DNA (245 μg) was incubated under the same conditions but in the absence of MT. Following incubation, the reaction mixtures were extracted sequentially with an equal volume of phenol (saturated with 10 mM Tris-HCl, pH 8.0, 1 mM EDTA), chloroform:isoamyl alcohol (24:1), and ether; the DNA was then ethanol precipitated.

Methylated Base Analysis

Chemically modified plasmid DNA was analyzed for the presence of methylated purines by hydrolyzing the DNA under mild acidic conditions [19]. The DNA hydrolysates were adjusted to pH 5 and injected onto a Durrum DC4A cation exchange HPLC column (0.2 × 25 cm) and eluted at 0.3 ml/min with 0.1 M ammonium formate, pH 5.1. After 30 min of isocratic elution, the composition of the mobile phase was programmed over 20 min to 0.1 M ammonium phosphate, pH 7.7, and maintained at this composition for 50 min. The UV absorbance of the chromatographic effluent was monitored at 254 nm, and fractions were collected for liquid scintillation counting.

Mutation Assay Based on Plasmid pSTR2

MM294A cells were transformed by chemically modified and unmodified plasmid DNAs by using a modification of the protocol of Mandel and Higa [20]. In general, MNU–treated and untreated plasmid DNAs (5–10 μg) were mixed with 2 ml competent MM294A cells (approximately 8 × 10^9 cells), and the mixture was placed on ice for 1 hr. The mixture was then heat shocked at 42°C for 90 sec and cooled on ice. The mixture was added to 20 ml Luria broth (LB) and incubated at 37°C for 90 min. Subsequently, a portion of the transformation mixture was removed for plating on LB plates containing 20 μg/ml tetracycline (Tc) to determine the number of cells transformed by the plasmid. The remainder of the mixture was allowed to incubate for 1 or 4 hr, at which time Tc was added to a final concentration of 20 μg/ml. Following a 30 min incubation period, 80 ml of LB containing 20 μg/ml Tc was added, and the culture was allowed to grow to stationary phase overnight. Plasmid DNA was isolated from the overnight culture and purified by CsCl-EtBr banding [21]. Five to 10 μg of the purified plasmid DNA was used to transform competent 6451 cells (approximately 8 × 10^9 cells). Following the transformation, cells were plated in the presence of Tc to determine the total number of transformed cells. By plating in the presence of both Tc and Str, the subpopulation of plasmid-transformed cells that possessed gene inactivation mutations in the *rpsL* gene were selected. The mutation frequency was calculated as the ratio of colonies arising in the presence of both Tc and Str to colonies forming in the presence of Tc alone.

Site-Specific Incorporation of a Tetranucleotide Containing O^6-Methylguanine Into a Viral Genome

The chemical synthesis of the tetranucleotide 5'-$_{HO}$Tpm^{6}GpCpA-3' has been previously described (m^{6}G = O^6-methyldeoxyguanosine) [22]. This oligonucleotide was incorporated as part of the unique *PstI* site in the genome of the virus M13mp8 [23], and the *in vivo* mutagenicity of O^6-MeGua present within the oligonucleotide was determined in MM294A cells [18]. In parallel, the mutagenic effects of O^6-MeGua were determined in MM294A cells that were depleted of MT by challenge with N-methyl-N'-nitro-N-nitrosoguanidine (MNNG) [18].

RESULTS

Plasmid pSTR2: A Forward Mutation Assay Providing a Positive Selection for the Mutant Phenotype

Plasmid pSTR2 (Fig. 1) contains the *E coli rpsL* gene, which encodes ribosomal protein S12 and represents the target used for detection of mutations induced by DNA damaging agents. Many mutations created in this genetic locus confer upon host cells the ability to survive in the presence of the antibiotic Str. In contrast, these selective conditions are lethal to cells containing nonmutant plasmids. Plasmid pSTR2 also contains the Tc^R gene, which was used to select all plasmid-transformed cells.

A generalized scheme illustrating how the mutation assay was performed is shown in Figure 2A. Plasmid pSTR2 DNA was treated *in vitro* with a chemical mutagen and then introduced into the *E coli* host cell MM294A (Str^S, recA$^+$) where lesions present in the DNA were acted upon by endogenous replication/repair systems. An aliquot of the cell suspension was plated in the presence of Tc to determine the efficiency of transformation, which is the indicator of plasmid survival after DNA damage. After growth of plasmid-transformed MM294A cells in the presence of Tc, plasmid DNA was isolated and then introduced into the *E coli* host cell 6451 (Str^R, recA$^-$). (For detection of mutant plasmids, the use of a Str^R second host was necessary, because the Str^S phenotype is dominant to Str^R.) Following transformation, one portion of the cell suspension was plated in the presence of Tc and a second in the presence of both Tc and Str. All transformed cells grew in the presence of Tc, whereas only cells containing plasmids mutated in the *rpsL* gene were capable of growing in the presence of both antibiotics. Acquisition of Str^R enables facile selection of a small number of mutants present in a large wild-type background.

Mutagenesis by N-Methyl-N-Nitrosourea

The use of the *rpsL* gene encoded on plasmid pSTR2 to detect mutation was evaluated by treating plasmid DNA with increasing doses of MNU (0, 15, 25, and 50 mM) and performing the mutation assay described above. A portion of the MNU-treated DNAs was acid hydrolyzed and analyzed by HPLC for the presence of Gua, Ade, and 7-MeGua. In this experiment, the level of 7-MeGua in hydrolysates of methylated DNA was determined by comparison with a known standard. The level of this base was used to estimate total DNA methylation (it was determined empirically that 7-MeGua represented 69% of the total methylation products under the conditions of these experiments; data not shown).

The results of the mutation assay are shown in Figure 3, in which plasmid survival and mutant fractions at increasing levels of plasmid DNA modification are

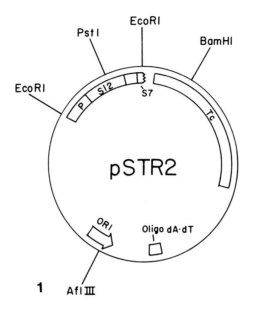

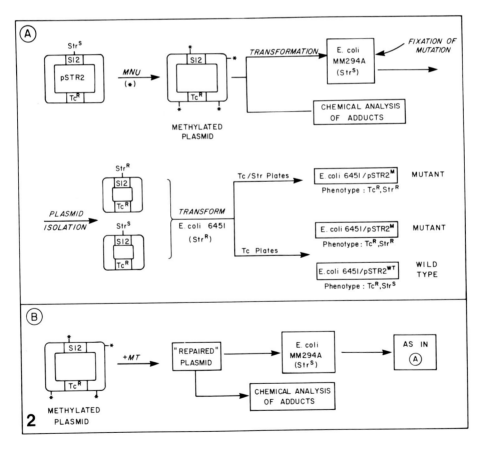

presented. A linear increase in mutation frequency was found with increasing methylation of plasmid DNA. A corresponding decrease in plasmid survival was also observed. A level of DNA modification of 81 adducts per pSTR2 genome resulted in 37% survival, which represented approximately one lethal hit. These results indicate that plasmid pSTR2 can be used to detect chemically induced mutagenesis in a dose-dependent manner. Reconstruction experiments (to be described elsewhere) were performed to determine if there was a bias in the quantitative determination of the Str^R mutants. A 13-fold bias in favor of cells containing mutant plasmids was found, and the data in Figure 3 and Table I were adjusted accordingly. The bias does not interfere with the interpretation of the data presented below.

Mutagenesis of MNU-Treated pSTR2 Following *In Vitro* Repair With O^6-Methylguanine DNA Methyltransferase

O^6-MeGua and O^4-MeThy are the principal lesions thought to be responsible for methylating agent-induced mutagenesis [6–16]. To investigate selectively the role of these lesions in mutagenesis, in our experiments methylated plasmid DNA was treated with MT, the DNA repair protein that removes the methyl group from O^6-MeGua and O^4-MeThy [24–27]. Plasmid pSTR2 DNA was treated with 25 mM ^{3}H-MNU, and then a portion of the treated DNA was incubated with MT (Fig. 2B). Both MT-treated and untreated DNAs were acid hydrolyzed and analyzed for the presence of methylated purines (with the exception of 1-methyl- and N^2-methylguanine) by HPLC. Hydrolysates of methylated DNA were coinjected with a mixture of methylated bases (7-MeAde, O^6-MeGua, 3-MeGua, 6-MeAde, 3-MeAde, and 1-MeAde), and chromatographic peaks corresponding to these bases were monitored by UV absorbance. Guanine, Ade, and 7-MeGua were monitored directly in hydrolysates of alkylated plasmid, without the addition of standards. Radioactivity coeluting at the position of the methylated bases was used to determine the binding level of each methylated base in MNU-treated DNA.

Both MT-treated and untreated plasmid DNAs were used in the pSTR2 mutation assay described above. Table I compares the level of methylated bases per pSTR2 genome with the observed mutant fractions. The data indicate that the only methylated base detectably affected by the MT treatment was O^6-MeGua. Specifically, the level of O^6-MeGua decreased by 99% (it is also expected that the MT protein removed the methyl group from O^4-MeThy [26,27], but this was not determined because the amount of radioactivity in the alkylated plasmid was insufficient to permit accurate measurement of this base). The loss of O^6-MeGua from methylated DNA correlated

---

Fig. 1. Plasmid pSTR2. This plasmid contains the gene encoding *E coli* ribosomal protein S12, DNA encoding the amino terminal portion of ribosomal protein S7, and the natural promoter of these genes. The gene encoding protein S12 is the marker used to detect chemically induced mutations. The plasmid also contains a gene that confers tetracycline (Tc) resistance to cells; this gene is the marker used to determine transformation.

Fig. 2. Mutation assay using plasmid pSTR2 as target for mutation. A. The steps involved in the mutation assay using plasmid pSTR2 as the mutagenic target are described in Materials and Methods. pSTR2^{WT} refers to wild-type pSTR2 plasmid DNA, and pSTR2^M refers to mutant pSTR2 plasmid DNA. B. "Repaired DNA" refers to plasmid DNA that contains all methylated bases produced by MNU except the DNA lesions removed by the O^6-methylguanine DNA methyltransferase (ie, O^6-MeGua and O^4-MeThy).

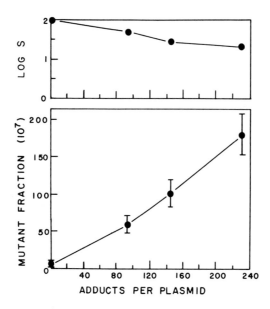

Fig. 3. Evaluation of plasmid pSTR2 as target for mutation. Plasmid pSTR2 was treated with increasing doses of MNU, as described in the text, and used in the mutation assay illustrated in Figure 2. Survival was measured as the total number of Tc[R] colonies following transformation of MM294A cells. Mutant fractions were determined by the ratio of Tc[R], Str[R] colonies to Tc[R] colonies following transformation of 6451 cells. Triplicate mutation assays were performed for each dose of MNU used. Mutation data represent mean $\pm$ 2 SD; S is the relative surviving fraction.

TABLE I. Effect of *In Vitro* Repair by O[6]-Methylguanine DNA Methyltransferase on MNU-Induced Mutagenesis*

DNA Treatment		Survival (%)	Mutant fraction (10^7)	Adducts per pSTR2 genome						
MNU	MT			7G	O[6]G	7A	3G	3A	1A	AP
0	–	100	9							
25	–	22	380 $\pm$ 28	100	13	1.5	1.2	10.6	0.3	19
25	+	22	8 $\pm$ 2	112	0.14	2.1	1.3	10	0.2	21

*Plasmid pSTR2 DNA was treated with 25 mM ^{3}H-MNU in 0.2 M Na cacodylate, pH 6.9, at 37°C for 1 hr. A portion of the methylated DNA was treated with O[6]-methylguanine DNA methyltransferase (MT). Both MT-treated and untreated DNAs were hydrolyzed and analyzed by HPLC for methylated purines. Analytical results are the average of duplicate chromatographic analyses. In parallel, MT-treated and untreated DNAs were used in a mutation assay, as described in the text. Mutation data are the average of duplicate (no MNU) or triplicate (25 mM MNU) mutation assays. These data have been corrected for a 13-fold bias in favor of mutant cells, which was detected in reconstruction experiments. Data reported are means $\pm$ 2SD.

almost exactly with the decrease in the mutability of the DNA. Without MT treatment, the mutation frequency of methylated plasmid DNA was 380×10^{-7}. However, methylated plasmid DNA that had been repaired *in vitro* by the MT protein had a mutation frequency approximately equal to background (8×10^{-7}). The decrease in the mutation frequency (98%) with MT treatment correlated with the decrease in the level of O[6]-MeGua in the DNA (99%). On the basis of this result, it was concluded from this experiment that lesions sensitive to the O^6-methylguanine repair protein (ie, O^6-MeGua and O^4-MeThy) are the principal mutagens in DNA treated with MNU.

Mutagenesis by O^6-Methylguanine

The studies described above suggest that two DNA adducts, O^6-MeGua and O^4-MeThy, are the likely precursor lesions to MNU-induced mutagenesis. To assess more specifically the role of these (and other) DNA lesions in chemical mutagenesis, we have developed a strategy for building individual adducts into known sites in the genomes of viruses and plasmids. By allowing these monoadducted genomes to replicate *in vivo*, pattern of mutagenesis created by normal biochemical processing of these adducts can be determined.

A complete characterization of the quantitative and qualitative nature of O^6-MeGua–induced mutagenesis was examined by building this adduct into a unique site in the genome of the *E coli* virus M13mp8 and introducing this vector into *E coli*, where mutations were fixed. A combination of chemical synthesis and recombinant DNA techniques [22,23] were used to construct genomes in which O^6-MeGua was situated at either of two positions within the unique *Pst*I recognition sequence of double-strand (ds) M13mp8 (positions 6255 or 6256) (Fig. 4A). (These DNA molecules are referred to herein as O^6-MeGua-M13mp8). A series of characterization experiments demonstrated that the O^6-MeGua residue was structurally intact and located within the *Pst*I site [23]. Double-strand O^6-MeGua-M13mp8 was constructed with a nick situated in the DNA strand opposite that containing the adduct and, upon alkali denaturation, ss, monoadducted genomes were formed. We elected to work initally with ss genomes, because the MT protein has been reported to act less effectively on ss DNA than on ds substrates [28,29].

Mutagenesis by O^6-MeGua was investigated by introducing ss O^6-MeGua-M13mp8 into *E coli* MM294A cells (Fig. 4B). A mixture of wild-type and mutant phage was produced, which was used to produce ds replicative form DNA. Mutations induced by O^6-MeGua targeted within the unique 6 base pair *Pst*I recognition site rendered the circular genomes insensitive to cleavage by this endonuclease. This property made it possible to isolate a pure mutant phage population for DNA sequencing and for calculation of mutation frequencies.

The mutation frequency of O^6-MeGua was expressed as the fraction of progeny phage possessing mutations in the *Pst*I site following transformation of *E coli* with monoadducted, ss genomes (ie, after step 2 in Fig. 4B) [18]. Because the lesion was located in either the $(+)$ or $(-)$ strand of O^6-MeGua-M13mp8, mutations were observed at positions 6255 and 6256, respectively (see Fig. 4A). As shown in Table II, the mutation frequencies of the adduct in the $(+)$ and $(-)$ strands (MF^+ and MF^-) were determined to be 0.36 and 0.08%, respectively. The sum of the values for the mutation frequencies in the individual strands is defined as the total mutation frequency of O^6-MeGua, MF^t, which was determined to be approximately 0.4%.

The mutation frequency we observed *in vivo* is several orders of magnitude less than that determined or predicted in previously published work. For example, *in vitro* studies measuring O^6-MeGua–directed misincorporation of noncomplementary nucleotides have shown that this lesion is misreplicated by DNA and RNA polymerases approximately one third of the time [12–14]. Similar and slightly higher mutagenic efficiencies of this lesion have been estimated from *in vivo* studies, in which O^6-MeGua was only one of many methylated bases present [30, 31]. The most likely

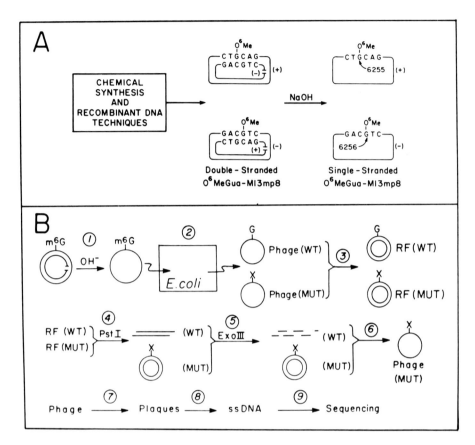

Fig. 4   A) Structures of M13mp8 genomes containing O^6-MeGua in the unique *Pst*I site. Numbers indicate positions within the phage genome modified by O^6-MeGua. B) Isolation of O^6-MeGua–derived mutants. Double-strand O^6-MeGua-M13mp8 was base denatured to give ss O^6-MeGua-M13mp8 (step 1), which then was used to transform *E coli* MM294A cells (step 2). A mixture of wild-type and mutant phage was produced (X denotes position of mutation) and used to infect JM103 cells. Replicative form DNA prepared from these phage (step 3) was treated with *Pst*I (step 4); mutant DNA remained circular, whereas wild-type molecules were linearized and subsequently selectively degraded with exonuclease III (step 5). Steps 4 and 5 were repeated, and the remaining DNA (an essentially pure mutant population) was retransfected into JM103 cells to produce phage (step 6). The ss phage genome was isolated for DNA sequencing (steps 7–9).

reason for the apparent discrepancy between our results and existing literature data is the fact that in our studies a single adduct was built into the genome, and this single lesion probably was removed quickly in *E coli* by the MT DNA repair protein.

There is an unusual characteristic of the MT protein that we were able to take advantage of to improve the likelihood that the adduct in O^6-MeGua-M13mp8 would escape repair. The MT protein acts by transferring the methyl group from O^6-MeGua in DNA to itself [25], becoming irreversibly inactivated in the process. In our studies, host cells were treated with MNNG 2 min before the O^6-MeGua-M13mp8 uptake step (step 2 of Fig. 4B). This treatment introduced O^6-MeGua residues into the host chromosome [6], and repair of these lesions depleted endogenous levels of the MT, thus diminishing the ability of the host to repair the single adduct in O^6-MeGua-

TABLE II. Mutation Frequency (%) Caused by O^6-MeGua in O^6-MeGua-M13

MNNG challenge $(\mu g/ml)^a$	O^6-MeGua-M13mp8[6]			M13mp8 MF^c
	MF^{-b}	MF^{+b}	MF^t	
0	0.08	0.36	0.4	$\leqslant 0.03$
17	1.3	4.1	5.4	$\leqslant 0.11$
33	3.6	4.7	8.3	$\leqslant 0.20$
50	4.1	13.7	17.8	$\leqslant 0.16$

[a]Some host cells for O^6-MeGua-M13mp8 replication were challenged with N-methyl-N'-nitro-N-nitrosoguanidine (MNNG) prior to DNA uptake; details are given in the text.
[b]MF^+ and MF^- are the percentage of progeny phage with O^6-MeGua-derived mutations that originated in the (+) and (−) strands, respectively; the sum of these quantities is MF^t.
[c]The upper limit of the mutation frequency of a control, which was the (+) strand of M13mp8 (this DNA did not contain O^6-MeGua at the PstI site).

M13mp8. (MNNG is known to induce several DNA repair systems, but we estimate that fixation of O^6-MeGua as a mutation occurred before their induction, and thus their effect on mutagenesis by this adduct should be small.) Pretreatment of cells with increasing doses of MNNG resulted in enhanced mutant fractions of O^6-MeGua-M13mp8 (Table II). At the highest level of MNNG treatment (50 $\mu g/ml$), MF^t had increased to almost 50 times the comparable value in unchallenged cells. The mutation frequency of this sample (approximately 20%) does not necessarily represent the inherent mutation efficiency of O^6-MeGua, because the function relating MNNG dose and mutagenesis (Table II) was still increasing at the maximum level of MNNG challenge; rather, this value represents the lower limit of the true mutation frequency of this lesion.

The nature of the mutations induced by O^6-MeGua was characterized by isolating and sequencing DNA from 60 individual mutant plaques. Figure 5 contains an autoradiogram of a DNA sequencing gel [32] and reveals the DNA sequences of the wild type and of the two mutant species in the vicinity of the PstI site of M13mp8. One mutant class showed a G to A transition mutation at genome position 6256 (shown in the leftmost lanes in Fig. 5); this class presumably arose from O^6-MeGua-M13mp8 molecules in which the adduct was located specifically in the (−) strand. The second class of O^6-MeGua–induced mutants arose presumably from the genomes in which the adduct was in the (+) strand; the data in the rightmost lanes in Figure 5 show that a C to T change had occurred and, since the sequence of the (−) strand appears in the autoradiogram, it is clear that a G to A change had occurred in the complementary (+) strand. Thus, the sequencing data are consistent with the original prediction based on model building [11] and *in vitro* data [12–14] that O^6-MeGua induces G to A transitions.

One factor that would facilitate the above type of analysis, in which mutagenesis by defined lesions is studied, would be a facile selection scheme by which mutant and wild-type genomes could be separated. We anticipate that plasmid pSTR2 will provide such a selection. One of the design features of this plasmid is a single PstI site in the coding region of the *rpsL* gene (Fig. 1). Adducts can be built directly into this site by the methodology described for M13mp8, and many mutations within this site may be selectable by virtue of their property of conferring Str^R to host cells (eg, a G to A change in the (−) strand would create an amber codon). An additional advantage of this approach over that described above is the fact that it may permit detection of

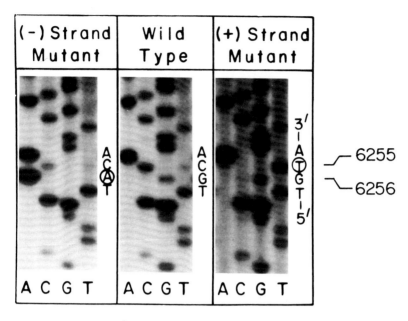

Fig. 5 DNA sequences of O⁶-MeGua–induced mutants. DNA of mutant phage was isolated and sequenced by the method of Sanger et al [32]. Shown here are autoradiograms of sequencing gels in the region of the M13mp8 genome containing the *Pst*I sites of (from left to right) (−) strand mutant, wild-type, and (+) strand mutant genomes.

mutations induced at locations distant from the site at which the adduct was originally located.

DISCUSSION

Analyses by several laboratories of the mutational specificity of S_N1-type methylating agents (eg, MNU and MNNG) have shown that these agents produce predominantly GC–AT transition mutations [33,34]. This type of analysis has aided in the development of concepts underlying the mechanism of action of these chemical agents, because it has helped to define the DNA lesions that are of potential importance in mutagenesis. However, because of the broad spectrum of DNA modifications following treatment by methylating agents, these analyses cannot permit unambiguous assignment of mutagenic effects to specific lesion(s). As reported here, we have developed two complementary experimental approaches to study the lesion(s) responsible for chemically induced mutagenesis and have described the use of these approaches to study the lesions responsible for MNU-induced mutagenesis. Our results have shown that MNU-induced mutagenesis *in vivo* is due to O⁶-MeGua and/or O⁴-MeThy and thus are in accord with the large literature in existence on alkylating agent-induced mutagenesis. In addition, we have shown that O⁶-MeGua, in isolation from all other DNA adducts, produces the same type of mutation that is predominantly observed after treatment of cells with MNU (ie, GC–AT transitions). Because methylation at the O⁴-position of thymine should result in mispairing to guanine [14,15], which should produce AT–GC but not GC–AT mutations, our results, in combination with those of Coulondre and Miller [33] and of Shinoura *et al* [34], suggest therefore that MNU-induced mutagenesis in *E coli* is likely to be due primarily to O^6-MeGua -and *not* to O^4-Methy. Moreover, because the levels of 7-MeGua, 7-MeAde, 3-MeAde, 3-MeGua and 1-MeAde did not change detectably upon MT treatment, we can rule out these lesions as having a significant role in mutagenesis.

From our work on site-specific mutagenesis, we have calculated a mutagenic efficiency for O^6-MeGua in ss DNA in the presence and in the absence of the MT repair protein. In the presence of a presumably fully competent DNA repair system, we observed approximately one mutagenic event for every 250 genomes containing O^6-MeGua residues. However, when host cells were depleted of MT, the mutation frequency increased 50-fold to about one mutagenic event for every five O^6-MeGua residues. We estimate that this value probably represents a lower limit of the true mutation efficiency of O^6-MeGua, because the mutation frequency observed at the highest level of MNNG challenge showed no evidence of leveling off (Table II). This value, however, is likely to be close to the true mutation frequency, because it is at the lower end of the range measured for mutagenesis of O^6-alkyl guanines *in vitro* [12–14], and it is within a factor of two or three of the level predicted by indirect *in vivo* measurements [30,31].

ACKNOWLEDGMENTS

For their contributions to this work, we express our gratitude to Brian Donahue, Bruce Demple, Kerry Fowler, and George Büchi. Financial support for this work was provided by grants 5 PO1 ES00597, T 32 ES07020, and CA 33821 from the NIH and by the Monsanto Fund.

REFERENCES

1. Singer B, Kusmierek JT: Annu Rev Biochem 52:655, 1982.
2. Miller EC: Cancer Res 38:1479, 1978.
3. Lawley PD: In Grover PL (ed): "Chemical Carcinogens and DNA." Boca Raton, FL: CRC Press, 1979, p 1.
4. Schendel PF, Defais M: Mol Gen Genet 177:661, 1980.
5. Shinoura Y, Ise T, Kato T, Glickman BW: Mutat Res 111:51, 1983.
6. Schendel PF, Robins PE: Proc Natl Acad Sci USA 75:6017, 1978.
7. Newbold RF, Warren W, Medcalf ASC, Amos J: Nature 283:596, 1980.
8. Beranek DT, Heflich RH, Kodel RL, Morris SM, Casciano DA: Mutat Res 110:171, 1983.
9. Dodson LA, Foote RW, Mitra S, Masker WE: Proc Natl Acad Sci USA 79:7440, 1982.
10. Eadie JS, Conrad M, Toorchen D, Topal MD: Nature 308:201, 1984.
11. Loveless A: Nature 223:205, 1969.
12. Gerchman LL, Ludlum DB: Biochim Biophys Acta 308:310, 1973.
13. Mehta JR, Ludlum DB: Biochim Biophys Acta 512:770, 1978.
14. Abbott PJ, Saffhill R: Biochim Biophys Acta 562:51, 1979.
15. Abbott PJ, Saffhill R: Nucleic Acids Res 4:761, 1977.
16. Singer B, Sagi J, Kusmierek JT: Proc Natl Acad Sci USA 80:4884, 1983.
17. Swenberg JA, Dyroff MC, Bedell MA, Popp JA, Huh N, Kirstein V, Rajewsky MF: Proc Natl Acad Sci, 81:1692, 1984.
18. Loechler EL, Green CL, Essigmann JM: Proc Natl Acad Sci USA 81:6271, 1984.
19. Lawley PD: In Montesano R, Bartsch H, Tomatis L (eds): "Screening Tests in Chemical Carcinogenesis." Lyon: IARC Scientific Publication No. 12, 1976, p 181.
20. Mandel M, Higa A: J Mol Biol 53:154, 1970.

21. Maniatis T, Fritsch EF, Sambrook J: In "Molecular Cloning, A Laboratory Manual." Cold Spring Harbor, NY: Cold Spring Harbor Laboratory, 1982, p 92.
22. Fowler KW, Büchi G, Essigmann JM: J Am Chem Soc 104: 1050, 1982.
23. Green CL, Loechler EL, Fowler KW, Essigmann JM: Proc Natl Acad Sci USA 81:13, 1984.
24. Karran P, Lindahl T, Griffin B: Nature 280:76, 1979.
25. Olsson M, Lindahl T: J Biol Chem 255:10569, 1980.
26. McCarthy TV, Karran P, Lindahl T: EMBO J 3:545, 1984.
27. Ahmmed Z, Laval J: Biochem Biophys Res Commun 120:1, 1984.
28. Lindahl T, Demple B, Robins P: EMBO J 1:1359, 1982.
29. Toorchen D, Lindamood C, Swenberg J, Topal MD: Carcinogenesis 5:1733, 1984.
30. Lawley P, Martin C: Biochem J 145:85, 1975.
31. Guttenplan J: Carcinogenesis 5:155, 1984.
32. Sanger F, Nicklen S, Coulson AR: Proc Natl Acad Sci USA 74:5463, 1977.
33. Coulondre C, Miller JH: J Mol Biol 117:577, 1977.
34. Shinoura Y, Kato T, Glickman BW: Mutat Res 111:43, 1983.

Biochemical and Molecular Epidemiology of Cancer 441–447 (1986)

Metabolic Activation of Mutagenic and Tumorigenic Dinitropyrenes

Zora Djurić, Robert H. Heflich, E. Kim Fifer, and Frederick A. Beland

National Center for Toxicological Research, Jefferson, Arkansas 72079 (Z.D., R.H.H., E.K.F., F.A.B.) and Department of Biochemistry, University of Arkansas for Medical Sciences, Little Rock, Arkansas 72205 (Z.D., F.A.B.)

Dinitropyrenes, environmental contaminants found in diesel emission, are tumorigenic in rats and mice and are among the most mutagenic compounds ever tested in the *Salmonella typhimurium* reversion assay. Incubation of *S typhimurium* TA1538 with 1,8-dinitropyrene resulted in the formation of one major DNA adduct, *N*-(deoxyguanosin-8-yl)-1-amino-8-nitropyrene. The same adduct was formed when the reduced intermediate *N*-hydroxy-1-amino-8-nitropyrene was reacted with DNA, which suggests that nitroreduction was involved in the metabolic activation of this dinitropyrene. Although 1,8-dinitropyrene was as much as 40-fold more mutagenic than 1-nitropyrene, the number of reversions per adduct induced by the C8-substituted deoxyguanosine adducts of either 1-nitropyrene or 1,8-dinitropyrene was similar. 1,8-Dinitropyrene may be more mutagenic than 1-nitropyrene because *N*-hydroxy-1-amino-8-nitropyrene served as a substrate for a bacterial transacetylase and therefore bound to DNA more efficiently than did *N*-hydroxy-1-aminopyrene, which did not appear to be a substrate for this enzyme. Similar routes of metabolic activation occurred with rat liver cytosol; 1,3-, 1,6-, and 1,8-dinitropyrene were reduced to metabolites, which were further activated by acetyl coenzyme A-dependent O-acetylation while 1-nitropyrene was not. These data indicate that nitrated pyrenes are metabolized to genotoxic products by nitroreduction and that dinitropyrenes are further activated by O-acetylation.

Key words: nitrated pyrenes, acetylation, DNA adducts, nitroreduction

Nitrated polycyclic aromatic hydrocarbons (PAHs) are ubiquitous environmental contaminants that arise from atmospheric reactions of PAHs with nitrogen oxides and from incomplete combustion processes [1,2]. Nitrated pyrenes are the predominant nitrated PAHs found in environmental samples and, among these, the dinitropyrenes (Fig. 1) are some of the most mutagenic compounds ever tested in the *Salmonella typhimurium* reversion assay [1–4]. The dinitropyrenes are also mutagenic to cultured mammalian cells [5–7] and elicit tumors in rodents [8–13].

Received May 16, 1985.

© **1986 Alan R. Liss, Inc.**

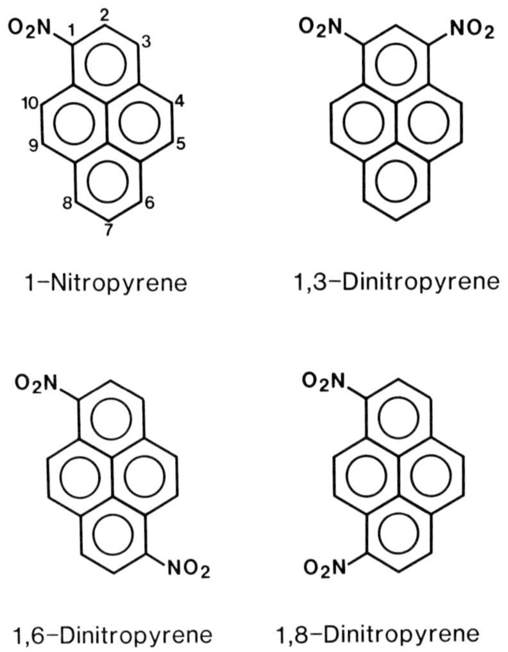

Fig. 1.   Structures of the nitrated pyrenes.

Mutagenicity testing of the dinitropyrenes in various strains of *S typhimurium* has revealed that both nitroreduction and esterification are involved in their activation to mutagens [14,15]. We have investigated this further by comparing the DNA adducts formed by 1,8-dinitropyrene in *S typhimurium* TA1538 with the adducts formed from reacting *N*-hydroxy-1-amino-8-nitropyrene with DNA. We have also compared the mutagenic efficiency of the 1,8-dinitropyrene adduct with the adduct formed from 1-nitropyrene, a related compound that is activated to a mutagen via nitroreduction but not acetylation. Finally, we have investigated the metabolic pathways in rat liver cytosol that lead to DNA-binding by dinitropyrenes.

MATERIALS AND METHODS

Tritiated nitrated pyrenes were obtained from Midwest Research Institute (Kansas City, MO), and mutagenicity testing with *S typhimurium* was performed as previously described [16]. *N*-Hydroxy-1-amino-8-nitropyrene was prepared in situ from 1-nitro-8-nitrosopyrene [17] by reaction with ascorbate using the method previously described for 1-nitrosopyrene [18]. Synthetic DNA adducts were identified by nuclear magnetic resonance and mass spectral analyses while cellular adducts were identified by their high pressure liquid chromatography (HPLC) retention times and pH partitioning profiles [19]. DNA was extracted from *S typhimurium* TA1538 after incubation with tritiated 1,8-dinitropyrene and hydrolyzed enzymatically to nucleosides as previously described [16,18]. The adducts were injected onto the HPLC column with unlabeled synthetic marker and eluted from a μBondapak-C_{18} reversed-phase column with a 30 min nonlinear gradient (Waters #2) of 20 to 65% methanol.

Rat liver cytosol, containing DNA and NADPH, was incubated with the nitrated pyrenes in the presence or absence of acetyl coenzyme A (AcCoA) as previously described [20]. Metabolites were quantified in incubations without added DNA. Briefly, 20 μM tritiated nitrated pyrene (1 Ci/mmole) was incubated under argon in a total volume of 1 ml with 50 mM sodium pyrophosphate (pH 7.4), 1 mM dithiothreitol, 1 mM NADPH, 1 mg/ml cytosolic protein, and 1 mM AcCoA. After 15 min, 1 ml of a 50/50 mixture of chloroform/methanol was added and a small aliquot of the chloroform layer, which contained $>95\%$ of the radioactivity in the incubation, was coinjected onto a μBondapak-C_{18} reversed-phase column. The metabolites were separated by HPLC using a 20 min nonlinear gradient (Waters #2) of 40 to 80% methanol and were identified by comparison of their retention times to synthetic standards and by UV and mass spectral analyses. Reactions conducted with 2 mg/ml calf thymus DNA were extracted with organic solvents, and the DNA was treated with RNases and proteases followed by additional organic extractions and precipitation. The recovered DNA was quantified by its absorbance at 260 nm and the level of binding was determined by liquid scintillation counting. Adducts formed by rat liver cytosol-catalyzed activation of the nitrated pyrenes were identified by comparison of HPLC retention times and pH partitioning profiles to synthetic standards.

RESULTS

Salmonella typhimurium TA1538 was incubated in suspension with 3 μM 1-nitropyrene or 3 μM 1,8-dinitropyrene for up to 2 hr. Under these conditions, 1,8-dinitropyrene was as much as 40-fold more mutagenic than 1-nitropyrene. Thus, after a 0.5 hr incubation, 1,8-dinitropyrene induced 681 revertants per 10^8 viable bacteria as compared to 16 revertants per 10^8 viable bacteria detected with 1-nitropyrene. The bacterial DNA was isolated, and, following enzymatic hydrolysis, the DNA adducts were analyzed by HPLC. One major adduct was observed in DNA from bacteria incubated with 1,8-dinitropyrene and this was identical to the adduct obtained from reacting *N*-hydroxy-1-amino-8-nitropyrene with DNA. The synthetic adduct was characterized by spectroscopic and chemical techniques as *N*-(deoxyguanosin-8-yl)-1-amino-8-nitropyrene. An analogous adduct has previously been identified in the DNA of *Salmonella* exposed to 1-nitropyrene [16]. When the reversion frequency was related to the adduct concentration, a linear relationship (Fig. 2) was observed and the mutagenic efficiency of the adduct derived from 1,8-dinitropyrene was similar to that previously found with the adduct from 1-nitropyrene [16].

Rat liver cytosol, containing NADPH as an electron donor, catalyzed the nitroreduction of 1-nitropyrene to 1-nitrosopyrene and 1-aminopyrene, and dinitropyrenes to nitronitrosopyrenes and aminonitropyrenes. In incubations with added AcCoA, *N*-acetyl-1-aminopyrene and *N*-acetylaminonitropyrenes were also formed. The *N*-acetylated metabolites were minor products for the dinitropyrenes, representing 10–20% of the amine formation, while with 1-nitropyrene, *N*-acetyl-1-aminopyrene was formed at levels threefold higher than 1-aminopyrene. *N*-Acetoxy derivatives were not detected in any of the AcCoA-fortified incubations, but this may be a result of their high chemical reactivity. Although nitroreduction alone resulted in DNA-binding, addition of AcCoA to these incubations greatly increased the DNA-binding of 1,8-dinitropyrene but not that of 1-nitropyrene (Fig. 3) even though 1-nitropyrene was more extensively *N*-acetylated than 1,8-dinitropyrene. The major adducts formed

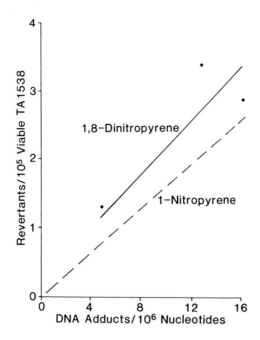

Fig. 2. Reversions induced in *Salmonella typhimurium* TA1538 by 1-nitropyrene and 1,8-dinitropyrene as a function of the number of adducts detected in the cellular genome. The solid line was calculated from a linear regression analysis of the data obtained from 1,8-dinitropyrene. The dashed line is from the data presented by Howard et al [16] for 1-nitropyrene.

via enzymatic activation of 1-nitropyrene and 1,8-dinitropyrene in rat liver cytosol were the same C8-substituted deoxyguanosine adducts found in *S typhimurium*. AcCoA also greatly increased the binding of 1,3- and 1,6-dinitropyrene to DNA and preliminary data indicate that they also formed C8-substituted deoxyguanosine adducts. This AcCoA-dependent DNA binding by the dinitropyrenes correlated with the amount of nitroreduction. Thus, the extent of 1,3-dinitropyrene nitroreduction was low and DNA-binding by 1,3-dinitropyrene in the presence of AcCoA was also low relative to 1,6- and 1,8-dinitropyrene.

DISCUSSION

Nitrated pyrenes are potent direct-acting mutagens in *S typhimurium* TA1538 because of efficient bacterial nitroreduction to their respective *N*-hydroxy aminopyrenes, which can then form DNA-reactive nitrenium ions [4,21,22]. Incubation of *S typhimurium* TA1538 with 1,8-dinitropyrene or 1-nitropyrene resulted in the formation of C8-substituted deoxyguanosine adducts, which are characteristic of nitrenium ion reactions [21,22]. However, although the number of mutations per 1,8-dinitropyrene adduct in the *S typhimurium* genome was similar to that of 1-nitropyrene (Fig. 2), 1,8-dinitropyrene was about 40-fold more mutagenic than 1-nitropyrene as a function of dose. This could be due to further activation of *N*-hydroxy-1-amino-8-nitropyrene by bacterial transacetylases [14,15] to form a reactive *N*-acetoxy arylamine, which results in more efficient DNA binding (Fig. 4).

A similar mechanism of activation was found in rat liver cytosol. The cytosolic enzymes were capable of reducing the nitrated pyrenes, but only the dinitropyrenes

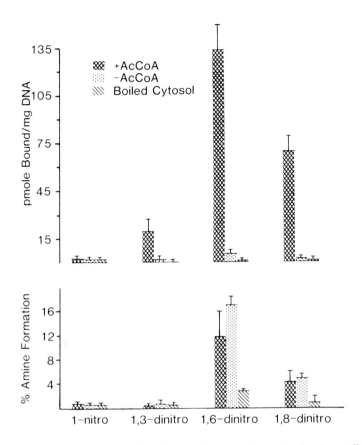

Fig. 3. DNA binding and nitroreduction of nitrated pyrenes after activation by rat liver cytosolic enzymes in the presence and absence of AcCoA. DNA was quantified by measuring its UV absorbance, and the level of binding was determined by liquid scintillation counting. HPLC was used to quantify the amount of 1-aminopyrene in 1-nitropyrene incubations and aminonitropyrenes in dinitropyrene incubations.

bound to DNA more efficiently in the presence of AcCoA (Fig. 3). This AcCoA-dependent binding may occur through formation of an arylhydroxamic acid that could be converted into a reactive N-acetoxy arylamine by N,O-acyltransferase [23] (Fig. 4). Alternatively, the N-acetoxy arylamine could be formed by direct O-acetylation, as has been observed with other N-hydroxy arylamines [24]. The failure of 1-nitropyrene to be activated by acetylases from either bacteria or rat liver cytosol may indicate that N-hydroxy-1-aminopyrene does not form an O-acetyl intermediate or that any N-acetoxy-1-aminopyrene formed may not have a sufficient lifetime to react with DNA.

1-Nitropyrene and 1,3-dinitropyrene were reduced to a similar extent by rat liver cytosol, and this was an order of magnitude less than that of either 1,6- or 1,8-dinitropyrene. Preliminary evidence indicates that this may be because reduced 1-nitropyrene and 1,3-dinitropyrene intermediates react more readily with oxygen to regenerate the parent nitrated pyrenes. This decreased nitroreduction of 1,3-dinitropyrene compared with 1,6- and 1,8-dinitropyrene appeared to limit the amount of AcCoA-dependent DNA binding. If bacterial nitroreduction of 1,3-dinitropyrene is

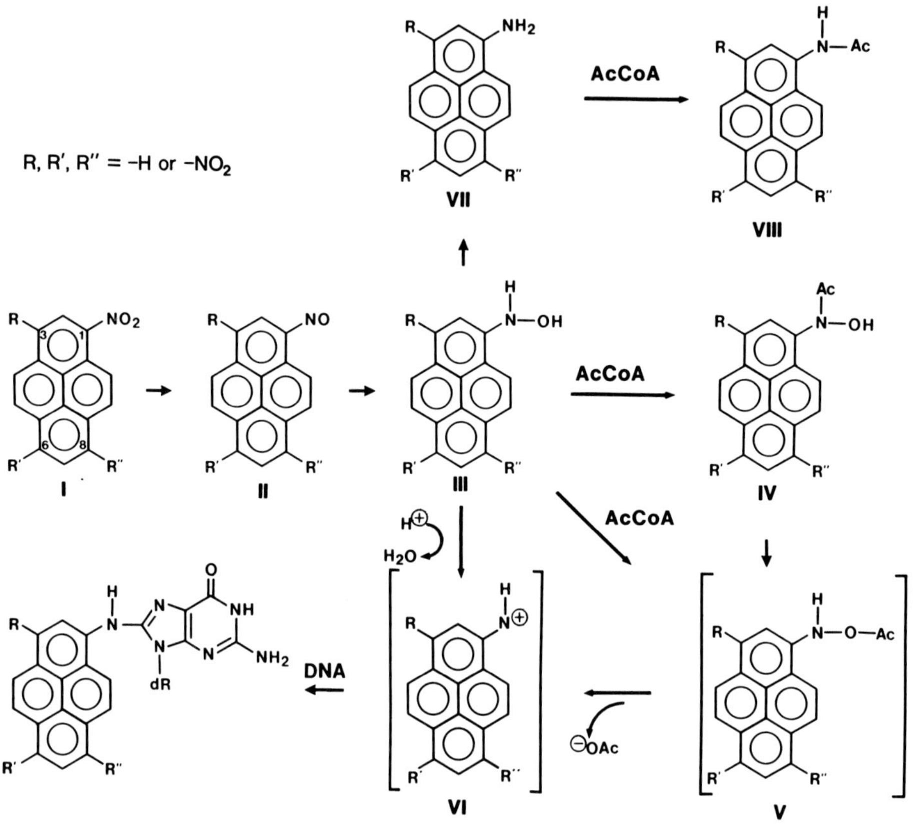

Fig. 4. Proposed mechanism for activation of nitrated pyrenes (I) to DNA-binding species. The compounds undergo sequential reduction to nitrosopyrenes (II) and N-hydroxy aminopyrenes (III). With 1-nitropyrene, the N-hydroxy amino metabolite reacts directly with DNA, while the analogous metabolites from the dinitropyrenes are further activated by AcCoA. This AcCoA-dependent binding may occur through the formation of an arylhydroxamic acid (IV), which can be converted into a reactive N-acetoxy arylamine (V) by N,O-acyltransferase. Alternatively, the N-acetoxy arylamine may be formed by direct O-acetylation of the N-hydroxy aminopyrene. In all cases, the predominant adducts formed are substituted at C8 of deoxyguanosine and arise through nitrenium ion intermediates (VI). N-Hydroxy aminopyrenes can also be further reduced to aminopyrenes (VII) and subsequently acetylated to N-acetylaminopyrenes (VIII).

similar to that in rat liver cytosol, this could explain why 1,3-dinitropyrene is less mutagenic than 1,6- or 1,8-dinitropyrene in S typhimurium TA98 [1,3]. In summary, these data indicate that metabolic activation of 1-nitropyrene and the dinitropyrenes by both S typhimurium and mammalian enzymes depends on nitroreduction and that the dinitropyrenes are further activated by acetylation.

ACKNOWLEDGMENTS

We thank Nancy F. Fullerton for technical assistance and Cindy Hartwick for helping to prepare this manuscript. Part of the research described in this article was conducted under contract to the Health Effects Institute (HEI), an organization jointly funded by the United States Environmental Protection Agency (EPA), under Assistance Agreement X812059, and automotive manufacturers. The contents of this article do not necessarily reflect the view of the HEI, and they do not necessarily reflect the policies of the EPA or automotive manufacturers. It is currently under review by the Institute. E.K.F. was supported in part by Interagency Agreement 224-82-002 with the Veterans Administration.

REFERENCES

1. Rosenkranz HS: Mutat Res 101:1, 1982.
2. Wei ET, Shu HP: Am J Public Health 73:1085, 1983.
3. Rosenkranz HS, Mermelstein R: Mutat Res 114:217, 1983.
4. Beland FA, Heflich RH, Howard PC, Fu PP: In Harvey RG (ed): "Polycyclic Hydrocarbons and Carcinogenesis." Washington, DC: American Chemical Society, 1985, pp 371–396.
5. Li AP, Dutcher JS: Mutat Res 119:389, 1983.
6. Cole J, Arlett CF, Lowe J, Bridges BA: Mutat Res 93:213, 1982.
7. Takayama S, Tanake M, Katoh Y, Terada M, Sugimura T: Gann 74:338, 1983.
8. Ohgaki H, Matsukura N, Morino K, Kawachi T, Sugimura T, Morita K, Tokiwa H, Hirota T: Cancer Lett 15:1, 1982.
9. Hirose M, Lee M-S, Wang CY, King CM: Cancer Res 44:1158, 1984.
10. El-Bayoumy K, Hecht SS, Sackl T, Stoner GD: Carcinogenesis 5:1449, 1984.
11. Nesnow S, Triplett LL, Slaga TJ: Cancer Lett 23:1, 1984.
12. Tokiwa H, Otofuji T, Horikawa K, Kitamori S, Otsuka H, Manabe Y, Kinouchi T, Ohnishi Y: JNCI 73:1359, 1984.
13. Ohgaki H, Hasegawa H, Kato T, Negishi C, Sato S, Sugimura T: Cancer Lett 25:239, 1985.
14. McCoy EC, McCoy GD, Rosenkranz HS: Biochem Biophys Res Commun 108:1362, 1982.
15. McCoy EC, Anders M, Rosenkranz HS: Mutat Res 121:17, 1983.
16. Howard PC, Heflich RH, Evans FE, Beland FA: Cancer Res 43:2052, 1983.
17. Fifer EK, Heflich RH, Djurić Z, Howard PC, Beland FA: Carcinogenesis 7:65, 1986.
18. Heflich RH, Howard PC, Beland FA: Mutat Res 149:25, 1985.
19. Moore PD, Koreeda M: Biochem Biophys Res Commun 73:459, 1976.
20. Djurić Z, Fifer EK, Beland FA: Carcinogenesis 6:941, 1985.
21. Kadlubar FF, Beland FA: In Harvey RG (ed): "Polycyclic Hydrocarbons and Carcinogenesis." Washington, DC: American Chemical Society, 1985, pp 341–370.
22. Beland FA, Beranek DT, Dooley KL, Heflich RH, Kadlubar FF: Environ Health Perspect 49:125, 1983.
23. Allaben WT, King CM: J Biol Chem 259:12128, 1984.
24. Flammang TJ, Kadlubar FF: In Boobis AR, Caldwell J, De Matteis F, Elcombe CR (eds): "Microsomes and Drug Oxidations." London: Taylor and Francis, 1985, pp 190–197.

Biochemical and Molecular Epidemiology of Cancer 449–457 (1986)

Detection of Rare Cells Expressing HTLV-III in Primary Lymphoid Tissue From Infected Individuals Using a Highly Sensitive In Situ Hybridization Method

Mary E. Harper, Lisa M. Marselle, Karen J. Chayt, Steven F. Josephs, Peter Biberfeld, Leon G. Epstein, James M. Oleske, Carl J. O'Hara, Jerome E. Groopman, Robert C. Gallo, and Flossie Wong-Staal

Laboratory of Tumor Cell Biology, National Cancer Institute, Bethesda, Maryland 20205 (M.E.H., L.M.M., K.J.C., S.F.J., R.C.G., F.W.-S.), Department of Pathology, Karolinska Institute and Hospital, Stockholm, Sweden (P.B.), Departments of Neuroscience and Pediatrics, University of Medicine and Dentistry of New Jersey, Newark, New Jersey, 07103 (L.G.E., J.M.O.) and Departments of Pathology and Medicine, New England Deaconess Hospital, Boston Massachusetts 02215 (C.J.O., J.E.G.)

A sensitive in situ hybridization method has been developed for detection and quantitation of human T-lymphotropic virus type III (HTLV-III) RNA expression in primary cells from infected individuals. Mononuclear cell cytospin preparations from lymph node, peripheral blood, and bone marrow of AIDS or ARC (AIDS-related complex) patients were hybridized with a [^{35}S] HTLV-III probe and exposed for 2 days. Infected cells expressing viral RNA were detected in 89% (8/9) of lymph node, 50% (7/14) of peripheral blood, and 17% (1/6) of bone marrow samples studied. However, in all positive preparations, cells containing HTLV-III RNA were observed at very low frequency, ie, <0.01% of total mononuclear cells. Positive cells generally exhibited morphological characteristics of lymphocytes and expressed viral RNA at relatively low abundancy (approximately 20–300 copies per cell). Similarly, hybridization to frozen tissue sections from infected individuals detected only rare cells expressing HTLV-III RNA in lymphoid tissue such as lymph node, thymus, and spleen. These results indicate that HTLV-III expression in lymphoid tissue is very low and likely cannot account for the T4 lymphocyte depletion characteristic of HTLV-III infection. Furthermore, the lymph node hyperplasia observed in HTLV-III–associated lymphadenopathy is not due to proliferation of HTLV-III–infected lymphocytes.

Key words: AIDS, viral RNA, HTLV-III expression, lymph node, peripheral blood, frozen sections

Human T-lymphotropic virus type III (HTLV-III), the etiologic agent of the acquired immunodeficiency syndrome (AIDS) as well as a variety of related disor-

Received December 13, 1985.

© **1986 Alan R. Liss, Inc.**

ders, is an exogenous retrovirus with tropism for helper T lymphocytes possessing the cell-surface antigen OKT4 [for review see 1,2]. Although HTLV-III shares many biological and biochemical properties with the other two members of this family, the transforming HTLV-I and HTLV-II viruses, it exhibits a cytopathic effect on OKT4 lymphocytes, leading to their depletion. The resulting immunosuppression, accompanied by opportunistic infections and/or Kaposi's sarcoma in frank AIDS [3–6], may also emcompass milder forms of the disease, which have been collectively grouped under the term AIDS-related complex (ARC). More recently, it has been recognized that HTLV-III may cause other disease manifestations as well, such as encephalopathy [7,8] and lymphocytic interstitial pneumonitis [9,10], even in the absence of immunodeficiency. Key questions in understanding the pathogenesis of HTLV-III infection include determination of the types of cells and tissues affected, which mechanisms are involved (either direct or indirect), and how host cellular responses relate to viral action.

To determine the presence of HTLV-III DNA sequences in primary tissue, uncultured biopsy or autopsy samples from AIDS and ARC patients have been assayed by Southern blot analysis. Although low levels of HTLV-III DNA were detected in some fresh lymphoid tissues, the majority of samples were negative [11]. On the other hand, it has been determined that HTLV-III can be isolated from approximately 50% of AIDS patients, 80% of ARC patients, and 30% of healthy individuals at risk for AIDS from a variety of tissues such as peripheral blood, bone marrow, and lymph node [12], suggesting the actual presence of virus in primary tissue.

To assay in a more sensitive manner for the presence of HTLV-III sequences and to quantitate expression levels within particular cells and tissues, we decided to utilize in situ hybridization because of advantages inherent in this method. In situ hybridization is direct, quantitative, and requires small tissue samples. Furthermore, this method can aid in identification of the types of cells infected with HTLV-III and localization of their distribution within particular tissues. Use of previously described methods for RNA in situ hybridization [13–16] did not detect HTLV-III RNA after short autoradiographic exposure times (several days). Therefore, we modified existing methodology to detect with high sensitivity and to quantitate HTLV-III RNA expression in primary tissue from infected individuals [17]. Using this method, we directly demonstrate that HTLV-III–infected cells expressing viral RNA can be detected in uncultured lymphoid tissue, but are present at very low frequency.

MATERIALS AND METHODS
Preparation of Cells and Tissue Sections

All specimens studied were obtained from HTLV-III seropositive individuals. Cytospin preparations were made on microscope slides from primary lymph node, peripheral blood, and bone marrow mononuclear cell fractions obtained by Ficoll separation [17]. Frozen tissue sections were prepared from samples snap-frozen at biopsy or autopsy and placed on polylysine-coated slides. All preparations were fixed by immersion in 4% paraformaldehyde in PBS for 1 min and then stored in 70% ethanol at 4°C until hybridized [17,18].

Preparation of [^{35}S]RNA Probes

HTLV-III–specific RNA was generated by transcription of pSP64 clone pBH10-R3, containing the 9-kb SSt I HTLV-III insert of BH10 [19], using [^{35}S] UTP and

SP6 polymerase [17]. Control RNA probes, specific for HTLV-I or bacteriophage lambda sequences, were also synthesized from the appropriate pSP64 clones. [^{35}S] RNAs, specific activity approximately 10^9 dpm/μg, were stored in aliquots at $-70°$C.

In Situ Hybridization

Hybridization was carried out as previously described [17]. Slide preparations were acetylated [20], immersed in 0.1 M Tris, pH 7.0, and 0.1 M glycine [18], and then hybridized with 10^8 dpm/ml (100 ng/ml) [^{35}S] RNA probe in 50% formamide–2 × SSC–10 mM dithiothreitol at 50°C for 3 hr. Following thorough rinsing in 50% formamide–2 × SSC at 52°C and ribonuclease digestion for 30 min, slides were autoradiographed with Kodak NTB2 emulsion and exposed at 4°C for 2 days. Preparations were developed and stained with Wright stain.

RESULTS

To study expression levels of HTLV-III in primary tissue from infected individuals, a highly sensitive in situ hybridization method was developed and utilized. Hybridization of the HTLV-III RNA probe described in Materials and Methods resulted in specific labeling of cells expressing viral RNA, as illustrated in the T-cell line H9, which supports HTLV-III replication [21]. Following a 2-day exposure, uninfected H9 cells exhibited no label (Fig. 1A). In contrast, the infected H9/HTLV-IIIB cells were heavily labeled, exhibiting an average of 100–150 grains per cell [17] (Fig. 1B). Comparison of grain count with Northern blot hybridization of isolated RNA from the same culture indicated that each grain following a 2-day exposure represents one to three copies of RNA [17]. In addition, prehybridization digestion of H9/HTLV-IIIB preparations with RNase or DNase indicated that grains were specific for viral RNA and not unintegrated HTLV-III DNA [17], which had been shown to be present in infected cells by Southern blot hybridization [10].

In situ hybridization of the HTLV-III probe to cytospin preparations of primary lymphoid cells from AIDS and ARC patients demonstrated that HTLV-III RNA expression levels in these tissues is very low. Lymph node mononuclear cell samples were found to contain only rare cells expressing viral RNA in 89% (8/9) samples studied (Table I; Fig. 1C). Labeled cells constituted less than 0.01% and in some cases 0.001% of the cell populations analyzed [17]. Hybridization of the HTLV-III probe to AIDS or ARC peripheral blood mononuclear cells also resulted in observation of very rare cells expressing viral RNA (Fig. 1D). Positive cells were generally present at a frequency similar to that in lymph node cell suspensions: less than 0.01% and usually less than 0.001% of mononuclear cells. However, a lower percentage of the peripheral blood samples studied were positive for labeled cells (7 of 14, or 50%; Table I) as compared to lymph node samples [17]. Bone marrow mononuclear cell preparations from AIDS and ARC patients exhibited even lower levels of HTLV-III RNA expression. Of six samples studied, only one (17%) contained cells expressing viral RNA (Table I). Again the frequency of cells positive for HTLV-III RNA was very low (approximately 0.001% of mononuclear cells).

In all HTLV-III-positive lymphoid tissues, labeled cells generally exhibited morphological features characteristic of lymphocytes. Grain counts showed that virus-positive cells contained from 20–100 grains per cell. Based on quantitative analysis

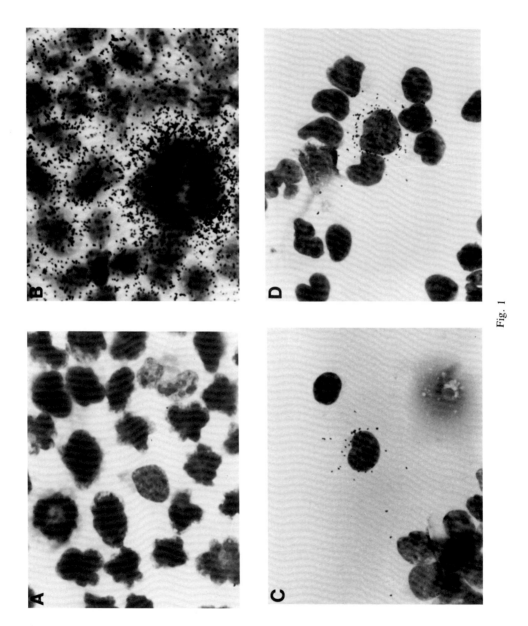

Fig. 1

TABLE I. Fresh Tissue Specimens From AIDS or ARC Patients Analyzed by In Situ Hybridization

Tissue tested[a]	Clinical diagnosis	No. of patients	
		Positive	Tested
LN mononuclear cells	ARC	3	4
	AIDS	3	3
PB mononuclear cells	ARC	2	2
	AIDS	5	12
BM mononuclear cells	ARC	0	3
	AIDS	1	3
LN frozen sections	PGL[b] prior to ARC	9	11
	ARC	4	4
	AIDS	1	1
Thymus frozen sections	AIDS	1	2
Spleen frozen sections	AIDS[c]	2	2

[a]LN, lymph node; PB peripheral blood, BM, bone marrow.
[b]PGL, persistent generalized lymphadenopathy.
[c]One patient developed Hodgkin's disease subsequent to AIDS.

of H9/HTLV-IIIB RNA described above, the HTLV-III-infected cells expressing viral RNA likely contained 20–300 copies of RNA per cell [17].

To confirm and extend the analysis of HTLV-III expression in lymphoid tissue, hybridization was also carried out to frozen tissue sections. Lymph nodes from HTLV-III-seropositive individuals with persistent generalized lymphadenopathy (PGL) were found to contain HTLV-III-positive cells in the majority of samples studied (14 of 16, or 88%; Table I; Fig 2A) [21]. Again, as in the lymph node cell suspensions, the number of cells expressing HTLV-III RNA was very low (0.001–0.01%). Similarly, spleen and thymus frozen sections from several AIDS patients were generally found to contain rare cells infected with HTLV-III and expressing viral RNA. In two cases of thymus obtained from pediatric AIDS patients, one specimen exhibited HTLV-III–positive cells (Fig. 2B) at a frequency of 0.001%, while the other specimen was negative for HTLV-III RNA. The two spleen specimens, one obtained from a pediatric AIDS case and the other from an adult patient with AIDS and Hodgkin's disease, were both found to exhibit cells expressing HTLV-III RNA (Fig. 2C) at a similarly low frequency. Morphologic analysis suggested that the virus-positive cells likely were lymphocytes.

DISCUSSION

In situ hybridization was used to detect cells expressing HTLV-III RNA in primary lymphoid tissue from AIDS and ARC patients. Of the tissues extensively tested, lymph nodes were most frequently found to contain virus-expressing cells:

Fig. 1. Detection of HTLV-III RNA in cytospin preparations by in situ hybridization of HTLV-III RNA probe. A) Uninfected H9 cell line, negative for HTLV-III RNA expression. B) Infected H9/HTLV-IIIB cell line, expressing an average of 100–400 copies of HTLV-III RNA per cell. C) Lymph node mononuclear cell preparation from patient with AIDS, demonstrating rare cell expressing HTLV-III RNA. D) Mononuclear cell preparation from primary peripheral blood of ARC patient, demonstrating rare cell containing HTLV-III RNA.

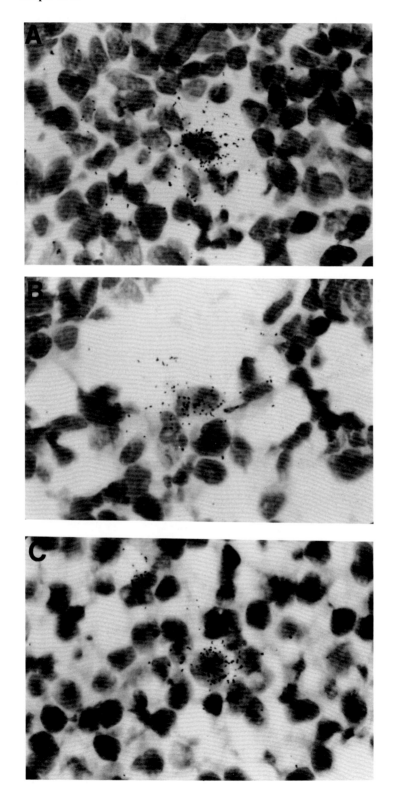

Fig. 2

89% of mononuclear cell preparations and 88% of frozen sections were positive. In contrast, mononuclear cell preparations from peripheral blood contained HTLV-III RNA-positive cells in approximately half of the samples tested, while only one bone marrow preparation of six studied was found to be positive. Because of the low number of thymus and spleen samples tested, it was not possible to compare levels of positivity with the other tissues.

In all samples found to contain cells expressing HTLV-III RNA, positive cells were detected at very low frequency, ie, 0.001–0.01% of total cells. This level of expression was relatively consistent among the various types of lymphoid tissue studied, as well as the type of preparation. However, our observation that a higher percentage of lymph node samples was positive compared to peripheral blood or bone marrow suggests the presence of more infected cells in lymph nodes. These results are supported by Southern blot hybridization experiments, which detected HTLV-III DNA in 7 of 34 lymph nodes, but in only 1 of 22 peripheral blood samples [11]. The overall low level of positive cells expressing RNA may be responsible in part for the lack of positive hybridization noted for some samples, and analysis of a higher number of cells may be required. Negative hybridization results could also be due to poor preservation of RNA during cell processing and slide preparation.

Detection of low abundancy RNA was made possible by several improvements in methodology that significantly increase sensitivity of detection. High specific activity [^{35}S]-labeled RNA probes were obtained by transcription of specific DNA fragments subcloned into vectors such as pSP64 [22]. Single-strand RNA probes offer several advantages, such as highly efficient hybridization [16], increased stability of hybrids, which allows more stringent hybridization and rinsing conditions [23], and use of ribonuclease digestion to remove unhybridized probe molecules, which contributes to low nonspecific labeling. Slide preparations were fixed with paraformaldehyde, found previously to result in efficient hybridization [18]. Comparison of this fixation method with ethanol-acetic acid fixation [13] by subsequent hybridization of H9/HTLV-IIIB cells with the HTLV-III probe indicated two to threefold higher grain counts on cells fixed with paraformaldehyde (results not shown). Moreover, storage in 70% ethanol following fixation provided excellent preservation of RNA, as evidenced by successful detection of cells expressing HTLV-III RNA on slide preparations stored for over 6 months.

One of several advantages of in situ hybridization is the potential for analysis of location of cells expressing HTLV-III within a particular tissue. Histopathological studies of lymph nodes from patients with PGL, which frequently accompanies or precedes other manifestations of AIDS, have described progressive changes in follicles [24,25], areas that normally contain a predominance of B cells. These stages, including hyperplasia, involution, atrophy, and depletion, show temporal and structural relationships with other follicular changes, such as invasion of T cells [26]. Interestingly, we found that most of the cells expressing HTLV-III RNA in lymph node frozen sections were present in follicles, suggesting a central role in the pathogenesis of HTLV-III–induced lymphadenopathy [21]. However, it is apparent from these studies, as well as from previous Southern blot hybridizations [11], that

Fig. 2. Detection of rare cells expressing HTLV-III RNA in frozen tissue sections from infected individuals. A) Lymph node tissue from a patient with lymphadenopathy. B) Thymus tissue from pediatric AIDS patient. C) Spleen tissue from patient with AIDS and Hodgkin's disease.

the lymph node hyperplasia observed in lymphadenopathy patients is not due to proliferation of HTLV-III–infected lymphocytes. In fact, immunocytochemical staining has shown the hyperplastic cells to be B cells [26], and follicles may be a site of antigenic stimulation of such cells by HTLV-III, leading to hyperplasia and/or the B-cell malignancies frequently seen in HTLV-III–infected individuals.

The actual number of cells infected with HTLV-III, including those cells not expressing RNA, cannot be determined by the in situ hybridization method as applied in this study. That some cells may contain the viral genome without expression of viral RNA has recently been shown (D. Zagury, personal communication). Our observation that expression of HTLV-III in primary lymphoid tissue of infected individuals is consistently very low in the presence of significantly decreased T4 lymphocytes suggests that viral replication may not account for depletion of the target T4 lymphocyte.

It has become increasingly apparent that HTLV-III may act through additional mechanisms in inducing other clinical manifestations. For example, HTLV-III RNA and DNA were detected at relatively high levels in brain tissue from patients with AIDS encephalopathy, suggesting a viral role in this disorder [27]. Based on cellular morphology, pattern of labeling, and histological examination, infected cells as visualized by in situ hybridization did not appear to be lymphocytes. More recently, we have detected the presence of significant numbers of cells expressing HTLV-III in lung tissue from a patient with lymphocytic interstitial pneumonitis [28]. Many of the positive cells did not exhibit morphological characteristics of lymphocytes and could represent cells of the monocyte-macrophage lineage. While it is likely that the rare cells expressing HTLV-III in lymphoid tissue are T4 lymphocytes, additional types of cells could also be infected, with or without viral expression. Continued application of in situ hybridization in combination with immunocytochemistry for identification of specific cell types (work in progress) should help to identify HTLV-III–infected cells at various stages of infection in our attempts to understand the diverse pathogenic effects of this virus.

REFERENCES

1. Wong-Staal F, Gallo RC: Nature 317:395, 1985.
2. Gallo RC, Wong-Staal F: Ann Intern Med 103:679, 1985.
3. Gottlieb MS, Schroff R, Schanker HM, Weisman JD, Fan PT, Wolf RA, Saxon A: N Engl J Med 305:1425, 1981.
4. Masur H, Michelis MA, Greene JB, Onorato I, Vande Stouwe RA, Holzman RS, Wormser G, Brettman L, Lange M, Murray HW, Cunningham-Rundles S: N Engl J Med 305:1431, 1981.
5. Siegal FP, Lopez C, Hammer GS, Brown AE, Kornfeld SJ, Gold J, Hassett J, Hirschman SZ, Cunningham-Rundles C, Adelsberg BR, Parham DM, Siegal M, Cunningham-Rundles S, Armstrong D: N Engl J Med 305:1439, 1981.
6. Friedman-Kien AE, Laubenstein LJ, Rubinstein P, Buimovici-Klein E, Marmor M, Stahl R, Spigland I, Kim KS, Zolla-Pazner S: Ann Intern Med 96:693, 1982.
7. Snider WD, Simpson DM, Nielsen S, Gold JWM, Metroka CE, Posner JB: Ann Neurol 14:403, 1983.
8. Epstein LG, Sharer LR, Joshi VV, Fojas MM, Koenigsberger MR, Oleske JM: Ann Neurol 17:488, 1985.
9. Scott G, Buck BE, Leterman JG, Bloom FL, Parks W: N Engl J Med 310:76, 1984.
10. Joshi VV, Oleske JM, Minnefor AB, Singh R, Bokhari T, Raphin RH: Pediatr Pathol 2:71, 1984.
11. Shaw GM, Hahn BH, Arya SK, Groopman JE, Gallo RC, Wong-Staal F: Science 226:1165, 1984.

12. Salahuddin SZ, Markham PD, Popovic M, Sarngadharan MG, Orndorff S, Fladagar A, Patel A, Gold J, Gallo RC: Proc Natl Acad Sci USA 82:5530, 1985.

13. Brahic M, Haase AT: Proc Natl Acad Sci USA 75:6125, 1978.

14. McDougall JK, Crum CP, Fenoglio CM, Goldstein LC, Galloway DA: Proc Natl Acad Sci USA 79:3853, 1982.

15. Singer RH, Ward DC: Proc Natl Acad Sci USA 79:7331, 1982.

16. Cox KH, DeLeon DV, Angerer LM, Angerer RC: Dev Biol 101:485, 1984.

17. Harper ME, Marselle LM, Gallo RC, Wong-Staal F: Proc Natl Acad Sci USA 83: 772–776, 1986.

18. Lawrence JB, Singer RH: Nucleic Acids Res 13:1777, 1985.

19. Hahn BH, Shaw GM, Arya SK, Popovic M, Gallo RC, Wong-Staal F: Nature 312:166, 1984.

20. Hayashi S, Gillam IC, Delaney AD, Tener, GM: J Histochem Cytochem 26:677, 1978.

21. Chayt KJ, Harper ME, Marselle LM, Biberfeld P, Biberfeld G, Gallo RC, Wong-Staal F: N Engl J Med (manuscript submitted).

22. Melton DA, Krieg PA, Rebagliati MR, Maniatis T, Zinn K, Green MR: Nucleic Acids Res 12:7035, 1984.

23. Berk AJ, Sharp PA: Cell 12:721, 1977.

24. Metroka CE, Cunningham-Rundles S, Pollack MS, Sonnabend JA, Davis JM, Gordon B, Fernandez RD, Mouradian J: Ann Intern Med 99:585, 1983.

25. Ioachim HL, Lerner CW, Tapper ML: Am J Surg Pathol 7:543, 1983.

26. Biberfeld P, Porwit-Ksiazek A, Bottiger B, Morfeldt-Mansson L, Biberfeld G: Cancer Res (Suppl) 45:4665s, 1985.

27. Shaw GM, Harper ME, Hahn BH, Epstein LG, Gajdusek DC, Price RW, Navia BA, Petito CK, O'Hara CJ, Groopman JE, Cho E-S, Oleske JM, Wong-Staal F, Gallo RC: Science 227:177, 1985.

28. Chayt KJ, Harper ME, Lewin EB, Rose R, Marselle LM, Oleske JM, Epstein LG, Wong-Staal F, Gallo RC: Ann Intern Med (manuscript submitted).

Index